Acute Leukemia: Outlook and Challenges

Acute Leukemia: Outlook and Challenges

Edited by **Matthew Griffin**

hayle medical

New York

Published by Hayle Medical,
30 West, 37th Street, Suite 612,
New York, NY 10018, USA
www.haylemedical.com

Acute Leukemia: Outlook and Challenges
Edited by Matthew Griffin

International Standard Book Number: 978-1-63241-008-5 (Hardback)

Printed in China.

Contents

Preface

This book has been a concerted effort by a group of academicians, researchers and scientists, who have contributed their research works for the realization of the book. This book has materialized in the wake of emerging advancements and innovations in this field. Therefore, the need of the hour was to compile all the required researches and disseminate the knowledge to a broad spectrum of people comprising of students, researchers and specialists of the field.

Acute leukemia refers to serious medical conditions related to cancerous growth of white blood cells. This book gives a broad overview of the elementary mechanisms underlying the extent of acute leukemia, current development, and future prospects in the management of this disease. The book talks about a categorization of acute leukemia, while considering the diagnoses reliant on methods that are crucial, and easily accessible, in the laboratory. It also discusses current advances in molecular biology, markers, receptors, and signaling molecules accountable for disease progression, diagnostics built upon biochips and other molecular genetic analysis. These developments equip clinicians with essential understanding and enhanced decision-making towards the most appropriate therapy for acute leukemia. Biochemical, structural, and genetic studies may import a new era of epigenetic based drugs besides supplementary molecular targets that will shape the basis for new treatment strategies. This book also includes pediatric acute leukemia, highlighting that children are not small adults when we talk about drug development. It also covers the topics like treatment of the disease, as chemotherapy- induced toxicity is yet an important clinical matter. The major challenge lies in minimizing the frequency and solemnity of unfortunate effects while managing efficacy and preventing over-treatment of patients.

At the end of the preface, I would like to thank the authors for their brilliant chapters and the publisher for guiding us all-through the making of the book till its final stage. Also, I would like to thank my family for providing the support and encouragement throughout my academic career and research projects.

Editor

Part 1

Introduction

1

Classification of Acute Leukemia

Gamal Abdul-Hamid
University of Aden/Hematology Unit
Yemen

1. Introduction

Acute leukemia is a proliferation of immature bone marrow-derived cells (blasts) that may also involve peripheral blood or solid organs. The percentage of bone marrow blast cells required for a diagnosis of acute leukemia has traditionally been set arbitrarily at 30% or more. However, more recently proposed classification systems have lowered the blast cell count to 20% for many leukemia types, and do not require any minimum blast cell percentage when certain morphologic and cytogenetic features are present.

2. Acute leukemia can be classified in many ways

(1) by morphology and cytochemistry supplemented by immunophenotyping, as proposed by French-American-British (FAB) group (Bennet et al 1976); (2) Proposed World Health Organization Classification of Acute Leukemia (Harris et al 1999); (3) by immunophenotyping alone, as proposed by the European Group for the immunological classification of leukemias (EGIL) (Bene et al 1995 & Hayhoe FG 1988).

The traditional classification of acute leukemia used criteria proposed by the French–American–British Cooperative Group (FAB) , using the 30% bone marrow blast cell cutoff (Bennett *et al*, 1985). This classification system originally distinguished different leukemia types by morphologic features and cytochemical studies, particularly myeloperoxidase (or Sudan black B) and non-specific esterase staining. It was revised to include leukemia types that could only be accurately identified with the addition of immunophenotyping or electron microscopic studies (Bennett *et al.*, 1991). Although the FAB classification failed to distinguish immunophenotypic groups of acute lymphoblastic leukemias, did not recognize the significance of myelodysplastic changes in acute myeloid leukemias or cytogenetic abnormalities in either leukemia type, and resulted in some subcategories of little clinical significance, this system provided very clear guidelines for classification. In addition, some distinct leukemia subtypes, particularly acute promyelocytic leukemia and acute myeloid leukemia with abnormal eosinophils, were found to correlate with specific cytogenetic aberrations and had unique clinical features, and those remain in recently proposed classification systems.

Acute myelogenous leukemia (AML) was based on how leukemic blasts, the predominant cell in the disease process, recapitulate normal hematopoiesis. Are blasts in a given case myeloblasts, monoblasts, megakaryoblasts, etc., and are they un-, minimally, or moderately differentiated.

The original classification scheme proposed by the French-American-British (FAB) Cooperative Group divides AML into 8 subtypes (M0 to M7) and ALL into 3 subtypes (L1 to L3). Although AML blasts evolve from common myeloid precursors, the 8 subtypes differ in degree of maturation (Table 1). As specified in the table, M0 designates AML with minimal morphologic or cytochemical differentiation, M1–2 AML with minimal or moderate granulocytic differentiation, M3 acute promyelocytic leukemia (APL), M4 AML with mixed myelomonocytic differentiation, M5a and M5b monoblastic leukemia with minimal or moderate differentiation, M6a myeloid leukemia with dysplastic background erythropoiesis, M6b acute erythroblastic leukemia, and M7 acute megakaryoblastic leukemia. The FAB classification of ALL includes 3 subtypes (L1 to L3), which are differentiated based on morphology, including cell size, prominence of nucleoli, and the amount and appearance of cytoplasm (Table 2). Approximately 75% of adult ALL cases have blasts with the B -cell phenotype, and 25% have blasts with the T-cell phenotype. The FAB classification of ALL and AML is based on morphology and cytochemical staining of blasts (Cheson et al 1990).

M0 AML with no Romanowsky or cytochemical evidence of differentiation
M1 Myeloblastic leukemia with little maturation
M2 Myeloblastic leukemia with maturation
M3 Acute promyelocytic leukemia (APL)
M3h APL, hypergranular variant
M3v APL, microgranular variant
M4 Acute myelomonocytic leukemia (AMML)
M4eo AMML with dysplastic marrow eosinophils
M5 Acute monoblastic leukemia (AMoL)
M5a AMoL, poorly differentiated
M5b AMoL, differentiated
M6 "Erythroleukemia"
M6a AML with erythroid dysplasia
M6b Erythroleukemia
M7 Acute megakaryoblastic leukemia (AMkL)

Table 1. French-American-British (FAB) Classification of Acute Myelogenous Leukemia

2.1 M0 Acute myeloblastic leukemia with minimally differentiated

AML-M0 is most common in adult patients. Accounts for approximately 5-10% of all AML patients. WBCs show Leukocytosis in 40% and > 50% with leukocytopenia. The diagnosis is made if less than 3% of the blasts are positive for peroxidase or the Sudan black B reaction and if the Blasts are positive for the myeloid-associated markers CD13, 14, CD15 or CD33, CD34 and negative for B or T lineage marker (CD3, CD10, CD19 and CD5). Bone marrow aspirated was hypercellular in all patients and contained a large number of leukemic blasts (Bennette JM 1991). Almost no mature myeloid cells were seen. The blasts were small to medium-sized round cells with an eccentric nucleus. The nucleus often had a flattened shape and was sometimes lobulated or cleaved and contained fine chromatin with several distinct nucleoli. The cytoplasm was lightly basophilic without granules. Auer rods are not found.

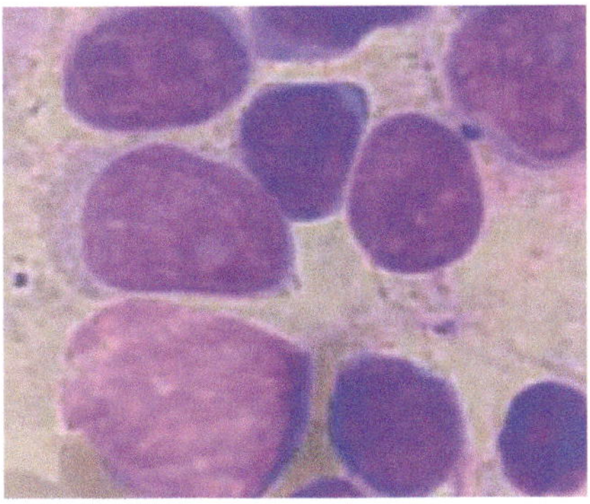

Fig. 1. Acute myeloblastic leukemia AML -M0

2.2 M1 Acute myeloblastic leukemia without maturation

It is found in all aged groups with highest incidence seen in adult and in infants less than a year old. Leukocytes in about 50% of patients at the time of diagnosis was increased. The predominant cell in the peripheral blood is usually a poorly differentiated myeloblast with finely reticulated chromatin and prominent nucleoli. Auer rods are found in the blast of 50% of the M1. If no evidence of granules or Auer rods is present, the blasts may resemble L2 lymphoblast. The myeloperoxidase or Sudan black B stains are positive in more than 3% of the blasts indicating granulocytes differentiation, the diagnosis is more likely AML-M1 than ALL (Bennett et al, 1976). PAS and alpha-naphthyl acetate esterase and naphthol AS-D-esterase are negative. About 50% of the patients will have acquired clonal chromosome aberrations in the leukemic cells. CD13, 14, 15, 33 and CD34 myeloid antigens are frequently positive in M1 leukemia. The most common cytogenetic abnormalities are: t (9; 22) (q34; q11)

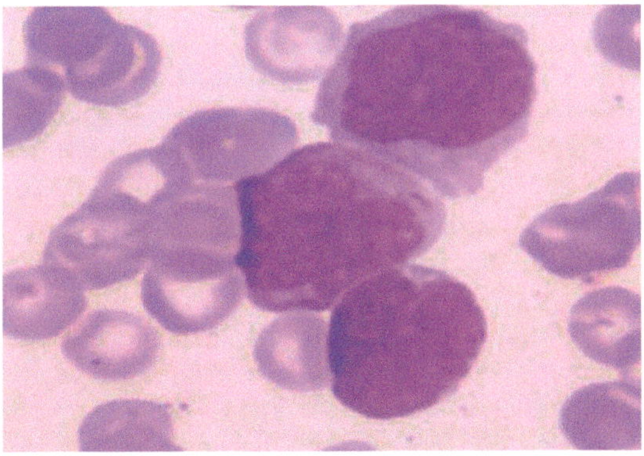

Fig. 2. Acute myeloblastic leukemia **AML-M1**

2.3 M2 Acute myeloblastic leukemia with maturation

The presenting symptoms for M2 AML are similar to those of the M1 type. Leukocytes increased in 50% of patients. Myeloblast can usually be found in the blood smears and may be the predominant cell type. Pseudopelger-Huet and hypogranular neutrophils being most common cells are seen in M2.

The bone marrow is hypercellular and types I and II myeloblasts make up from 30-83% of the promyelocytes to mature segmented cells. The monocytic component is less than 20%, differentiating M2 from M4. Basophils in some patient (M2 baso) was increased. Eosinophils and their precursors may be abundant, and in some cases accounts for up to 15% of myelogram (Berger and Flandrin, 1984). The characteristic that distinguishes AML-M2 from AML-M1 is the presence of maturation at or beyond the promyelocyte stage. Abnormal neutrophil maturation appears to be an integral part of AML-M2 with t(8;21) translocation. The neutrophils may show many abnormal nuclear segmentations and Auer rods.
Cytochemistry; Myeloperoxidase (MPO) reaction in blast cells gives the same result as in AML-M1, but the reaction is often of little practical value because the granulocytic nature of AML-M2 is usually demonstrated clearly by the presence of maturing cells in the granulocytic series. Sodium fluoride does not inhibit esterase. PAS and nonspecific esterase are negative. Positive reaction with CD13 and CD15 antigens are frequently seen in cases of M2.

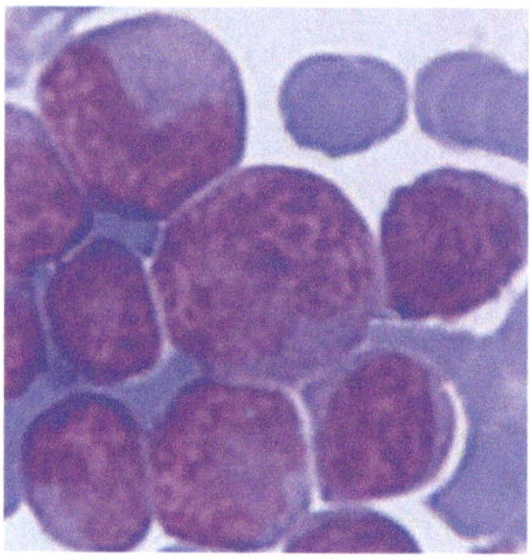

Fig. 3. Acute myeloblastic leukemia **AML-M2**

2.4 M3 Acute promyelocytic leukemia (APL)

The median age and survival average of APL is about 18 months and occurred in younger adult. M3 is of particular interest because it results in the fusion of a truncated retinoic acid receptor alpha (RAR-alpha) gene on chromosome 17 to a transcription unit called PML (for promyelocytic leukemia) on chromosome 15. It is interesting to note that high doses of the vitamin A derivative all-trans-retinoic acid are able to overcome thus block in differentiation both in vitro and in vivo and this agent has been successfully used to induce remission in patients.
A "variant" form of M3 (Bennett et al, 1980) is characterized by paucity of granules within the promyelocytic blasts and should not be confused with monocytic leukemia. The blasts are large with abundant cytoplasm, and the nucleus is usually irregular. The nucleus is often bilobed or markedly indented and a nucleolus can be seen in each lobe. The cytoplasm is completely occupied by closely packed large granules, staining bright pink, red or purple. Cells containing bundles of Auer rods "faggots" randomly distributed in the cytoplasm are characteristic, but are not present in all cases.
It is believed that the release of large numbers of promyelocytic granules containing a procoagulant initiate disseminated intravascular clotting (DIC). This is the most serious complication of M3 AML occurs frequently in both AML-M3 as well as AML-M3 variant (McKenna et al, 1982) . Initial therapy with the differentiating agent all-trans-retinoic acid

(ATRA) has improved significantly the treatment of AML-M3 in this regard; early mortality as a result of DIC is substantially reduced.
Cytochemistry: Peroxidase (MPO) and Sudan black B are strong positive. The periodic acid Schiff (PAS) is negative and Nonspecific esterase is also weak positive . The MPO reaction is also strong positive in the AML-M3 variant.
Immunological studies demonstrate positivity with CD13, CD15, CD1 and CD33 myeloid antigens. Cytogenetic studies have revealed a high prevalence (almost 50%) of the chromosomal translocation t(15; 17) associated with both AML M3 and M3 variant . **M3** AML with t(15;17) is usually characterized by the association of the lymphoid marker, CD2 and CD19, with myeloid markers and the negativity of HLA-DR and CD34.

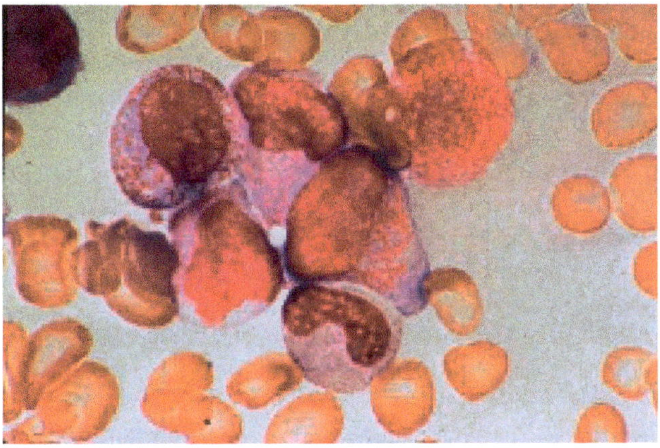

Fig. 4. Promyelocytic leukemia AML-M3

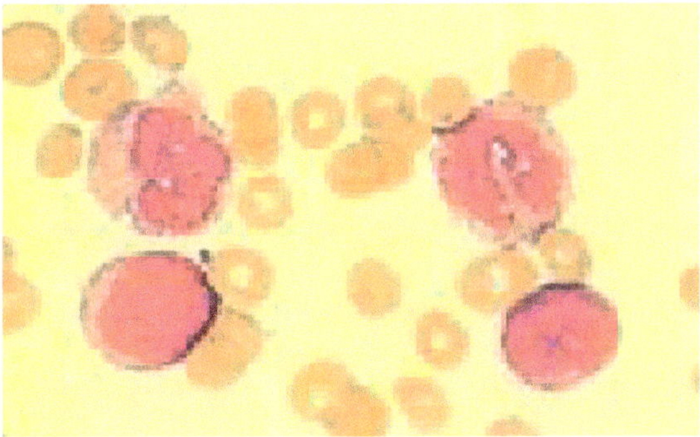

Fig. 5. Acute myelomonocytic leukemia M4

2.5 M4 Acute myelomonocytic leukemia (AMML)

It is distinguished from M1, M2, and M3 by an increased proportion of leukemia monocytic cells in the bone marrow or blood or both. Gingival hyperplasia with gingival bleeding is present. Serum and urine levels of muramidase (lysozyme) are usually elevated because of the monocytic proliferation. The leukocyte count is usually increased monocytic cells (monoblast, promoncytes, monocytes), are increased to 5000/μL or more. Anemia and thrombocytopenia are present in almost all cases. The marrow differs from M1, M2 and M3 in those monocytic cells exceed 20% of the nonerythroid nucleated cells. The sum of the myelocytic cells including myeloblasts, promyelocytes and later granulocytes is >20% and <80% of nonerythroid cells. This bone marrow picture together with a peripheral blood monocyte count of 5000/μL or more is compatible with a diagnosis of M4.

Confirmation of the monocytic component of this subgroup requires cytochemistry. The profile includes positive reactions for sudan black B or peroxidase and both specific and non-specific esterase. A few cases of M4 AML are characterized by increased marrow eosinophils and classified as M4e (Berger et al 1985) . Immunological studies demonstrate positivity with CD13, CD33, CD11b and CD14. Cytogenetic: inv(16) (p13; q22) and del (16)(q22) .

2.6 M5 Acute monoblastic leukemia (AMoL)

Common findings are weakness, bleeding and a diffuse erythematous skin rash. There is a high frequency of extramedulary infiltration of the lungs, colon, meninges, lymphnodes, bladder and larynx and gingival hyperplasia. Serum and urinary muramidase levels are often extremely high. The one criterion for a diagnosis of M5 is that 80% or more of all nonerythroid cells in the bone marrow are monocytic cells. There are two distinct forms 5a (maturation index <4%) and 5b (maturation index > 4%).M5a: Granulocyte <20% and Monocyte >80% >80% monoblast. M5b: Granulocyte <20% and Monocyte >80% <80% monoblast (Characterized by the presence of all developmental stages of monocytes; monoblast, promonocyte, monocyte)

Cytochemistry: Non-specific esterase stains and alpha-naphthyl esterase are positive and PAS is negative. Myeloperoxidase and Sudan black are weak diffuse activity in the monoblast. The use of alph-naphthyl butyrate esterase (ANBE) is advantageous because of its greater degree of specificity and stronger reaction, and also because sodium fluoride inhibition is not required (Shibata et al, 1985). Immunological studies demonstrate positivity with CD11b and CD14. There is a strong association between AML M5/M4 and deletion and translocations involving band 11q23.

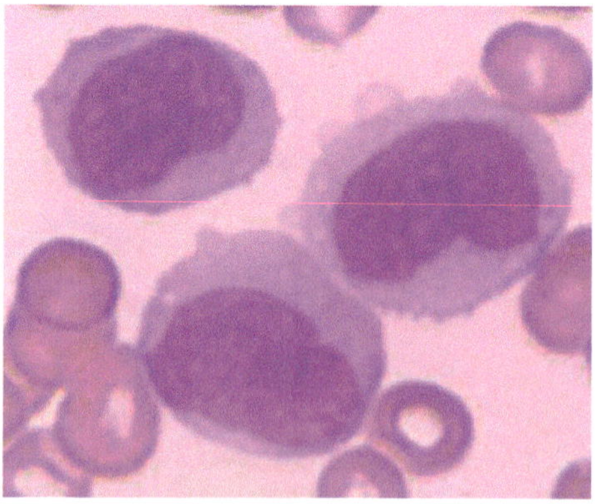

Fig. 6. M5 Acute monoblastic leukemia (AMoL)

2.7 M6 "Erythroleukemia"

M6 is a rare form of leukemia that primarily affects the peripheral cells. It is nonsexist in children. The clinical manifestations are similar to other types of AML. The most frequent presentation is bleeding. The most dominant changes in the peripheral blood are anemia with sticking poikilocytosis and anisocytosis. Nucleated red cells demonstrate abnormal nuclear configuration. The leukocytes and platelets are usually decreased. The diagnosis of erythroleukemia can be made when more than 50% of all nucleated bone marrow cells are erythroid and 30% or more of all remaining nonerythroid cells are type I or type II blast cells (Bennett et al, 1985). The erythroblast is abnormal with bizarre morphologic features. Giant multilobular or multinucleated forms are common. Other features are; fragmentation, Howell-Jolly bodies, ring sideroblast, megaloblastic and dyserythropoiesis changes are common. The cytochemistry of erythroblasts are normally PAS negative but in AML-M6, erythroblasts especially pronormoblast demonstrates coarse positivity of PAS. Blast cells express a variety of myeloid associated antigens such as CD13, CD33, anti-MPO with or without expression of precursor-cell markers as CD34, HLA-Dr determinants as for blast cells from other AML subtypes. In M6-variant forms, the more differentiated cells can be detected by the expression of glycophorin A and the absence of myeloid markers.

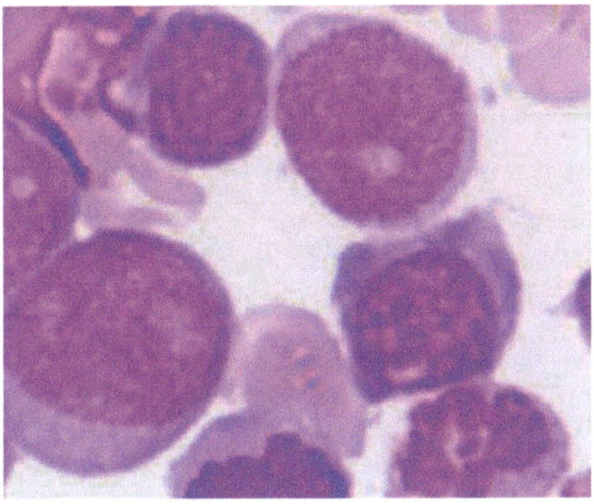

Fig. 7. M6 "Erythroleukemia"

2.8 M7 Acute megakaryoblastic leukemia (AMkL)

M7 is rare. It occurs as a leukemia transformation of chronic granulocytic leukemia (CGL) and myelodysplastic syndrome (MDS). Pancytopenia is characteristic at initial diagnosis. Peripheral blood shows micromegakaryocytes and undifferentiated blasts. Bone marrow dry tap is common. Bone marrow biopsy show increased fibroblasts and/or increased reticulin and presence of greater than 30% blast cells. The diagnosis of M7 should be suspected when the blast cells show cytoplasmic protrusion or budding. As bone marrow smears obtained by aspiration may not be adequate to make a diagnosis, the peripheral blood films must be examined carefully for the presence of micromegakaryoblasts. Bone marrow biopsy sections are usually necessary and show a prominent reticulin fibrosis and excessive numbers of small blasts.

Cytochemistry: Peroxidase is negative, PAS +/-, Esterase +/- and positive acid phospatase. Cytochemical positivity for α-naphthyl acetate esterase reaction and negative reaction with α-naphthyl butyrate esterase is unique to megakaryoblast. (Monocytes react positively with both esterase substrates).

The monoclonal antibodies that reacts with platelet glycoprotein Ib, IIb/IIIa and IIIb, using immunologic technique as well as CD41, CD42 and CD61 positivity.
There is no unique chromosomal abnormality associated with acute megakaryoblastic leukemia, with the exception of t(1;22)(p13;q13), which has been found almost exclusively in young children, less than 18 months old who do not have Downís syndrome.

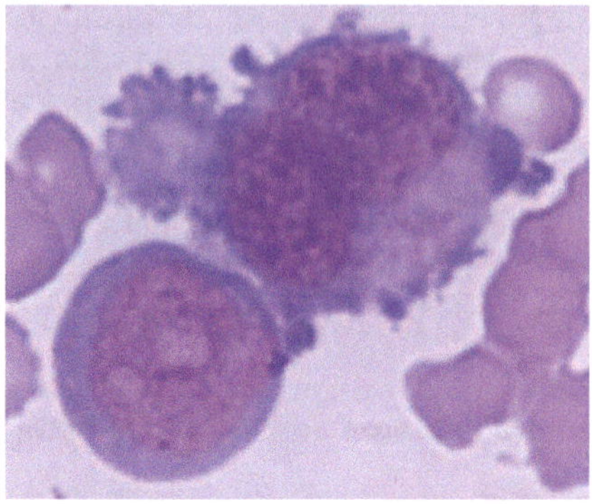

Fig. 8. M7 Acute megakaryoblastic leukemia (AMkL)

Morphologic Classification	
FAB Type	**Features of Blasts**
L1	Small cells with scant cytoplasm; nucleoli indistinct and not visible
L2	Large, heterogeneous cells with moderately abundant cytoplasm; clefting and indentation of nucleus; large and prominent nucleoli
L3	Large cells with moderately abundant cytoplasm; regular, oval-to-round nucleus; prominent nucleoli; prominent cytoplasmic basophilia and cytoplasmic vacuoles

Table 2. Morphologic Classification of Acute Lymphocytic Leukemia

Acute lymphoblastic leukemia (ALL) is divided in FAB L1 (children), L2 (older children and adult), and L3 (patients with leukemia secondary to Burkitt's lymphoma. These types are defined according to two criteria (1) the occurrence of individual cytologic features and (2) the degree of heterogeneity among the leukemic cells. These features considered are cell size, chromatin, nuclear shape, nucleoli, and degree of basophilia in the cytoplasm and the presence of cytoplasmic vacuolation (Bennett et al 1976).
ALL-L1: Homogenous cells **(Small cell):** One population of cells within the case. Small cells predominant, nuclear shape is regular with occasional cleft. Nuclear contents are rarely visible. Cytoplasm is moderately basophilic. L1 accounts 70% of patients. The L1 type is the acute leukemia that is common in childhood, with 74% of these cases occurring in children 15 years of age or younger.
ALL-L2: Heterogeneous cells: Large cells with an irregular nuclear shape, cleft in the nucleus are common. One or more large nucleoli are visible. Cytoplasm varies in colour and nuclear membrane irregularities. L2 accounts 27% of ALL patients. The FAB-L2 blast may be

confused with the blasts of acute myeloid leukemia. Approximately 66% of these cases of ALL in patients older than 15 years are of type 2.

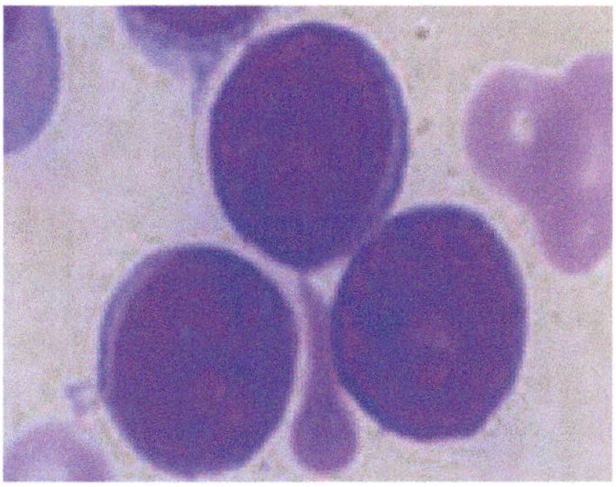

Fig. 9. Acute lymphoblastic leukemia L1

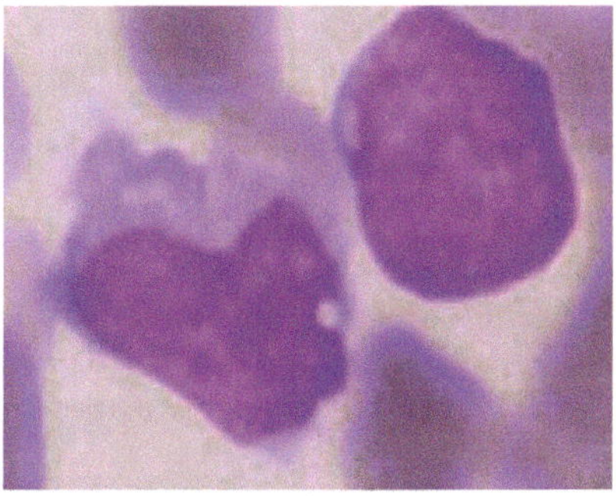

Fig. 10. Acute lymphoblastic leukemia L2

ALL-L3: Burkitt's lymphoma type: Cells are large and homogenous in size, nuclear shape is round or oval. One to three prominent nucleoli and sometimes to 5 nuleoli are visible. Cytoplasm is deeply basophilic with vacuoles often prominent. Intense cytoplasmic basophilia is present in every cell, with prominent vacuolation in most. A high mitotic index is characteristic with presence of varying degrees of macrophage activity. Mature B-lymphoid markers are expressed by most cases.

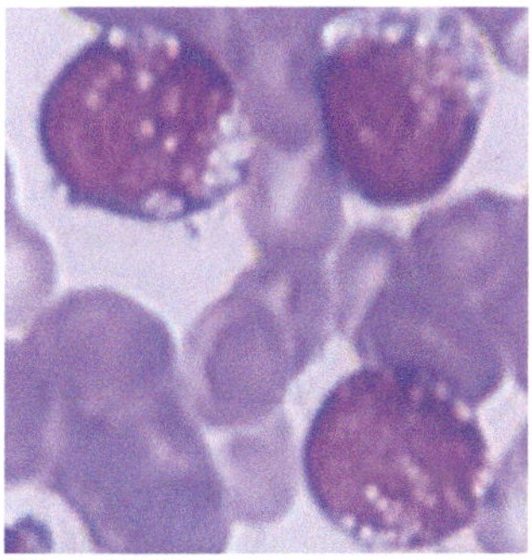

Fig. 11. Acute lymphoblastic leukemia L3

Acute Myeloid Leukemia (AML) and Related Precursor Neoplasm
AML with recurrent genetic abnormalities
AML with t(8;21)(q22;q22); RUNX1-RUNX1T1
AML with inv(16)(p13.1q22) or t(16;16)(p13.1;q22); CBFB-MYH11
Acute promyelocytic leukemia with t(15;17)(q22;q12); PML-RARA
AML with t(9 ;11)(p22;q23); MLLT3-MLL
AML with t(6;9)(p23;q34); DEK-NUP214
AML with inv(3)(q21q26.2) or t(3;3)(q21;q26.2); RPN1-EVI1
AML with mutated NPM1
AML with mutated CEBPA
AML with myelodysplasia-related changes
Therapy-related myeloid neoplasms
Myeloid sarcoma
Myeloid proliferations related to Down syndrome
Transient abnormal myelopoiesis
Myeloid leukemia associated with Down syndrome
Blastic plasmacytoid denderitic cell neoplasm

Table 3. World Health Organization Classification of Acute Myelogenous Leukemia (2008)

AML defined as ≥20% blasts in blood or bone marrow; however, clonal, recurring cytogenetic abnormalities should be considered AML regardless of blast percentage. Ongoing clinical trials may continue to use French-American-British (FAB) criteria of ≥30% blasts until completion of trial. FAB classification identified as M0 through M7.

The classification schemes by the World Health Organization (WHO) require the additional evaluation of the leukemic blasts by molecular analysis and flow cytometry (Harris NL 1997 & Brunangelo Falini 2010, Sachdeva et al 2006). The results of these 4 methods of evaluation (i.e, morphology, staining, molecular analysis, flow cytometry) not only differentiate ALL from AML, but also categorize the subtypes of acute leukemia. Table 3 summarizes the new classification of AML as proposed by WHO, Knowing the subtype of a patient's leukemia helps in predicting the clinical behavior of the disease and the prognosis, and in making treatment recommendations. This classification also improves the reproducibility of diagnoses and stresses the heterogeneity of the subtypes of AML and ALL (Vardiman 2009). Recent advances in molecular biology have shown that various subtypes of AML and ALL behave differently and should not be treated similarly. For example, the identification of M3 AML (acute promyelocytic leukemia) is crucial because it is associated with disseminated intravascular coagulation (DIC), and retinoic acid, in addition to chemotherapy, is the treatment of choice.

The two most significant differences between the FAB and the WHO classifications are:

(a) A lower blast threshold for the diagnosis of AML: The WHO defines AML when the blast percentage reaches 20% in the bone marrow.

(b) Patients with recurring clonal cytogenetic abnormalities should be considered to have AML regardless of the blast percentage (8;21)(q22;q22), t(16;16)(p13;q22), inv(16)(p13;q22), or t(15;17)(q22;q12) (Arber DA et al 2008abc, Weinberg OK et al 2009).

The world Health Organization (WHO) classification has changed the grouping of ALL to reflect increased understanding of the biology and molecular pathogenesis of the diseases. In addition to discarding the L1-L3 terms, the new classification characterizes these heterogenous diseases based upon immunophenotype into 3 basic categories: precursor B-cell ALL, precursor T-cell ALL, and mature B-cell ALL (Burkitt lymphoma/leukemia) (Jaffe et al 2001)

WHO classification
Precursor B-cell ALL/LBL
Cytogenetic subgroups
t(9;22)(q34,q11),BCR/ABL
t(v;11q23);MLL rearranged
t(1;19)(q23;p13);PBX1/E2A
t(12;21)(p13;q22);TEL/AML1
Hypodiploid
Hyperdiploid, >50
Precursor T-cell ALL/LBL
Mature B-cell leukemia/lymphoma
ALL= acute lymphoblastic leukemia; LBL= lymphoblastic lymphoma; MLL= mixed lineage leukemia

Table 4. World Health Organization classification of acute lymphoblastic leukemia

Abnormalities in chromosome number as well as structural rearrangements (translocations) occur commonly in ALL. Important cytogenetic abnormalities in precursor B-cell ALL that are associated with a poor prognosis include t(9;22) or Philadelphia chromosome-positive (Ph+) ALL, which increases in frequency with age; t(4;11); hypodiploidy, especially if <45% chromosomes ; and trisomy 8 in adult ALL. The t(4;11) results from a balanced translocation involving a gene on the long arm of chromosome 11 at band q23 (11q23), known as the mixed lineage leukemia (MLL) gene. MLL gene translocations occur most commonly in infancy and are associated with both acute lymphoid and myeloid leukemias.

3. European Group for the Immunological classification of Leukemias (EGIL)

The European Group for the Immunological Classification of Leukemias (EGIL)(Bene MC et al 1995 & Hoelzer et al 2002)) has proposed that acute leukaemia be classified on the basis of immunophenotype alone. This classification has the strength that it suggests standardized criteria for defining a leukaemia as myeloid, T lineage, B lineage, or biphenotypic. It also suggests criteria for distinguishing biphenotypic leukaemia from AML with aberrant expression of lymphoid antigens, and from ALL with aberrant expression of myeloid antigens. However, a purely immunological classification has the disadvantage that discrete entities may fall into one of two categories; for example some cases of AML of FAB M2 subtype associated with t(8;21)(q22;q22) would be classified as "AML of myelomonocytic lineage", while others would be classified as "AML with lymphoid antigen expression," depending on whether or not a case showed aberrant expression of CD19. In addition, rare cases of acute leukaemia have been described which were clearly myeloid when assessed by cytology and cytochemistry but which did not express any of the commonly investigated myeloid antigens.

Precursor B-lymphoblastic leukemia (HLA-DR+, TdT+, CD19+, and/or CD79a+, and/or CD22+, and/or CD34+). This type of ALL accounts for around 75% of adult cases and is subdivided into the following groups:

a. Pro B-ALL expresses HLA-DR, TdT, and CD19. CD10-, cytoplasmic immunoglobulin negative; represents approximately 10% of adult ALL.
b. Common ALL is characterized by the presence of CD10, cytoplasmic immunoglobulin negative; comprises greater than 50% of adult cases of ALL.
c. Pre B-ALL is characterised by the expression of cytoplasmic immunoglobulin and CD10; this subtype of ALL is identified in nearly 10% of adult cases.
d. Mature B-ALL is found in approximately 4% of adult ALL patients. The blast cells express surface antigens of mature B cells, including surface membrane immunoglobulin (SmIg+). They are typically TdT and CD34 negative and have L3 morphology. This category overlaps with Burkitt lymphoma, which is included under the mature B-cell neoplasms.

Precursor T-lymphoblastic leukemia

Cells are TdT+ in addition to cytoplasmic CD3+ and CD34+. This type of ALL accounts for around 25% of adult cases and is subdivided into:

a. Pro T-ALL CD2-, CD7+, CD4-, CD8- seen in around 7% of adult ALL.
b. Pre T-ALL CD2+, CD7+, CD4-, CD8-.
c. Cortical T-ALL or Thymic ALL (Thy ALL) is CD1a+ and accounts for 17% of adult ALL CD7+, CD2+, CD5+, CD4+, CD8+
d. Mature T-ALL are surface CD3+, CD2+, CD7+, CD4 or 8, and TdT/CD34/CD1a- and make up approximately 1% of adult ALL.

Table 5. European Group for the Immunological Characterization of Leukemias (EGIL) classification of acute lymphocytic leukemia (Hoelzer 2002)

The consensus considers a 20% minimum threshold to define a positive reaction of blast cells to a given monoclonal antibody. Roughly 75% of cases of adult ALL are of B-cell lineage. B-lineage markers are CD19, CD20, CD22, CD24, and CD79a (Huh 2000).

The earliest B-lineage markers are CD19, CD22 (membrane and cytoplasm) and CD79a (Campana 1988). A positive reaction for any two of these three markers, without further differentiation markers, identifies pro-B ALL. The presence of CD10 antigen (CALLA) defines the "common" ALL subgroup. Cases with additional identification of cytoplasmatic IgM constitute the pre-B group, whereas the presence of surface immunglobulin light chains defines mature B-ALL.

T-cell ALL constitutes approximately 25% of all adult cases of ALL. T-cell markers are CD1a, CD2, CD3 (membrane and cytoplasm), CD4, CD5, CD7 and CD8. CD2, CD5 and CD7 antigens are the most immature T-cell markers, but none of them is absolutely lineage-specific, so that the unequivocal diagnosis of T-ALL rests on the demonstration of surface/cytoplasmic CD3.

ALL of B or T lineage can additionally express myeloid antigens or stem-cell antigen CD34. The latter has little diagnostic relevance but can be prognostically important (De Waele 2001) The scoring system recently proposed by the EGIL group addressed the characterization of the acute leukemia as B or T lineage ALL, or AML by including the most specific markers for the lymphoid and myeloid lineages among those of earlier stages of cell differentiation, plus some non-specific but stem-cell markers. The system introduced a modified terminology specific to each 'maturation' step within the B- or T-cell lineage (EGIL 1995) and was confirmed as adequate for both diagnosis and subclassification of ALL (Thalhammer-Scherrer 2002).

4. European Group for the Immunological characterization of Leukemias (EGIL) classification for biphenotypic acute leukemia

Biphenotypic acute leukemia (BAL), or acute leukemia with a single population of blasts coexpressing markers of two different lineages, is a rare clinical entity.
The scoring systems proposed by Catovsky *et al.* and by the EGIL (Bene 1995) allowed for a better definition of biphenotypic acute leukemia (BAL), clearly distinguishing them from classical AL expressing aberrantly one or two markers of another lineage. However, increasing evidence suggests that this system has limitations, as acknowledged by the 2008 World Health Organization (WHO) Classification of Tumors of Hematopoietic and Lymphoid Tissues. Although substantially improved in relation to the EGIL, the new WHO Classification is still not optimal for guiding the clinical management of patients with BAL. Typical examples of such aberrations are the expression of CD15 on B-ALL(Maynadie et al 1997), or of CD2 on acute promyelocytic -AML(Albano 2006). In 1998, the EGIL further refined this scoring system by attributing one point for the expression of CD117, after showing the strong relationship of this marker with engagement in the myeloid lineage (Bene MC et al 1998) . To identify BAL, it is therefore necessary to consider aberrant co-expression of markers usually associated to different lineages, with a score higher than 2 in more than one lineage (Zhao XF et al 2009)

	B-lineage	T-lineage	Myeloid lineage
2 point	CD79	CD3	MPO
	IgM	Anti TCR	Lisozyme
	CD22		
1 point	CD19	CD2	CD13
	CD10	CD5	CD33
	CD20	CD8	CD65
		CD10	
0.5 point	TdT	TdT	CD14
	CD24	CD17	CD15
		CD10	CD64, CD117

Table 6. EGIL Scoring system for biphenotypic acute leukemia

Biphenotypic acute leukemia is defined when scores are >2 for the myeloid lineage and >1 for the lymphoid lineage. In some T-ALL cases, clonality of TCR alphabeta rearrangements can now be assessed cytoflourmetrically (Langerak 2001, Xu XQ et al 2009).
The prognosis of biphenotypic acute leukemia patients is poor when compared with de novo acute myeloid leukemia or acute lymphoblastic leukemia. Biphenotypic acute leukemia patients showed a much higher incidence of CD34 antigen expression, complex abnormal karyotype, extramedullary infiltration, relapse, and resistance to therapy after relapse (Xu XQ et al 2009).

5. Conclusion

Acute leukaemia can be classified in many ways. An ideal classification is one which recognizes real entities with fundamental biological differences. The FAB classification of ALL and AML is based on morphology and cytochemical staining of blasts. However, the recent classification schemes proposed by the World Health Organization (WHO) require the additional evaluation of the leukemic blasts by molecular analysis and flow cytometry. The results of these 4 methods of evaluation (ie, morphology, staining, molecular analysis, flow cytometry) not only differentiate ALL from AML, but also categorize the subtypes of acute leukemia . Recent advances in molecular biology have shown that various subtypes of AML and ALL behave differently and should not be treated similarly. For example, the identification of M3 AML (acute promyelocytic leukemia) is crucial because it is associated with disseminated intravascular coagulation (DIC), and retinoic acid, in addition to chemotherapy, is the treatment of choice.

The European Group for the Immunological Classification of Leukemias (EGIL) has proposed that acute leukaemia be classified on the basis of immunophenotype alone. This classification has the strength that it suggests standardized criteria for defining a leukaemia as myeloid, T lineage, B lineage, or biphenotypic. It also suggests criteria for distinguishing biphenotypic leukaemia from AML with aberrant expression of lymphoid antigens, and from ALL with aberrant expression of myeloid antigens.

6. References

Albano F, Mestice A, Pannunzio A, Lanza F, Martino B, Pastore D, et al. The biological characteristics of CD34+ CD2+ adult acute promyelocytic leukemia and the CD34 CD2 hypergranular (M3) and microgranular (M3v) phenotypes. *Haematologica.* 2006;91:311-6.

Arber DA, Brunning RD, Le Beau MM, Falini B, Vardiman JW, Porwit A, Thiele J, Bloomfield CD. Acute myeloid leukaemia with recurrent genetic abnormalities. In: *WHO Classification of Tumours of Haematopoietic and Lymphoid Tissues.* 4th edition. pp. 110-123. Swerdlow SH, Campo E, Harris NL et al. (eds.). International Agency for Research on Cancer (IARC), Lyon, France, 2008a.

Arber DA, Brunning RD, Orazi A, Bain BJ, Porwit A, Vardiman JW, Le Beau MM, Greenberg PL. Acute myeloid leukaemia with myelodysplasia-related changes. In: *WHO Classification of Tumours of Haematopoietic and Lymphoid Tissues.* 4th edition. pp. 124-126. Swerdlow SH, Campo E, Harris NL et al. (eds.). International Agency for Research on Cancer (IARC), Lyon, France, 2008b.

Arber DA, Brunning RD, Orazi A, Porwit A, Peterson L, Thiele J, Le Beau MM. Acute myeloid leukemia, not otherwise specified. In: *WHO Classification of Tumours of Haematopoietic and Lymphoid Tissues.* 4th edition. pp. 130-139. Swerdlow SH, Campo E, Harris NL et al. (eds.). International Agency for Research on Cancer (IARC), Lyon, France, 2008c.

Bene MC, Castoldi G, Knapp W, et al. Proposals for the immunological classification of acute leukemias. Leukemia 1995;9:1783-6

Bennett JM, Catovsky D, Daniel MT, et al. Proposals for the classification of the acute leukaemias (FAB cooperative group). Brj Haematol 1976;33:451-8.

Benett JM, Catovsky D, Daniel MT et al(1980) The French-American-British (FAB) Cooperative Group. Corresponence; a variant form of hypergranular promyelocytic leukemia (M3). Br J Haematol 44: 169-70

Benette JM, CatoSky D, Daniel MT et al(1982) Proposals for the classification of myelodsplastic syndromes. Br J Haematol 51; 189-99

Bennett JM, Catovsky D, Daniel M-T, et al. Criteria for the diagnosis of acute leukemia of megakaryocytic lineage (M7): a report of the French-American-British cooperative group. Ann Intern Med 1985;103:460-2.

Bennett JM, Catovsky D, Daniel MT, et al. Proposal for the recognition of minimally differentiated acute myeloid leukaemia (AML MO). Brj Haematol 1991;78:325-9.

Berger R, Flandrin G (1984) Determining the nature of cells studied cytogenetically. Cancer Surveys 3:423-38

Berger R, Bernheim A, Daniel MT, et al(1985) Cytogenetic studies on acute myelomonocytic leukemia (M4) with eosinophilia. Leuk Res 9: 279-88

Campana D, Janossy G. Proliferation of normal and malignant human immature lymphoid cells. Blood 1988; 71: 1201-1210

Catovsky D, Matutes E, Buccheri V, Shetty V, Hanslip J, Yoshida N, Morilla R. A classification of acute leukaemia for the 1990s. *Ann Hematol.* 1991;62:16–21.

Cheson BD, Cassileth PA, Head DR, et al. Report of the National Cancer Institute-sponsored workshop on definitions of diagnosis and response in acute myeloid leukemia. J Clin Oncol 1990;8:813–9.

De Waele M, Renmans W, Vander GK, Jochmans K, Schots R, Otten J, et al. Growth factor receptor profile of CD34+ cells in AML and B-lineage ALL and in their normal bone marrow counterparts. Eur J Haematol 2001; 66: 178-187

European Group for the Immunological Characterization of leukemia (EGIL), Bene MC, Castoldi G, Knapp W, et al. Proposals for the immunological classification of acute leukemias. Leukemia 1995;9:1783-6.

Falini B, Tiacci E, Martelli MP, Ascni S, Pileri SA. New classification of acute myeloid leukemia and precursor-related neoplasms: changes and unsolved issues. Discov Med. 2010 Oct;10(53):281-92.

First MIC Cooperative Study Group. Morphologic, immunologic, and cytogenetic (MIC) working classification of acute lymphoblastic leukaemias. Cancer Genet Cytogenetic 1986;23:189-97.

Harris NL, Jaffe ES, Diebold J, et al. World Health Organization classification of neoplastic diseases of the hematopoietic and lymphoid tissues: report of the ClinicalAdvisory Committee meeting—Airlie House, Virginia, November 1997. J Clin Oncol 1999;17:3835–49.

Hayhoe FG. The classification of acute leukaemia. Blood Rev 1988;2:186-93.

Hoelzer D., GokbugerN: Diagnostik und Therapie der akuten lymphatischen Leukaemia des Erwachsenen. Onkologie 8 (7) (2002) 672-85

Huh YO, Ibrahim S. Immunophenotypes in adult acute lymphocytic leukemia. Role of flow cytometry in diagnosis and monitoring of disease. Hematol Oncol Clin North Am 2000; 14: 1251-1265

Jaffe ES, Harris NL, Stein H et al: *World Health Organization Classification of Tumours of haematopoietic and lymphoid tissue f.* Lyon, IARC Press, 2001.

Langerak AW, van Den BR, I.L., Boor PP, van Lochem EG, Hooijkaas H, et al. Molecular and flow cytometric analysis of the Vbeta repertoire for clonality assessment in mature TCRalphabeta T-cell proliferations. Blood 2001; 98: 165-173

Maynadié M, Campos L, Moskovtchenko P, Sabido O, Aho S, Lenormand B, et al. Heterogenous expression of CD15 in acute lymphoblastic leukemia: a study of ten anti-CD15 monoclonal antibodies in 158 patients. *Leuk Lymphoma.* 1997;25:135–43.

McKenna RW, Parkin J, Bllomfield CD et al (1982)Acute promyelocytic leukemia: a study of 39 caes with identification of a hyperbasophilic microgranular variant. Br J Haematol 50:201-14

Sachdeva MU, Ahluwalia J, Das R, et al (2006) Role of FAB classification of acute leukemias in era of immunophenotyping.Indian J Pathol Microbiol: 2006 Oct;49(4):524-7.

Shibata A, Bennett JM, Castoldi GL et al (1985) Recommended methods for cytological procedures in haematology. Clin Lab Haematol 7:55-74

Thalhammer-Scherrer R, Mitterbauer G, Simonitsch I, Jaeger U, Lechner K, Schneider B, et al. The immunophenotype of 325 adult acute leukemias: relationship to morphologic and molecular classification and proposal for a minimal screening program highly predictive for lineage discrimination. Am J Clin Pathol 2002; 117: 380-389

Vardiman JW. The World Health Organization (WHO) classification of tumors of the hematopoietic and lymphoid tissues: an overview with emphasis on the myeloid neoplasms. Chem Biol Interact 2010 Mar 19;184(1-2):16-20.

Weinberg OK, Seetharam M, Ren K, Seo K, Merker JD, Gotlib J, Zehnder JL, Arber DA. Clinical characterization of acute myeloid leukemia with myelodysplasia-related changes as defined by the 2008 WHO classification system. Blood. 2009 Feb 26;113(9):1906-8.

Xu XQ, Wang JM, Lu SQ, Chen L, Yang JM, Zhang WP, Song XM, Hou J, Ni X, Qiu HY. Clinical and biological characteristics of adult biphenotypic acute leukemia in comparison with that of acute myeloid leukemia and acute lymphoblastic leukemia: a case series of a Chinese population. Haematologica. 2009 Jul;94(7):919-27.

2

Diagnosis of Acute Leukemia in Under-Resourced Laboratories

Abbas H. Abdulsalam
Al-Yarmouk Teaching Hospital, Baghdad
Iraq

1. Introduction

Laboratory diagnosis of acute leukemia in modern hematology practice is increasingly relying on guidelines that require the availability of relatively expensive machines with consistent need for continuous quality control, kits supply and maintenance.

In under-resourced hematology laboratories there is usually a missing step in the battery of required investigations. Moreover, when some of the advanced diagnostic instruments can be found then the problem of chronic inadequate and irregular supply of kits and services would supervene. Therefore, the laboratory diagnosis would mostly depend on the more basic, but consistently available and well controlled, laboratory techniques that should at least include complete blood count (CBC) and peripheral blood morphology, after which a bone marrow study with aspirate and sometimes a trephine biopsy will follow.

Moreover, in specialized hematology centers there may be a routine availability of few special stains, a very limited immunophenotyping CD markers panel, cytogenetics and PCR or FISH testing mostly for BCR-ABL1 oncogene.

The aim of diagnosis, lineage assignment and sub-classification of acute leukemia in these laboratories should immediately serve a clear therapeutic goal.

Sketching rational systematic schemes for optimum use of the locally available investigation options would usually permit the diagnosis of most varieties of acute leukemias with a very acceptable level of reliability. Also these schemes may provide invaluable information regarding the prospect of update and future plans for laboratory development as it can show clearly where the weak joints are (Abdulsalam, 2010).

2. Basis of diagnosis of myelodysplastic syndrome (MDS)

The WHO classification of this pre-AML disorder (Table 1) can be applied in most under-resourced laboratories as it only entails the use of peripheral blood morphology and bone marrow aspirate morphology with Perl's reaction (diagnosis of rare hypoplastic and myelofibrotic MDS would require also bone marrow trephine biopsy) with the sole addition of cytogenetics, preferably performed on marrow aspirate sample.

Even when cytogenetic testing is not available, still the WHO classification can be reliably applied for the diagnosis of most of the MDS subcategories, with the exceptions of the otherwise provisional diagnosis of MDS-5q- syndrome (which is characteristically found in a middle age or an elderly female with peripheral blood macrocytic anemia and upper

Type	Peripheral blood	Bone marrow aspirate
Refractory cytopenia with unilineage dysplasia: - Refractory anemia (RA) - Refractory neutropenia - Refractory thrombocytopenia	Uni- or bi-cytopenia and <1% blasts	Unilineage dysplasia* with <5% blasts
Refractory anemia with ring sideroblasts (RARS)	Anemia and <1% blasts	Erythroid dysplasia only with <5% blasts and >15% ring sideroblasts
Refractory cytopenia with multilineage dysplasia	Bi- or pan-cytopenia and <1% blasts	Bi- or tri-dysplasia with <5% blasts and <15% ring sideroblasts
Refractory cytopenia with multilineage dysplasia and ring sideroblasts	Bi- or pan-cytopenia and <1% blasts	Bi- or tri-dysplasia with <5% blasts and >15% ring sideroblasts
Refractory anemia with excess blasts-1 (RAEB-1)	1-4% blasts	5-9% blasts and no Auer rods
Refractory anemia with excess blasts-2 (RAEB-2)	5-19% blasts	10-19% blasts, or <19% blasts plus Auer rods**
MDS-Unclassified	Uni-, bi- or pan-cytopenia and <1% blasts	Cytogenetic diagnosis of MDS with uni-, bi- or tri-lineage dysplasia in <10% of the cells and <5% blasts
Isolated $5q^-$ syndrome	Anemia with upper normal or increase platelet count	Isolated del(5q) on cytogenetic study, prominent large megakaryocytes with hypolobated nuclei and <5% blasts***

* Dysplasia is considered significant only if it is present in >10% of the cells.
** If Auer rods or pseudo-Chediak Higashi inclusions are present then MDS RAEB-2 is diagnosed even when the peripheral blood and bone marrow blasts are <5% and <10% respectively.
*** If blasts > 5% then it is classified as RAEB, although still lenalidomide treatment should be tried.

Table 1. WHO classification of MDS, 2008 (Vardiman, et al, 2009)

normal platelet count or even thrombocytosis, bone marrow megakaryocytes of normal overall size but with a relatively small mono- or bi-lobed nucleus and a very good response to a therapeutic trial of lenalidomide) (Kelaidi et al, 2008) and MDS-Unclassified (which can be diagnosed on follow up when the disease persists or even progress). This classification, unlike the late FAB classification, would keep with the newest 20% blasts cut-off point to diagnose acute leukemia, coping with the worldwide standards of MDS literatures and provide much more relevant prognostic groups.

3. Diagnosis of acute leukemia in under-resourced laboratories

FAB classification (Table 2) of acute leukemia should be applied in under-resourced laboratories where the only available routine techniques for diagnosis are morphology and special stains (Abdulsalam, 2010). The scheme in (Figure 1) may be used as a general guideline for the diagnosis of acute leukemia in under-resourced laboratories; however, it should be modified to optimally fit into the locally available techniques.

The practical application of WHO classification for acute leukemia (Tables 3 and 4) requires both diagnosis and risk stratification. The diagnosis can be based on morphology, special stains and immunophenotyping (preferably using flowcytometry, or if it is not available then one can rely on either immunocytochemistry with/without immunohistochemistry). Laboratory risk stratification relies on cytogenetics and multiplex conventional PCR.

Later on, a follow up for minimal residual disease can be performed using the same genetic abnormality found at diagnosis, i.e., cytogenetic remission, or more accurately, real time quantitative (RQ) PCR for quantization of the characteristic translocation that was found positive (but without quantization using conventional "qualitative" PCR) at diagnosis.

Acute leukemia	Subtype	Morphology	Additional tests
ALL	L1	Small, homogeneous with high N:C ratio blasts	TdT, CD3, CD79a, CD20, CD10
	L2	Larger, heterogeneous, nucleolated with low N:C ratio blasts	
	Leukemic phase of Burkitt's lymphoma (L3)	Large, homogeneous and nucleolated blasts with basophilic and vacuolated cytoplasm	Cytogenetics, ISH or PCR
AML	M0	Undifferentiated blasts	Anti-MPO, CD117, CD33, CD68 or Lysozyme
	M1	Undifferentiated blasts ± dysplastic myeloid differentiation	SBB stain
	M2	Myeloblasts with myeloid maturation	
	M3	Characteristic morphology, Faggot cells	
	M3 variant	Characteristic morphology, bilobed nuclei	
	M4	Peripheral blood monocytes ≥5.0 $*10^9/l$ ± bone marrow monocytic lineage ≥20%	NSE confirmation of monocytic lineage
	M5a (Monoblastic), M5b (Monocytic) and M5c (Histiocytic)	Bone marrow monocytic lineage ≥80%	
	M6	Trilineage dysplasia and >50% erythroblasts	SBB, Glycophorin + anti-MPO, avoid CD34 as it would stain both myeloblasts and proerythroblasts
	M7	Blast with cytoplasmic blebs and bone marrow fibrosis	CD41

Table 2. Diagnosis of acute leukemia based on FAB groups

Follow up for minimal residual disease using a multi-color flowcytometry can be adequately performed (Thorn et al, 2011) but is usually more demanding than the genetic techniques, and therefore, it may not be the best choice in a resource-poor laboratory.

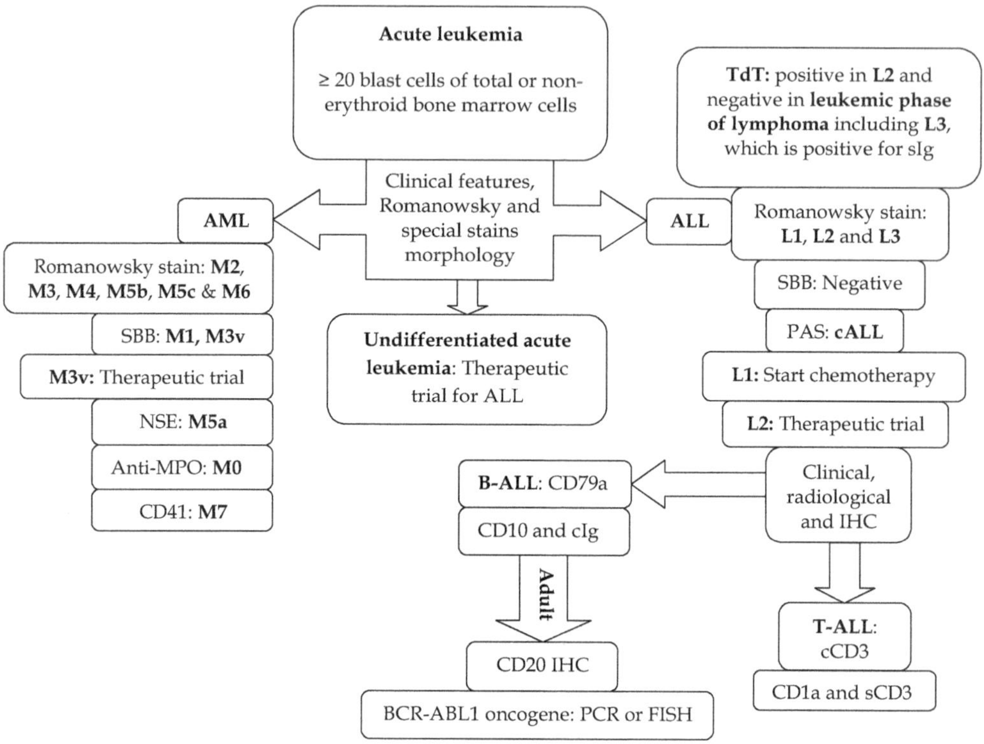

Fig. 1. Options for diagnosis of acute leukemia in resource-poor laboratories: FAB-based classification serving a clear therapeutic target.

3.1 Basis of diagnosis of acute leukemia

In the WHO classification of acute leukemia (Jaffe, et al, 2001) the diagnosis is based on an arbitrary cut-off point of 20% blasts as a percentage of bone marrow total or non-erythroid cells or as a percentage of peripheral blood cells. This exact percent is also applied nowadays in under-resourced laboratories were the FAB classification should be used (Bain, 2010a).

This 20% myeloblasts cut-off point seems to be universally accepted and for the time being it represents the best known tool for defining acute leukemia. However, the word "arbitrary" may still precede it and this may be attributed to (Abdulsalam, 2011):

1. This precise percent does not represent some specific biological event in the continuum of increasing blast count, but it is merely, to the best to our current knowledge, a cut-off point that permits a relatively clear classification and therapeutic aim. However, the fact that some high risk MDS patients are being treated actively with only 10% bone marrow blasts should be remembered.

--- Therapy- related myeloid neoplasms
--- De novo myeloid neoplasms
- AML with *recurrent genetic abnormalities* including

  t(8;21)(q22;q22); RUNX1-RUNX1T1
  inv(16)(p13.1q22) or t(16;16)(p13.1;q22); CBFB-MYH11
  t(15;17)(q22;q12); PML-RARA
  t(9;11)(p22;q23); MLLT3-MLL
  t(6;9)(p23;q34); DEK-NUP214
  inv(3)(q21q26.2) or t(3;3)(q21;q26.2); RPN1-EVI1
  t(1;22)(p13;q13); RBM15-MKL1
  Provisional entity: AML with mutated NPM1
  Provisional entity: AML with mutated CEBPA
- AML with myelodysplasia-related changes
- AML not otherwise categorized
- Myeloid sarcoma
- Myeloid proliferation related to Down syndrome
- Transient abnormal myelopoiesis
- Myeloid leukemia associated with Down syndrome
- Blastic plasmacytoid dendritic cell neoplasm

Table 3. WHO classification of AML, 2008 (Vardiman, et al, 2009)

--- B lymphoblastic leukemia/lymphoma
- B lymphoblastic leukemia/lymphoma, not otherwise specified
- B lymphoblastic leukemia/lymphoma with *recurrent genetic abnormalities* including

  t(9;22)(q34;q11.2) and BCR-ABL1
  translocation involving 11q23 and MLL rearrangement
  t(12;21)(p13;q22) and ETV6-RUNX1
  hyperdiploidy (> 50 chromosomes)
  hypodiploidy (< 46 chromosomes)
  t(5;14)(q31;q32) and IL3-IGH
  t(1;19)(q23;p13.3) and TCF3-PBX1

--- T lymphoblastic leukemia/lymphoma

Table 4. WHO classification of ALL, 2008 (Vardiman, et al, 2009)

2. The significant difference in the cut-off point of blast percent between peripheral blood and bone marrow is well established in MDS as the two groups RAEB-1 (blast count less than 5% in peripheral blood and 5-9% in bone marrow) and RAEB-2 (blast count 5-9% in peripheral blood and 10-19% in bone marrow). In acute leukemia no such discrimination is available.
3. The morphological finding of pathological "clonal" blast, type II that contains Auer rods, Pseudo-Chédiak-Higashi (Abdulsalam & Sabeeh, 2011) (Image 1) or other specific inclusions that are not seen in reactive marrow, is referring to the diagnosis of RAEB-2 or AML, here again the arbitrary cut-off point of 20% blasts will decide the specific diagnosis.
4. The original FAB classification was based for many years on the arbitrary cut-off point of 30% bone marrow blasts and previously some patients with 20-29% blasts remained stable over months without chemotherapy. However, this major percent change was driven by the survival studies which revealed that patients with 20-29% myeloblasts have a similar survival pattern as those with 30% and more in the bone marrow (Jaffe et al, 2001).
5. Although myeloblasts recognition criteria as agranular and granular blasts achieved a reasonable consensus, there are minor discordances in their definitions and in practice it may be a matter of convention (subjective method) to discriminate it from the continuum of cells, as in deciding whether this cell is a blast type III or a promyelocyte.
6. The "blasts" refer to myeloblasts, lymphoblasts, monoblasts, promonocytes and megakaryoblasts.
7. Diagnosis of AML-M3 and its variant is not related to the blast percent.
8. Cases with blast cells less than 20% may still be diagnosed as acute leukemia if they present with certain recurrent cytogenetic abnormalities as in AML M4 with inv(16) or t(16;16)(p13;q22) and AML M2 with t(8;21) (Jaffe et al, 2001).
9. The utilization of 20% lower blast threshold is not really an issue in ALL because most patients at diagnosis already have more than 50% blasts. Moreover, a patient with normal or reduced peripheral blood count and bone marrow lymphoblasts about or slightly above 20% would usually be classified as lymphoblastic lymphoma rather than ALL. A 25% cut-off point has been suggested to arbitrarily differentiate between the two conditions.
10. In AML-M0 and M1 the 20% blasts cut-off point is also of no use in practice.

Laboratory diagnosis of acute leukemia in modern hematology practice is increasingly relying on objective techniques to detect a specific ultrastructural or genetic abnormality. Therefore, the era of 20% blasts to diagnose acute leukemia may not stand the time any longer than that of the old FAB group 30% blasts lower threshold. However, at least in the present and the near future the morphology will remain the initial diagnostic test of acute leukemia and the abovementioned blast threshold will still be useful as a tool for classification (Abdulsalam, 2011).

The presence or absence of myeloblasts has a central role in diagnosis of AML and suspicion of ALL respectively. The blasts are divided into agranular (type I) and granular (type II and III) blasts based on Romanowsky stain morphology. However, when using SBB stain many of the "apparently" agranular blasts turn to be granular. Pathognomonic signs of AML that can be seen with Romanowsky stain and more frequently with SBB stain include SBB-positive granules, Auer rods, atypical "thick" Auer rods, pseudo-Chediak-Higashi inclusions (Abdulsalam et al, 2011a) (Image 1) and rectangular crystalline structures (Merino & Esteve, 2005) .

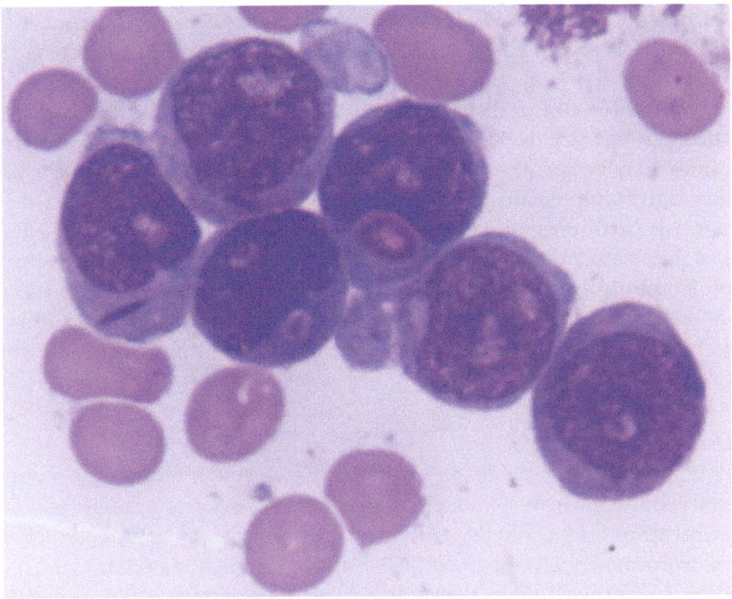

Image 1. Pseudo-Chédiak-Higashi inclusions together with atypical "thick" Auer rods in AML.

3.2 Clinical features

At diagnosis, acute leukemia should, in most of the cases, be clinically manifested within the last month with non-specific features like lethargy and fatigue or more commonly with specific features related to organ infiltration including bone marrow which results in anemia-related features, infections and bleeding. Other organ infiltration may refer not only to broad suspicion of acute leukemia but more likely to lineage assignment or even to a specific diagnosis, e.g., hepatosplenomegaly, lymphadenopathy, CNS symptoms and testicular involvement are in favor of ALL, severe bone pain in lower extremities would refer to B-ALL, thymic mediastinal mass and pleural effusion to T-ALL, bleeding tendency with overt coagulation tests defect can refer to AML-M3 and its variant and gum hypertrophy, skin involvement and hepatosplenomegaly in M4 and, more commonly, in M5.

3.3 Complete blood count (CBC)

Acute leukemia in most of the cases would present with one, or more often more abnormalities of the CBC, including anemia, leucocytosis (or less common leucopenia) and thrombocytopenia. Even when the WBC count is within normal limits the anemia, thrombocytopenia and WBC flags (in most automated cell counters) would raise fair enough suspicion.

Clinical features combined with CBC should be very sensitive in directing acute leukemia cases to be studied by peripheral blood smear.

3.4 Peripheral blood smear

Should be the backbone for the diagnosis of acute leukemia when there is leucocytosis or when leucocyte count is within reference range, as in most of the cases it provides a specific

diagnosis (ALL-L3 and AML-M3), a provisional diagnosis (ALL-L1 and AML M2, M3 variant, M4, M5b, M5c and M6) or at least a limited differential diagnosis (ALL-L2 and AML-M0, M1, M5a and M7).
When blasts are numerous in peripheral blood then special stains like SBB can be applied directly to it, this can be very useful for emergency diagnosis of AML-M3 variant especially within short time like before the weekend (Abdulsalam & Sabeeh, 2010). In cases with leucopenia, although frank blast cells may not be easily found, still there should be at least a clue to the diagnosis (including anemia, thrombocytopenia and myeloid dysplasia).
The presence of nucleated red cells and myeloid dysplasia mainly in the form of Pelger-Huet neutrophils should be investigated as the former can refer to AML-M6 and the later can suggest an AML with myelodysplasia. A bone marrow study should follow including aspirate and biopsy (when there is peripheral blood pancytopenia, and dry tap, hypocellular, diluted or difficult aspirate).

3.5 Bone marrow aspirate (BMA)

The diagnosis of acute leukemia in many instances is evident from the peripheral blood film; however, the bone marrow aspirate examination is always essential for confirmation of diagnosis, classification and application of special techniques including cytochemical stains, genetic studies, Immunocytochemistry (ICC) and immunohistochemistry (IHC).
IHC staining can be applied using the clotted marrow aspirate as a regular tissue sample after fixation and without decalcification (Bain, 2001a), to avoid bone marrow biopsy when there is no need for this procedure apart from the intention to apply immunophenotyping; however, it should be noted that the only use of clotted aspirate is for immunophenotyping, i.e., it should not be used as a regular morphology sample or any other application.
Apart from AML-M3 and its variant, the provisional and final diagnosis of the subtype of acute leukemia should not be issued before a proper BMA is performed. The classification of AML FAB groups is based on the percentages of blasts, maturing myeloid series (promyelocytes to neutrophils), monocytic series and erythroblasts from the total nucleated marrow cells. Also in some occasions many vital signs may be seen only in marrow aspirate like few Faggot cells in AML-M3 variant and even Auer rods. This phenomenon is aggravated when there is a peripheral leucopenia.
Diagnosis of acute leukemia is based on the presence of at least 20% blasts of total nucleated marrow cells, this condition may not be applicable especially in some AML cases, then 20% blasts limit should be obtained from the non-erythroid non-lymphoid marrow cells, otherwise the case would be labelled as MDS (Table 1). The reason for setting two lower thresholds is to simplify the morphology counts in practice, where in the first type of threshold the hematologist needs only to count the blast cells from all the nucleated cells in the field, this is much easier in practice but it would certainly require much higher blast threshold (which is available in almost all cases of ALL and many AML patients) than what would be required in the second form, which would be much more effort demanding and time consuming as one has to exclude erythroblasts, lymphocytes, plasma cells, macrophages and mast cells from the count.
Diagnosis of AML with myelodysplasia can only be confirmed by studying the bone marrow aspirate morphology with trilineage dysplasia. Dyserythropoiesis alone can be seen in many malignancies and is multifactorial, dysmyelopoiesis is supportive to the diagnosis of AML; however in cases where neutrophils and maturing myeloid cells are few then

absence of dysmyelopoiesis does not affect the diagnosis. Dysmegakaryopoiesis, especially in the form of micromegakaryocytes is in favour of diagnosis of AML with a preceding myelodysplastic syndrome.

3.6 Bone marrow biopsy

Is indicated when failed to obtain an adequate marrow aspirate, which may result from improper aspiration technique, presence of fibrosis (especially in ALL and AML-M7; in both conditions there may be a leucoerythroblastic anemia and tear drop poikilocytes in peripheral blood), aleukemic or subleukemic peripheral blood and bone marrow aspirate smears due to heavily packed marrow (especially in ALL) or presence of hypoplastic acute leukemia (especially in AML). It is also indicated when there is an intention to apply routine immunophenotyping (although this can be adequately applied on clotted marrow sections, see paragraph 3.5). It can be stated that the bone marrow biopsy is not an essential investigation in acute leukemia diagnosis when obtaining an adequate marrow aspirate (Bain, 2001b).

The presence of peripheral blood leucocyte count above or within the upper normal count can be used as an indicator that a bone marrow biopsy would not be essential; in contrast, leucopenia or pancytopenia suggest the need for bone marrow biopsy.

3.7 Acute Myeloid Leukemia (AML)

With Romanowsky stain morphology AML- M2, M3, M4, M5b, M5c and M6 can be recognized readily.

By adding few special stains such as Sudan black B, and not myeloperoxidase (MPO) as SBB has a little more sensitivity in detecting myeloblasts which is crucial for diagnosis of AML, plus a non-specific esterase (NSE) stain as ANAE it becomes possible to recognize AML-M1 and most cases of AML-M5a respectively (Bain, 2006).

Rare types of AML like M5c require a higher degree of morphology experience, in which malignant cells appearance is reminiscent of tissue histiocytes (Image 2) (Abdulsalam & Sabeeh, 2009a).

The AML cases that cannot be distinguished by Romanowsky and special stains morphology are M0 and M7, for which the presence of myeloid dysplasia (abnormal nuclear morphology and cytoplasm hypogranularity using a Romanowsky stain or absence of SBB stained granules from maturing myeloid cells and neutrophils) (Image 7) in the former and the blasts' cytoplasmic blebs and bone marrow fibrosis in the latter may give a hint for the probable diagnosis, however there is still the need for more positive diagnostic technique and as the flow cytometry immunophenotyping may not be available then the use of a limited number of CD markers study by ICC/IHC is the option, these include mainly anti-myeloperoxidase for M0 and CD41 for M7.

When resources are limited then it is for the best to concentrate on cytoplasmic ICC/IHC CD markers with the highest lineage sensitivity and specificity.

There is a small proportion of cases that would be only certainly subclassified after the response to treatment as in rare forms of AML-M3v in spite that SBB stain is usually of help in this form (Images 5 and 6).

Risk stratification of AML is based on genetic studies.

3.8 Acute Lymphoblastic Leukemia (ALL)

Consideration of clinical as well as hematological features permits a strong presumptive diagnosis of ALL (Bain, 2010). ALL-L3 diagnosis (which should be referred to as the

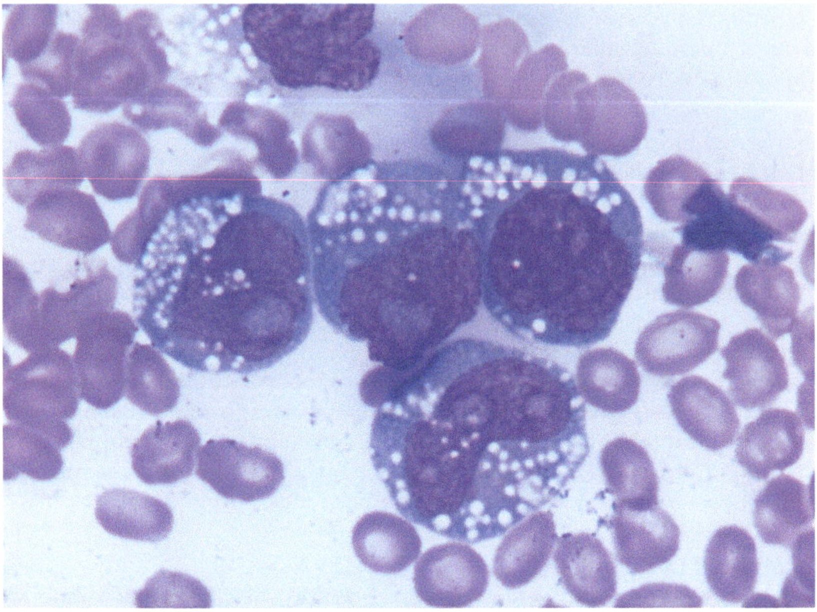

Image 2. Blast cells appearance in AML-M5c.

leukemic phase of Burkitt's lymphoma as it arises from mature B-cells) would be obvious by morphology alone and it is convenient to rely on morphological diagnosis of ALL-L1 and start treatment. Also if a patient with an acute leukemia showing heterogeneous blasts that has no morphological markers of myeloid differentiation, negative staining with SBB with unavailability of further differentiating procedures then it may be treated initially as ALL-L2, as statistically speaking it would be much more possible than AML-M0. The negative result in staining with SBB is very helpful, while the addition of the special stain PAS would improve the chances of the correct diagnosis of common ALL. However, a case with positive staining results for both SBB and PAS is an acute myeloid leukemia (Image 3).

Clinical features as bone pain and radiological sign of mediastinal mass may presumptively aid in differentiating between B- and T-ALL, however, using ICC/IHC antibodies including CD79a for B lineage and CD3 for T lineage are necessary. After setting the diagnosis of B-ALL in adults then ICC/IHC CD20 typing and PCR or FISH for BCR-ABL1 fusion gene would affect the treatment options.

In children (neonate up to 15 years) there is some reluctance for BCR-ABL1 testing due to its low frequency, only about 3%. However, it may be prudent to test for this transcript in children who have some lymphoblasts with large azurophilic granules (represent approximately 10% of cases) (Jaffe, et al, 2001) as this, beside cutting short additional costs, can offer a safer limit.

Rare cases of ALL-L2 that are confused with leukemic phase of large cell lymphoma can be differentiated through the use of TdT immunohistochemistry typing on bone marrow biopsy slide, which would be positive in ALL but not in lymphoma.

Risk stratification of ALL is based on immunophenotypic and genetic studies.

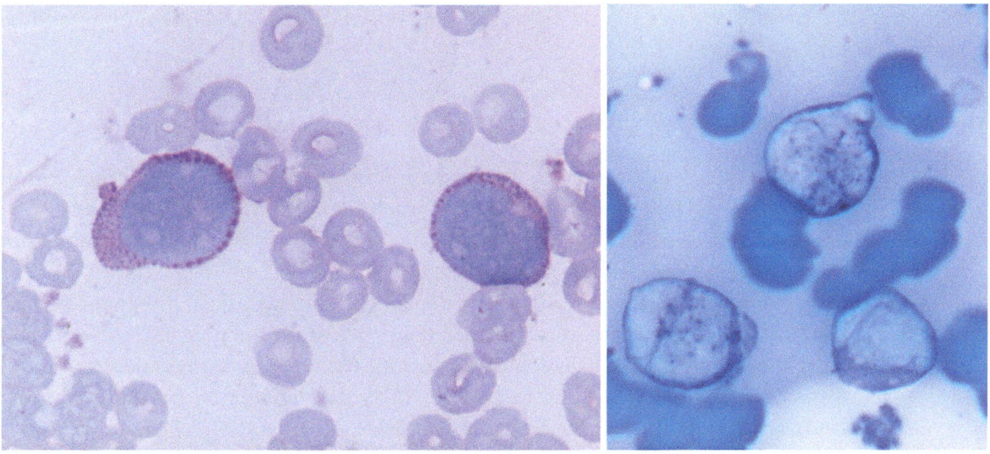

Image 3. Composite photograph of a patient with AML-M1 who had a 95% PAS-positive blasts (left image) and SBB positive blasts (right image).

3.9 Biphenotypic acute leukemia

The diagnosis of this acute leukemia requires a simultaneous application of several myeloid and lymphoid CD markers, or at least a request for the main lymphoid markers (CD3 and CD79a) after finding a SBB positive result (Matutes et al, 1997).

In resource-poor laboratories a step-by-step algorithm is followed in order to use the least possible resources, therefore, the identification of a mixed acute leukemia can be missed, as when some clinical, morphological, cytochemical or immunological markers refer to one diagnosis then the other lines of investigations are usually skipped to save expenses. However, misdiagnosis of this rare type of acute leukemia to only one of its components may, in some cases, not adversely affect the patient.

3.10 Rare types of acute leukemia

In a resource-poor laboratory these types of acute leukemia can be identified only if it happened to show some characteristic features using one of the essential techniques including, e.g., AML-M5c characteristic peripheral blood and bone marrow morphology, while others like biphenotypic acute leukemia may be misdiagnosed to only one of its components as described in paragraph 3.9. Natural killer-cell leukemia can be confused initially with reactive lymphocytosis as it results in CD3 negative and its characteristic CD56 marker is not usually tested for in an under-resourced laboratory.

3.11 Special stains

For diagnosis of AML, especially M1 and M5, the addition of Sudan black B (SBB) and a non-specific esterase stain as α-naphthyl acetate esterase is respectively essential. While for ALL a negative result (0-2%, these rare SBB positively stained blasts represent remnant normal myeloblasts) with SBB staining is crucial to support the diagnosis. The addition of PAS stain would not add a lot to support the diagnosis of ALL as it can, at least occasionally, be equally positive in AML; however, a positive PAS stained vacuolated blasts can be useful to refer to cALL in 98% of cases (Bain, 2010a), here again CD10 ICC/IHC staining would be more meaningful.

3.11.1 Sudan Black B (SBB) stain

It is one of the few, but very useful, cytochemical stains to choose in a resource-poor laboratory. Care should always be paid for counting blasts with the right black color, intensely stained granules. The appealing characters that entail the use of SBB stain are:

i. The reaction and non-reaction with SBB stain are both significant, as the former refer practically to AML and the latter supports the diagnosis of ALL or AML-M0.
ii. The intensity of a positive reaction with SBB in general parallels myeloperoxidase activity. Generally local experience would decide which stain to choose. However, SBB gives a slightly more intense reaction and sensitivity than myeloperoxidase staining in the detection of myeloblasts and is safer than the older technique of MPO staining (using carcinogenic benzidine or its derivatives).
iii. Better demonstration of Auer rods by using SBB stain than any of the usual Romanowsky stains. This would be of utmost benefit to identify all MDS cases with Auer rods, to differentiate some AML from ALL cases (Image 4) and also to follow up AML cases for morphological remission after induction chemotherapy.

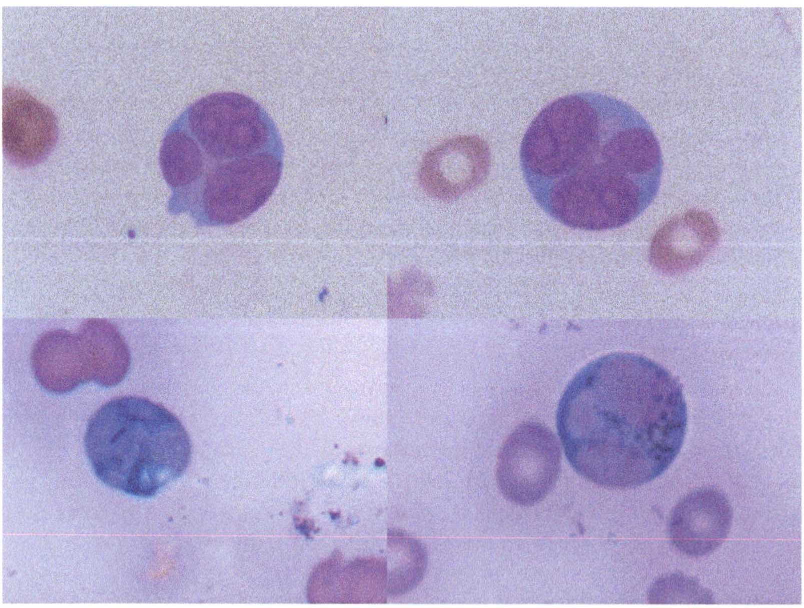

Image 4. Composite photograph of the peripheral blood film of a patient with AML-M2, the blasts showed unusual nuclear lobulation, these blasts contained SBB positive granules and Auer rods (Abdulsalam et al, 2011b)

In all AML subtypes, except for AML-M3, the presence of even one blast cell with Auer rod would refer to failure to achieve remission and indicate the need for a second induction chemotherapy course, while in AML-M3 finding an Auer rod after induction is usually a part of response to treatment as it appears in more maturing myeloid cells (Wong, 2010) (Image 5).

iv. The presence of 3% or more SBB stain positive blasts would characteristically refer to the diagnosis of AML-M1 rather than ALL.
    Although it is now about 30 years since first reporting that in very rare cases even ALL blasts may show SBB positivity (Tricota, et al, 1982); however characters like being of less intensity than the control (remnant normal cells of the myeloid series), non-granular and diffuse reaction help to indicate that these are not myeloblasts. Also lymphoblasts would universally stain negative with MPO which can then be used to confirm the nature of the blasts.

v. Increased SBB stain positivity at diagnosis is associated with better prognosis.

vi. Speedy and firm enough diagnosis of AML-M3 variant cases (Image 6) to start ATRA treatment in the same day (Abdulsalam & Sabeeh, 2010).

vii. Demonstration of myeloid series dysplasia (Image 7) (Bain, 2010b).

viii. The stain can be easily applied to peripheral blood as well as bone marrow aspirate smears.

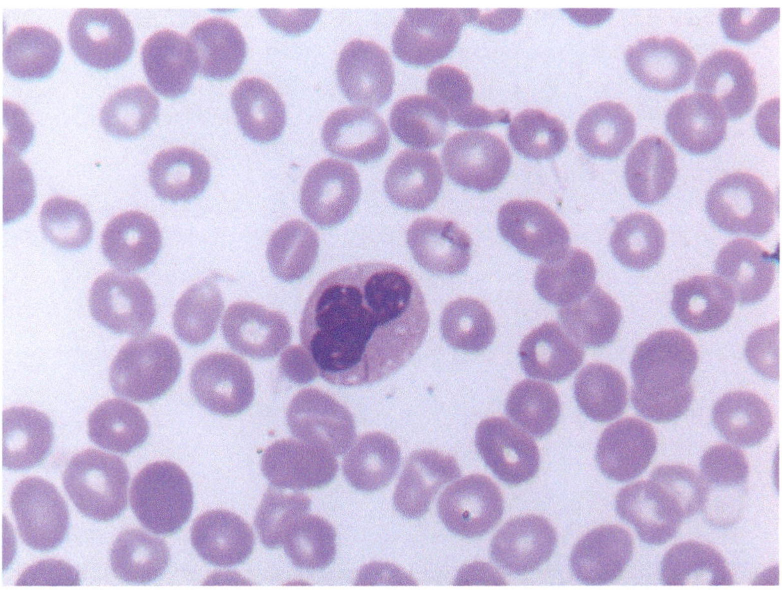

Image 5. Peripheral blood film of a patient with AML-M3 on ATRA treatment showing a dysplastic neutrophil that contains an Auer rod (Abdulsalam and Sabeeh, 2009b)

3.11.1.1 How to count the percentage of SBB positively stained blasts

The literatures are always referring to directly counting the blasts from the SBB stain slide, which is the best technique if the blasts can be easily recognized, but in practice and especially with AML-M1 this is not always feasible due to the nature of the stain which renders many blasts indistinguishable from other less immature cells. Therefore, there should be a second best technique to count the percent of smear positive SBB blasts, because it is not always possible to differentiate all the blasts directly from the SBB slide.

In the author's hematology laboratory practice the following procedure is applied by first utilizing the Leishman stain slide for counting cells into 3 categories as fractions from all the total marrow cells: 1st the blast cells; 2nd the maturing myeloid cells, which would be all assumed to stain positive, although some may actually be negative as a feature of myelodysplasia but nevertheless in calculations this would provide a higher safety threshold to avoid inappropriately classifying a case as AML and 3rd category for lymphocytes and nucleated red cells, which would be negatively stained. Then from the SBB stain slide count all the SBB positive cells and deducing the relative percentage of the SBB positive blasts.

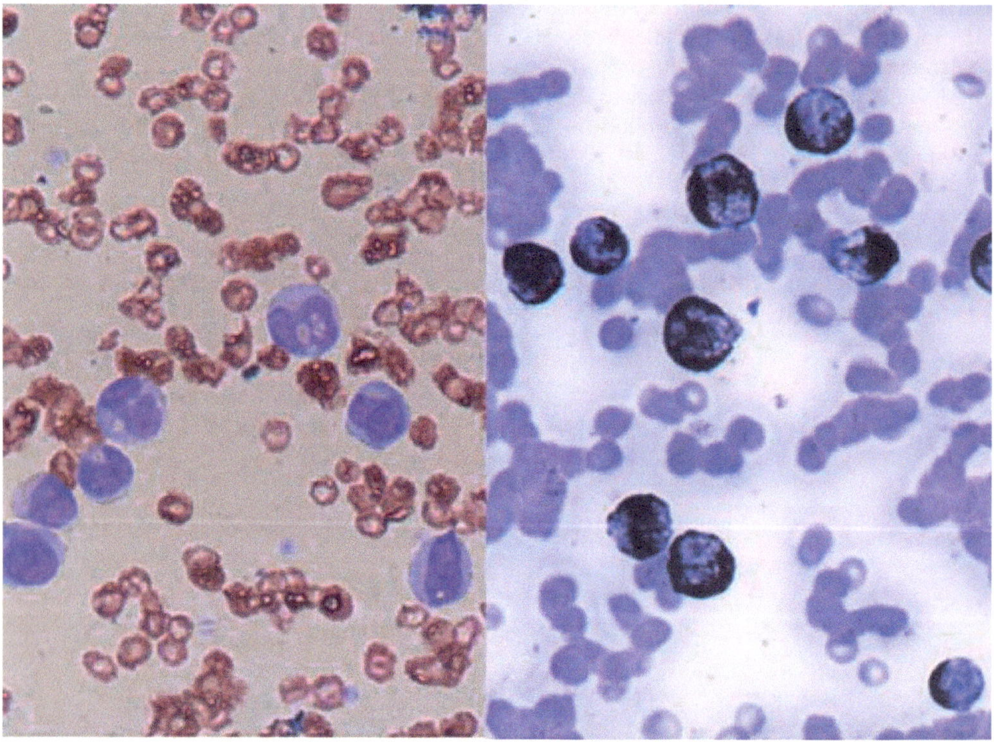

Image 6. Composite photograph showing Leishman staining (*left*) and SBB, cytochemical, staining (*right*) diagnosis of the variant form of AML-M3 (Abdulsalam & Sabeeh, 2010).

3.11.2 NSE

Including α-naphthyl acetate esterase (ANAE), or preferably, α-naphthyl butyrate esterase (ANBE) which is more specific than the acetate stain for the monocytic lineage, either stain is required to confirm the morphological diagnosis of AML-M4, M5a and M5b.

In some occasions there might be a differential diagnosis between M3v and M5b, in which cases it is best to avoid discrimination between them based only on NSE as it may be positive in both leukemias, instead a strong reaction with SBB in M3v can be used.

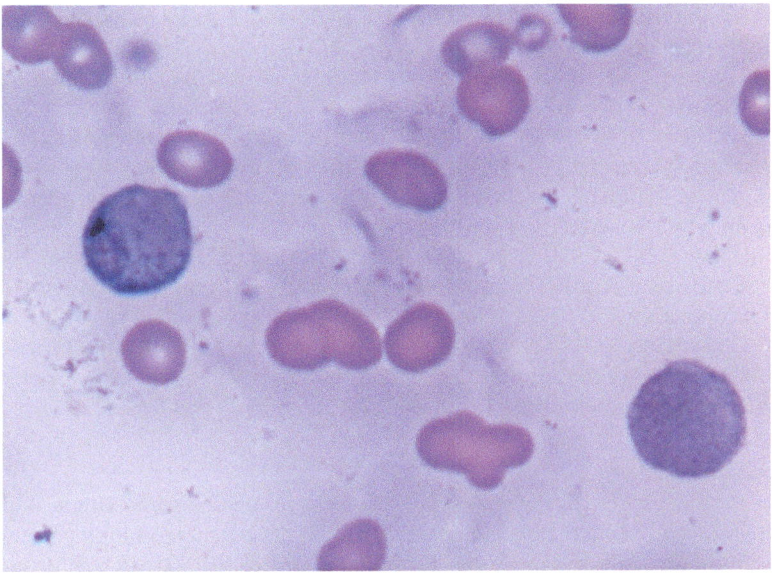

Image 7. Dysplastic metamyelocyte (bottom right) that is completely agranular with SBB staining. {Same patient in Image 4}

3.11.3 Periodic Acid Schiff (PAS)

It adds a minor support to diagnosis of ALL as a similar reaction can be seen, although less frequently in AML. Although the pattern of reaction was considered important in some literatures (Lewis et al, 2006) to differentiate between ALL (with clear cytoplasm between the positive granules) and AML (with cytoplasmic smudge positivity between the positive granules) but in practice relying on such a difference is very difficult, therefore, PAS use is considered non-essential and should be replaced by CD3 and CD79a ICC/IHC.

The other late advantage of PAS was to refer to possible cases of c-ALL; again this use has been superseded by CD10.

3.12 Immunophenotyping

Refers to identification of antigens within or on the surface of cells for the purpose of lineage assignment. It is not a proof for clonality instead of the genetic study.

In AML patients it is essential for proper diagnosis of M0 and M7. In ALL it is essential for diagnosis and risk stratification including T and B lineage assignment (as there is no reliable morphological features to differentiate between them), and subclassification into pro-, common (c), pre- and mature B-ALL and early, cortical and mature T-ALL.

A suggested list of ICC and IHC CD markers that should be available for diagnosis of acute leukemia can include: CD3 for T-ALL (CD7 is more sensitive than CD3, it almost reach 100% sensitivity for T-ALL but is not specific as it is also positive in 20% of AML cases; however, CD7 is still an excellent substitute for T-lineage assignment in rare cases of CD3 negative T-ALL where with the proper clinical and radiological features, Romanowsky and special stains morphology and other CD markers, as negative anti-MPO, then the diagnosis of ALL is evident) and CD79a for B-ALL.

When B-ALL diagnosis is confirmed then CD20 would help to decide for anti-CD20 (Rituximab) treatment option.
TdT would help to differentiate ALL-L2 (where it is positive) from leukemic phase of lymphoma (where it is negative).
For B-ALL CD10 is negative in pro-B-ALL and positive in common-ALL (c-ALL) which confers better prognosis. In pre-B-ALL cytoplasmic immunoglobulin (cIg) is positive while surface Ig (sIg) is positive only in mature B-ALL (ALL-L3 or leukemic phase of Burkitt's lymphoma, in which case TdT is negative).
Only cytoplasmic CD3 (cCD3) is positive in early T-ALL, cCD3 and CD1a are both positive in thymic or cortical T-ALL which confers better prognosis, while in mature T-ALL surface CD3 (sCD3) is positive and CD1a is negative.
Anti-myeloperoxidase, CD117 or CD33 can be used for AML-M0 and CD41 for AML-M7.
The availability of CD45 can be useful in rare occasions to ensure the hemopoietic nature of a poorly differentiated malignancy (Bain et al, 2002).

3.12.1 Flowcytometry

The newer multicolor (detecting many CD markers in/on the same single malignant cell) and multiparametric (a character comparative to that of automated blood counters studying characters like cell size and granularity) flowcytometer is one of the ultimate routine techniques in diagnosis of AML and ALL, primary risk stratification of ALL and follow up for MRD. When there is leucocytosis due to leukemic blasts then the flowcytometry study can be done on peripheral blood, otherwise, a bone marrow aspirate is the specimen of choice. However, the current price of the flowcytometer, cost of operating kits and maintenance make it unsuitable for laboratories with small budget.

3.12.2 Immunocytochemistry (ICC)

This technique should be consistently used in resource-poor laboratories for lineage and sub-lineage assignment of acute leukemia. It is applied on the bone marrow aspirate smear or, less conveniently on the peripheral blood after removal of plasma or on buffy coat (only if the blast percent is high). Sample spread can be done on a regular glass-slide (it is not essential to use a positively charged slide as in IHC) and after fixation in alcohol, ICC can be applied directly or after storage.
In acute leukemia the results of ICC (Image 8) can be interpreted in much more logical sense than IHC as the remaining normal or reactive cells can express some diagnosis-unrelated but confusing CD marker that in the aspirate can be easily detected to appear only for non-blast cells.

3.12.3 Immunohistochemistry (IHC)

Can be used as a substitute for ICC as the second best test for immunophenotyping of acute leukemia in the resource-poor laboratories if the blast percent is high, and if the results are unequivocally positive or negative or when the bone marrow aspirate is inadequate, otherwise when the blast percent is low or when the IHC positive result is in the borderline zone (20-30%) the judgment on the result of IHC can be difficult. For paraffin embedded IHC the designation between marker-positive blasts or reactive cells can be very difficult and in almost all conditions the total positivity per all marrow cells is expressed.

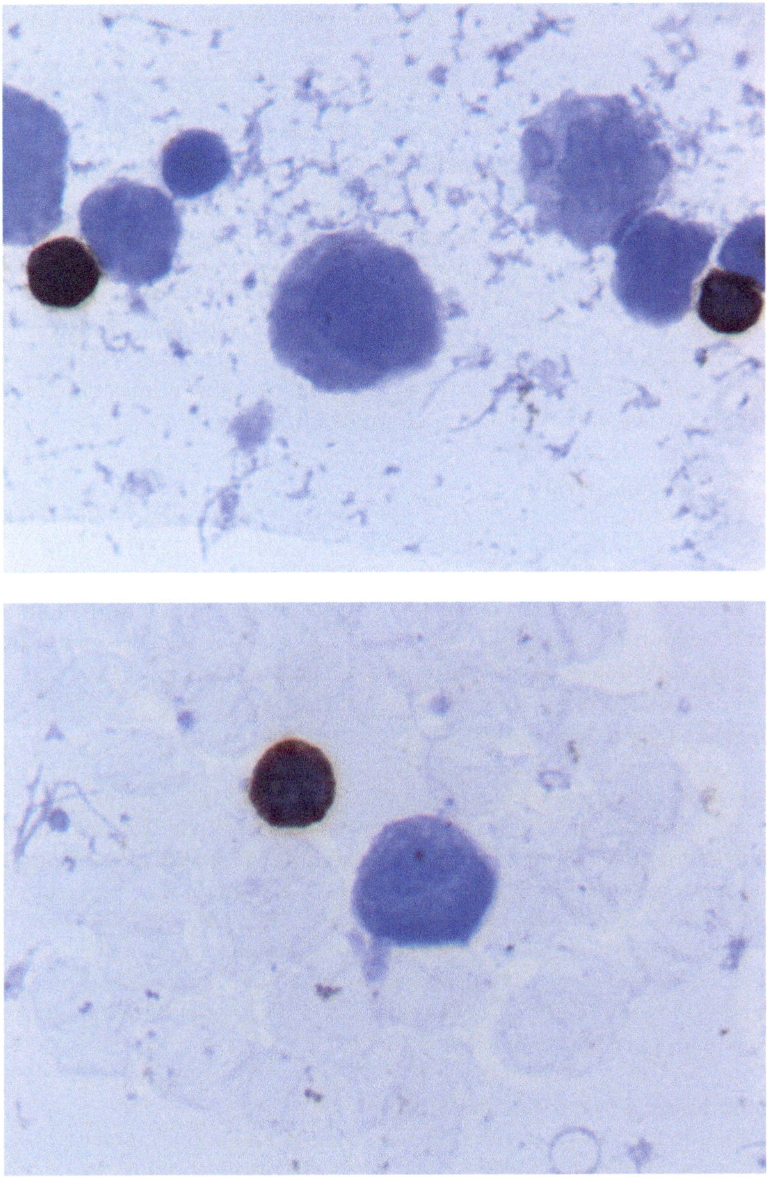

Fig. 8. Composite photograph of the same AML-M1 patient in (Image 2) showing CD 3 negative blasts (top image) with 28% "uncounted" positive small lymphocytes, and CD20 negative blasts (bottom image) with 5% "uncounted" positive small lymphocytes.

3.13 Genetic studies

Including mainly cytogenetics, InSitu Hybridization (ISH) and PCR. All of these techniques have advantages and limitations and the choice in acute leukemia should be based on at

least two different techniques that would give complementary information especially for risk stratification and follow up for MRD.
Older techniques, like Feulgen stain for quantization of DNA contents should be avoided even in under-resourced laboratories because these techniques are non-standard and confusing.

3.13.1 Cytogenetics

It should be routinely applied for every suspected case of acute leukemia. Cytogenetics would represent to genetic studies what a blood smear represents to hematology, i.e., study of morphology of chromosomes and blood cells respectively. However, it has major limitations as the procedure-inherent failure rate and inability to detect small size aberrations or cryptic translocations.
Cytogenetics, beside a molecular study, is essential for the application of the WHO classification of acute leukemia and its risk stratification.

3.13.2 InSitu Hybridization (ISH)

Including Flourescent InSitu Hybridization (FISH) and Chromogenic InSitu Hybridization (CISH). Each technique has its advantages and limitations. FISH would represent a molecular genetic study plus demonstration of some chromosomal morphology. While CISH would represent a molecular genetic study plus demonstration of tissue morphology. In the author's opinion both techniques are not ideal for diagnosis, risk stratification and follow up of acute leukemia in an under-resourced laboratory.

3.13.3 Polymerase Chain Reaction (PCR)

Using only one detection kit multiplex RT-PCR assay is an effective, sensitive, accurate and cost-effective one-step multiple molecular re-arrangements diagnostic and risk-stratification tool. It is a complementary technique to conventional cytogenetics for risk stratification of acute leukemia and it provides a platform for the later on possibility of RQ-PCR detection of minimal residual disease (MRD) as multiplex RT-PCR is a qualitative procedure and is not used by itself as a mean for detection of MRD. For ALL, ETV6-RUNX1 and TCF3-PBX1 (both confer good prognosis), and MLL-MLLt2 and BCR-ABL1 (both confer poor prognosis) (Cerveira at al, 2000 and Shai, 2010); and for AML, FLT3 and MLL (both confer poor prognosis), and NPM1 and CEBPA (both confer good prognosis) (Strehl et al, 2001) paired primers are useful options (Salto-Tellez et al, 2003).

3.14 Chemotherapeutic trial for acute leukemia

A chemotherapeutic trial for those who cannot afford to seek a more precise diagnosis with genetic study and lineage specification abroad is a realistic option, as the response to treatment could be a very useful confirmation of the provisional diagnosis. The two examples already the author had faced are AML-M3v diagnosed provisionally only by morphology but with a dramatic response to ATRA trial, confirming the diagnosis (Image 9) and a few cases of morphologically undifferentiated acute leukemia in which the induction therapy for ALL is tried first (using vincristine and prednisolone only). If the patient responds, then a diagnosis of ALL can be deduced; if not, the regimen should be shifted to chemotherapy of AML (Abdulsalam, 2009).

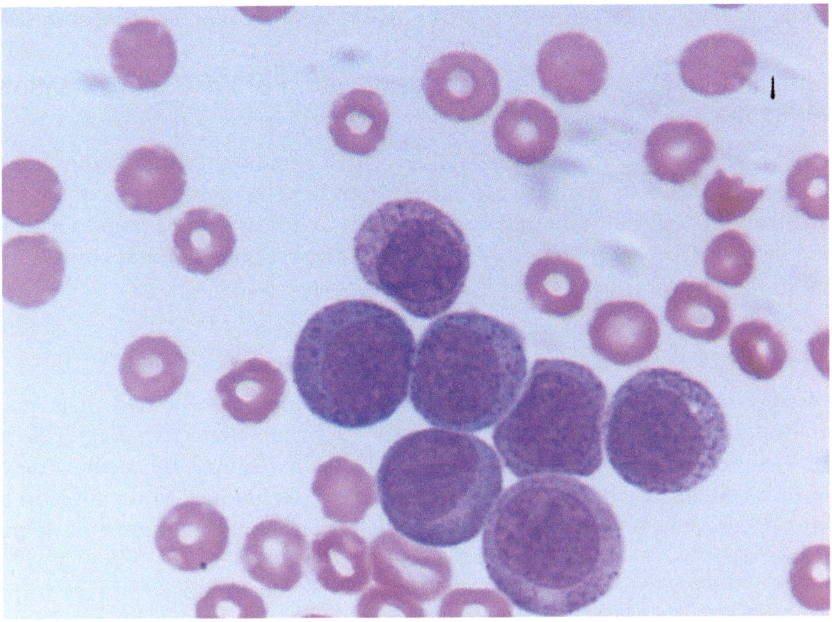

Image 9. Peripheral blood film showed 94% abnormal granulated promyelocytes. In the absence of any specialized tests, the diagnosis was made from cytological features. There was a dramatic response to ATRA, confirming the morphological diagnosis of AML-M3v (Abdulsalam & Nafila, 2009).

3.15 Lumbar puncture

Looking for cerebrospinal fluid (CSF) involvement with acute leukemia is advised in all patients with ALL, while for patients with AML it is only indicated for patients with neurological symptoms.

3.16 Remission

Durable remission in acute leukemia is based on clinical and morphological evidences. Clinical remission includes absence of symptoms and signs of leukemia. Complete blood count consistent with remission would include absence of severe anemia, neutrophil count more than 1 $\times 10^9/l$ and platelet count more than 100 $\times 10^9/l$ (Bain, 2010). Morphological remission of acute leukemia from peripheral blood involves absence of blasts, immature myeloid cells and nucleated red cells. Bone marrow aspirate consistent with morphological remission would include blast cells being less than 5% with absence of Auer rods. The presence of even one Auer rod on SBB stain would refer to failure to achieve remission.

Flowcytometry, cytogenetics or molecular genetics may be used to validate a morphological remission if any of these techniques were already utilized at diagnosis.

3.17 Minimal residual disease (MRD)

Detection of MRD entails the availability of either RQ-PCR or multi-color flowcytometry. Both techniques may not be routinely feasible for a laboratory with poor-resources.

4. Minimal technical requirements for application of WHO classification of acute leukemia

There should be at least a routine availability of CBC (manual or, preferably, automated), peripheral blood and bone marrow aspirate smears (and in some occasions bone marrow biopsy), SBB and a NSE stains, immunocytochemistry with/without immunohistochemistry (including at least CD3, CD79a, anti-MPO and CD41), cytogenetics and conventional PCR for the multiplex primers already mentioned in paragraph 3.13.3.

5. Conclusion

In hematology laboratories where the diagnostic resources are limited, it is essential to establish local guidelines that are practical in developing cost-effective diagnostic protocols for conditions for which the treatment is available, plus leaving the door wide open for future improvements, as to the introduction of newer techniques to the already available procedures once a newer therapeutic agent with certain lineage assignment demands has been introduced.

6. Acknowledgement

I would like to thank Dr. Nafila Sabeeh, laboratory hematologist at Al-Yarmouk Teaching hospital, for her invaluable notes.

7. References

Abdulsalam, A. 2009. Chemotherapeutic trial for acute leukemia in Iraq. *Turkish Journal of Hematology*, 264, 216.

Abdulsalam, A. 2010. Laboratory diagnosis of acute leukemia in Iraq, the available options. *Turkish Journal of Hematology*, 27, 320-321.

Abdulsalam, A. 2011. "Arbitrary" criterion for the diagnosis of acute leukemia. *Turkish Journal of Hematology*, 28 (2): 149-150.

Abdulsalam, A., Sabeeh, N. 2009a. Acute myeloid leukemia with histiocytic differentiation. *American Society of Hematology image bank*, 9, 80.

Abdulsalam, A., Sabeeh, N. 2009b. Auer rod in a neutrophil following ATRA treatment of acute promyelocytic leukemia. *Slide atlas, BloodMed, British Society of Haematology*. Wiley-Blackwell.

Abdulsalam, A., Sabeeh, N. 2010. Cytological/cytochemical diagnosis of the variant form of acute promyelocytic leukaemia. *Slide atlas, BloodMed, British Society of Haematology*. Wiley-Blackwell.

Abdulsalam, A., Sabeeh, N., Bain, B. 2011a. Pseudo-Chédiak-Higashi inclusions together with Auer rods in acute myeloid leukemia. *American Journal of Hematology*, 86 (7): 602.

Abdulsalam, A., Sabeeh, N., Bain, B. 2011b. Myeloblasts with unusual morphology. *American Journal of Hematology*, 86 (6): 499.

Bain, B. 2001a. Bone marrow aspiration. *Journal of Clinical Pathology*, 54: 657-663.

Bain, B. 2001b. Bone marrow trephine biopsy. *Journal of Clinical Pathology*, 54: 737-742.

Bain, B. 2006. *Blood cell, a practical guide*. 4th ed. Blackwell publishing, Singapore.

Bain, B. 2010a. *Leukaemia diagnosis* 4th ed. Wiley-Blackwell, Singapore.

Bain, B. 2010b. Neutrophil dysplasia demonstrated on Sudan black B staining. *American Journal of Hematology*, 85, 9, 707.

Bain, B., Barnett, D., Linch, D., Matutes, E., Reilly, J.T. 2002. Revised guideline on immunophenotyping in acute leukaemias and chronic lymphoproliferative disorders. Clinical and Laboratory Haematology, 24: 1-13.

Cerveira, N., Ferreira, S., DoÂ ria, S., Veiga, I., Ferreira, F., Mariz, J., Marques, M., Castedo, S. 2000. Detection of prognostic significant translocations in childhood acute lymphoblastic leukaemia by one-step multiplex reverse transcription polymerase chain reaction. *British Journal of Haematology*, 109: 638-640.

Jaffe, E., Harris, N., Stein, H., Variman, J. 2001. *World Health Organization classification of tumors, Tumors of Haemopoietic and Lymphoid tissues*. IARC press, Lyon.

Kelaidi, C., Eclache, V., Fenaux, P. 2008. The role of lenalidomide in the management of myelodysplasia with del 5q. *British Journal of Haematology*, 140: 267-278.

Lewis, M., Bain, B., Bates, I. 2006. Dacie and Lewis practical haematology 10th ed. Churchill Livingstone, Germany.

Matutes, E., Morilla, R., Farahat, N., Carbonell, F., Swansbury, J., Dyer, M., Catovsky, D. 1997. Definition of acute biphenotypic leukemia. *Haematologica*, 82: 64-66.

Merino, A., Esteve, J. 2005. Acute myeloid leukaemia with peculiar blast cell inclusions and pseudo-eosinophilia. *British Journal of Haematology*, 131, 286.

Salto-Tellez, M., Shelat, S., Benoit, B., Rennert, H., Carroll, M., Leonard, D., Nowell, P., Bagg, A. 2003. Multiplex RT-PCR for the Detection of Leukemia-Associated Translocations. *Journal of Molecular Diagnostics*, 5 (4): 231-236.

Shai, I. 2010. Application of genomics for risk stratification of childhood acute lymphoblastic leukaemia: from bench to bedside? *British Journal of Haematology*, 151: 119-131.

Strehl, S., Konig, M., Mann, G., Haas, O. 2001. Multiplex reverse transcriptase-polymerase chain reaction screening in childhood acute myeloblastic leukemia. *Blood*, 97 (3): 805-808.

Thörn, I., Forestier, E., Botling, J., Thuresson, B., Wasslavik, C., Björklund, E., Aihong, L., Eleonor L.E., Malec, M., Grönlund, E., Torikka, K., Heldrup, J., Abrahamsson, J., Behrendtz, M., Söderhäll, S., Jacobsson, S., Olofsson, T., Porwit, A., Lönnerholm, G., Rosenquist, R., Sundström, C. 2011. Minimal residual disease assessment in childhood acute lymphoblastic leukaemia: a Swedish multi-centre study comparing real-time polymerase chain reaction and multicolour flow cytometry. *British Journal of Haematology*, 152 (6): 743-753.

Tricota, G., Broeckaert, A., Van Hoof, A., Verwilgdhen RL. 1982. Sudan Black B positivity in acute lymphoblastic leukaemia. *British Journal of Haematology*, 51, 615-621.

Vardiman, J., Thiele, J., Arber, D., Brunning, R., Borowitz, M., Porwit, A., Harris, N., Le Beau, M., Lindberg, E., Tefferi, A., Bloomfield, C. 2009. The 2008 revision of the World Health Organization (WHO) classification of myeloid neoplasms and acute leukemia: rationale and important changes. *Blood,* 114, 937-951.

Wong, F. 2010. All-*trans*-retinoic acid therapy. *British Journal of Haematology,* 149: 309.

Part 2

Molecular Mechanisms and Markers

3

Lymphocyte Commitment and Ikaros Transcription Factors

Mariastefania Antica
Rudjer Boskovic Institute
Croatia

1. Introduction

T lymphocytes like all blood cells are progenies of a single multipotent hematopoietic stem cell (HSC). The existence of HSCs was proven by Till and McCulloch in 1961 when bone marrow cells injected into irradiated mice formed multilineage colonies in their spleens. These cells were called colony forming units (CFU-S) and they have potential for self-renewal and differentiation into all types of blood cells(Till and McCulloch 1961; Wu et al. 1968). For lymphocyte development HSCs migrate from the bone marrow, differentiate in the thymus into immunocompetent cells and seed the peripheral lymphatic organs. This process occurs during fetal development (for review see (Godin and Cumano 2002), but also during the adult life of an individual since T lymphocytes have to be continuously replenished. Transplantation experiments proved that thirty hematopoietic stem cells are sufficient to save 50 percent of lethally irradiated mice, and to reconstitute all blood cell types in vivo (Spangrude et al. 1988). Because it is extremely important to produce immunocompetent T cells the process of their maturation and development is strictly regulated and is succumb to very strict check points at several stages of differentiation. In this context we'll discuss Ikaros family transcription factors as major regulators of T lymphocyte development.

2. Committed lymphocyte precursor

For a long time it has been postulated analogously to committed myeloid precursors that there is a committed lymphocyte precursor. However the first experiments that showed the existence of a committed lymphocyte precursor was described in the early 90tis when a new population of cells in the thymus was found and its features described (Wu 1991; Wu et al. 1991). These cells expressed most markers of the multipotent hematopoietic stem cells like Thy-$1^{low}$$CD44^{+}$$H2k^{+}$Sca-$1^{+}$ but they expressed Sca-2 and low levels of CD4. These cells were negative for all mature blood cells markers lymphocytes ($CD8^{-}CD3^{-}Ig^{-}$), macrophages (Mac-1^{-}), granulocytes (Gr-1^{-}) and erhytrocytes ($TER119^{-}$), lineage negative, (Lin^{-} cells). Their Ig and TCR receptor genes were in germline configuration. The described precursors represent 0.05% of the cells in an adult mouse thymus. If the cells were sorted and transferred by intrathymic injections (*i.t.*) into lethally irradiated congenic mice they developed into all thymic subpopulations, first $CD4^{-}CD8^{-}$ (double negatives, DN) thymocytes, than into

CD4$^+$CD8$^+$ double positives which give rise to mature CD4$^+$ and CD8$^+$ lymphocytes. Mature cells derived from the CD4^{low} precursors seeded the spleen, lymph nodes and bone marrow. The reconstitution potential of the described precursors was lower and the time for development was shorter when compared to the multipotent hematopoietic stem cells from the bone marrow. These experiments proved that the CD4^{low} precursors in the thymus can develop into T lymphocytes. Because of their resemblance to the multipotent progenitors from the bone marrow it was important to answer the question whether their potential was restricted only to develop into T lymphocytes. Therefore we transplanted these cells into the periphery by injecting them intravenously (*i.v.*) into lethally irradiated congenic animals. Their progenies were found to develop into T lymphocytes similarly to the results obtained by direct *i.t.* transplantation experiments. When injected intravenously they also developed into B lymphocytes but there were no myeloid progenies. During fetal development these cells were detected from day 14 in the fetal thymus but only after birth their function was comparable to the adult ones(Antica et al. 1993). In the bone marrow the CD4^{low} precursor cells were described, but their function was not lymphocyte restricted (Antica et al. 1994a). Further studies showed that in the bone marrow the marker that could differentiate the lymphoid precursor cells from the multipotent precursors was IL7Rα (Kondo et al. 1997). This population, called common lymphoid precursor (CLP) is characterized by Lin$^-$ Thy-1$^-$Sca-1^{lo}c-Kit^{lo} IL-7R$^+$ and possess rapid and prominent short-term lymphoid-restricted (T, B, and NK cells) reconstitution activity. However, this progenitor population clonally produces both B and T lymphocytes, but have little myeloid potential *in vivo.* A recently developed bioinformatics method, called Mining Developmentally Regulated Genes, which mines the publically available microarray data to identify genes that are up- or down-regulated within a developmental pathway was applied to identify surface proteins that distinguish functional CLPs from other progenitors (Inlay et al. 2009; Sahoo et al. 2010). A surface marker Ly6d dissects the CLP population in two and shows that it consists of a mixture of all lymphoid progenitor cells (ALP) which retain B and T lymphoid potential, and BLP (B cell biased lymphoid progenitors). This manuscript offers strong support for the validity of our earlier conclusions. However, ALPs still keep low myeloid potential indicating that ALPs are either a mixture of the CD4^{low} precursor cells and myeloid progenitors or is a single population but at an earlier developmental stage and still multipotent(Wu et al. 1991; Antica et al. 1993; Antica et al. 1994b; Inlay et al. 2009). Here we also stress the necessity and importance of *in vivo* assays for the determination of physiologic lineage potentials since it has been recently shown that *in vitro* assays can misrepresent *in vivo* lineage potentials of murine lymphoid progenitors(Richie Ehrlich et al. 2011).

From the clinical point of view defining the earliest lymphoid precursor is important for a rapid engraftment and protection from infections after hematopoietic stem cell transplantation in chemotherapy or irradiation compromised patients (Arber et al. 2003; Holländer et al. 2010).

3. Ikaros transcription factors

Mechanisms and factors that regulate lymphocyte development from stem cells have to be very accurate since any alteration of this process may lead to serious diseases like leukemia.

Transcription factors from the Ikaros family play an essential role in the commitment of hematopoietic progenitors into the lymphoid lineage as well as in the choice of effector functions at later stages of development(Georgopoulos 1994; Sun et al. 1996; Wang et al. 1998; Cortes et al. 1999). Their role has been addressed by gene targeting and such gene inactivation studies have identified Ikaros, Aiolos and Helios as transcription factors required for the maturation of lymphocytes(Morgan 1997; Hahm 1998; Kelley 1998). It has been shown that mice homozygous for a deletion in these genes undergo remarkable changes in their lymphocyte populations and also those ageing animals with the same mutation develop lymphoproliferative disorders. A number of studies show that Ikaros genes in both mice and human malignancies might be deregulated (Winandy et al. 1995; Nichogiannopoulou et al. 1999; Nakase et al. 2000; Nakayama et al. 2000; Nakase et al. 2002; Rebollo and Schmitt 2003; Dovat et al. 2005; Mullighan et al. 2008; Matulic et al. 2009; Billot et al. 2010). Therefore we addressed the question whether a combination of transcription factor failures may contribute to the development of human lymphoma. We amplified human mRNA from formalin fixed paraffin embedded tissues from lymphoma patients in order to have consistent and well defined groups of patients. Hence, we were able to analyze Ikaros, Aiolos and Helios mRNA from archive tissue specimens from patients with Hodgkin's and non- Hodgkin's lymphoma and follicular hyperplasia (Antica et al. 2008; Antica et al. 2010). Further we and others show a deregulation in human leukemia. Acute lymphoblastic leukemia (ALL) is characterized by the Philadelphia chromosome (Ph) which encodes the BCR-ABL1 tyrosine kinase, the most frequent cytogenetic abnormality (~25–30% of cases)(Mancini et al. 2005). Deletion of the IKAROS gene (*IKZF1*) was found in 83.7% cases of BCR-ABL1 ALL, but not in chronic-phase CML(Mullighan et al. 2008). Posttranscriptional regulation of alternative splicing of Ikaros was associated with resistance to tyrosine kinase inhibitors (TKIs) in Ph/positive acute lymphoblastic leukemia (ALL) patients (Iacobucci et al. 2008). Further, *IKZF1* deletions are likely to be a genomic alteration that significantly affects the prognosis of Ph-positive ALL in adults (Martinelli et al. 2009). Further, when Ikaros expression was analyzed by real time RT-PCR the quantitative distribution of mRNA level in hematopoietic cells of patients with lymphocytic leukemia was similar but a clear difference among groups was due to Aiolos lower expression in all types of acute leukemia(Antica et al. 2007). The mechanisms involved have been tested in the mouse model. It has been found that pre-BCR induces Ikaros to inhibit the proliferation of Philadelphia chromosome-positive B-ALL cells (Trageser et al. 2009). Pre–B cell receptor/*IKAROS*-induced cell cycle arrest can be reversed by dominant-negative Ikaros splicing variant IK6(Trageser et al. 2009). A possible mechanism of Ikaros suppression has been described by Ma et al. Their experiments on mice show that Ikaros inhibits c-Myc as a direct target, resulting in inhibition of pre B-lymphocyte proliferation (Ma et al 2010).

In the last ten years a new system, besides fetal thymic organ cultures (FTOC) or reaggregation cultures, for T cell growth *in vitro* has been developed. It has been shown that OP9 stromal cells transfected with the Notch ligand delta like 1 DL1 (OP9-DL1) can support T lymphocyte differentiation *in vitro* (Schmitt and Zúñiga-Pflücker 2002). This new technology provided a powerful tool for analyzing developmental phases from multipotent stem cells to mature T lymphocytes at single cell level *in vitro* and allowed a better understanding of the processes underlying development. However, there are still a lot of unanswered and exciting questions to be solved. Who is regulating Ikaros and

Notch? How transcription factors regulate development with their partners and DNA where and how do they interfere with their partners, and DNA, how can we identify targets for new drugs and finally how can we produce T cells *in vitro* for practical applications and regenerative medicine?

4. References

Antica, M., Cicin-Sain, L., Kapitanovic, S., Matulic, M., Dzebro, S., and Dominis, M. 2008. Aberrant Ikaros, Aiolos, and Helios expression in Hodgkin and non-Hodgkin lymphoma. *Blood* 111(6): 3296-3297.

Antica, M., Dubravcic, K., Weber, I., Rasic, L., Labar, B., and Batinic, D. 2007. A search for a mutation of the Aiolos phosphorylation domain in lymphocytes from patients with leukemia. *Haematologica* 92(2): 260-261.

Antica, M., Paradzik, M., Novak, S., Dzebro, S., and Dominis, M. 2010. Gene expression in formalin-fixed paraffin-embedded lymph nodes. *Journal of Immunological Methods* 359(1-2): 42-46.

Antica, M., Wu, L., Shortman, K., and Scollay, R. 1993. Intrathymic lymphoid precursor cells during fetal thymus development. *Journal of Immunology* 151(11): 5887-5895.

Antica, M., Wu, L., Shortman, K., and Scollay, R. 1994. Thymic stem cells in mouse bone marrow. *Blood* 84(1): 111-117.

Arber, C., BitMansour, A., Sparer, T.E., Higgins, J.P., Mocarski, E.S., Weissman, I.L., Shizuru, J.A., and Brown, J.M.Y. 2003. Common lymphoid progenitors rapidly engraft and protect against lethal murine cytomegalovirus infection after hematopoietic stem cell transplantation. *Blood* 102(2): 421-428.

Billot, K., Soeur, J., Chereau, F., Arrouss, I., Merle-Beral, H., Huang, M.-E., Mazier, D., Baud, V., and Rebollo, A. 2010. Deregulation of Aiolos expression in chronic lymphocytic leukemia is associated to epigenetic modifications. *Blood 117(6): 1917-1927*

Cortes, M., Wong, E., Koipally, J., and Georgopoulos, K. 1999. Control of lymphocyte development by the Ikaros gene family. *Current Opinion in Immunology* 11(2): 167-171.

Dovat, S., Montecino-Rodriguez, E., Schuman, V., Teitell, M.A., Dorshkind, K., and Smale, S.T. 2005. Transgenic Expression of Helios in B Lineage Cells Alters B Cell Properties and Promotes Lymphomagenesis. *J Immunol* 175(6): 3508-3515.

Georgopoulos, K. 1994. The Ikaros gene is required for the development of all lymphoid lineages. *Cell* 79: 143-156.

Godin, I. and Cumano, A. 2002. The hare and the tortoise: an embryonic haematopoietic race. *Nat Rev Immunol* 2(8): 593-604.

Hahm, K. 1998. Helios, a T-cell restricted Ikaros family member that quantitatively associates with Ikaros at centromeric heterochromatin. *Genes Dev* 12: 782-796.

Holländer, G.A., Krenger, W., and Blazar, B.R. 2010. Emerging strategies to boost thymic function. *Current Opinion in Pharmacology* 10(4): 443-453.

Iacobucci, I., Lonetti, A., Messa, F., Cilloni, D., Arruga, F., Ottaviani, E., Paolini, S., Papayannidis, C., Piccaluga, P.P., Giannoulia, P. et al. 2008. Expression of spliced oncogenic Ikaros isoforms in Philadelphia-positive acute lymphoblastic leukemia patients treated with tyrosine kinase inhibitors: implications for a new mechanism of resistance. *Blood* 112(9): 3847-3855.

Inlay, M.A., Bhattacharya, D., Sahoo, D., Serwold, T., Seita, J., Karsunky, H., Plevritis, S.K., Dill, D.L., and Weissman, I.L. 2009. Ly6d marks the earliest stage of B-cell specification and identifies the branchpoint between B-cell and T-cell development. *Genes & Development* 23(20): 2376-2381.

Kelley, C.M. 1998. Helios, a novel dimerization partner of Ikaros expressed in the earliest hematopoietic progenitors. *Curr Biol* 8: 508-515.

Kondo, M., Weissman, I.L., and Akashi, K. 1997. Identification of clonogenic common lymphoid progenitors in mouse bone marrow. *Cell* 91: 661-672.

Ma, S., Pathak, S., Mandal, M., Trinh, L., Clark, M.R., and Lu, R. 2010. Ikaros and Aiolos Inhibit Pre-B-Cell Proliferation by Directly Suppressing c-Myc Expression. *Mol Cell Biol* 30(17): 4149-4158.

Mancini, M., Scappaticci, D., Cimino, G., Nanni, M., Derme, V., Elia, L., Tafuri, A., Vignetti, M., Vitale, A., Cuneo, A. et al. 2005. A comprehensive genetic classification of adult acute lymphoblastic leukemia (ALL): analysis of the GIMEMA 0496 protocol. *Blood* 105(9): 3434-3441.

Martinelli, G., Iacobucci, I., Storlazzi, C.T., Vignetti, M., Paoloni, F., Cilloni, D., Soverini, S., Vitale, A., Chiaretti, S., Cimino, G. et al. 2009. IKZF1 (Ikaros) Deletions in BCR-ABL1 Positive Acute Lymphoblastic Leukemia Are Associated With Short Disease-Free Survival and High Rate of Cumulative Incidence of Relapse: A GIMEMA AL WP Report. *Journal of Clinical Oncology* 27(31): 5202-5207.

Matulic, M., Paradzik, M., Cicin-Sain, L., Kapitanovic, S., Dubravcic, K., Batinic, D., and Antica, M. 2009. Ikaros family transcription factors in chronic and acute leukemia. *American Journal of Hematology* 84(6): 375-377.

Morgan, B. 1997. Aiolos, a lymphoid restricted transcription factor that interacts with Ikaros to regulate lymphocyte differentiation. *EMBO J* 16: 2004-2013.

Mullighan, C.G., Miller, C.B., Radtke, I., Phillips, L.A., Dalton, J., Ma, J., White, D., Hughes, T.P., Le Beau, M.M., Pui, C.-H. et al. 2008. BCR-ABL1 lymphoblastic leukaemia is characterized by the deletion of Ikaros. *Nature* 453(7191): 110-114.

Nakase, K., Ishimaru, F., Avitahl, N., Dansako, H., Matsuo, K., Fujii, K., Sezaki, N., Nakayama, H., Yano, T., Fukuda, S. et al. 2000. Dominant Negative Isoform of the Ikaros Gene in Patients with Adult B-Cell Acute Lymphoblastic Leukemia. *Cancer Res* 60(15): 4062-4065.

Nakase, K., Ishimaru, F., Fujii, K., Tabayashi, T., Kozuka, T., Sezaki, N., Matsuo, Y., and Harada, M. 2002. Overexpression of novel short isoforms of Helios in a patient with T-cell acute lymphoblastic leukemia. *Experimental Hematology* 30(4): 313-317.

Nakayama, H., Ishimaru, F., Katayama, Y., Nakase, K., Sezaki, N., Takenaka, K., Shinagawa, K., Ikeda, K., Niiya, K., and Harada, M. 2000. Ikaros expression in human hematopoietic lineages. *Experimental Hematology* 28(11): 1232-1238.

Nichogiannopoulou, N., Trevisan, M., Naben, S., Friedrich, C., and Georgopoulos, K. 1999. Defects in the activity of hemopoietic stem cells in Ikaros mutant mice. *J Exp Med* 190: 1201-1214.

Rebollo, A. and Schmitt, C. 2003. Ikaros, Aiolos and Helios: Transcription regulators and lymphoid malignancies. *Immunology and Cell Biology* 81(3): 171-175.

Richie Ehrlich, L.I., Serwold, T., and Weissman, I.L. 2011. In vitro assays misrepresent in vivo lineage potentials of murine lymphoid progenitors. *Blood* 117(9): 2618-2624.

Sahoo, D., Seita, J., Bhattacharya, D., Inlay, M.A., Weissman, I.L., Plevritis, S.K., and Dill, D.L. 2010. A method of mining developmentally regulated genes using Boolean implications. *Proceedings of the National Academy of Sciences* 107(13): 5732-5737.

Schmitt, T.M. and Zúñiga-Pflücker, J.C. 2002. Induction of T Cell Development from Hematopoietic Progenitor Cells by Delta-like-1 In Vitro. *Immunity* 17(6): 749-756.

Spangrude, G.J., Heimfeld, S., and Weissman, I.L. 1988. Purification and characterization of mouse hematopoietic stem cell. *Science* 241: 58-92.

Sun, L., Liu, A., and Georgopoulos, K. 1996. Zinc finger-mediated protein interactions modulate Ikaros activity, a molecular control of lymphocyte development. *EMBO J* 15: 5358-5369.

Till, J.E. and McCulloch, C.E. 1961. A direct measurement of the radiation sensitivity of normal mouse bone marrow cells. *Radiation Research* 14: 213-222.

Trageser, D., Iacobucci, I., Nahar, R., Duy, C., von Levetzow, G., Klemm, L., Park, E., Schuh, W., Gruber, T., Herzog, S. et al. 2009. Pre B cell receptor mediated cell cycle arrest in Philadelphia chromosome positive acute lymphoblastic leukemia requires IKAROS function. *The Journal of Experimental Medicine* 206(8): 1739-1753.

Wang, J.-H., Avitahl, N., Cariappa, A., Friedrich, C., Ikeda, T., Renold, A., Andrikopoulos, K., Liang, L., Pillai, S., Morgan, B.A. et al. 1998. Aiolos Regulates B Cell Activation and Maturation to Effector State. *Immunity* 9(4): 543-553.

Winandy, S., Wu, P., and Georgopoulos, K. 1995. A dominant mutation in the Ikaros gene leads to rapid development of leukemia and lymphoma. *Cell* 83(2): 289-299.

Wu, A.M., Siminovitch, L., Till, J.E., and McCulloch, E.A. 1968. Evidence for a relationship between mouse hemopoietic stem cells and cells forming colonies in culture. *Proceedings of the National Academy of Sciences* 59: 1209-1215.

Wu, L. 1991. CD4 expressed on earliest T-lineage precursor cells in the adult murine thymus. *Nature* 349: 71-74.

Wu, L., Antica, M., Johnson, G.R., Scollay, R., and Shortman, K. 1991. Developmental potential of the earliest precursor cells from the adult mouse thymus. *J Exp Med* 174(6): 1617-1627.

4

Molecular Markers for Risk Stratification in Adult Acute Myeloid Leukemia with Normal Cytogenetics

Ota Fuchs
Institute of Hematology and Blood Transfusion, Prague,
Center of Experimental Hematology, First Medical Faculty, Charles University, Prague,
Czech Republic

1. Introduction

Acute myeloid leukemia (AML) is a broad range of disorders that are all characterized by a block in the differentiation and by uncontrolled proliferation of hematopoietic progenitor cells. AML is the most frequent hematological malignancy in adults, with an annual incidence of three to four cases per 100 000 individuals. Specific recurrent chromosomal abnormalities can be identified in approximately 55% of cases by cytogenetic analysis. These detected chromosomal aberrations are the most important tool to classify patients at their initial diagnosis and to divide them into favorable, intermediate and unfavorable subgroups. The age of the patient is also an important prognostic factor (Juliusson et al., 2009; Szotkowski et al., 2010). However, approximately 45% of adult patients with AML have normal karyotype (cytogenetically normal /CN/-AML patients) and are usually classified as an intermediate risk group (Mrozek et al., 2007; Smith et al., 2011). These patients have a 5-year overall survival rate between 24% and 42%, but clinical outcome may vary greatly.

The prognosis of AML with normal cytogenetics may be further subdivided based on genetic lesions. Even though a growing number of genetic lesions have been identified in CN-AML, about 25% CN-AML patients do not carry any of the currently known mutations. Therefore, many research groups conducted retrospective studies to find some candidate molecular markers that could identify good and poor risk AML patients with normal karyotype. In recent years, a number of gene mutations (*NPM1* /nucleophosmin/, *FLT3* /Fms-like tyrosine kinase 3/, *MLL*-PTD /mixed lineage leukemia-partial tandem duplications/, *C/EBPα* /CCAAT/enhancer-binding protein alpha/CEBPA/, *WT1* /Wilms tumor 1/, *DNMT3A* /DNA methyltransferase 3A/, *IDH1* and *IDH2* /isocitrate dehydrogenase/, *CBL* /Casitas B-lineage lymphoma/and others), as well as deregulated expression of genes (*BAALC* /brain and acute leukemia cytoplasmic/, *ERG* /ETS-related gene/, *MN1* /meningioma 1/, *EVI1* /ecotropic virus integration 1/, *AF1q* /ALL1-fused gene chromosome 1q/, *PRAME* /preferentially expressed antigen in melanoma/, *WT1*) have been found and further molecular markers (gene expression profiles and microRNA expression signatures) are studied and incorporated into clinical practice (Baldus & Bullinger, 2008; Bullinger & Valk, 2005; Bullinger 2006; Kohlmann et al, 2010; Marcucci et al., 2009, 2011a,b; Motyckova & Stone, 2010; Ramsingh et al., 2010; Schlenk et al., 2008; Wouters et al., 2009). It is necessary to improve current classification systems in order to reflect better the molecular heterogeneity of CN-AML (Döhner et al., 2010; Vardiman et al., 2009).

In addition, some of the genetic abnormalities have also been found to be useful for minimal residual disease (MRD) monitoring and as potential therapeutic targets in the development of new agents for AML therapy. The aim of monitoring of MRD is the identification of cases with a very high risk of relapse who then can be treated much earlier and more effectively (Jaeger & Kainz, 2003; Schnittger et al., 2009; Shook et al., 2009).

Knowing the status of *FLT-3* and other molecular markers (mutations and gene expression described above together with gene expression profiling) in CN-AML patients has not only prognostic significance but is important in the treatment based on these molecular markers. For example, patients with *FLT3*-ITD (an internal tandem duplication of the FLT3 receptor tyrosine kinase gene), who are not candidates for induction therapy and allogeneic stem cell transplantation may respond to an FLT3 inhibitor used in combination with chemotherapy or without chemotherapy. Deregulation of microRNA (miR) in CN-AML patients may act as complementary hit in the multisteps mechanism of leukemogenesis and has been not only used to identify subsets of CN-AML patients with diversified outcome but will certainly play a role in the future of treatment in new therapeutic strategies. Thus, miR expression profiling has diagnostic and prognostic significance.

2. Methods for the detection of gene mutations and expression

2.1 Sample material

After informed consent patient- or healthy individual-derived mononuclear cells were isolated from bone marrow (BM) or peripheral blood cells by a ficoll (for example Ficoll-Paque PLUS, GE Healthcare Bio-Sciences AB, Uppsala, Sweden) density gradient centrifugation. Total RNA and genomic DNA were isolated. Yield and quality of the RNA were measured by spectrophotometric analysis. Each sample was assessed for the integrity of RNA by discrimination of 18S and 28 S ribosomal RNA on 1% agarose gels using ethidium bromide for visualization. Complementary DNA was synthetised from total RNA using reverse transcriptase (for example SuperScript II reverse transcriptase (Invitrogen Corporation, Carlsbad, CA, USA).

2.2 Detection of gene mutations

Most mutation detection methods use PCR (polymerase chain reaction) to amplify the region of DNA of interest. Mutant DNA has a different secondary structure (conformation) compared with that of the normal DNA. Frequently, this difference in conformation results in altered gel electrophoresis mobility of the mutant DNA species. Single-strand conformation polymorphism (SSCP) method (Orita et al., 1989; Perry, 1999) based on this conformation change is a fast and efficient method for detecting many types of aberrations, including point mutations, insertions, deletions and rearrangements (Frayling, 2002; Kutach et al., 1999). SSCP has the sensitivity to identify single nucleotide changes in the DNA sequence. Thermally denaturated DNA is electrophoresed and mutation is detected as aberrantly migrating bands on the electrophoresis gel. Analyzed PCR products must be less than 300 bp and preferably less than 200 bp in size because the method is increasingly inefficient with increasing size of the PCR product. Another technique, related to SSCP is

DNA heteroduplex analysis (Frayling, 2002). Both SSCP and heteroduplex analysis can be carried on fluorescent DNA analysers at a controlled temperature. The related techniques DGGE (denaturing gradient gel electrophoresis) and TGGE (thermal gradient gel electrophoresis) arevery efficient, but they require specially designed PCR primers of increased length (Frayling, 2002). Sequencing of the mutated PCR product is almost universally carried out using dideoxy terminator chemistry .

High resolution melting (HRM) analysis is rapidly becoming the most important initial screen procedure for potential mutations (Razga et al., 2009; Tan et al., 2008; Vaughn & Elenitoba-Johnson, 2004; Wittwer, 2009). PCR amplification and subsequent HRM analysis are sequentially performed in the one tube. HRM is more simple than denaturing high - performance liquid chromatography (DHPLC), which can be also used after PCR amplification for mutation detection (Bianchini et al., 2003; Kosaki et al., 2005; Roti et al., 2006). Real-time PCR machine with HRM capability, for example LightCycler 480 High - Resolution Melting Master (Roche Diagnostics) has been successfully used for PCR amplification and HRM analysis. PCR reactions must be designed in the maner to avoid primer dimers and non-specific amplification. DNA has to be prepared in a uniform fashion to avoid variation in salt concentration with effect on the melting. HRM significantly reduces the quantity of samples that is necessary for sequencing with consequent reduction of cost and labour and enables rapid detection of mutations. The melting curves are normalized and temperature shifted to allow samples to be directly compared. Difference plots are generated by selecting a negative (nonmutated) control as the base-line and the fluorescence of all other samples is plotted relative to this negative control. Significant differences in fluorescence are indicative of mutations which must be detected by sequencing. Noordermer et al. (2010) used HRM curve analysis for rapid identification of *IDH1* and *IDH2* mutations in AML.

Currently, identification of mutations by PCR and direct nucleotide sequencing is used as the gold standard. The great progress was achieved in DNA sequencing technology in last ten years after the end of Human Genome Project (Mardis, 2011). The Roche/454, Life Technologies SOliD and Illumina instruments have been used to sequence the complete tumor and normal genomes in order to identify mutations that alter the protein-coding genes. Whole genome sequencing is now possible at a reasonable cost per tumor and normal genome of around $ 30,000 and can be completed in about 8 days. A pilot study of high-throughput, sequence-based mutational profiling of primary AML cell genomes was done eight years ago (Ley et al., 2003). Whole genomic DNA sequencing of a cytogenetically normal FAB M1 AML patient was done three years ago and discovered ten genes with acquired mutations (Ley et al., 2008). Eight novel somatic mutations were described in genes not previously implicated in AML pathogenesis. Two well-known AML-associated mutations, including *FLT3-ITD*, which constitutively activates kinase signaling and a four base insertion in exon 12 of the *NPM1* gene were also detected. Mardis et al. (2009) identified twelve somatic mutations within the coding sequences of genes and 52 somatic point mutations in conserved or regulatory portions of the AML genome. Two known mutations in NRAS and NPM1 and ten novel mutations were detected. One of these mutations (missense R132C mutation in *IDH1* gene) is today included in many mutational screening of AML patients. The more efficient, faster and cheaper approach will be sequencing of coding regions (the cDNA transcriptome) but the abundance of transripts can vary and some mutations can be missed (Greif et al., 2011). The size of the transcriptome is about ten times shorter than a diploid human genome

Mutations in molecular markers can be present in low abundance within a high background of wild type sequence that may only differ from mutant at a single nucleotide. Several methods exist for detection of somatic mutations by real-time PCR. These methods include use of allele-specific competitive blocker PCR (Orou et al., 1995), blocker-PCR (Seyama et al., 1992), real-time genotyping with locked nucleic acids (Ugozzoli et al., 2004), the amplification refractory mutation system (Newton et al., 1989), and fluorescent amplicon generation as a novel real-time PCR technology (Amicarelli et al., 2007).
Mutated NPM1 is localised in the cytoplasm and not in the nucleus (Bolli et al., 2007; Falini et al., 2006; Liso et al., 2008; Oelschlaegel et al., 2010). Immunohistochemical detection of cytoplasmic nucleophosmin is performed with monoclonal antibody or by Western blotting (Falini et al., 2006, 2009, 2010a; Martelli et al. 2008).

2.3 Technique of real-time PCR (RQ-PCR) for marker gene expression evaluation

RQ-PCR permits accurate quantification of PCR products during the exponential phase of the PCR amplification process. Three main types of this analysis are used: (1) RQ-PCR using the hydrolysis probe format ("TaqMan probe"); (2) RQ-PCR using the hybridization probe format; and (3) RQ-PCR using SYBR Green Dye (Kern et al., 2005). Analysis with TaqMan probe uses 5´-3´ exonuclease activity of the *Thermus aquaticus* (Taq) polymerase to detect and quantify the PCR product. The hydrolysis probe is positioned within the target sequence and is conjugated with a reporter fluorochrome at the 5´ end and a quencher fluorochrome at the 3´ end. The quencher avoids the reporter from emission of a fluorescence signal as long as the probe is intact and both fluorochromes are in the close proximity. Upon amplification of the target sequence, the hydrolysis probe is displaced from the DNA strand by the Taq polymerase and subsequently hydrolysed by the 5´-3´ exonuclease activity of the Taq polymerase. This results in displacement of of the reporter from the quencher and the fluorescence of the reporter becomes detectable.
Generally two quantification types (relative or absolute) in RQ-PCR are possible. A relative quantification based on relative expression of a target gene versus a reference gene is adequate for the most purposes. For absolute quantification, based either on an internal or an external calibration curve (Bustin et al., 2005; Ptaffl, 2001, Ptaffl et al. 2002), the methodology must be highly validated and the identical LightCycler PCR amplification efficiencies for standard material and target cDNA must be confirmed.

2.4 Genes and microRNAs microarrays

RNA was extracted using Trizol reagent and processed for Affymetrix U133 plus 2.0 GeneChip (Affymetrix, Santa Clara, CA) hybridizations. Briefly, from 5 µg total RNA, double-stranded cDNA was prepared with the use of the T7-Oligo(dT) primer (Affymetrix). *In vitro* transcription for amplification and biotinylation of the RNA transcript was performed with the BioArray HighYield RNA Transcript Labeling Kit (T7; Enzo Life Science, Farmingdale, NY). Biotin-cRNA (10 µg) was fragmented and hybridized onto the U133 plus 2.0 GeneChip for 16 hours at 45°C and labelled with Cy-3-streptavidin conjugate according to manufacturer protocols. Scanned images were converted to CEL files using GCOS software (Affymetrix). For the miRNA microarray chips, biotinylated first-strand cDNA was synthesized in reverse transcription from 2.5 to 5.0 µg total RNA using biotin-labeled random octamer oligo primer from pretreatment BM and blood mononuclear cell samples and hybridized to miRNA microarray chip KCC/TJU containing 368 probes in triplicate, corresponding to 245 human miRNA genes. After hybridization for 18 hours at 25°C and washing, direct detection of the biotin-containing transcripts by streptavidin-Alexa647 conjugate was done and processed slides were scanned. Expression profiles were analyzed in GENESPRING software(Silicon Genetics, Redwood City, CA).

3. Mutations in the molecular markers

3.1 Mutations in the *NPM1* gene

Nucleophosmin (NPM1, also called nucleolar protein B23, numatrin or NO38) is a multifunctional phosphoprotein which contains 294 amino acids (Okuwaki et al., 2006). NPM1 is one of the three nucleophosmin isoforms which are generated through alternative splicing. NPM1 resides predominantly in the nucleoli, but also continuously shuttles between nucleus and cytoplasm (Frehlick et al., 2006). The *NPM1* gene is located on chromosome 5q35 in humans and is composed of 12 exons (Chan et al., 1989). NPM1 is essential for processing and transportation of ribosomal RNA and proteins, molecular chaperoning, and regulation of the stability of tumor suppressors, such as p53 and ARF (Borer et al., 1989; Colombo et al., 2002; Enomoto et al., 2006; Herrera et al., 1995; Li & Hann, 2009; Maggi et al., 2008; Savkur & Olson, 1998; Yu et al., 2006). The ARF tumor suppressor is a protein that is transcribed from an alternate reading frame of the inhibitor of cyclin-dependent kinase CDK4. NPM1 can affect DNA replication, repair and transcription by interacting with the components of chromatin such as histones and chromatin remodeling proteins (Amin et al., 2008a,b; Angelov et al., 2006; Koike et al., 2010). NPM1 plays important roles in cell cycle (Ugrinova et al., 2007; Xiao et al., 2009). NPM1 may preferentially promote ribosome biogenesis in G1, facilitate DNA replication during S-phase while supporting chromosome segregation in mitosis (Hisaoka et al., 2010).

Almost 40% of CN-AML patients have mutations in exon 12 of the *NPM1* gene which result in loss of tryptophan residues normally required for NPM1 binding to the nucleoli and in the generation of an additional nuclear export signal motif at the C-terminus of NPM1 which causes its abnormal cytoplasmic localization (Bolli et al., 2007; Falini et al., 2006; Liso et al., 2008; Oelschlaegel et al., 2010). These mutations are the most common genetic alterations in adult CN-AML patients and are associated with female sex, higher white blood count, increased blast percentage, and low or absent CD34 expression. Cytoplasmic nucleophosmin leukemic mutant is also rarely generated by a exon-11 NPM1 mutation (Albiero et al., 2007). Acute myeloid leukemias with mutated NPM1 (NPM1c+) have distinct characteristics, including a significant association with a normal karyotype, involvement of different hematopoietic lineages, a specific gene-expression profile and clinically, a better response to induction therapy and a favorable prognosis (Meani & Alcalay, 2009; Rau & Brown, 2009, Falini et al., 2010). NPM1c+ maintains the capacity of wild-type NPM to interact with a variety of cellular proteins, and impairs their activity by delocalizing them to the cytoplasm. NPM1c+ specifically inhibits the activities of the cell-death proteases, caspase-6 and -8, through direct interaction with their cleaved, active forms, but not the immature procaspases. NPM1c+ not only affords protection from death ligand-induced cell death but also suppresses caspase-6/-8-mediated myeloid differentiation (Leong et al., 2010).

After the discovery of NPM1-mutated AML in 2005 and its subsequent inclusion as a provisional entity in the 2008 World Health Organization classification of myeloid neoplasms, several controversial issues remained to be clarified (Falini, 2011). It was unclear whether the NPM1 mutation was a primary genetic lesion and whether additional chromosomal aberrations and multilineage dysplasia (MLD) had any impact on the biologic and prognostic features of NPM1-mutated AML. Moreover, it was uncertain how to classify AML patients who were double-mutated for NPM1 and CEBPA. Recent studies have shown that: (1) the NPM1 mutant perturbs hemopoiesis in experimental models; (2) leukemic stem cells from NPM1-mutated AML patients carry the mutation; and (3) the NPM1 mutation is usually mutually exclusive of biallelic CEPBA mutations. Moreover, the biologic and clinical features of NPM1-mutated AML do not seem to be significantly influenced by concomitant chromosomal aberrations or multilineage dysplasia. NPM1-mutated AML with and without MLD showed overlapping immunophenotype (CD34 negativity) and gene expression profile (CD34 down-regulation, homeobox (*HOX*) genes up-regulation). Altogether, these pieces of evidence point to NPM1-mutated AML as a founder genetic event that defines a distinct leukemia entity accounting for approximately one-third of all AML. Distinctive gene expression and microRNA signatures were found associated with AML bearing cytoplasmic mutated NPM1 (Becker et al., 2010; Garzon et al., 2008, Verhaak et al., 2005).

Approximately 40% of patients with *NPM1* mutations also carry *FLT3* internal tandem duplications (*FLT3-ITD*). Patients with *NPM1* mutations, who did not also have *FLT3* mutation have generally more favorable prognosis (Gale et al., 2008; Scholl et al., 2008; Luo et al., 2009). The favourable prognosis of NPM1-mutated/FLT3-ITD negative patients might be explained by a higher bax/bcl-2 ratio (Del Poeta et al., 2010). These patients respond to induction therapy and stay in remission more likely. These patients may be exempted from allogenic hematopoietic stem cell transplantation during the first complete remission because their outcome after conventional consolidation chemotherapy is the same as after allogenic transplantation. However, patients with *NPM1* mutations who also carry *FLT3* mutation have bad prognosis.

Moreower, *NPM1* mutations due to their frequency and stability, may be used for minimal residual disease monitoring in AML patients with a normal karyotype (Bacher et al., 2009; Schnittger et al., 2009; Dvorakova et al., 2010).

3.2 FLT3 mutations

The feline c-fms proto-oncogene product is a 170 kd glycoprotein with associated tyrosine kinase activity. Fms-like tyrosine kinase 3 (FLT3) and its ligand (FL) are important in hematopoietic progenitor cell proliferation and differentiation (Gilliland & Griffin, 2002). As a result of ligand binding, FLT3 receptor on the cell surface of hematopoietic progenitors dimerizes, resulting in activation of its tyrosine kinase domain, receptor autophosphorylation, and recruitment of downstream signaling molecules such as signal transducer and activator of transcription 5a (STAT5a), and the MAPK (mitogen activated protein kinases) pathways leading to proliferative and pro-survival effects.

Internal tandem duplication (ITD) of base pairs within the juxtamembrane coding portion or point mutations in the second kinase domain occur in approximately 30% of patients with newly diagnosed AML and result in constitutive activation of the *FLT3* gene on chromosome 13q12 (Nakao et al., 1996; Naoe & Kiyoi, 2004; Yamamoto et al., 2001). *FLT3* mutations in the case of ITDs are associated with chemoresistance in the leukemic stem cells, shorter disease-free survival and overall survival and higher rate of relapse (Frohling et al., 2002; Ravandi et al., 2010; Whitman et al., 2010). Specific gene expression signature associated with *FLT3*-ITD was described (Bullinger et al., 2008; Whitman et al., 2010).

Overexpression of *FLT3,* homeobox genes and immunotherapeutics targets and decreased expression of erythropoiesis-associated genes is connected with *FLT3*-ITD. The prognostic significance of *FLT3* point mutations is less clear with conflicting results (Mead et al., 2008). In clinical practice, a frequent approach to patients with poor prognostic AML is to offer allogenic stem cell transplantation (SCT). Gale et al. (2005) found no benefit from any form of transplantation consolidation for patients with *FLT3-ITD*. Several inhibitors of FLT3 have entered clinical trials and are studied alone or mainly in combination with chemotherapy (Kindler et al., 2010; Small, 2008; Weisberg et al., 2009; Wiernik, 2010).

3.3 CCAAT/enhancer binding protein alpha (*CEBPA*) mutations

The CCAAT/enhancer binding protein alpha (C/EBPα) is the founding member of a family of related leucine zipper transcription factors that play important roles in myeloid differentiation (Friedman et al., 2007; Keeshan et al., 2003; Pabst & Mueller, 2007; Suh et al, 2006; Tenen et al. 1997). Members of this family consist of N-terminal transactivation domains, a DNA-binding basic domain, and a C-terminal leucine rich dimerization region (Fig. 1).

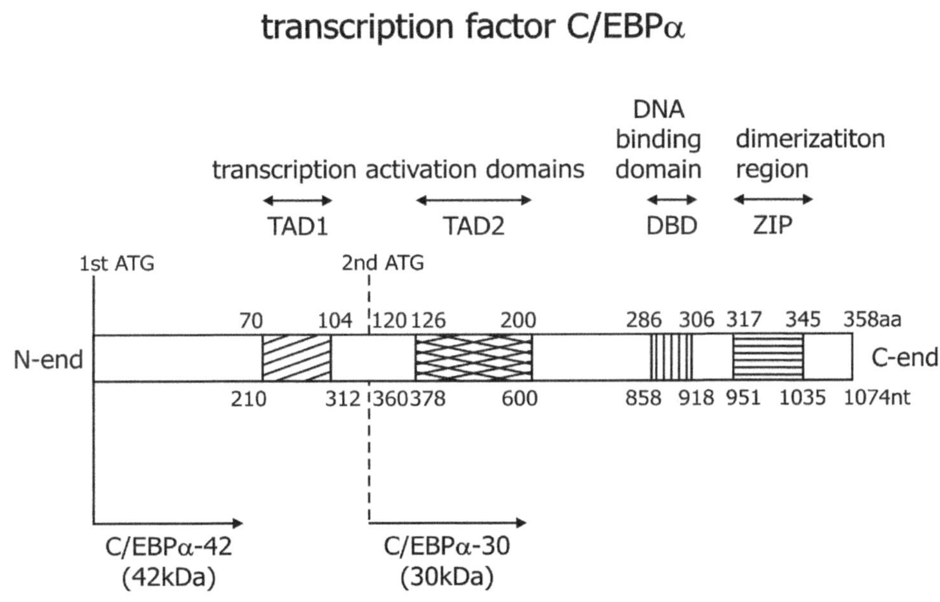

Fig. 1. The location of functional domains within the C/EBPα protein. Numbers directly above the schema indicate the amino acids of the human C/EBPα. Numbers directly under the schema indicate nucleotides (GenBank Accession No. NM_004364.2). The full-length 42 kDa form of C/EBPα protein and the shorter, dominant negative 30 kDa form of this protein are also shown.

The dimerization domain, known as "leucine zipper", contains leucine repeats that intercalate with leucine repeats of the dimer partner forming a coiled coil of α helices in parallel orientation. C/EBPα mRNA is translated into two major proteins, C/EBPα p42 (42 kDa) and C/EBPα p30 (30 kDa) by ribosomal scanning mechanism in which a fraction of ribosomes ignore the first two AUG codons and initiate translation at the third AUG codon located 357 nucleotides downstream of the first one (Fig. 1). The 30 kDa protein lacks the transactivating domain TAD1 (Fig. 1) and was shown to inhibit DNA binding and transactivation by C/EBPα p42 (Pabst et al., 2001). C/EBPα p30 fails to induce myeloid differentiation (D'Alo' et al., 2003; Friedman et al., 2007). Targeted inactivation of C/EBPα in mice demonstrates its importance in the proper development and function of liver, adipose tissue, lung and hematopoietic tissues (Flodby et al., 2006; Wang et al., 1995; Zhang et al., 1997). C/EBPα is highly expressed in these differentiated tissues where it controls differentiation-dependent gene expression and inhibits cell proliferation (Fuchs 2007). Learning more about the precise molecular functions of the C/EBPα protein and how these are affected by leukemogenic mutations should lead to an improved understanding of the cellular functions that are disrupted in patients with AML.

CEBPA mutations were found in 10-19% of CN-AML patients (Gombart et al., 2002; Fröhling et al., 2004; Fuchs et al., 2008, 2009; Lin et al., 2005; Pabst et al., 2001; Preudhomme et al., 2002). Two kinds of mutations were mainly described: 1) truncating, frameshift mutations occuring near the N-terminus in one of the two transcription activations domais (TAD1 and TAD2) on one allele and 2) in-frame insertions or deletions clustering within the C-terminal basic domain- leucine zipper (DBD and ZIP) on the other allele. Often, CN-AML patients with *CEBPA* mutations belong to FAB (French -American -British) subtypes M1 or M2 and have one mutation towards N-end and one towards C-end but other cases of mutations were also detected. Kato et al. (2011) showed that a mutation of *CEBPA* in one allele was observed in AML after MDS while the two alleles are mutated in de novo AML. Favourable impact of *CEBPA* mutations was mainly observed in patients with biallelic mutation and with lack of *FLT3*-ITD (Dufour et al., 2010; Hou et al., 2009; Pabst et al., 2009; Radomska et al. 2006; Taskesen et al., 2011; Wouters et al., 2009).

3.4 Partial tandem duplications of the *MLL* gene

The mixed lineage leukemia gene (*MLL*, also known as *ALL-1* or *HRX*), located on chromosome 11q23, encodes a histone methyltransferase and is frequently rearranged in AML. Wild-type *MLL* is schematicly presented in Fig. 2. To date, *MLL* has been found in more than sixty different translocations with different fusion partners (Basecke et al., 2006; De Braekeleer et al., 2005). Partial tandem duplications of the *MLL* gene were first observed in CN-AML by Caligury et al., 1994. These duplications consist of an in-frame repetition of *MLL* exons in a 5´-3´ direction and lead to the change of the resulting transcript and protein. *MLL*-PTD are named according to the fused exons (mainly e9/e3, e10/e3, e11/e3).

MLL-PTD are detectable in 5%-11% of patients with CN-AML (Döhner et al., 2002; Döhner & Döhner 2008; Schnittger et al., 2000; Steudel et al., 2003). *MLL*-PTD have been found also in peripheral blood and bone marrow samples of healthy adults. However in contrast to the *MLL*-PTD in AML, *MLL*-PTD in healthy adults had often unusual exon fusions and showed an ladder on gel electrophoresis after the nested RT-PCR (Basecke et al., 2006; Marcucci et al., 1998; Schnittger et al., 1998). *MLL*-PTD cooperate with silencing of the *MLL* wild-type allele by epigenetic mechanisms. *MLL*-PTD contribute to leukemogenesis through hypermethylation of DNA and epigenetic silencing of tumor suppressor genes (Dorrance et al., 2006; Whitman et al., 2008a). Inhibitors of DNA methyltransferase and histone acetylase inhibitors and their combination can re-activate the wild-type allele in *MLL*-PTD-positive blasts (Whitman et al., 2005).

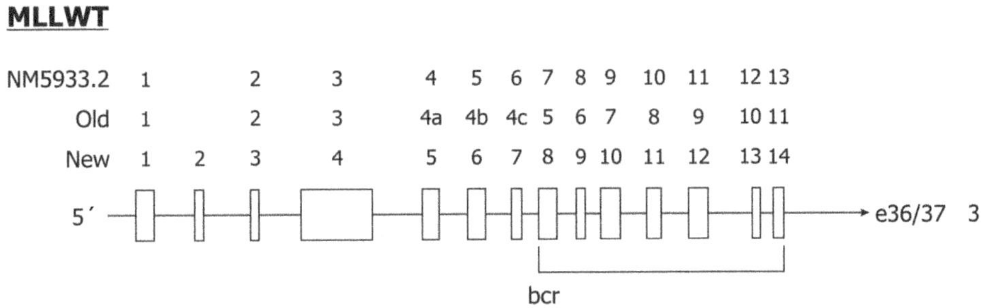

Fig. 2. Exon-intron structure of the wild-type *MLL* gene involved in tandem and nontandem duplications. The nomenclature is different in various studies (Nilson et al., 1996; Strout et al., 1998, Šárová et al., 2009). The *MLL* gene as a whole contains 36 or 37 exons according to the different nomenclatures and the resulting product of its expression contains 3969 amino acids. In the case of *MLL*-PTD e9/e3 are exons and introns between exons 3 and 9 inserted between exons 9 and 10 of the wild-type *MLL* and are duplicated by this way (the fusion of introns 2 and 9).

MLL-PTD are associated with shorter duration of the complete remission, shorter relapse-free survival and event-free survival, but *MLL*-PTD have no effect on overall survival Döhner & Döhner.

3.5 Wilms´ tumor 1 (WT1) mutations

The Wilms tumor 1 (*WT1*) gene is located on chromosome 11p13 and encodes a zinc-finger transcriptional regulator that can function as tumor suppressor in patients with the WAGR (Wilms´ tumor predisposition, aniridia, genitourinary abnormalities, and mental retardation) tumor predisposition syndrome (Haber et al., 1990) and as an oncogene in various leukemias, as well as other cancers (Ariyaratana & Loeb, 2007; King-Underwood et al., 1996; Miwa et al., 1992; Yang et al., 2007). Mutations in *WT1* gene were found in approximately 10% of AML patients (Hou et al., 2010; Gaidzik et al., 2009; Owen et al., 2010; Paschka et al., 2008; Virappane et al. 2008). Mutations are mainly localized in zinc-finger domains in exons 7 and 9 but can be also found in exons 1,2,3, and 8. The truncated WT1 protein is the result of frameshift mutations in exon 7. Truncated WT1 is without nuclear localization signal and does not bind to other interacting proteins as p53 and its homologue p73. Frameshift mutations in exon 9 are less frequent but there are also missense mutations. *WT1* mutations have been reported as an adverse prognostic factor in adult CN-AML and independently predict for poor outcome (Hou et al., 2010; Gaidzik et al., 2009; Owen et al., 2010; Paschka et al., 2008; Renneville et al., 2009; Virappane et al. 2008). *WT1* mutations lead to inferior rate of complete remission, higher incidence of relapse abd to shorter relapse-free survival and overall survival. A recent study demonstrated that a single nucleotide polymorphism SNP rs16754 in the WT1 mutational hotspot predicted favorable outcome in CN-AML (Damm et al. 2010).

3.6 Isocitrate dehydrogenase 1 and 2 (*IDH1*, *IDH2*) gene mutations

Mardis et al. (2009) found recurring mutations in codon 132 of the *IDH1* gene by sequencing a whole AML genome as described in paragraph 2.2. The protein encoded by this gene is the enzyme that catalyzes the oxidative carboxylation of isocitrate to α-ketoglutarate leading to nicotinamide adenine dinucleotide phosphate production in Krebs cycle and was found in the cytoplasm and peroxisomes (Geisbrecht & Gould, 1999). Three classes of IDH isoenzymes exist in mammalian cells (two forms of mitochondrial IDH and cytosolic IDH). *IDH1* gene is localized to chromosome band 2q33.3 and *IDH2* gene to chromosome band 15q26.1 (Narahara et al.,1985; Oh et al.,1996). *IDH2* encodes the mitochondrial isoform that uses nicotinamide adenine dinucleotide phosphate as a cofactor. The same cofactor is also used by IDH1.

Most cancer-associated enzyme mutations result in constitutive activation or inactivation of the mutated enzyme. *IDH1* and *IDH2* mutations result in the new enzyme activity, production of 2-hydroxyglutarate, not shared by wild type enzymes (Ward et al., 2010). This accumulation of 2-hydroxyglutarate induces global DNA hypermethylation, disrupts TET2 function because this enzyme is α-ketoglutarate-dependent, and impairs hematopoietic differentiation (Figueroa et al., 2010). *TET2* is a homolog of the gene originally discovered at the chromosome ten-eleven translocation (TET) site in a subset of patients with AML. TET2 catalyzes the conversion of methylcytosine to 5-hydroxymethylcytosine, suggesting a potential role for TET proteins in epigenetic regulation. Blocking the accumulation of 2-hydroxyglutarate through the inhibition of mutant IDH enzymes could represent a therapeutic target (Dang et al. , 2010; Cazola 2010).

IDH1 mutations at codon R132 occur in CN-AML patients with a frequency of 5.5% to 11% (Boissel et al., 2010; Gross et al., 2010; Patel et al., 2011; Schnittger et al., 2010; Wagner et al., 2010). A strong association between *IDH1* mutations and the *NPM1* mutation and M1 FAB subtype was observed. On the other hand, *IDH1* mutations are inversely associated with the M4 FAB subtype and expression of HLA-DR, CD13 and CD14 antigens. The prognostic impact of *IDH1* mutations in CN-AML is associated with a higher risk of relapse and a shorter overall survival (Abbas et al., 2010; Boissel et al., 2010; Marcucci et al., 2010; Paschka et al., 2010; Schnittger et al., 2010). Others (Chou et al., 2010a; Patel et al., 2011; Wagner et al., 2010), however, found no significant impact of *IDH1* mutations on CN-AML patients outcome. *IDH2* mutations in exon 4, including mainly codon R140 and in rare cases codon R172, had no prognostic impact (Thol et al., 2010). Recent study of Chou et al. (2011) showed high stability of *IDH2* mutations during disease evolution and their connection with favorable prognosis. Contrary to this observation, Boissel et al. (2010) found *IDH2* mutations independently associated with a higher risk of relapse and shorter overall survival. The prognostic impact of *IDH1* mutations and *IDH2* mutations needs further study as very controversial results were obtained. Green et al. (2010) observed no difference in outcome between *IDH1* mutated and nonmutated patients when the results were stratified by an *NPM1* mutation status but an adverse outcome for *IDH1* mutated patients when the results were correlated with *FLT3*-ITD mutation.

3.7 Mutations in gene for DNA methyltransferase 3A (*DNMT3A*)

About 22% of CN-AML patients have *DNMT3A* mutations. The most common *DNMT3A* mutation affects amino acid R882 but other parts of *DNMT3A* gene are also affected by mutations in CN-AML patients (Ley et al., 2010). Aberrant DNA methylation contributes to the pathogenesis of cancer (Rodríguez-Paredes & Esteller 2011; Taberlay & Jones, 2011; Watanabe & Maekawa, 2010). Clusters of CpG dinucleotides in promoters of tumor-supppressor genes are hypermethylated in cancer genomes and this hypermethylation results in reduced expression of the downstream gene. However, inhibition of DNA methyltransferases is only one potential mechanism of function of demethylating agents (5-azacytidine and decitabine). *DNMT3A* mutations do not change 5-methylcytosine content in AML genomes but are associated with poor survival. *DNMT3A* mutations are in many cases found together with *FLT3* mutations, *NPM1* mutations and *IDH1* mutations. All these combinations of mutations have a significantly worse outcome.

3.8 *RAS* mutations in CN-AML

Ras-signaling cascade contributes to the molecular pathogenesis of myeloproliferative disorders (Chan et al., 2004). Ras oncogenes (small GTPases) regulate mechanism of proliferation, differentiation, and apoptosis. *NRAS* (neuroblastoma RAS) mutations were detected in 9% of adult CN-AML patients and 14% of CN-AML patients younger than 56 or 60 years (Bacher et al., 2006; Bowen et al., 2005). There was no prognostic impact of these mutations in most studies (Gaidzik & Döhner, 2008; Ritter et al., 2004; Schlenk & Döhner, 2009). Mutations in other members of *Ras* family are rare in CN-AML and there was also no consistent effect on prognosis but the presence of *Ras* mutations appears to sentisize AML blasts to high dose cytarabine *in vivo* (Motyckova & Stone 2010).

3.9 Other gene mutations in CN-AML

Mutations in *RUNX1* have been shown in approximately 10%-13% of CN-AML (Döhner & Döhner, 2008, Tang et al., 2009). These mutations were positively associated with *MLL*-PTD and negatively associated with *NPM1* and *CEBPA* mutations. They predict ed a lower complete remission rate and shorter disease-free and overall survival .

TET2 (ten-eleven-translocation) first described in 2008, include frameshift, nonsense and missense mutations lying across several of its 12 exons located on chromosome 4q24 (Abdel-Wahab et al., 2009; Bacher et al., 2010; Mohr et al., 2011; Nibourel et al., 2010). The direct influence of mutations in *TET2* on patient survival in CN-AML remains a disputable issue. *TET2* mutations were revealed in 10%-25% of CN-AML patients. Abdel-Wahab et al. (2009) showed a decreased survival rate in mutated *TET2* in comparison with wild-type *TET2* group of CN-AML. However, Nibourel et al. (2010) did not find significant impact of *TET2* mutation on clinical outcome of CN-AML patients but they observed mutated *TET2* strongly associated with mutated *NPM1*. Recently, Metzeler et al. (2011) have found *TET2* mutations in 23%of CN-AML patients and these mutations were associated with older age. In favorable–risk group of CN-AML patients with *CEBPA* mutation and/or mutated *NPM1* without *FLT3*-ITD, *TET2*-mutated patients had shorter event-free survival, lower complete remission rate and shorter disease-free and overal survival. In CN-AML patients with intermediate risk with wild-type *CEBPA* and wild-type *NPM1* without *FLT3*-ITD, *TET2* mutations were not associated with outcomes.

CBL (Casitas B-cell lymphoma) mutations were identified in rare cases of CN-AML (Bacher et al., 2010; Makishima et al., 2009; Reindl et al., 2009). Cbl is E3 ubiquitin ligase involved in degradation of activated receptor tyrosine kinases, including Src kinases (Makishima et al., 2009). Presence of these mutations was suggested to be involved in aberrant *FLT3* expression. FLT3 ligand–dependent hyperproliferation of *CBL* mutant cells could be abrogated by treatment with the specific inhibitor, midostaurin (PKC412).

Mutations in the additional sex comb-like 1 (*ASXL1)* gene were analyzed in exon 12 in CN-AML patients and 8.9% mutations were detected (Chou et al., 2010b). This mutation was closely associated with older age, male sex, *RUNX1* mutation and expression of human leukocyte-antigen-DR and CD34 (Chou et al., 2010b; Rocquain et al., 2010). Association with *FLT3*-ITD, *NPM1* mutation, *WT1* mutation, and expression of CD33 and CD15 was not detected. *ASXL1* mutated patients had a shorter overall survival than patients without this mutation, but the mutation was not an independent adverse prognostic factor in multivariete analysis.

Phosphoinositide phospholipase Cβ1 (*PI-PLCβ1*) gene mutations are very rare in CN-AML (Damm et al., 2010). Follo et al. (2009) described greater representation of these mutations (monoallelic deletions) in AML and their association with a worse clinical outcome.

4. Overexpression of marker genes with prognostic relevance

Alterations in the expression of genes belonging to signal transduction pathways as well as transcription factors are known to play a functional role in the pathogenesis of AML. Therefore, these marker genes are implicated in the process of leukemogenesis and their overexpression may be useful to predict outcome in CN-AML patients.

4.1 *WT1* gene expression

The *WT1* gene overexpression was found in several leukemias, including AML (Cilloni et al., 2009). WT1 mRNA levels in the peripheral blood can predict relapse after achieving complete remission, and its levels after consolidation therapy are closely correlated with disease-free and overall survival, and with early relapse (Cilloni et al., 2009; Gianfaldoni et al., 2010; Miyawaki et al., 2010). Monitoring of *WT1* expression is significant predictor of relapse in AML patients after hematopoietic cell transplantation (Lange et al., 2011).

4.2 *BAALC* (brain and acute leukemia, cytoplasmic) expression

The *BAALC* gene, located on chromosome 8q22.3, is primarily expressed in neuroectoderm-derived tissues and in hematopoietic precursors and encodes a protein with unknown function (Baldus et al., 2003, 2006; Langer et al., 2008; Santamaria et al., 2010). High level of *BAALC* expression showed a higher refractoriness to induction treatment , lower complete remission rate after salvage therapy and lower overall survival and relapse - free survival in intermediate-risk AML (Santamaria et al., 2010). The *BAALC* expression is considered an independent prognostic factor in CN-AML. High *BAALC* expression was associated with *FLT3*-ITD, and high *ERG* expression in multivariable analysis (Baldus et al., 2006). High *BAALC* expression is also connected with overexpression of genes involved in drug resistance (*MDR1*) and stem cell markers (*CD133, CD34, KIT*). In low *BAALC* expressers, genes associated with undifferentiated hematopoietic precursors and unfavorable outcome predictors were downregulated, while *HOX*-genes and *HOX*-gene-embedded-miR were upregulated (Schwind et al., 2010). Global *miR* expression analysis did not reveal significant differences between different rate *BAALC* expression groups (Langer et al., 2008). Inverse association between the expression of *miR148a* and *BAALC* was revealed.

4.3 *ERG* (v-ets erythroblastosis virus E26 oncogene homolog) expression

ETS-related gene (*ERG*), located at chromosome band 21q22, is downstream effector of signaling transduction pathways involved in the regulation of cell proliferation, differentiation, and apoptosis (Marcucci et al., 2005,2007; Mrózek et al., 2007; Metzeler et al. 2009, Schwind et al., 2010). CN-AML patients with overexpression of *ERG* have been reported to have a poor clinical outcome. When combined with other known prognostic markers, *ERG* expression can improve the molecular risk-based stratification of patients with CN-AML. Low *ERG* expression is associated with downregulation of genes involved in the DNA-methylation machinery, upregulation of *miR148a,* which targets DNA methyltransferase 3B (*DNMT3B*) and with better outcome (Schwind et al., 2010).

4.4 *MN1* (meningioma 1) expression

MN1 is located at 22q11 and its overexpression is associated with lower response rate after first course of induction therapy and poor clinical outcome for CN-AML patients. Moreover, high *MN1* expression was connected with a higher relapse rate and worse relapse-free and overall survival (Grosveld, 2007; Heuser et al., 2006; Langer et al., 2009). *MN1* expression levels were directly correlated with *BAALC* expression levels and with the expression of genes reported as associated with a *BAALC* expression signature, specifically with expression of *CD34* and *ABCB1* (*MDR1*) and several other genes (Langer et al., 2008, 2009). *MN1* expression levels were negatively connected with expression of *HOX* genes and with *NPM1* mutated CN-AML (Langer et al., 2009). *MN1*-associated miR-expression signature comprises 15 miR, expression of 8 miR (*hsa-miR-126* family) was positively correlated and expression of 7 miR (*hsa-miR-16, hsa-miR-19a* and *hsa-miR-20a,* all members of *miR-17-92* polycistron) negatively correlated with *MN1* expression (Langer et al., 2009). *MN1* overexpression confered resistance to the differentiation activity of all-trans-retinoic acid (ATRA) in AML (Heuser et al., 2007).

4.5 *EVI1* (ecotropic viral integration site 1) expression

Human *EVI1* is localized to chromosome 3 band q26, spans 60kb, and contains 16 exons (Goyama &Kurokawa, 2009). High *EVI1* expression occurs in approximately 8% of patients with *de novo* AML (Barjesteh van Waalwijk van Doom-Khosrovani et al., 2003). High *EVI1* expression was observed not only in AML carrying the chromosome 3 abnormalities, but also in CN-AML (Gröschel et al., 2010; Lugthart et al., 2008; Santamaria et al., 2009) and is in both groups connected with poor treatment response.

4.6 Other molecular marker genes expression

The *PRAME* (preferentially expressed antigen of melanoma) gene was shown to be expressed in high levels in AML. PRAME mRNA was observed in about one-third of AML cases and there was a good correlation between PRAME mRNA level and hematological remission and relapse. It may be also useful marker to detect minimal residual disease after allogenic transplantation (Paydas et al., 2005; Qin et al. ., 2009). Epping et al. (2005) showed that PRAME is a repressor of retinoic acid signaling but Steinbach et al. (2007) did not confirm this mechanism in the pathogenesis of AML. Specific immunotherapies for patients with AML using leukemia-associated antigens (LAA) as target structures might be a therapeutic option. Expression of genes for these antigens have prognostic importance (Greiner et al., 2008).

AF1q (ALL1 fused gene from chromosome 1q) gene overexpression in CN-AML patients is associated with a significantly greater incidence of concurrent *FLT3*-ITD and with a poor outcome (Strunk et al., 2009). NC-AML patients with low *AF1q* expression had better overall survival and complete remission rate than patients with high AF1q mRNA level.

High *MLL5* (mixed lineage leukemia 5) expression is associated with a favorable outcome of CN-AML patients and enables identification of a significant proportion of patients with favorable prognosis that are not identified by other markers analyses (Damm et al., 2011).
Increased expression of the phosphoinositide phospholipase Cβ1 (*PI-PLC β1*) gene is an independent prognostic factor in CN-AML and is associated with a significantly shorter overall survival but with no difference for relapse-free survival (Damm et al., 2010).
The Rho family of small GTPases, including Rho, Rac and Cdc42, functions as critical mediators of signaling pathways from plasma membrane regulating actin assembly, migration, proliferation and survival in hematopoietic cells. *RhoH* gene, also known as Translocation Three Four (*TTF*), encodes a 191-amino acid protein belonging to the Rho family (Gu et al., 2005; Iwasaki et al., 2008). Rho H functions as a negative regulator for interleukin 3 (IL3) - induced signals through modulation of the JAK-STAT (Janus Kinase-Signal Transducer and Activator of Transcription)- signaling pathway (Gűndogdu et al., 2010). Low RhoH levels are connected with an upregulation of IL3- dependent cell growth, STAT5 activity and an increase of CD123 surface expression that has been described in AML patients (Gűndogdu et al., 2010). Multivariate analysis demonstrated that low expression of *RhoH* was an independent unfavorable prognostic factor for both overall and disease-free survival of AML in the intermediate risk group (Iwasaki et al., 2008).
Activation of Notch signal pathway (expression of *Notch1*, *Jagged1* and *Delta1* as members of this pathway) is associated with a poorer prognosis for AML patients with intermediate risk (Xu et al., 2010).
The Forkhead transcription factors (FOXO) are direct target of the PI3K/AKT (protein kinase B) signaling and they integrate the signals of several other transduction pathways at the transcriptional level. The PI3K/AKT/FOXO signaling pathway is up-regulated in AML. High *FOXO3a* expression is associated with a poorer prognosis in CN-AML (Santamaria et al., 2009) and the increased levels of both total and of highly phosphorylated FOXO3a correlate with higher proliferation and blood blasts and these high levels of FOXO3a are an adverse prognostic factor in AML (Kornblau et al., 2010).
Bone marrow neoangiogenesis plays an important pathogenetic and possible prognostic role in AML (Hou et al., 2008; Lee et al., 2007; Loges et al., 2005; Mourah et al. 2009). Multivariable analysis showed that the levels of vascular endothelial growth factor (VEGF) transcript isoform 121 (VEGF121) remained an independent prognostic factor for either event-free survivasl or overall survival (Mourah et al., 2009). High levels of VEGF121 were significantly related to a worse prognosis. Angiopoietin-2 (*Ang2*) gene expression represents also an independent prognostic factor in AML with intermediate risk and high *Ang2* expression is associated with an unfavorable prognosis (Hou et al., 2008; Lee et al., 2007; Loges et al., 2005). High *VEGFC* expression appeared strongly associated with reduced complete remission rate, reduced overall and event-free survival in adult AML independent of cytogenetic risk and white blood cell count (de Jonge et al., 2010). High *VEGFC* expression was related to enhanced chemoresistance and predicted adverse long-term prognosis.
TGFβ (transforming growth factor beta) superfamily receptors ALK-1 (activin receptor like kinase) and ALK-5 have an important role in endothelial cells behavior and might be involved in the pathogenesis of AML. *ALK-1* and *ALK-5* are both expressed by the majority of AML patients. *ALK-5* expression has a significant negative impact on complete remission achievment and overall survival of AML patients (Otten et al., 2011).

Dysregulation of the Wnt/β-catenin pathway has been observed in various malignancies, including AML. Overexpression of β-catenin is an independent adverse prognostic factor in AML (Chen et al., 2009; Ysebaert et al., 2006).
Chemokine (C-X-C motif) receptor 4 (CXCR4) retains hematopoietic progenitors and leukemia cells within the marrow microenvironment. Multivariate analysis revealed *CXCR4* expression as an independent prognostic factor for disease relapse and survival (Konoplev et al., 2007; Spoo et al., 2007; Tavernier-Tardy et al., 2009). Low *CXCR4* expression correlated with a better prognosis, resulting in a longer relapse-free and overall survival.
Many studies of AML have linked the overexpression of ABCB1 (also named permeability glycoprotein, Pgp), a member of ATP-binding proteins coded by the multi-drug resistance gene (*MDR1*), to poor prognosis (Leith et al., 1997; Steinbach & Legrand, 2007; Trnkova et al., 2007). Other drug-resistance proteins BCRP (breast cancer resistance protein, also named ABCG2) and LRP (lung resistance protein) have also an adverse impact (Dimiani et al., 2010; Huh et al., 2006).

5. Gene expression profiling in CN-AML

Gene expression profiling (GEP) was described twelve years ago by Golub et al. (1999). GEP analyses on the basis of microarrays allow the simultaneous characterization of thousands of genes. GEP is useful for the classification of leukemias. In CN-AML, microarray GEP has been applied to identify expression signatures in order to predict clinical outcome within this very heterogeneous group of patients.
Bullinger et al. (2004) and Radmacher et al. (2006) defined by GEP two novel molecular subclasses of CN-AML with significant differences in survival times with respect to the presence or absence of *FLT3* mutations and the FAB subtypes.
NPM1 gene mutations are connected with specific gene expression pattern in CN-AML (Alcalay et al., 2005; Becker et al., 2010; Garzon et al., 2008; Verhaak et al., 2005; Wilson et al., 2006). This specific gene expression signature was characterised by the activation of homeobox (*HOX*) genes including a particular subset of homeobox *TALE* (three amino acid loop extension) genes distinguish themselves from typical homeodomains containing genes. Downregulated in the *NPM1* mutations group were genes whose low expression is associated with better prognosis in CN-AML as *BAALC, MN1, ERG*, and multidrug resistance genes.
Comparison of gene expression between biallelic *CEBPA* mutation and monoallelic *CEBPA* mutation AML was described by Dufour et al. (2010). Expression of multiple members of the homeobox gene family (*HOXA5, HOXA9, HOXA10, HOXB2*, and *HOXB6*), *CD34*, and lymphoid markers *CD6, CD52*, and *TSPO* (gene for translocator protein, benzodiazepine receptor) is downregulated in CN-AML patients with biallelic *CEBPA* mutation.
Specific gene expression signatures associated with *FLT3*-ITD and *FLT3*-TKD (mutations in the tyrosine kinase domain) were described (Bullinger et al., 2008; Neben et al., 2005; Whitman et al., 2008b, 2010). Overexpression of *FLT3*, homeobox genes (*HOXB3, HOXB5, PBX3, MEIS1*), and immunotherapeutic targets (*WT1, CD33*) and underexpression of leukemia associated (*MLLT3, TAL1*) and erythropoiesis-associated genes (*GATA3, EPOR, ANK1, HEMGN*) is typical for *FLT3*-ITD, whereas overexpression of gene for transcription factor FOXA1 containing forkhead box was observed in *FLT3*-TKD (Neben et al., 2005, Whitman et al., 2010). Whereas the predictive value for *FLT3*-ITD was relatively high (77%), the high number of false predictions eliminates GEP as an investigational tool for research

studies waiting on an entrance to clinical practice and decision making (Marcucci et al., 2011a; Verhaak et al., 2009; Wouters et al., 2009). GEP technique seems not to be in future a primary diagnostic tool but will be used in many cases as a confirmative method.

6. MicroRNA expression profiling

MicroRNAs (miRs) are small noncoding RNAs of 19 to 25 nucleotides which function as negative regulators of gene expression by causing target mRNA cleavage or by interfering with target mRNA translation. Dysregulation of miRs plays an important role in the pathogenesis of many cancers based on their involvement in basic cellular functions (Nana-Sinkam & Croce, 2010). In addition, miRs have the capacity to target tens to hundreds of genes simultaneously. Thus, they are attractive candidates as prognostic biomarkers and therapeutic targets in cancer.

MiR expression signatures have been correlated with recurrent molecular aberrations in AML. *NPM1* mutations associate with upregulation of *miR10a, miR10b, and miR196a,* all lying in the genomic cluster of *HOX* genes that are overexpressed (Becker et al., 2010, Garzon et al., 2008). Upregulation of *miR181a* and *miR181b* expression is associated with *CEBPA* mutations in CN-AML (Marcucci et al., 2008; 2009; 2011b). *FLT3*-ITD was observed to be associated with *miR155* upregulation and *miR144* and *miR451* downregulation (Whitman et al., 2010). Genome-wide profiling identified aberrantly expressed miR associated with R172 *IDH2* mutated CN-AML patients (Marcucci et al., 2010). The most upregulated *miR* genes were genes of *miR125* family (*miR125a* and *miR125b*), *miR1* and *miR133*. The most downregulated *miR* genes were *miR194-1, miR526, miR520a-3p,* and *miR548b*.

Recent studies have also shown that clinical outcome in CN-AML is affected by changes in miR expression. Overexpression of *miR20a, miR25, miR191, miR199a* and *miR199b* adversely affected overall survival (Garzon et al., 2008).

7. DNA methylation arrays

DNA cytosine methylation in CpG islands regulates gene expression. Aberrant methylation of specific genes was observed in cancer including leukemia, although little is known about the mechanisms of this specific gene sets methylation. Genome-wide promoter DNA methylation profiling revealed unique AML subgroups and methylation patterns that are associated with clinical outcome (Bullinger & Armstrong, 2010; Figueroa et al., 2010). DNA methylation profiles segregates patients with *CEBPA* mutations from other subtypes of leukemia and defined four epigenetically distinct forms of AML with *NPM1* mutations. Epigenetic modification of the *CEBPA* promoter regions was also described and *CEBPA* hypermethylation appeared to be favorable prognostic marker in addition to *NPM1* mutation with lack of *FLT3*-ITD and *CEBPA* bi-allelic, double mutations (Hackanson et al., 2008; Lin et al., 2010; Szankasi et al., 2011). Lugthart et al. (2011) found that the promoter DNA methylation signature of *EVI1* AML blast cells differed from normal bone marrow cells and other AMLs and contained many hypermethylated genes. EVI1 was observed to physically interact with DNA methyltransferases 3A and 3B and colocalize with them in nuclei and complex is involved in EVI1-mediated transcriptional repression. Cases with the significantly higher levels of EVI1 are associated with many more methylated genes (Lugthart et al., 2011).

8. Conclusion and future directions

CN-AML is very heterogeneous on the molecular level and harbours many genetic alterations that define new molecular subgroups. This molecular heterogeneity of CN-AML is not fully reflected in current classification systems (Vardiman et al. 2008, Döhner et al., 2010). Molecular markers with prognostic significance are very important for future therapies. Decision over whether to allograft a patient in first complete remission depends on the evaluation in a risk/benefit analysis in prognostic scoring system (Smith et al., 2011). The favorable cytogenetic risk group is now supplemented by CN-AML with mutant *NPM1* or biallelic *CEBPA* mutations in the absence of *FLT3*-ITD (Döhner et al., 2010). These CN-AML patients may not need to be referred for allogenic stem cell transplantation in first complete remission (Burnett et al., 2011). Low expression of *BAALC* is also associated with favorable outcome in CN-AML (Santamaria et al., 2010), but not in association with *FLT3, NPM1,* and *CEBPA* mutations and may not be prognostic in older patients (Langer et al., 2008). Low *BAALC* expression is an important factor for complete remission achievment and longer disease-free survival. Even better overall survival is reached in CN-AML patients who had low *ERG* expression in addition to low *BAALC* expression (Burnett et al., 2011). The similarity of *BAALC* and *ERG* expression signatures between younger and older CN-AML patients and the fact that these molecular markers affect similarly outcomes in the group of younger and older than 60 years CN-AML patients sugest that older patients with favorable molecular risk factors, such as low *BAALC* and *ERG* expression , if treated more intensively, might have outcomes comparable with those of younger CN-AML patients with the same molecular markers (Schwind et al., 2010). Patients with low *ERG,* low *EVI1,* and high *PRAME* expression levels were also shown to have a good prognosis (Santamaria et al., 2009). Recently, Damm et al. (2011) proposed an integrative prognostic risk score (IPRS) for CN-AML patients based on clinical and molecular markers. Nine clinical, hematological and molecular factors including age, white blood cell count, mutation status of *NPM1, FLT3*-ITD, *CEBPA, WT1* single nucleotide polymorphism SNP rs16754, and expression levels of *BAALC, ERG, MN1,* and *WT1* (Damm et al., 2011). Other molecular markers like *NRAS, MLL-PTD, WT1, IDH1,* or *IDH2* mutations were not significant and thus not included in the IPRS.

Genomewide search and new technologies will help to subcategorize CN-AML. Gene and microRNA signatures and DNA methylation signatures obtained in these studies may detect potential targets for new therapies.

9. Acknowledgment

This work was supported by the research intention VZ 00023736 from the Ministry of Health of the Czech Republic, grant MSM 0021620808 and grant LC 06044 from the Ministry of Education, Youth and Sport of the Czech Republic.

10. References

Abbas, S.; Lugthart, S.; Kavelaars, F.G.; Schelen, A.; Koenders, J.E.; Zeilemaker, A.; van Putten, W.J.; Rijneveld, A.W.; Löwenberg, B. & Valk, P.J. (2010) Acquired mutations in the genes encoding IDH1 and IDH2 both are recurrent aberrations in acute myeloid leukemia: prevalence and prognostic value. *Blood,* Vol. 116, No. 12, (September), pp. 2122-2126, ISSN 0006-4971

Abdel-Wahab, O.; Mullally, A.; Hedvat, C.; Garcia-Manero, G.; Patel, J.; Wadleigh, M.; Malinge, S.; Yao, J.; Kilpivaara, O.; Bhat, R.; Huberman, K.; Thomas, S.; Dolgalev, I.; Heguy, A.; Paietta, E.; Le Beau, M.M.; Beran, M.; Tallman, M.S.; Ebert, B.L.; Kantarjian, H.M.; Stone, R.M.; Gilliland, D.G.; Crispino, J.D. & Levine, R.L. (2009) Genetic characterization of TET1, TET2, and TET3 alterations in myeloid malignancies. *Blood*, Vol. 114, No. 1, (July), pp. 144-147, ISSN 0006-4971

Amicarelli G, Shehi E, Makrigiorgos GM, Adlerstein D (2007). FLAG assay as a novel method for real-time signal generation during PCR: application to detection and genotyping of KRAS codon 12 mutations. *Nucleic Acids Research* Vol. 35, No. 19, e131, ISSN 0305-1048

Amin, M. A.; Matsunaga, S.; Uchiyama, S. & Fukui, K. (2008a) Depletion of nucleophosmin leads to distortion of nucleolar and nuclear structures in HeLa cells. *Biochemical Journal*, Vol. 415, No. 3, (November), pp. 345–351, ISSN 0264-6021

Amin, M.A.; Matsunaga, S.; Uchiyama, S. & Fukui, K. (2008b) Nucleophosmin is required for chromosome congression, proper mitotic spindle formation, and kinetochore-microtubule attachment in HeLa cells. *FEBS Letters*, Vol. 582, No. 27, (November), pp. 3839-3844, ISSN 0014-5793

Angelov, D. ; Bondarenko, V.A.; Almagro, S.; Menoni, H.; Mongélard, F.; Hans, F.; Mietton, F.; Studitsky, V.M.; Hamiche, A.; Dimitrov, S. & Bouvet P. (2006) Nucleolin is a histone chaperone with FACT-like activity and assists remodeling of nucleosomes. *EMBO Journal*, Vol. 25, No. 8, (April), pp. 1669–1679, ISSN 0261-4189

Ariyaratana, S. & Loeb, D.M. (2007) The role of the Wilms tumour gene (WT1) in normal and malignant haematopoiesis. *Expert Reviews in Moecular Medicine*, Vol. 9, No. 14, (May), pp. 1-17, ISSN 1462-3994

Bacher, U.; Badbaran, A.; Fehse, B.; Zabelina, T.; Zander, A.R. & Kröger, N. (2009) Quantitative monitoring of NPM1 mutations provides a valid minimal residual disease parameter following allogeneic stem cell transplantation. *Experimental Hematology*, Vol. 37, No. 1, (January), pp. 135-142. ISSN 0301-472X

Bacher, U.; Haferlach, C.; Schnittger, S.; Kohlmann, A.; Kern, W. & Haferlach, T. (2010) Mutations of the TET2 and CBL genes: novel molecular markers in myeloid malignancies. *Annals of Hematology*, Vol. 89, No. 7, (July), pp. 643-652, ISSN 0939-5555

Bacher, U.; Haferlach, T.; Schoch, C.; Kern, W. & Schnittger, S. (2006) Implications of NRAS mutations in AML: a study of 2502 patients. *Blood*, Vol. 107, No. 10, (May), pp. 3847-3853, ISSN 0006-4971

Bacher U, Kohlmann A, Haferlach C, Haferlach T. (2009) Gene expression profiling in acute myeloid leukaemia (AML). *Best Practice & Research Clinical Haematology*, Vol. 22, No. 2, (June), pp. 169-180, ISSN 1521-6926

Baldus, C.D. & Bullinger, L. (2008). Gene expression with prognostic implications in cytogenetically normal acute myeloid leukemia. *Seminars in Oncology*, Vol. 35, No. 4, (August), pp. 356-364, ISSN 0093-7754

Baldus, C.D.; Tanner, S.M.; Ruppert, A.S.; Whitman, S.P.; Archer, K.J.; Marcucci, G.; Caligiuri, M.A.; Carroll, A.J.; Vardiman, J.W.; Powell, B.L.; Allen, S.L.; Moore, J.O.; Larson, R.A.; Kolitz, J.E.; de la Chapelle, A. & Bloomfield, C.D. (2003) BAALC expression predicts clinical outcome of de novo acute myeloid leukemia patients with normal cytogenetics: a Cancer and Leukemia Group B Study. *Blood*, Vol. 102, No. 5, (September), pp. 1613-1618, ISSN 0006-4971

Baldus, C.D.; Thiede, C.; Soucek, S.; Bloomfield, C.D. ; Thiel, E. & Ehninger, G. (2006) BAALC expression and FLT3 internal tandem duplication mutations in acute myeloid leukemia patients with normal cytogenetics: prognostic implications. *Journal of Clinical Oncology*, Vol. 24, No. 5, (February), pp. 790-797, ISSN 0732-183X

Barjesteh van Waalwijk van Doorn-Khosrovani, S.; Erpelinck, C.; van Putten, W.L.; Valk, P.J.; van der Poel-van de Luytgaarde, S.; Hack, R.; Slater, R.; Smit, E.M.; Beverloo, H.B.; Verhoef, G.; Verdonck, L.F.; Ossenkoppele, G.J.; Sonneveld, P.; de Greef, G.E.; Löwenberg, B. & Delwel, R. (2003) High EVI1 expression predicts poor survival in acute myeloid leukemia: a study of 319 de novo AML patients. *Blood*, Vol. 101, No. 3, (February), pp. 837-845, ISSN 0006-4971

Basecke, J.; Whelan, J.T.; Griesinger, F. & Bertrand, F.E. (2006) The MLL partial tandem duplication in acute myeloid leukaemia. *British Journal of Haematology*, Vol. 135, No. 4, (November), pp. 438-449, ISSN 0007-1048

Becker, H.; Marcucci, G.; Maharry, K.; Radmacher, M.D.; Mrózek, K.; Margeson, D.; Whitman, S.P.; Wu, Y.Z.; Schwind, S.; Paschka, P.; Powell, B.L.; Carter, T.H.; Kolitz, J.E.; Wetzler, M.; Carroll, A.J.; Baer, M.R.; Caligiuri, M.A.; Larson, R.A. & Bloomfield, C.D. (2010) Favorable prognostic impact of NPM1 mutations in older patients with cytogenetically normal de novo acute myeloid leukemia and associated gene- and microRNA-expression signatures: a Cancer and Leukemia Group B study. *Journal of Clinical Oncology*, Vol. 28, No. 4, (February), pp. 596-604, ISSN 0732-183X

Bianchini, M.; Ottaviani, E.; Grafone, T.;, Giannini, B.; Soverini, S.; Terragna, C.; Amabile, M.; Piccaluga, P.P.; Malagola, M.; Rondoni, M.; Bosi, C.; Baccarani, M. & Martinelli, G. (2003) Rapid detection of Flt3 mutations in acute myeloid leukemia patients by denaturing HPLC. *Clinical Chemistry*, Vol. 49, No. 10, (October), pp. 1642-1650, ISSN 0009-9147

Boissel, N.; Nibourel, O.; Renneville, A.; Gardin, C.; Reman, O.; Contentin, N.; Bordessoule, D.; Pautas, C.; de Revel, T.; Quesnel, B.; Huchette, P.; Philippe, N.; Geffroy, S.; Terre, C.; Thomas, X.; Castaigne, S.; Dombret, H. & Preudhomme, C. (2010) Prognostic impact of isocitrate dehydrogenase enzyme isoforms 1 and 2 mutations in acute myeloid leukemia: a study by the Acute Leukemia French Association group. *Journal of Clinical Oncology*, Vol. 28, No. 23, (August), pp. 3717-3723, ISSN 0732-183X

Bolli, N.; Nicoletti, I.; De Marco, M.F.; Bigerna, B.; Pucciarini, A.; Mannucci, R.; Martelli, M.P.; Liso, A.; Mecucci, C.; Fabbiano, F.; Martelli, M.F.; Henderson, B.R. & Falini, B. (2007) Born to be exported: COOH-terminal nuclear export signals of different strength ensure cytoplasmic accumulation of nucleophosmin leukemic mutants. *Cancer Research*, Vol. 67, No. 13, (July), pp. 6230-623, ISSN 0008-5472

Borer, R.A.; Lehner, C.F.; H. M. Eppenberger, H.M. & Nigg, E.A. (1989) Major nucleolar proteins shuttle between nucleus and cytoplasm. *Cell*, Vol. 56, No. 3, (February), pp. 379–390, ISSN 0092-8674

Bowen, D.T.; Frew, M.E.; Hills, R.; Gale, R.E.; Wheatley, K.; Groves, M.J.; Langabeer, S.E.; Kottaridis, P.D.; Moorman, A.V.; Burnett, A.K. & Linch, D.C. (2005) RAS mutation in acute myeloid leukemia is associated with distinct cytogenetic subgroups but does not influence outcome in patients younger than 60 years. *Blood*, Vol. 106, No. 6, (September), pp. 2113-2119, ISSN 0006-4971

Bullinger, L. (2006) Gene expression profiling in acute myeloid leukemia. *Haematologica*, Vol. 91, No. 6, (June), pp. 733-738, ISSN 0390-6078

Bullinger, L. & Armstrong, S.A. (2010) HELP for AML: methylation profiling opens new avenues. *Cancer Cell*, Vol. 17, No. 1, (January), pp. 1-3, ISSN 1535-6108

Bullinger, L.; Döhner, K.; Bair, E.; Fröhling, S.; Schlenk, R.F.; Tibshirani, R.; Döhner, H. & Pollack, J.R. (2004) Use of gene-expression profiling to identify prognostic subclasses in adult acute myeloid leukemia. *New England Journal of Medicine*, Vol. 350, No. 16, (April), pp. 1605-1616, ISSN 0028-4793

Bullinger, L.; Döhner, K.; Kranz, R.; Stirner, C.; Fröhling, S.; Scholl, C.; Kim, Y.H.; Schlenk, R.F.; Tibshirani, R.; Döhner, H. & Pollack, J.R. (2008) An FLT3 gene-expression signature predicts clinical outcome in normal karyotype AML. *Blood*, Vol. 111, No. 9, (May), pp. 4490-4495. ISSN 0006-4971

Bullinger, L. & Valk, P.J. (2005) Gene expression profiling in acute myeloid leukemia. *Journal of Clinical Oncology*, Vol. 23, No. 26, (September), pp. 6296-6305, ISSN 0732-183X

Burnett, A.; Wetzler, M. & Löwenberg, B. (2011) Therapeutic advances in acute myeloid leukemia. *Journal of Clinical Oncology*, Vol. 29, No. 5, (February), pp. 487-494, ISSN 0732-183X

Bustin, S.A.; Benes, V.; Nolan, T. & Pfaffl, M.W. (2005) Quantitative real-time RT-PCR--a perspective. *Journal of Molecular Endocrinology*, Vol. 34, No. 3, (June), pp. 597-601, 0952-5041

Caligiuri, M.A.; Schichman, S.A.; Strout, M.P.; Mrózek, K.; Baer, M.R.; Frankel, S.R.; Barcos, M.; Herzig, G.P.; Croce, C.M. & Bloomfield, C.D. (1994) Molecular rearrangement of the ALL-1 gene in acute myeloid leukemia without cytogenetic evidence of 11q23 chromosomal translocations. *Cancer Research*, Vol. 54, No. 2, (January), pp. 370-373, ISSN 0008-5472

Cazzola, M. (2010) *IDH1* and *IDH2* mutations in myeloid neoplasms-Novel paradigmsand cliunical implications. *Haematologica*, Vol. 95, No. 10, pp. 1623-1627, ISSN 0390-6078

Cilloni, D.; Renneville, A.; Hermitte, F.; Hills, R.K.; Daly, S.; Jovanovic, J.V.; Gottardi, E.; Fava, M.; Schnittger, S.; Weiss, T.; Izzo, B.; Nomdedeu, J.; van der Heijden, A.; van der Reijden, B.A.; Jansen, J.H.; van der Velden, V.H.; Ommen, H.; Preudhomme, C.; Saglio, G. & Grimwade, D. (2009) Real-time quantitative polymerase chain reaction detection of minimal residual disease by standardized WT1 assay to enhance risk stratification in acute myeloid leukemia: a European LeukemiaNet study. *Journal of Clinical Oncology*, Vol. 27, No. 31, (November), pp. 5195-5201, ISSN 0732-183X

Chan, I.T.; Kutok, J.L.; Williams, I.R.; Cohen, S.; Kelly, L.; Shigematsu, H.; Johnson, L.; Akashi, K.; Tuveson, D.A.; Jacks, T. & Gilliland, D.G. (2004) Conditional expression of oncogenic K-ras from its endogenous promoter induces a myeloproliferative disease. *Journal of Clinical Investigation*, Vol. 113, No. 4, (February), pp. 528-538, ISSN 0021-9738

Chan, W.Y.; Liu, Q.R; Borjigin, J.; Busch, H.; Rennert O.M. ; Tease, L.A. & Chan, P.K. (1989) Characterization of the cDNA encoding human nucleophosmin and studies of its role in normal and abnormal growth. *Biochemistry*, Vol. 28, No. 3, (February), pp. 1033- 1039, ISSN 0006-2960

Chen, C.C.; Gau, J.P.; You, J.Y.; Lee, K.D.; Yu, Y.B.; Lu, C.H.; Lin, J.T.; Lan, C.; Lo, W.H.; Liu, J.M. & Yang, C.F. (2009) Prognostic significance of beta-catenin and topoisomerase IIalpha in de novo acute myeloid leukemia. *American Journal of Hematology*, Vol. 84, No. 2, (February), pp. 87-92, ISSN 0361-8609

Chou, W.C.; Hou, H.A.; Chen, C.Y.; Tang, J.L.; Yao, M.; Tsay, W.; Ko, B.S.; Wu, S.J.; Huang, S.Y.; Hsu, S.C.; Chen, Y.C.; Huang, Y.N.; Chang, Y.C.; Lee, F.Y.; Liu, M.C.; Liu, C.W.; Tseng, M.H.; Huang, C.F. & Tien, H.F. (2010a) Distinct clinical and biologic characteristics in adult acute myeloid leukemia bearing the isocitrate dehydrogenase 1 mutation. *Blood*, Vol. 115, No. 14, (April), pp. 2749-2754, ISSN 0006-4971

Chou, W.C.; Huang, H.H.; Hou, H.A.; Chen, C.Y.; Tang, J.L.; Yao, M.; Tsay, W.; Ko, B.S.; Wu, S.J.; Huang, S.Y.; Hsu, S.C.; Chen, Y.C.; Huang, Y.N.; Chang, Y.C.; Lee, F.Y.; Liu, M.C.; Liu, C.W.; Tseng, M.H.; Huang, C.F. & Tien, H.F. (2010b) Distinct clinical and biological features of de novo acute myeloid leukemia with additional sex comb-like 1 (ASXL1) mutations. *Blood*, Vol. 116, No. 20, (November), pp. 4096-4094, ISSN 0006-4971

Chou, W.C.; Lei, W.C.; Ko, B.S.; Hou, H.A.; Chen, C.Y.; Tang, J.L.; Yao, M.; Tsay, W.; Wu, S.J.; Huang, S.Y.; Hsu, S.C.; Chen, Y.C.; Chang, Y.C.; Kuo, K.T.; Lee, F.Y.; Liu, M.C.; Liu, C.W.; Tseng, M.H.; Huang, C.F. & Tien, H.F. (2011) The prognostic impact and stability of Isocitrate dehydrogenase 2 mutation in adult patients with acute myeloid leukemia. *Leukemia*, Vol. 25, No. 2, (February), pp. 246-253, ISSN 0887-6924

Colombo, E.; Bonetti, P.; Lazzerini Denchi, E.; Martinelli, P.; Zamponi, R.; Marine, J.C.; Helin, K.; Falini, B. &. Pelicci, P.G. (2005) Nucleophosmin is required for DNA integrity and p19Arf protein stability. *Molecular and Cellular Biology*, Vol. 25, No. 20, (October), pp. 8874–8886, ISSN 0270- 7306

Colombo, E.; Marine, J.C.; Danovi, D.; Falini, B. & Pelicci, P.G. (2002) Nucleophosmin regulates the stability and transcriptional activity of p53. *Nature Cell Biology* Vol. 4, No. 7, (July), pp. 529 – 533, ISSN 1465-7392

D'Alo', F.; Johansen, L.M.; Nelson, E.A.; Radomska, H.S.; Evans, E.K.; Zhang, P.; Nerlov, C. & Tenen, D.G. (2003). The amino terminal and E2F interaction domains are critical for C/EBP alpha-mediated induction of granulopoietic development of hematopoietic cells. *Blood*, Vol. 102, No. 9, pp. 3163-3171, ISSN 0006-4971

Damm,F.; Heuser, M.; Morgan, M.; Yun, H.; Grosshennig, A.; Göhring, G.; Schlegelberger, B.; Döhner, K.; Ottmann, O.; Lübbert, M.; Heit, W.; Kanz, L.; Schlimok, G.; Raghavachar, A.; Fiedler, W.; Kirchner, H.; Döhner, H.; Heil, G.; Ganser, A. & Krauter, J. (2010a) Single nucleotide polymorphism in the mutational hotspot of WT1 predicts a favorable outcome in patients with cytogenetically normal acute myeloid leukemia. *Journal of Clinical Oncology*, Vol. 28, No. 4 (February), 578-585, ISSN 0732-183X

Damm F, Heuser M, Morgan M, Wagner K, Görlich K, Grosshennig A, Hamwi I, Thol F, Surdziel E, Fiedler W, Lübbert M, Kanz L, Reuter C, Heil G, Delwel R, Löwenberg B, Valk PJ, Krauter J, Ganser A. (2011a) Integrative prognostic risk score in acute myeloid leukemia with normal karyotype. *Blood*, Mar 3. [Epub ahead of print], ISSN 0006-4971

Damm, F.; Lange, K.; Heuser, M.; Oberacker, T.; Morgan, M.; Wagner, K.; Krauter, J.; Schlegelberger, B.; Ganser, A. & Göhring, G. (2010b) Phosphoinositide phospholipase Cbeta1 (PI-PLCbeta1) gene in myelodysplastic syndromes and cytogenetically normal acute myeloid leukemia: not a deletion, but increased PI-PLCbeta1 expression is an independent prognostic factor. *Journal of Clinical Oncology*, Vol. 28, No. 22 (August), e384-387, ISSN 0732-183X

Damm, F.; Oberacker, T.; Thol, F.; Surdziel, E.; Wagner, K.; Chaturvedi, A.; Morgan, M.; Bomm, K.; Göhring, G.; Lübbert, M.; Kanz, L.; Fiedler, W.; Schlegelberger, B.; Heil, G.; Schlenk, R.F.; Döhner, K.; Döhner, H.; Krauter, J.; Ganser, A. & Heuser, M. (2011b)Prognostic importance of histone methyltransferase MLL5 expression in acute myeloid leukemia. *Journal of Clinical Oncology*, Vol. 29, No. 6 (February), pp. 682-689, ISSN 0732-183X

Dang, L.; Jin, S. & Su, S.M. (2010) IDH mutations in glioma and acute myeloid leukemia. *Trends in Molecular Medicine*, Vol. 16, No. 9, (September), pp. 387-397, ISSN 1471-4914

De Braekeleer, M.; Morel, F.; Le Bris, M.J.; Herry, A. & Douet-Guilbert, N. (2005) The MLL gene and translocations involving chromosomal band 11q23 in acute leukemia. *Anticancer Research*, Vol. 25, No. 3B, (May-June), pp. 1931-1944, ISSN 0250-7005

De Jonge, H.J.M.; Valk, P.J.; Veeger, N.J.; ter Elst, A.; den Boer, M.L.; Cloos, J.; de Haas, V.; van den Heuvel-Eibrink, M.M.; Kaspers. G.J.; Zwaan, C.M.; Kamps, W.A.; Löwenberg, B. & de Bont, E.S. (2010) High VEGFC expression is associated with unique gene expression profiles and predicts adverse prognosis in pediatric and adult acute myeloid leukemia. *Blood*, Vol. 116, No. 10, pp. 1747-1754, ISSN 0006-4971

Del Poeta, G.; Ammatuna, E.; Lavorgna, S.; Capelli, G.; Zaza, S.; Luciano, F.; Ottone, T.; Del Principe, M.I.; Buccisano, F.; Maurillo, L.; Panetta, P.; de Fabritiis, P.; Stasi, R.; Venditti, A.; Amadori, S. & Lo Coco, F. (2010) The genotype nucleophosmin mutated and FLT3-ITD negative is characterized by high bax/bcl-2 ratio and favourable outcome in acute myeloid leukaemia. *British Journal of Haematology*, Vol. 149, No. 3, (May), pp. 383-387, ISSN 0007-1048

Damiani, D.; Tiribelli, M.; Michelutti, A.; Geromin, A.; Cavallin, M.; Fabbro, D.; Pianta, A.;Malagola, M.; Damante, G.; Russo, D. & Fanin, R. (2010) Fludarabine-based induction therapy does not overcome the negative effect of ABCG2 (BCRP) over-expression in adult acute myeloid leukemia patients. *Leukemia Research*, Vol. 34, No. 7, (July), pp. 942-945,ISSN 0145-2126

Döhner, K. & Döhner, H. (2008) Molecular characterization of acute myeloid leukemia. *Haematologica*, Vol. 93, No. 7, (July), pp. 976-982, ISSN 0390-6078

Döhner, H.; Estey, E.H.; Amadori, S.; Appelbaum, F.R.; Büchner, T.; Burnett, A.K.; Dombret, H.; Fenaux, P.; Grimwade, D.; Larson, R.A., Lo-Coco, F.; Naoe, T.; Niederwieser, D.; Ossenkoppele, G.J.; Sanz, M.A.; Sierra, J.; Tallman, M.S.; Löwenberg, B.; Bloomfield, C.D. & European LeukemiaNet (2010) Diagnosis and management of acute myeloid leukemia in adults: recommendations from an international expert panel, on behalf of the European LeukemiaNet. *Blood*, Vol. 115, No. 3, (January), pp. 453-474, , ISSN 0006-4971

Döhner, K.; Tobis, K.; Ulrich, R.; Fröhling, S.; Benner, A.; Schlenk, R.F. & Döhner, H. (2002) Prognostic significance of partial tandem duplications of the MLL gene in adult patients 16 to 60 years old with acute myeloid leukemia and normal cytogenetics: a study of the Acute Myeloid Leukemia Study Group Ulm. *Journal of Clinical Oncology*, Vol. 20, No. 15, (August), pp. 3254-3261, ISSN 0732-183X

Dorrance, A.M.; Liu, S.; Yuan, W.; Becknell, B.; Arnoczky, K.J.; Guimond, M.; Strout, M.P.; Feng, L.; Nakamura, T.;Yu, L.; Rush, L.J.; Weinstein, M.; Leone, G.; Wu, L.; Ferketich, A.; Whitman, S.P.; Marcucci, G. & Caligiuri, M.A. (2006) Mll partial tandem duplication induces aberrant Hox expression in vivo via specific epigenetic alterations. *Journal of Clinical Investigation*, Vol. 116, No. 10, (October), pp. 2707-2716, ISSN 0021-9738

Dvorakova, D.; Racil, Z.; Jeziskova, I.; Palasek, I.; Protivankova, M.; Lengerova, M.; Razga, F. & Mayer, J. (2010) Monitoring of minimal residual disease in acute myeloid leukemia with frequent and rare patient-specific NPM1 mutations. *American Journal of Hematology*,Vol. 85, No. 12, (December), pp. 926-929, ISSN 0361-8609

Dufour, A.; Schneider, F.; Metzeler, K.H.; Hoster, E.; Schneider, S.; Zellmeier, E.; Benthaus, T.; Sauerland, M.C.; Berdel, W.E.; Büchner, T.; Wörmann, B.; Braess, J.; Hiddemann, W.; Bohlander, S.K. & Spiekermann, K. (2010) Acute myeloid leukemia with biallelic CEBPA gene mutations and normal karyotype represents a distinct genetic entity associated with a favorable clinical outcome. *Journal of Clinical Oncology*, Vol. 28, No. 4, (February), pp. 570-577, ISSN 0732-183X

Enomoto, T.; Lindström, M.S.; Jin, A.; Ke, H. & Zhang, Y. (2006) Essential role of the B23/NPM core domain in regulatingARF binding and B23 stability. *Journal of Biological Chemistry*, Vol. 281, No. 27, (May), pp. 18463–18472, ISSN 0021-9258

Epping, M.T.; Wang, L.; Edel, M.J.; Carlée, L.; Hernandez, M. & Bernards, R. (2005) The human tumor antigen PRAME is a dominant repressor of retinoic acid receptor signaling. *Cell*, Vol. 122, No. 6, (September), pp. 835-847, ISSN 0092-8674

Falini, B. (2010b) Acute myeloid leukemia with mutated nucleophosmin (NPM1): molecular,pathological, and clinical features. *Cancer Treatment and Research*, Vol. 145, pp. 149-168, ISSN 0927-3042

Falini, B.; Bolli, N.; Liso, A.; Martelli, M.P.; Mannucci, R.; Pileri, S. & Nicoletti, I. (2009) Altered nucleophosmin transport in acute myeloid leukaemia with mutated NPM1: molecular basis and clinical implications. *Leukemia*, Vol. 23, No.10, (October),pp. 1731-1743, ISSN 0887-6924

Falini, B.; Bolli, N.; Shan, J.; Martelli, M.P.; Liso, A.; Pucciarini, A.; Bigerna, B.; Pasqualucci, L.; Mannucci, R.; Rosati, R.; Gorello, P.; Diverio, D.; Roti, G.; Tiacci, E.; Cazzaniga, G.; Biondi, A.; Schnittger, S.; Haferlach, T.; Hiddemann, W.; Martelli, M.F.; Gu, W.; Mecucci, C. & Nicoletti, I. (2006b) Both carboxy-terminus NES motif and mutated tryptophan(s) are crucial for aberrant nuclear export of nucleophosmin leukemic mutants in NPMc+ AML. *Blood*, Vol. 107, No. 11, (June), pp. 4514-4523, ISSN 0006-4971

Falini, B.; Mecucci, C.; Tiacci, E.; Alcalay, M.; Rosati, R.; Pasqualucci, L.; La Starza, R.; Diverio, D.; Colombo, E.; Santucci, A.; Bigerna, B.; Pacini, R.; Pucciarini, A.; Liso, A.; Vignetti, M.; Fazi, P.; Meani, N.; Pettirossi, V.; Saglio, G.; Mandelli, F.; Lo-Coco, F.; Pelicci, P.G.; Martelli, M.F. & GIMEMA Acute Leukemia Working Party. (2005) Cytoplasmic nucleophosmin in acute myelogenous leukemia with a normal karyotype. *The New England Journal of Medicine*, Vol. 352, No. 3, (January), pp. 254–266, ISSN 0028-4793

Falini, B.; Martelli, M.P.; Bolli, N.;, Bonasso, R.; Ghia, E.; Pallotta, M.T.; Diverio, D.; Nicoletti, I.; Pacini, R.; Tabarrini, A.; Galletti, B.V.; Mannucci, R.; Roti, G.; Rosati, R.; Specchia, G.; Liso, A.; Tiacci, E.; Alcalay, M.; Luzi, L.; Volorio, S.; Bernard, L.; Guarini, A.; Amadori, S.; Mandelli, F.; Pane, F.; Lo-Coco, F.; Saglio, G.; Pelicci, P.G.; Martelli, M.F. & Mecucci, C. (2006) Immunohistochemistry predicts nucleophosmin (NPM) mutations in acute myeloid leukemia. *Blood*, Vol. 108, No. 6, (September), pp. 1999-2005, ISSN 0006-4971

Falini, B.; Martelli, M.P.; Bolli, N.; Sportoletti, P.; Liso, A.; Tiacci, E. & Haferlach, T. (2011) Acute myeloid leukemia with mutated nucleophosmin (NPM1): is it a distinct entity? *Blood*, Vol. 117, No. 4, (January), pp. 1109-1120, ISSN 0006-4971

Falini, B.; Martelli, M.P.; Pileri, S.A. & Mecucci, C. (2010a) Molecular and alternative methods for diagnosis of acute myeloid leukemia with mutated NPM1: flexibility may help. *Haematologica*, Vol. 95, No. 4, (April), pp. 529-534, ISSN 0390-6078

Figueroa, M.E.; Abdel-Wahab, O.; Lu, C.; Ward, P.S.; Patel, J.; Shih, A.; Li, Y.; Bhagwat, N.; Vasanthakumar, A.; Fernandez, H.F.; Tallman, M.S.; Sun, Z.; Wolniak, K.; Peeters, J.K.; Liu, W.; Choe, S.E.; Fantin, V.R.; Paietta, E.; Löwenberg, B.; Licht, J.D.; Godley, L.A.; Delwel, R.; Valk, P.J.; Thompson, C.B.; Levine, R.L. & Melnick, A. (2010) Leukemic IDH1 and IDH2 mutations result in a hypermethylation phenotype, disrupt TET2 function, and impair hematopoietic differentiation. *Cancer Cell*, Vol. 18, No. 6, (December), pp. 553-567, ISSN 1535-6108

Figueroa, M.E.; Lugthart, S.; Li, Y.; Erpelinck-Verschueren, C.; Deng, X.; Christos, P.J.; Schifano, E.; Booth, J.; van Putten, W.; Skrabanek, L.; Campagne, F.; Mazumdar, M.; Greally, J.M.; Valk, P.J.; Löwenberg, B.; Delwel, R. & Melnick, A. (2010) DNA methylation signatures identify biologically distinct subtypes in acute myeloid leukemia. *Cancer Cell*, Vol. 17, No. 1, (January), pp. 13-17, ISSN 1535-6108

Flodby, P.; Barlow, C.; Kylefjord, H.; Ahrlund-Richter, L. & Xanthopoulos, K.G. (1996) Increased hepatic cell proliferation and lung abnormalities in mice deficient in CCAAT/enhancer binding protein alpha. *Journal of Biological Chemistry*, Vol. 271, No. 40, (October), pp. 24753-24760, ISSN 0021-9258

Frayling, I.M. (2002) Methods of molecular analysis: mutation detection in solid tumours. *Molecular Pathology*, Vol. 55, No. 2, (April), ISSN 1366-8714

Frehlick, L.J.; Eirín-López, J.M. & Ausió, J. (2007). New insights into the nucleophosmin/ nucleoplasmin family of nuclear chaperones. *BioEssays*, Vol. 29, No.1, (January), pp. 49-59, ISSN 1521-1878

Friedman, A.D. (2007) C/EBPalpha induces PU.1 and interacts with AP-1 and NF-kappaB to regulate myeloid development. *Blood Cells, Moecules and Diseases*, Vol. 39, No. 3, (November-December), pp. 340-343, ISSN 1079-9796

Fröhling, S.; Schlenk, R.F.; Breitruck, J.; Benner, A.; Kreitmeier, S.; Tobis, K.; Döhner, H. & Döhner, K. (2002) AML Study Group Ulm. Acute myeloid leukemia. Prognostic significance of activating FLT3 mutations in younger adults (16 to 60 years) with acute myeloid leukemia and normal cytogenetics: a study of the AML Study Group Ulm. *Blood*, Vol. 100, No. 13, (December), pp. 4372-4380, ISSN 0006-4971

Fröhling, S.; Schlenk, R.F.; Stolze, I.; Bihlmayr, J.; Benner, A.; Kreitmeier, S.; Tobis, K.; Döhner, H. & Döhner, K. (2004) CEBPA mutations in younger adults with acute myeloid leukemia and normal cytogenetics: prognostic relevance and analysis of cooperating mutations. *Journal of Clinical Oncology*, Vol. 22, No. 4, (February), pp. 624-633, ISSN 0732-183X

Fuchs, O. (2007) Growth-inhibiting activity of transcription factor C/EBPalpha, its role in haematopoiesis and its tumour suppressor or oncogenic properties in leukaemias. *Folia Biologica* (Praha), Vol. 53, No. 3, pp. 97-108, ISSN 0015-5500

Fuchs, O.; Provaznikova, D.; Kocova, M.; Kostecka, A.; Cvekova, P.; Neuwirtova, R.; Kobylka, P.; Cermak, J.; Brezinova, J.; Schwarz, J.; Markova, J.; Salaj, P.; Klamova, H.; Maaloufova, J.; Lemez, P.; Novakova, L. & Benesova, K. (2008) CEBPA polymorphisms and mutations in patients with acute myeloid leukemia, myelodysplastic syndrome, multiple myeloma and non-Hodgkin's lymphoma. *Blood Cells, Moecules and Diseases*, Vol. 40, No. 3, (May-June), pp. 401-405, ISSN1079-9796

Fuchs, O.; Kostecka, A.; Provaznikova, D.; Krasna, B.; Brezinova, J.; Filkukova, J.; Kotlin, R.; Kouba, M.; Kobylka, P.; Neuwirtova, R.; Jonasova, A.; Caniga, M.; Schwarz, J.; Markova, J.; Maaloufova, J.; Sponerova, D.; Novakova, L. & Cermak, J. (2009) Nature of frequent deletions in CEBPA. *Blood Cells, Molecules and Diseases*, Vol. 43, No. 3 (November-December), pp. 260-263, ISSN1079-9796

Gaidzik, V. & Döhner , K. (2008) Prognostic implications of gene mutations in acute myeloid leukemia with normal cytogenetics. *Seminars in Oncology*, Vol. 35, No. 4, (August), pp. 346-355, ISSN 0093-7754

Gaidzik, V.I.; Schlenk, R.F.; Moschny, S.; Becker, A.; Bullinger, L.; Corbacioglu, A.; Krauter, J.;Schlegelberger, B.; Ganser, A.; Döhner, H.; Döhner, K. & German-Austrian AML Study Group. Prognostic impact of WT1 mutations in cytogenetically normal acute myeloid leukemia: a study of the German-Austrian AML Study Group. *Blood*, Vol. 113, No. 19, (May), pp. 4505-11, ISSN 0006-4971

Gale, R.E.; Green, C.; Allen, C.; Mead, A.J.; Burnett, A.K.; Hills, R.K.; Linch, D.C. & Medical Research Council Adult Leukaemia Working Party (2008) The impact of FLT3 internal tandem duplication mutant level, number, size, and interaction with NPM1 mutations in a large cohort of young adult patients with acute myeloid leukemia. *Blood*, Vol. 111, No. 5,(March), pp. 2776-2784, ISSN 0006-4971

Garzon, R.; Garofalo, M.; Martelli, M.P.; Briesewitz, R.; Wang, L.; Fernandez-Cymering, C.; Volinia, S.; Liu, C.G.; Schnittger, S.; Haferlach, T.; Liso, A.; Diverio, D.; Mancini, M.; Meloni, G.; Foa, R.; Martelli, M.F.; Mecucci, C.; Croce, C.M. & Falini, B. (2008) Distinctive microRNA signature of acute myeloid leukemia bearing cytoplasmic mutated nucleophosmin. *The Proceedings of the National Academy of Sciences of the USA*, Vol. 105, No. 10, pp. 3945-3950, ISSN 0027-8424

Geisbrecht, B.V., Gould, S.J.(1999) The human PICD gene encodes a cytoplasmic and peroxisomal NADP(+)-dependent isocitrate dehydrogenase. *Journal of Biological Chemistry*, Vol. 274, No. 43, (October), pp. 30527-30533, ISSN 0021-9258

Gianfaldoni, G.; Mannelli, F.; Ponziani, V.; Longo, G.; Bencini, S.; Bosi, A. & Vannucchi, A.M. (2010) Early reduction of WT1 transcripts during induction chemotherapy predicts for longer disease free and overall survival in acute myeloid leukemia. *Haematologica*, Vol. 95, No. 5, (May), pp. 833-836, ISSN 0390-6078

Gilliland, D.G. & Griffin, J.D. (2002) The roles of FLT3 in hematopoiesis and leukemia. *Blood*, Vol. 100, No. 5, (September), pp. 1532-1542, ISSN: 0006-4971

Golub,T.; Slonim, D.K.; Tamayo, P.; Huard, C., Gaasenbeek M, Mesirov JP, Coller H, Loh ML, Downing JR, Caligiuri MA, Bloomfield CD, Lander ES. (1999) Molecular classification of cancer: class discovery and class prediction by gene expression monitoring. *Science*, Vol. 286, No. 5439, (October), pp.531-537, ISSN 0036-8075

Gombart, A.F.; Hofmann, W.K.; Kawano, S.; Takeuchi, S.; Krug, U.; Kwok, S.H.; Larsen, R.J.; Asou, H.; Miller, C.W.; Hoelzer, D. & Koeffler, H.P. (2002) Mutations in the gene encoding the transcription factor CCAAT/enhancer binding protein alpha in myelodysplastic syndromes and acute myeloid leukemias. *Blood*, Vol. 99, No. 4, (February), pp. 1332-1340, ISSN 0006-4971

Green, C.L.; Evans, C.M.; Hills, R.K.; Burnett, A.K.; Linch, D.C. & Gale, R.E. (2010) The prognostic significance of IDH1 mutations in younger adult patients with acute myeloid leukemia is dependent on FLT3/ITD status. *Blood*, Vol. 116, Vol. 15, (October), pp. 2779-2782, ISSN 0006-4971

Greif, P.A.; Eck, S.H.; Konstandin, N.P.; Benet-Pagès, A.; Ksienzyk, B.; Dufour, A.; Vetter, A.T.; Popp, H.D.; Lorenz-Depiereux, B.; Meitinger, T.; Bohlander, S.K. & Strom, T.M. (2011) Identification of recurring tumor-specific somatic mutations in acute myeloid leukemia by transcriptome sequencing. *Leukemia*, Feb 22. [Epub ahead of print], ISSN 0887-6924

Greiner, J.; Bullinger, L.; Guinn, B.A.; Döhner, H. & Schmitt, M. (2008) Leukemia-associated antigens are critical for the proliferation of acute myeloid leukemia cells. *Clinical Cancer Research*, Vol. 14, No. 22, (November), pp. 7161-7166, ISSN 1078-0432

Grisendi, S.; Mecucci, C.; Falini, B. &. Pandolfi, P.P. (2006) Nucleophosmin and cancer. *Nature Reviews Cancer*, Vol. 6, No. 7, (July), pp. 493–505, ISSN 1474-175X

Gröschel, S.; Lugthart, S.; Schlenk, R.F.; Valk, P.J.; Eiwen, K.; Goudswaard, C.; van Putten, W.J.; Kayser, S.; Verdonck, L.F.; Lübbert, M.; Ossenkoppele, G.J.; Germing, U.; Schmidt-Wolf, I.; Schlegelberger, B.; Krauter, J.; Ganser, A.; Döhner, H.; Löwenberg, B.; Döhner, K. & Delwel, R. (2010) High EVI1 expression predicts outcome in younger adult patients with acute myeloid leukemia and is associated with distinct cytogenetic abnormalities. *Journal of Clinical Oncology*, Vol. 28, No. 12, (April), pp. 2107-2107, ISSN 0732-183X

Gross, S.; Cairns, R.A.; Minden, M.D.; Driggers, E.M.; Bittinger, M.A.; Jang, H.G.; Sasaki, M.; Jin, S.; Schenkein, D.P.; Su, S.M.; Dang, L.; Fantin, V.R. & Mak, T.W. (2010) Cancer-associated metabolite 2-hydroxyglutarate accumulates in acute myelogenous leukemia with isocitrate dehydrogenase 1 and 2 mutations. *Journal of Experimental Medicine*, Vol. 207, No. 2, (February), pp. 339-344, ISSN 0022-1007

Grosveld, G.C. (2007) MN1, a novel player in human AML. *Blood Cells Molecules and Diseases*, Vol. 39, No. 3, November- December), pp. 336-339, ISSN 1079-9796

Gu, Y.; Jasti, A.C.; Jansen, M. & Siefring, J.E. RhoH, a hematopoietic-specific Rho GTPase, regulates proliferation, survival, migration, and engraftment of hematopoietic progenitor cells. *Blood*, Vol. 105, Vol. 4, (February), pp. 1467-1475, ISSN 0006-4971

Gündogdu, M.S.; Liu, H.; Metzdorf, D.; Hildebrand, D.; Aigner, M.; Aktories, K.; Heeg, K. & Kubatzky, K.F. (2010) The haematopoietic GTPase RhoH modulates IL3 signalling through regulation of STAT activity and IL3 receptor expression. *Molecular Cancer*, Vol. 25, No. 9, (August), p. 225, ISSN 1476-4598

Haber, D.A.; Buckler, A.J.; Glaser, T.; Call, K.M.; Pelletier, J.; Sohn, R.L.; Douglass, E.C. & Housman, D.E. (1990) An internal deletion within an 11p13 zinc finger gene contributes to the development of Wilms' tumor. *Cell*, Vol. 61, No. 7, (June), pp. 1257-1269, ISSN 0092-8674

Hackanson, B.; Bennett, K.L.; Brena, R.M.; Jiang, J.; Claus, R.; Chen, S.S.; Blagitko-Dorfs, N.; Maharry, K.; Whitman, S.P.; Schmittgen, T.D.; Lübbert, M.; Marcucci, G.; Bloomfield, C.D. & Plass, C. (2008) Epigenetic modification of CCAAT/enhancer binding protein alpha expression in acute myeloid leukemia. *Cancer Research*, Vol. 68, No. 9, (May), pp. 3142-3151, ISSN 0008-5472

Harada, Y. & Harada, H. (2009) Molecular pathways mediating MDS/AML with focus on AML1/RUNX1 point mutations. *Journal of Cellular Physiology*, Vol. 220, No. 1, (July), pp. 16-20, ISSN 0021-9541

Heesch. S.; Schlee, C.; Neumann, M.; Stroux, A.; Kühnl, A.; Schwartz, S.; Haferlach, T.; Goekbuget, N.; Hoelzer, D.;, Thiel, E.; Hofmann, W.K. & Baldus, C.D. (2010) BAALC-associated gene expression profiles define IGFBP7 as a novel molecular marker in acute leukemia. *Leukemia*, Vol. 24, No. 8, (August), pp. 1429-1436, ISSN 0887-6924

Herrera, J. E.; Savkur, R. & Olson, M. O. (1995) The ribonuclease activity of nucleolar protein B23. *Nucleic Acids Research*, Vol. 23, No. 19, (October), pp. 3974–3979, ISSN 0305-1048

Heuser, M.; Argiropoulos, B.; Kuchenbauer, F.; Yung, E.; Piper, J.; Fung, S.; Schlenk, R.F.; Dohner, K.; Hinrichsen, T.; Rudolph, C.; Schambach, A.; Baum, C.; Schlegelberger, B.; Dohner, H.; Ganser, A. & Humphries, R.K. (2007) MN1 overexpression induces acute myeloid leukemia in mice and predicts ATRA resistance in patients with AML. *Blood*, Vol. 110, No. 5, (September), pp. 1639-1647, ISSN 0006-4971

Heuser, M.; Beutel, G.; Krauter, J.; Döhner, K.; von Neuhoff, N.; Schlegelberger, B. & Ganser, A. (2006) High meningioma 1 (MN1) expression as a predictor for poor outcome in acute myeloid leukemia with normal cytogenetics. *Blood*, Vol. 108, No. 12, (December), pp. 3898-3905, ISSN 0006-4971

Hisaoka, M.; Ueshima, S.; Murano, K.; Nagata, K. & Okuwaki, M. (2010) Regulation of nucleolar chromatin by B23/nucleophosmin jointly depends upon its RNA binding activity and transcription factor UBF. *Molecular and Cellular Biology*, Vol. 30, No. 20, (October), pp. 4952-4964, ISSN 0270- 7306

Hou, H.A.; Chou, W.C.; Lin, L.I.; Tang, J.L.; Tseng, M.H.; Huang, C.F.; Yao, M.; Chen, C.Y.; Tsay, W. & Tien, H.F. (2008) Expression of angiopoietins and vascular endothelial growth factors and their clinical significance in acute myeloid leukemia. *Leukemia Research*, Vol. 32, No. 6, (June), pp. 904-912, ISSN0145-2126

Hou, H.A.; Huang, T.C.; Lin, L.I.; Liu, C.Y.; Chen, C.Y.; Chou, W.C.; Tang, J.L.; Tseng, M.H.; Huang, C.F.; Chiang, Y.C.; Lee, F.Y.; Liu, M.C.; Yao, M.; Huang, S.Y.; Ko, B.S.; Hsu, S.C.; Wu, S.J.; Tsay, W.; Chen, Y.C. & Tien, H.F. (2010) WT1 mutation in 470 adult patients with acute myeloid leukemia: stability during disease evolution and implication of its incorporation into a survival scoring system. *Blood*, Vol. 115, No. 25, (June), pp. 5222-5231, ISSN 0006-4971

Hou, H.A.; Lin, L.I.; Chen, C.Y. & Tien, H.F. (2009) Reply to 'Heterogeneity within AML with CEBPA mutations; only CEBPA double mutations, but not single CEBPA mutations are associated with favorable prognosis'. *British Journal of Cancer*, Vol. 101, No. 4, (August), pp. 738-740, ISSN 0007-0920

Huh, H.J.; Park, C.J.; Jang, S.; Seo, E.J.; Chi, H.S.; Lee, J.H.; Lee, K.H.; Seo, J.J.; Moon, H.N. & Ghim T. (2006) Prognostic significance of multidrug resistance gene 1 (MDR1), multidrug resistance-related protein (MRP) and lung resistance protein (LRP) mRNA expression in acute leukemia. *Journal of Korean Medical Science*, Vol. 21, No. 2, (April), pp. 253-258, ISSN 1011-8934

Iwasaki, T.; Katsumi, A.; Kiyoi, H.; Tanizaki, R.; Ishikawa, Y.; Ozeki, K.; Kobayashi, M.; Abe, A.; Matsushita, T.; Watanabe, T.; Amano, M.; Kojima, T.; Kaibuchi, K. & Naoe, T. (2008) Prognostic implication and biological roles of RhoH in acute myeloid leukaemia. *European Journal of Haematology*, Vol. 81, No. 6, (December), pp. 454-460, ISSN 0902-4441

Jaeger, U. & Kainz. B. (2003) Monitoring minimal residual disease in AML: the right time for real time. *Annals of Hematology*, Vol. 82, No. 3, (March), pp.139-147, ISSN 0939-5555

Juliusson, G.; Antunovic, P.; Derolf, A.; Lehmann, S.; Möllgård, L.; Stockelberg, D.; Tidefelt, U.; Wahlin, A. & Höglund, M. (2009) Age and acute myeloid leukemia: real world data on decision to treat and outcomes from the Swedish Acute Leukemia Registry. *Blood*, Vol. 113, No. 18, (April), pp. 4179-4187, ISSN 0006-4971

Kato, N.; Kitaura, J.; Doki, N.; Komeno, Y.; Watanabe-Okochi, N.; Togami, K.; Nakahara, F.; Oki, T.; Enomoto, Y.; Fukuchi, Y.; Nakajima, H.; Harada, Y.; Harada, H. & Kitamura, T. (2011) Two types of C/EBPα mutations play distinct but collaborative roles in leukemogenesis: lessons from clinical data and BMT models. *Blood*, Vol. 117, No. 1, (January), pp. 221-233, ISSN 0006-4971

Keeshan, K.; Santilli, G.; Corradini, F.; Perrotti, D. & Calabretta, B. (2003) Transcription activation functionof C/EBPα is required for induction of granulocyte differentiation. *Blood*, Vol. 102, No. 4, (August), pp. 1267-1275, ISSN 0006-4971

Kern, W.; Schoch, C.; Haferlach, T. & Schnittger, S. (2005) Monitoring of minimal residual disease in acute myeloid leukemia. *Critical Reviews in Oncology / Hematology*, Vol. 56, No. 2, (November), pp. 283-309, ISSN 1040-8428

Kindler, T.; Lipka, D.B. & Fischer, T. (2010) FLT3 as a therapeutic target in AML: still challenging after all these years. *Blood*, Vol. 116, No. 24, (December), pp. 5089-5102, ISSN 0006-4971

King-Underwood, L.; Renshaw, J. & Pritchard-Jones, K. (1996) Mutations in the Wilms' tumor gene WT1 in leukemias. *Blood*, Vol. 87, No. 6, (March), pp. 2171-2179, ISSN 0006-4971

Kohlmann, A.; Bullinger, L.; Thiede, C.; Schaich, M.; Schnittger, S.; Döhner, K.; Dugas, M.; Klein, H.U.; Döhner, H.; Ehninger, G. & Haferlach, T. (2010) Gene expression profiling in AML with normal karyotype can predict mutations for molecular markers and allows novel insights into perturbed biological pathways. *Leukemia*, Vol. 24, No. 6, (June), pp. 1216-1220, ISSN 0887-6924

Koike, A.; Nishikawa, H.;, Wu, W.; Okada, Y.; Venkitaraman, A.R. & Ohta, T. (2010) Recruitment of phosphorylated NPM1 to sites of DNA damage through RNF8-dependent ubiquitin conjugates. *Cancer Research*, Vol. 70, No. 17 (September), pp. 6746-6756, ISSN 0008-5472

Konoplev, S.; Rassidakis, G.Z.; Estey, E.; Kantarjian, H.; Liakou, C.I.; Huang, X.;, Xiao, L.; Andreeff, M.; Konopleva, M. & Medeiros, L.J. (2007) Overexpression of CXCR4 predicts adverse overall and event-free survival in patients with unmutated FLT3 acute myeloid leukemia with normal karyotype. *Cancer*, Vol. 109, No. 6, (March), pp. 1152-1156, ISSN 1097-0142

Kornblau, S.M., Singh, N.; Qiu, Y.; Chen, W.; Zhang, N. & Coombes, K.R. (2010) Highly phosphorylated FOXO3A is an adverse prognostic factor in acute myeloid leukemia. *Clinical Cancer Research*, Vol.16, No. 6, (March), pp. 1865-1874, ISSN 1078-0432

Kosaki, K.; Udaka, T. & Okuyama, T. (2005) DHPLC in clinical molecular diagnostic services. *Molecular Genetics and Metabolism*, Vol. 86, No. 1-2, (September-October), pp. 117-123, ISSN 1096-7192

Kutach, L.S., Bolshakov, S., Ananthaswamy, H.N. (1999) Detection of mutations and polymorphisms in the p53 tumor suppressor gene by single-strand conformation polymorphism analysis. *Electrophoresis*, Vol. 20, No. 6, (June), pp. 1204-1210, ISSN 0173-0835

Lange, T.; Hubmann, M.; Burkhardt, R.; Franke, G.N.; Cross, M.; Scholz, M.; Leiblein, S.; Al-Ali, H.K.; Edelmann, J.; Thiery, J. & Niederwieser, D. (2011) Monitoring of WT1 expression in PB and CD34(+) donor chimerism of BM predicts early relapse in AML and MDS patients after hematopoietic cell transplantation with reduced-intensity conditioning. *Leukemia*, Vol. 25, No. 3, (March), pp. 498-505, ISSN 0887-6924

Langer, C.; Marcucci, G.; Holland, K.B.; Radmacher, M.D.; Maharry, K.; Paschka, P.; Whitman, S.P.; Mrózek, K.; Baldus, C.D.; Vij, R.; Powell, B.L.; Carroll, A.J.; Kolitz, J.E.; Caligiuri, M.A.; Larson, R.A. & Bloomfield, C.D. (2009) Prognostic importance of MN1 transcript levels, and biologic insights from MN1-associated gene and microRNA expression signatures in cytogenetically normal acute myeloid leukemia: a cancer and leukemia group B study. *Journal of Clinical Oncology*, Vol. 27, No. 19, (July), pp. 3198-3204, ISSN 0732-183X

Langer, C.; Radmacher, M.D.; Ruppert, A.S.; Whitman, S.P.; Paschka, P.; Mrózek, K.; Baldus, C.D.; Vukosavljevic, T.; Liu, C.G.; Ross, M.E.; Powell, B.L.; de la Chapelle, A.; Kolitz, J.E.; Larson, R.A.; Marcucci, G. & Bloomfield, C.D. Cancer and Leukemia Group B (CALGB) (2008) High BAALC expression associates with other molecular prognostic markers, poor outcome, and a distinct gene-expression signature in cytogenetically normal patients younger than 60 years with acute myeloid leukemia: a Cancer and Leukemia Group B (CALGB) study. *Blood*, Vol. 111, No. 11, (June), pp. 5371-5379, ISSN 0006-4971

Lee, C.Y.; Tien, H.F.; Hu, C.Y.; Chou, W.C. & Lin, L.I. (2007) Marrow angiogenesis-associated factors as prognostic biomarkers in patients with acute myelogenous leukaemia. *British Journal of Cancer*, Vol. 97, No. 7, (October), pp. 877-882, ISSN

Leith, C.P.; Kopecky, K.J.; Chen, I.M.; Eijdems, L.; Slovak, M.L.; McConnell, T.S.; Head, D.R.; Weick, J.; Grever, M.R.; Appelbaum, F.R. & Willman, C.L. (1999) Frequency and clinical significance of the expression of the multidrug resistance proteins MDR1/P-glycoprotein, MRP1, and LRP in acute myeloid leukemia: a Southwest Oncology Group Study. *Blood*, Vol. 94, No. 3, (August), pp. 1086-1099, ISSN 0006-4971

Leong, S.M.; Tan, B.X.; Bte Ahmad, B.; Yan, T.; Chee, L.Y.; Ang, S.T.; Tay, K.G.; Koh, L.P.; Yeoh, A.E.; Koay, E.S.; Mok, Y.K. & Lim, T.M. (2010) Mutant nucleophosmin deregulates cell death and myeloid differentiation through excessive caspase-6 and -8 inhibition. *Blood*, Vol. 116, No. 17, (October), pp. 3286-3296, ISSN 0006-4971

Ley, T.J.; Ding, L.; Walter, M.J.; McLellan, M.D.; Lamprecht, T.; Larson, D.E.; Kandoth, C.; Payton, J.E.; Baty, J.; Welch, J.; Harris, C.C.; Lichti, C.F.; Townsend, R.R.; Fulton, R.S.; Dooling, D.J.; Koboldt, D.C.; Schmidt, H.; Zhang, Q.; Osborne, J.R.; Lin, L.; O'Laughlin, M.; McMichael, J.F.; Delehaunty, K.D.; McGrath, S.D.; Fulton, L.A.; Magrini, V.J.; Vickery, T.L.; Hundal, J.; Cook, L.L.; Conyers, J.J.; Swift, G.W.; Reed, J.P.; Alldredge, P.A.; Wylie, T.; Walker, J.; Kalicki, J.; Watson, M.A.; Heath, S.; Shannon, W.D.; Varghese, N.; Nagarajan, R.; Westervelt, P.; Tomasson, M.H.; Link, D.C.; Graubert, T.A.; DiPersio, J.F.; Mardis, E.R. & Wilson, R.K. (2010) DNMT3A mutations in acute myeloid leukemia. *The New England Journal of Medicine*, Vol. 363, No. 25, (December), pp. 2424-2433, ISNN 0028-4793

Ley, T.J.; Mardis, E.R.; Ding, L.; Fulton, B.; McLellan, M.D.; Chen, K.; Dooling, D.; Dunford-Shore, B.H.; McGrath, S.; Hickenbotham, M.; Cook, L.; Abbott, R.; Larson, D.E.; Koboldt, D.C.; Pohl, C.; Smith, S.; Hawkins, A.; Abbott, S.; Locke, D.; Hillier, L.W.; Miner, T.; Fulton, L.; Magrini, V.; Wylie, T.; Glasscock, J.; Conyers, J.; Sander, N.; Shi, X.; Osborne, J.R.; Minx, P.; Gordon, D.; Chinwalla, A.; Zhao, Y.; Ries, R.E.; Payton, J.E.; Westervelt, P.; Tomasson M.H.; Watson, M.; Baty, J.; Ivanovich, J.; Heath, S.; Shannon, W.D.; Nagarajan, R.; Walter, M.J.; Link, D.C.; Graubert, T.A.; DiPersio, J.F. & Wilson, R.K. (2008) DNA sequencing of a cytogenetically normal acute myeloid leukaemia genome. *Nature*, Vol. 456, No. 7218, (November), pp. 66-72, ISSN 0028-0836

Ley, T.J.; Minx, P.J.; Walter, M.J.; Ries, R.E.; Sun, H.; McLellan, M.; DiPersio, J.F.; Link, D.C.; Tomasson, M.H.; Graubert, T.A.; McLeod, H.; Khoury, H.; Watson, M.; Shannon, W.; Trinkaus, K.; Heath, S.; Vardiman, J.W.; Caligiuri, M.A.; Bloomfield, C.D.; Milbrandt, J.D.; Mardis, E.R. & Wilson, R.K. (2003) A pilot study of high-throughput, sequence-based mutational profiling of primary human acute myeloid leukemia cell genomes. *The Proceedings of the National Academy of Sciences of the USA*, Vol. 100, No. 24, (November), pp. 14275-14280, ISSN 0027-8424

Li, Z.; Hann, S.R. (2009) The Myc-nucleophosmin-ARF network: a complex web unveiled. *Cell Cycle*, Vol. 8, No.17, (September), pp. 2703-2707, ISSN 1551-4005

Lin, L.I.; Chen, C.Y.; Lin, D.T.; Tsay, W.; Tang, J.L.; Yeh, Y.C.; Shen, H.L.; Su, F.H.; Yao, M.; Huang, S.Y. & Tien, H.F. (2005). Characterization of CEBPA mutations in acute myeloid leukemia: most patients with CEBPA mutations have biallelic mutations and show a distinct immunophenotype of the leukemic cells. *Clinical Cancer Research*, Vol. 11, No. 4, (February), pp. 1372-1379, ISSN 1078-0432

Lin, T.C.; Hou, H.A.; Chou, W.C.; Ou, D.L.; Yu, S.L.; Tien, H.F. & Lin, L.I. (2011) CEBPA methylation as a prognostic biomarker in patients with de novo acute myeloid leukemia. *Leukemia*, Vol. 25, No. 1, (January), pp. 32-40, ISSN 0887-6924

Liso, A.; Bogliolo, A.; Freschi, V.;, Martelli, M.P.;, Pileri, S.A.; Santodirocco, M.; Bolli, N.; Martelli, M.F. & Falini, B. (2008) In human genome, generation of a nuclear export signal through duplication appears unique to nucleophosmin (NPM1) mutations and is restricted to AML. *Leukemia*, Vol. 22, No. 6, (June), pp. 1285-1289, ISSN 0887-6924

Loges, S.; Heil, G.; Bruweleit, M.; Schoder, V.; Butzal, M.; Fischer, U.; Gehling, U.M.; Schuch, G.; Hossfeld, D.K. & Fiedler, W. (2005) Analysis of concerted expression of angiogenic growth factors in acute myeloid leukemia: expression of angiopoietin-2 represents an independent prognostic factor for overall survival. *Journal of Clinical Oncology*, Vol. 23, No. 6, (February), pp. 1109-1117, ISSN 0732-183X

Lugthart, S.; Figueroa, M.E.; Bindels, E.; Skrabanek, L.; Valk, P.J.; Li, Y.; Meyer, S.; Erpelinck-Verschueren, C.; Greally, J.; Löwenberg, B.; Melnick, A. & Delwel, R. (2011) Aberrant DNA hypermethylation signature in acute myeloid leukemia directed by EVI1. *Blood*, Vol. 117, No. 1, (January), pp. 234-241, ISSN 0006-4971

Luo, J.; Qi, C.; Xu, W.; Kamel-Reid, S.; Brandwein, J. & Chang, H. (2010) Cytoplasmic expression of nucleophosmin accurately predicts mutation in the nucleophosmin gene in patients with acute myeloid leukemia and normal karyotype. *American Journal of Clinical Pathology*, Vol. 133, No. 1, (January), pp. 34-40, ISSN 0002-9173

Maggi Jr., L. B.; Kuchenruether, M.; Dadey, D.Y.; Schwope, R.M.; Grisendi, S.; Townsend, R.R.; Pandolfi, P.P. & Weber, J.D. (2008) Nucleophosmin serves as a rate-limiting nuclear export chaperone for the mammalian ribosome *Molecular and Cellular Biology*, Vol. 28, No. 23, (December), pp. 7050–7065, ISSN 0270- 7306

Makishima, H.; Cazzolli, H.; Szpurka, H.; Dunbar, A.; Tiu, R.; Huh, J.; Muramatsu, H.; O'Keefe, C.; Hsi, E.; Paquette, R.L.; Kojima, S.; List, A.F.; Sekeres, M.A.; McDevitt, M.A. & Maciejewski, J.P. (2009) Mutations of e3 ubiquitin ligase cbl family members constitute a novel common pathogenic lesion in myeloid malignancies. *Journal of Clinical Oncology*, Vol. 27, No. 36, (December), pp. 6109-6116, ISSN 0732-183X

Marcucci, G.; Baldus, C.D.; Ruppert, A.S.; Radmacher, M.D.; Mrózek, K.; Whitman, S.P.; Kolitz, J.E.; Edwards, C.G.; Vardiman, J.W.; Powell, B.L.; Baer, M.R.; Moore, J.O.; Perrotti, D.; Caligiuri, M.A.; Carroll, A.J.; Larson, R.A.; de la Chapelle, A. & Bloomfield, C.D. (2005) Overexpression of the ETS-related gene, ERG, predicts a worse outcome in acute myeloid leukemia with normal karyotype: a Cancer and Leukemia Group B study. *Journal of Clinical Oncology*, Vol. 23, No. 36, (December), pp. 9234-9242, ISSN 0732-183X

Marcucci, G.; Haferlach, T. & Döhner, H. (2011a) Molecular genetics of adult acute myeloid leukemia: prognostic and therapeutic implications. *Journal of Clinical Oncology*, Vol. 29, No. 5, Feb 10; 29(5):475-486, ISSN 0732-183X

Marcucci, G.; Maharry, K.; Radmacher, M.D.; Mrózek, K.; Vukosavljevic, T.; Paschka, P.; Whitman, S.P.; Langer, C.; Baldus, C.D.; Liu, C.G.; Ruppert, A.S.; Powell, B.L.; Carroll, A.J.; Caligiuri, M.A.; Kolitz, J.E.; Larson, R.A. & Bloomfield, C.D. (2008) Prognostic significance of, and gene and microRNA expression signatures associated with, CEBPA mutations in cytogenetically normal acute myeloid leukemia with high-risk molecular features: a Cancer and Leukemia Group B Study. *Journal of Clinical Oncology*, Vol. 26, No. 31, (November), pp. 5078-5087, ISSN 0732-183X

Marcucci, G.; Maharry, K.; Whitman, S.P.; Vukosavljevic, T.; Paschka, P.; Langer, C.; Mrózek, K.; Baldus, C.D.; Carroll, A.J.; Powell, B.L.; Kolitz, J.E.; Larson, R.A.; Bloomfield, C.D. & Cancer and Leukemia Group B Study (2007) High expression levels of the ETS-related gene, ERG, predict adverse outcome and improve molecular risk-based classification of cytogenetically normal acute myeloid leukemia: a Cancer and Leukemia Group B Study. *Journal of Clinical Oncology*, Vol. 25, No. 22, (August), pp. 3337-3343, ISSN 0732-183X

Marcucci, G.; Maharry, K.; Wu, Y.Z.; Radmacher, M.D.; Mrózek, K.; Margeson, D.; Holland, K.B.; Whitman, S.P.; Becker, H.; Schwind, S.; Metzeler, K.H.; Powell, B.L.; Carter, T.H.; Kolitz, J.E.; Wetzler, M.; Carroll, A.J.; Baer, M.R.; Caligiuri, M.A; Larson, R.A. & Bloomfield, C.D. (2010) IDH1 and IDH2 gene mutations identify novel molecular subsets within de novo cytogenetically normal acute myeloid leukemia: a Cancer and Leukemia Group B study. *Journal of Clinical Oncology*, Vol. 28, No. 14 (May), pp. 2348-2355, ISSN 0732-183X

Marcucci, G.; Mrózek, K.; Radmacher, M.D.; Bloomfield, C.D. & Croce, C.M. (2009) MicroRNA expression profiling in acute myeloid and chronic lymphocytic leukaemias. *Best Practice & Research Clinical Haematology*, Vol. 22, No. 2, (June), pp. 239-248, ISSN 1521-6926

Marcucci, G.; Mrózek, K.; Radmacher, M.D.; Garzon, R. & Bloomfield, C.D. (2011b) The prognostic and functional role of microRNAs in acute myeloid leukemia. *Blood*, Vol. 117, No. 4, (January), pp. 1121-1129, ISSN 0006-4971

Marcucci, G.; Strout, M.P.; Bloomfield, C.D. & Caligiuri, M.A. (1998) Detection of unique ALL1 (MLL) fusion transcripts in normal human bone marrow and blood: distinct origin of normal versus leukemic ALL1 fusion transcripts. *Cancer Research*, Vol. 58, No. 4, (February), pp. 790-793, ISSN 0008-5472

Mardis, E.R. (2011) A decade's perspective on DNA sequencing technology. *Nature*, Vol. 470, No. 7333, (February), pp. 198-203, ISSN 0028-0836

Mardis, E.R.; Ding, L.; Dooling, D.J.; Larson, D.E.; McLellan M.D.; Chen, K.; Koboldt, D.C.; Fulton, R.S.; Delehaunty, K.D.; McGrath, S.D.; Fulton, L.A.; Locke, D.P.; Magrini, V.J.; Abbott, R.M.; Vickery, T.L.; Reed, J.S., Robinson, J.S.; Wylie, T.; Smith, S.M.; Carmichael, L.; Eldred, J.M.; Harris, C.C.; Walker, J.;, Peck, J.B.; Du, F.; Dukes, A.F.; Sanderson, G.E.; Brummett, A.M.; Clark, E.; McMichael, J.F.; Meyer, R.J.; Schindler, J.K.; Pohl, C.S.; Wallis, J.W.; Shi, X.; Lin, L.; Schmidt, H.;, Tang, Y.; Haipek, C.; Wiechert, M.E.; Ivy, J.V.; Kalicki, J.; Elliott, G.; Ries, R.E.; Payton, J.E.; Westervelt, P.; Tomasson, M.H.; Watson, M.A.; Baty, J.; Heath, S.; Shannon, W.D.; Nagarajan, R.; Link, D.C.; Walter, M.J.; Graubert, T.A.; DiPersio, J.F.; Wilson, R.K. & Ley, T.J. (2009) Recurring mutations found by sequencing an acute myeloid leukemia genome. *The New England Journal of Medicine*, Vol. 361, No. 11, (September), pp. 1058-1066, ISSN 0028-4793

Mariano, A.R.;, Colombo, E.; Luzi, L.; Martinelli, P.; Volorio, S.; Bernard, L.; Meani, N.; Bergomas, R.; Alcalay, M. & Pelicci, P.G. (2006) Cytoplasmic localization of NPM in myeloid leukemias is dictated by gain-of-function mutations that create a functional nuclear export signal. *Oncogene*, Vol. 25, No. 31, (July), pp. 4376–4380, ISSN 0950-9232

Martelli, M.P.; Manes, N.; Liso, A.; Pettirossi, V.; Verducci Galletti, B.; Bigerna, B.; Pucciarini, A.; De Marco, M.F.; Pallotta, M.T.; Bolli, N.; Sborgia, M.; di Raimondo, F.; Fabbiano, F.; Meloni, G.; Specchia, G.; Martelli, M.F. & Falini, B. (2008) A western blot assay for detecting mutant nucleophosmin (NPM1) proteins in acute myeloid leukaemia. *Leukemia*, Vol. 22, No.12, pp. 2285-2288, ISSN 0887-6924

Mead, A.J.; Gale, R.E.; Hills, R.K.; Gupta, M.; Young, B.D.; Burnett, A.K. & Linch, D.C. (2008) Conflicting data on the prognostic significance of FLT3/TKD mutations in acute myeloid leukemia might be related to the incidence of biallelic disease. *Blood*, Vol. 112, No. 2, (July), pp. 444-445, ISSN 0006-4971

Meani, N. & Alcalay, M. (2009) Role of nucleophosmin in acute myeloid leukemia. *Expert Review of Anticancer Therapy*, Vol. 9, No. 9, (September), pp. 1283-1294, ISSN 1473-7140

Metzeler, K.H., Dufour, A.; Benthaus, T.; Hummel, M.; Sauerland, M.C.; Heinecke, A.; Berdel, W.E.; Büchner, T.; Wörmann, B.; Mansmann, U.; Braess, J.; Spiekermann, K.; Hiddemann, W.; Buske, C. & Bohlander, S.K. (2009) ERG expression is an independent prognostic factor and allows refined risk stratification in cytogenetically normal acute myeloid leukemia: a comprehensive analysis of ERG, MN1, and BAALC transcript levels using oligonucleotide microarrays. *Journal of Clinical Oncology*, Vol. 27, No. 30, (October), pp. 5031-5038, ISSN 0732-183X

Metzeler, K.H.; Maharry, K.; Radmacher, M.D.; Mrózek, K.; Margeson, D.; Becker, H.; Curfman, J.; Holland, K.B.; Schwind, S.; Whitman, S.P.; Wu, Y.Z.; Blum, W.; Powell, B.L.; Carter, T.H.; Wetzler, M.; Moore, J.O.; Kolitz, J.E.; Baer, M.R.; Carroll, A.J.; Larson, R.A.; Caligiuri, M.A.; Marcucci, G. & Bloomfield, C.D. (2011) TET2 Mutations Improve the New European LeukemiaNet Risk Classification of Acute Myeloid Leukemia: A Cancer and Leukemia Group B Study. *Journal of Clinical Oncology*, Feb 22, [Epub ahead of print], ISSN 0732-183X

Miwa, H.; Beran, M. & Saunders, G.F. (1992) Expression of the Wilms' tumor gene (WT1) in human leukemias. *Leukemia*, Vol. 6, No. 5, (May), pp. 405-409, ISSN 0887-6924

Miyawaki, S.; Hatsumi, N.; Tamaki, T.; Naoe, T.; Ozawa, K.; Kitamura, K.; Karasuno, T.; Mitani, K.; Kodera, Y.; Yamagami, T. & Koga, D. (2010) Prognostic potential of detection of WT1 mRNA level in peripheral blood in adult acute myeloid leukemia. *Leukemia & Lymphoma*, Vol. 51, No. 10, (October), pp. 1855-1861, ISSN 1042-8194

Mohr, F.; Döhner, K.; Buske, C. & Rawat, V.P. (2011) TET Genes: new players in DNA demethylation and important determinants for stemness. *Experimental Hematology*,Vol. 39, No. 3, (March), pp. 272-281, ISSN 0301-472X

Motyckova, G. & Stone R.M. (2010) The role of molecular tests in acute myeloid leukemia treatment decisions. *Current Hematology Malignancies Report*, Vol. 5, pp. 109-117, ISSN 1558-822X

Mourah, S.; Porcher, R.; Lescaille, G.; Rousselot, P.; Podgorniak, M.P.; Labarchede, G.; Naimi, B.;Medioni, J.; Dombret, H. & Calvo, F. (2009) Quantification of VEGF isoforms and VEGFR transcripts by qRT-PCR and their significance in acute myeloid leukemia. *The International Journal of Biological Markers*, Vol. 24, No. 1, (January-March), pp. 22-31, ISSN 1724-6008

Mrózek, K.; Döhner, H. & Bloomfield, C.D. (2007) Influence of new molecular prognostic markers in patients with karyotypically normal acute myeloid leukemia: recent advances. *Current Opinion in Hematology*, Vol. 14, No. 2, (March), pp. 106-114, ISSN 1065-6251

Nakao, M.; Yokota, S.; Iwai, T.; Kaneko, H.; Horiike, S.; Kashima, K.; Sonoda, Y.; Fujimoto, T. & Misawa, S. (1996) Internal tandem duplication of the flt3 gene found in acute myeloid leukemia. *Leukemia*, Vol. 10, No. 12, (December), pp. 1911-1918, ISSN 0887-6924

Nana-Sinkam, P. & Croce, C.M. (2010) MicroRNAs in diagnosis and prognosis in cancer: what does the future hold? *Pharmacogenomics*, Vol. 11, No. 5, (May), pp. 667-669, ISSN 1462-2416

Naoe, T. & Kiyoi, H. (2010) Normal and oncogenic FLT3. *Cellular and Molecular Life Sciences*, Vol. 61, No. 23, (December), pp. 2932-2938, ISSN 1420-682X

Narahara K, Kimura S, Kikkawa K, Takahashi Y, Wakita Y, Kasai R, Nagai S, Nishibayashi Y, Kimoto H. (1985) Probable assignment of soluble isocitrate dehydrogenase (IDH1) to 2q33.3. *Human Genetics*, Vol. 71, No.1, pp. 37-40, ISSN 0340-6717

Newton, C.R.; Graham, A.; Heptinstall, L.E.; Powell, S.J.; Summers, C.; Kalsheker, N.; Smith, J.C. & Markham, A.F. (1989) Analysis of any point mutation in DNA. The amplification refractory mutation system (ARMS). *Nucleic Acids Research*, Vol. 17, No. 7, (April), pp. 2503-2516, ISSN 0305-1048

Nibourel, O.; Kosmider, O.; Cheok, M.; Boissel, N.; Renneville, A.; Philippe, N.; Dombret, H.; Dreyfus, F.; Quesnel, B.; Geffroy, S.; Quentin, S.; Roche-Lestienne, C.; Cayuela, J.M.; Roumier, C.; Fenaux, P.; Vainchenker, W.; Bernard, O.A.; Soulier, J.; Fontenay, M. & Preudhomme, C. (2010) Incidence and prognostic value of TET2 alterations in de novo acute myeloid leukemia achieving complete remission. *Blood*, Vol. 116, No. 7, (August), pp. 1132-1135, ISSN 0006-4971

Nilson, I.; Löchner, K.; Siegler, G.; Greil, J.; Beck, J.D.; Fey, G.H. & Marschalek, R. (1996) Exon/intron structure of the human ALL-1 (MLL) gene involved in translocations to chromosomal region 11q23 and acute leukaemias. *British Journal of Haematology*, Vol. 93, No. 4, (June), pp. 966-972, ISSN 0007-1048

Noordermeer, S.M.; Tönnissen, E.; Vissers, I.; van der Heijden, A.; van de Locht, L.T.; Deutz-Terlouw, P.P.; Marijt, E.W.; Jansen, J.H. & van der Reijden, B.A. (2011) Rapid identification of IDH1 and IDH2 mutations in acute myeloid leukaemia using high resolution melting curve analysis. *British Journal of Haematology*, Vol. 152, No. 4, (February), pp. 493-496, ISSN 0007-1048

Oelschlaegel, U.; Koch, S.; Mohr, B.; Schaich, M.; Falini, B.; Ehninger, G. & Thiede, C. (2010) Rapid flow cytometric detection of aberrant cytoplasmic localization of nucleophosmin (NPMc) indicating mutant NPM1 gene in acute myeloid leukemia. *Leukemia*, Vol. 24, No.10, (October), pp. 1813-1816, ISSN 0887-6924

Oh, I.U.; Inazawa, J.; Kim, Y.O.; Song, B.J. & Huh, T.L. (1996) Assignment of the human mitochondrial NADP(+)-specific isocitrate dehydrogenase (IDH2) gene to 15q26.1 by in situ hybridization. *Genomics*, Vol. 38, No. 1, (November), pp.104-106, ISSN 0888-7543

Orita, M.; Iwahana, H.; Kanazawa, H.; Hayashi, K. & Sekiya, T. (1989) Detection of polymorphisms of human DNA by gel electrophoresis as single-strand conformation polymorphisms. *The Proceedings of the National Academy of Sciences of the USA*, Vol. 86, No. 8, (April), pp. 2766-2770, ISSN 0027-8424

Orou, A.; Fechner, B.; Utermann, G. & Menzel, H.J. (1995) Allele-specific competitive blocker PCR: a one-step method with applicability to pool screening. *Human Mutation*, Vol. 6, No. 2, (February), pp. 163-169, ISSN1059-7794

Otten, J.; Schmitz, L.; Vettorazzi, E.; Schultze, A.; Marx, A.H.; Simon, R.; Krauter, J.; Loges, S.; Sauter, G.; Bokemeyer, C. & Fiedler, W. (2011) Expression of TGF-β receptor ALK-5 has a negative impact on outcome of patients with acute myeloid leukemia. *Leukemia*, Vol. 25, No. 2, (February), pp. 375-379, ISSN 0887-6924

Owen, C.; Fitzgibbon, J. & Paschka, P. (2010) The clinical relevance of *Wilms Tumor I* (WT1) gene mutations in acute leukaemia. *Hematological Oncology*, Vol. 28, (December), pp. 13-19, ISSN 1099-1069

Pabst, T.; Eyholzer, M.; Fos, J. & Mueller, B.U. (2009) Heterogeneity within AML with CEBPA mutations; only CEBPA double mutations, but not single CEBPA mutations are associated with favourable prognosis. *British Journal of Cancer*, Vol. 100, No. 8, (April), pp. 1343-1346, ISSN 0007-0920

Pabst, T. & Mueller, B.U. (2007) Transcriptional dysregulation during myeloid transformation in AML. *Oncogene*, Vol. 26, No. 47, (October), pp. 6829-6837, ISSN 0950-9232

Pabst, T.; Mueller, B.U.; Zhang, P.; Radomska, H.S.; Narravula, S.; Schnittger, S.; Behre, G.; Hiddemann, W. & Tenen, D.G. (2001) Dominant-negative mutations of CEBPA, encoding CCAAT/enhancer binding protein-alpha (C/EBPalpha), in acute myeloid leukemia. *Nature Genetics*, Vol. 27, No. 3, (March), pp. 263-270, ISSN 1061-4036

Paschka, P.; Marcucci, G.; Ruppert, A.S.; Whitman, S.P.; Mrózek, K.; Maharry, K.; Langer, C.; Baldus, C.D.; Zhao, W.; Powell, B.L.; Baer, M.R.; Carroll, A.J.; Caligiuri, M.A.;, Kolitz, J.E.; Larson, R.A. & Bloomfield, C.D. (2008) Wilms' tumor 1 gene mutations independently predict poor outcome in adults with cytogenetically normal acute myeloid leukemia: a cancer and leukemia group B study. *Journal of Clinical Oncology*, Vol. 26, No. 28 (October), pp. 4595-4602, ISSN 0732-183X

Paschka, P.; Schlenk, R.F.; Gaidzik, V.I.; Habdank, M.; Krönke, J.; Bullinger, L.; Späth, D.; Kayser, S.; Zucknick, M.; Götze, K.; Horst, H.A.; Germing, U.; Döhner, H. & Döhner, K. (2010) IDH1 and IDH2 mutations are frequent genetic alterations in acute myeloid leukemia and confer adverse prognosis in cytogenetically normal acute myeloid leukemia with NPM1 mutation without FLT3 internal tandem duplication. *Journal of Clinical Oncology*, Vol. 28, No. 22 (August), pp. 3636-3643, ISSN 0732-183X

Patel, K.P.; Ravandi, F.; Ma, D.; Paladugu, A.; Barkoh, B.A.; Medeiros, L.J. & Luthra, R. (2011) Acute myeloid leukemia with IDH1 or IDH2 mutation: frequency and clinicopathologic features. *American Journal of Clinical Pathology*, Vol. 135, No. 1, (January), pp. 35-45, ISSN 0002-9173

Paydas, S.; Tanriverdi, K.; Yavuz, S.; Disel, U.; Baslamisli, F. & Burgut, R. (2005) PRAME mRNA levels in cases with acute leukemia: clinical importance and future prospects. *American Journal of Hematology*, Vol. 79, No. 4, (August), pp. 257-261, ISSN 0361-8609

Perry, D.J. (1999) Screening for Mutations in DNA by Single-Stranded Conformation Polymorphism (SSCP) Analysis. *Methods in Molecular Medicine*, Vo1. 31, pp. 105-10, ISSN 1543-1894

Pfaffl, M.W. (2001) A new mathematical model for relative quantification in real-time RT-PCR. *Nucleic Acids Research*, Vol. 29, No. 9, (May), e45, ISSN 0305-1048

Pfaffl, M.W., Horgan, G.W. & Dempfle, L. (2002) Relative expression software tool (REST) for group-wise comparison and statistical analysis of relative expression results in real-time PCR. *Nucleic Acids Research* May 1; 30(9):e36. ISSN 0305-1048

Preudhomme, C.; Sagot, C.; Boissel, N.; Cayuela, J.M.; Tigaud, I.; de Botton, S.; Thomas, X.; Raffoux, E.; Lamandin, C.; Castaigne, S.; Fenaux, P.; Dombret, H. & ALFA Group. (2002) Favorable prognostic significance of CEBPA mutations in patients with de novo acute myeloid leukemia: a study from the Acute Leukemia French Association (ALFA). *Blood*, Vol. 100, No. 8, (October), pp. 2717-2723, ISSN 0006-4971

Qin, Y.; Zhu, H.; Jiang, B.; Li, J.; Lu, X.; Li, L.; Ruan, G.; Liu, Y.; Chen, S. & Huang, X. (2009) Expression patterns of WT1 and PRAME in acute myeloid leukemia patients and their usefulness for monitoring minimal residual disease. *Leukemia Research*, Vol. 33, No. 3, (March), pp. 384-390, ISSN 0145-2126

Radmacher, M.D.; Marcucci, G.; Ruppert, A.S.; Mrózek, K.; Whitman, S.P.; Vardiman, J.W.; Paschka, P.; Vukosavljevic, T.; Baldus, C.D.; Kolitz, J.E.; Caligiuri, M.A.; Larson, R.A.; Bloomfield, C.D. & Cancer and Leukemia Group B. (2006) Independent confirmation of a prognostic gene-expression signature in adult acute myeloid leukemia with a normal karyotype: a Cancer and Leukemia Group B study. *Blood*, Vol. 108, No. 5, (September), pp. 1677-1683, ISSN 0006-4971

Radomska, H.S.; Bassères DS, Zheng R, Zhang P, Dayaram T, Yamamoto Y, Sternberg DW, Lokker N, Giese NA, Bohlander SK, Schnittger S, Delmotte MH, Davis RJ, Small D, Hiddemann W, Gilliland DG, Tenen DG. (2006) Block of C/EBP alpha function by phosphorylation in acute myeloid leukemia with FLT3 activating mutations. *The Journal of Experimental Medicine*, Vol. 203, No. 2, (February), pp. 371-381, ISSN 0022-1007

Ramsingh, G.; Koboldt, D.C.; Trissal, M.; Chiappinelli, K.B.; Wylie, T.; Koul, S.; Chang, L.W.; Nagarajan, R.; Fehniger, T.A.; Goodfellow, P.;, Magrini, V.; Wilson, R.K.; Ding, L.; Ley, T.J.; Mardis, E.R. & Link, D.C. (2010) Complete characterization of the microRNAome in a patient with acute myeloid leukemia. *Blood*, Vol. 116, No. 24, (December), pp. 5316-5326, ISSN 0006-4971

Rau, R. & Brown, P. (2009) Nucleophosmin (NPM1) mutations in adult and childhood acute myeloid leukaemia: towards definition of a new leukaemia entity. *Hematological Oncology*, Vol. 27, No. 4, (December), pp. 171-181, ISSN 1099-1069

Ravandi, F.; Kantarjian, H.; Faderl, S.; Garcia-Manero, G.; O'Brien, S.; Koller, C.; Pierce, S.; Brandt, M.; Kennedy, D.; Cortes, J. & Beran, M. (2010) Outcome of patients with FLT3-mutated acute myeloid leukemia in first relapse. *Leukemia Research*, Vol. 34, No. 6, (June), pp. 752-756, ISSN 0145-2126

Rázga, F.; Dvořáková, D., Jurček, T., Ježíšková, I., Křístková, Z. & Mayer, J. (2009) CEBPA gene mutational status: a complete screening using high-resolution melt curve analysis. *Molecular Diagnosis & Therapy*, Vol. 13, No. 3, pp. 195-200, ISSN 1177-1062

Reindl, C.; Quentmeier, H.; Petropoulos, K.; Greif, P.A.; Benthaus, T.; Argiropoulos, B.; Mellert, G.; Vempati, S.; Duyster, J.; Buske, C.; Bohlander, S.K.; Humphries, K.R.; Hiddemann, W. & Spiekermann, K. (2009) CBL exon 8/9 mutants activate the FLT3 pathway and cluster in core binding factor/11q deletion acute myeloid leukemia/myelodysplastic syndrome subtypes. *Clinical Cancer Research*, Vol. 15, No. 7, (April), pp. 2238-2247, ISSN 1078-0432

Renneville, A.; Boissel, N.; Zurawski, V.; Llopis, L.; Biggio, V.; Nibourel, O.; Philippe, N.; Thomas, X.; Dombret, H. & Preudhomme, C. (2009) Wilms tumor 1 gene mutations are associated with a higher risk of recurrence in young adults with acute myeloid leukemia: a study from the Acute Leukemia French Association. *Cancer*, Vol. 115, No. 16, (August), pp. 3719-3727, ISSN 1097-0142

Ritter, M.; Kim, T.D.; Lisske, P.; Thiede, C.; Schaich, M. & Neubauer, A. (2004) Prognostic significance of N-RAS and K-RAS mutations in 232 patients with acute myeloid leukemia. *Haematologica*, Vol. 89, No. 11, pp. 1397-1399, ISSN 0390-6078

Rocquain, J.; Carbuccia, N.; Trouplin, V.; Raynaud, S.; Murati, A.;, Nezri, M.; Tadrist, Z.; Olschwang, S.; Vey, N.; Birnbaum, D.; Gelsi-Boyer, V. & Mozziconacci, M.J. (2010) Combined mutations of ASXL1, CBL, FLT3, IDH1, IDH2, JAK2, KRAS, NPM1, NRAS, RUNX1, TET2 and WT1 genes in myelodysplastic syndromes and acute myeloid leukemias. *BMC Cancer*, Vol. 10, (August), p. 401, ISSN 1471-2407

Rodríguez-Paredes, M. & Esteller,M. (2011) Cancer epigenetics reaches mainstream oncology. *Nature Medicine*, Vol. 17, No. 3, (March), pp. 330-339, ISSN 1546-170X

Roti, G.; Rosati, R.; Bonasso, R.; Gorello, P.; Diverio, D.; Martelli, M.F.; Falini, B.; Mecucci, C. & Gruppo Italiano Malattie Ematologiche dell' Adulto Working Party. (2006) Denaturing high-performance liquid chromatography: a valid approach for identifying NPM1 mutations in acute myeloid leukemia. *Journal of Molecular Diagnostics*, Vol. 8, No. 2, (May), pp. 254-259, ISSN 1525-1578

Santamaría, C.; Chillón, M.C.; García-Sanz, R.; Pérez, C.; Caballero, M.D.; Mateos, M.V.; Ramos, F.; de Coca, A.G.; Alonso, J.M.; Giraldo, P.; Bernal, T.; Queizán, J.A.; Rodríguez, J.N.; Puig, N.; Balanzategui, A.; Sarasquete, M.E.; Alcoceba, M.; Díaz-Mediavilla, J.; San Miguel, J. & González, M. (2010) BAALC is an important predictor of refractoriness to chemotherapy and poor survival in intermediate-risk acute myeloid leukemia (AML). *Annals of Hematology*, Vol. 89, No. 5, (May), pp. 453-458, ISSN 0939-5555

Santamaría, C.M.; Chillón, M.C.; García-Sanz, R.; Pérez, C.; Caballero, M.D.; Ramos, F.; de Coca, A.G.; Alonso, J.M.; Giraldo, P.; Bernal, T.; Queizán, J.A.; Rodriguez, J.N.; Fernández-Abellán, P.; Bárez, A.; Peñarrubia, M.J.; Balanzategui, A.; Vidriales, M.B.; Sarasquete, M.E.; Alcoceba, M.; Díaz-Mediavilla, J.; San Miguel, J.F. & Gonzalez, M. (2009) Molecular stratification model for prognosis in cytogenetically normal acute myeloid leukemia. *Blood*, Vol. 114, No. 1, (July), pp. 148-152, ISSN 0006-4971

Sárová, I.; Brezinová, J.; Zemanová, Z.; Lizcová, L.; Berková, A.; Izáková, S.; Malinová, E.; Fuchs, O.; Kostecka, A.; Provazníková, D.; Filkuková, J.; Maaloufová, J.; Starý, J. & Michalová, K. (2009) A partial nontandem duplication of the MLL gene in four patients with acute myeloid leukemia. *Cancer Genetics and Cytogenetics*, Vol. 195, No. 2, (December), pp. 150-156, ISSN 0165-4608

Savkur, R. S. & Olson, M. O. (1998) Preferential cleavage in pre-ribosomal RNA by protein B23 endoribonuclease. *Nucleic Acids Research*, Vol. 26, No. 19, (October), pp. 4508–4515, ISSN 0305-1048

Schlenk, R.F. & Döhner, K. (2009) Impact of new prognostic markers in treatment decisions in acute myeloid leukemia. *Current Opinion in Hematology*, Vol. 16, pp. 98-104, ISSN 1065-6251

Schlenk, R.F.; Döhner, K.; Krauter, J.; Fröhling, S.; Corbacioglu, A.; Bullinger, L.; Habdank, M.; Späth, D.; Morgan, M.; Benner, A.; Schlegelberger, B.; Heil, G.; Ganser, A.; Döhner, H. & German-Austrian Acute Myeloid Leukemia Study Group. (2008) Mutations and treatment outcome in cytogenetically normal acute myeloid leukemia. *The New England Journal of Medicine*, Vol. 358, No. 18, (May), pp. 1909-1918, ISSN 0028-4793

Schnittger, S.; Haferlach, C.; Ulke, M.; Alpermann, T.; Kern, W. & Haferlach, T. (2010) IDH1 mutations are detected in 6.6% of 1414 AML patients and are associated with intermediate risk karyotype and unfavorable prognosis in adults younger than 60 years and unmutated NPM1 status. *Blood*, Vol. 116, No. 25, (December), pp. 5486-5496, ISSN 0006-4971

Schnittger, S.; Kern, W.; Tschulik, C.; Weiss, T.; Dicker, F.; Falini, B.; Haferlach, C. & Haferlach, T. (2009) Minimal residual disease levels assessed by NPM1 mutation-specific RQ-PCR provide important prognostic information in AML. Blood, Vol.114, No. 11, (September),pp. 2220-2231, ISSN 0006-4971

Schnittger, S.; Kinkelin, U.; Schoch, C.; Heinecke, A.; Haase, D.; Haferlach, T.; Büchner, T.; Wörmann, B.; Hiddemann, W. & Griesinger, F. (2000) Screening for MLL tandem duplication in 387 unselected patients with AML identify a prognostically unfavorable subset of AML. *Leukemia*, Vol. 14, No. 5, (May), pp. 796-804, ISSN 0887-6924

Schnittger, S.; Wörmann, B.; Hiddemann, W. & Griesinger, F. (1998) Partial tandem duplications of the MLL gene are detectable in peripheral blood and bone marrow of nearly all healthy donors. *Blood*, Vol. 92. No. 5, (September), pp. 1728-1734, ISSN 0006-4971

Scholl, S.; Theuer, C.; Scheble, V.; Kunert, C.; Heller, A.; Műgge, L.O.; Fricke, H.J.; Höfken, K. & Wedding, U. (2008) Clinical impact of nucleophosmin mutations and Flt3 internal tandem duplications in patients older than 60 yr with acute myeloid leukaemia. *European Journal of Haematology*, Vol. 80, No. 3, (March), pp. 208-215, ISSN 0902-4441

Schwind, S.; Marcucci, G.; Maharry, K.; Radmacher, M.D.; Mrózek, K.; Holland, K.B.; Margeson, D.; Becker, H.; Whitman, S.P.; Wu, Y.Z.; Metzeler, K.H.; Powell, B.L.; Kolitz, J.E.; Carter, T.H.; Moore, J.O.; Baer, M.R.; Carroll, A.J.; Caligiuri, M.A.; Larson, R.A. & Bloomfield, C.D. (2010) BAALC and ERG expression levels are associated with outcome and distinct gene and microRNA expression profiles in older patients with de novo cytogenetically normal acute myeloid leukemia: a Cancer and Leukemia Group B study. *Blood*, Vol. 116. No. 25, (December), pp. 5660-5669, ISSN 0006-4971

Seyama, T.; Ito, T.; Hayashi, T.; Mizuno, T.; Nakamura, N. & Akiyama, M. (1992) A novel blocker-PCR method for detection of rare mutant alleles in the presence of an excess amount of normal DNA. *Nucleic Acids Research*, Vol. 20, No. 10, (May), pp. 2493-2496, ISSN 0305-1048

Shook, D.; Coustan-Smith, E.; Ribeiro, R.C.; Rubnitz, J.E. & Campana, D. (2009) Minimal residual disease quantitation in acute myeloid leukemia. *Clinical Lymphoma & Myeloma*, Vol. 9, Suppl. 3, pp. S281-S285, ISSN 1557-9190

Small, D. (2008) Targeting FLT3 for the treatment of leukemia. *Seminars in Hematology*, Vol. 45, No. 3, Suppl. 2 (July), pp. S17-S21, ISSN 0037-1963

Smith, M.L.; Hills, R.K. & Grimwade, D. (2011) Independent prognostic variables in acute myeloid leukaemia. *Blood Reviews*, Vol. 25, No. 1, (January), pp. 39-51, ISSN 0268-960X

Spoo, A.C.; Lübbert, M.; Wierda, W.G. & Burger, J.A. (2007) CXCR4 is a prognostic marker in acute myelogenous leukemia. *Blood*, Vol. 109, No. 2, (January), pp. 786-791, ISSN 0006-4971

Steinbach, D. & Legrand, O. (2007) ABC transporters and drug resistance in leukemia: was P-gp nothing but the first head of the Hydra? *Leukemia*, Vol. 21, No. 6, (June), pp. 1172-1176, ISSN 0887-6924

Steinbach, D.; Pfaffendorf, N.; Wittig, S.& Gruhn, B. (2007) PRAME expression is not associated with down-regulation of retinoic acid signaling in primary acute myeloid leukemia. *Cancer Genetics and Cytogenetics*, Vol. 177, No. 1, (August), pp. 51-54, ISSN 0165-4608

Steudel, C.; Wermke, M.; Schaich, M.; Schäkel, U.; Illmer, T.; Ehninger, G. & Thiede, C. (2003) Comparative analysis of MLL partial tandem duplication and FLT3 internal tandem duplication mutations in 956 adult patients with acute myeloid leukemia. *Genes Chromosomes Cancer*, Vol. 37, No. 3, (July), pp. 237-251, ISSN 1045-2257

Strout, M.P.; Marcucci, G.; Bloomfield, C.D. & Caligiuri, M.A. (1998) The partial tandem duplication of ALL1 (MLL) is consistently generated by Alu-mediated homologous recombination in acute myeloid leukemia. *The Proceedings of the National Academy of Sciences of the USA*, Vol. 95, No. 5, pp. 2390-2395, ISSN 0027-8424

Suh, H.C.; Gooya, J.; Renn, K.; Friedman, A.D.; Johnson, P.F. & Keller, J.R. (2006) C/EBPalpha determines hematopoietic cell fate in multipotential progenitor cells by inhibiting erythroid differentiation and inducing myeloid differentiation. *Blood*, Vol. 107, No. 11, (June), pp. 4308-4316, ISSN 0006-4971

Szankasi, P.; Ho, A.K.; Bahler, D.W.; Efimova, O. & Kelley, T.W. (2011) Combined testing for CCAAT/enhancer-binding protein alpha (CEBPA) mutations and promoter methylation in acute myeloid leukemia demonstrates shared phenotypic features. *Leukemia Research*, Vol. 35, No. 2, (February), pp. 200-207, ISSN 0145-2126

Szotkowski, T.; Muzik, J.; Voglova, J.; Koza, V.; Maaloufova, J.; Kozak, T.; Jarosova, M.; Michalova, K.; Zak, P.; Steinerova, K.; Vydra, J.; Lanska, M.; Katrincsakova, B.; Sicova, K.; Pavlik, T.; Dusek, L. & Indrak, K. (2010) Prognostic factors and treatment outcome in 1,516 adult patients with de novo and secondary acute myeloid leukemia in 1999-2009 in 5 hematology intensive care centers in the Czech Republic. *Neoplasma*, Vol. 57, No. 6, pp. 578-589, ISSN 0028-2685

Tan, A.Y.; Westerman, D.A.; Carney, D.A.; Seymour, J.F.; Juneja, S. & Dobrovic, A. (2008) Detection of NPM1 exon 12 mutations and FLT3 - internal tandem duplications by high resolution melting analysis in normal karyotype acute myeloid leukemia. *Journal of Hematology & Oncology*, Vol. 1 , (July), pp. 10, ISSN 1756-8722

Taberlay, P.C. & Jones, P.A. (2011) DNA methylation and cancer. Prog Drug Res. 2011;67:1-23

Tang, J.L.; Hou, H.A.; Chen, C.Y.; Liu, C.Y.; Chou, W.C.; Tseng, M.H.; Huang, C.F.; Lee, F.Y.; Liu, M.C.; Yao, M.; Huang, S.Y.; Ko, B.S.; Hsu, S.C.; Wu, S.J.; Tsay, W.; Chen, Y.C.; Lin, L.I. &, Tien, H.F. (2009) AML1/RUNX1 mutations in 470 adult patients with de novo acute myeloid leukemia: prognostic implication and interaction with other gene alterations. *Blood*, Vol. 114, No. 26, (December), pp. 5352-5361, ISSN 0006-4971

Taskesen, E.; Bullinger, L.; Corbacioglu, A.; Sanders, M.A.; Erpelinck, C.A.; Wouters, B.J., van der Poel-van de Luytgaarde, S.C.; Damm, F.; Krauter, J.; Ganser, A.; Schlenk, R.F.; Löwenberg, B.; Delwel, R.; Döhner, H.; Valk, P.J. & Döhner, K. (2011) Prognostic impact, concurrent genetic mutations, and gene expression features of AML with CEBPA mutations in a cohort of 1182 cytogenetically normal AML patients: further evidence for CEBPA double mutant AML as a distinctive disease entity. *Blood*, Vol. 117, No. 8, (February), pp. 2469-2475, ISSN 0006-4971

Tavernier-Tardy, E.; Cornillon, J.; Campos, L.; Flandrin, P.; Duval, A.; Nadal, N. & Guyotat, D. (2009) Prognostic value of CXCR4 and FAK expression in acute myelogenous leukemia. *Leukemia Research*, Vol. 33, No. 6, (June), pp. 764-768, ISSN 0145-2126

Tenen, D.G.; Hromas, R.; Licht, J.D. & Zhang, D.E. (1997) Transcription factors, normal myeloid development, and leukaemia, *Blood*, Vol. 90, No. 2, (July), pp. 489-519, ISSN 0006-4971

Thol, F.; Damm, F.; Wagner, K.; Göhring, G.; Schlegelberger, B.; Hoelzer, D.; Lübbert, M.; Heit, W.; Kanz, L.; Schlimok, G.; Raghavachar, A.; Fiedler, W.; Kirchner, H.; Heil, G.; Heuser, M.; Krauter, J. & Ganser,A. (2010) Prognostic impact of IDH2 mutations in cytogenetically normal acute myeloid leukemia. *Blood*, Vol. 116, No. 4, (July), pp. 614-616, ISSN 0006-4971

Trnková, Z.; Bedrlíková, R.; Marková, J.; Michalová, K.; Stöckbauer, P. & Schwarz, J. (2007) Semiquantitative RT-PCR evaluation of the MDR1 gene expression in patients with acute myeloid leukemia. *Neoplasma*, Vol. 54, No. 5, pp. 387-390, ISSN 0028-2685

Ugozzoli, L.A.; Latorra, D.; Puckett, R.; Arar, K. & Hamby, K. (2004) Real-time genotyping with oligonucleotide probes containing locked nucleic acids. *Analytical Biochemistry*, Vol. 324, No. 1, (January), pp. 143-152, ISSN 0003-2697

Ugrinova, I.; K. Monier, K.; Ivaldi, C.; Thiry, M.; Storck, S.; Mongelard, F. & Bouvet, P. (2007) Inactivation of nucleolin leads to nucleolar disruption, cell cycle arrest and defects in centrosome duplication. *BMC Molecular Biology*, Vol. 8, (August) article 66, ISSN 1471-2199

Vardiman, J.W.; Thiele, J.; Arber, D.A.; Brunning, R.D.; Borowitz, M.J.; Porwit, A.; Harris, N.L.; Le Beau, M.M.; Hellström-Lindberg, E.; Tefferi, A. & Bloomfield, C.D. (2009) The 2008 revision of the World Health Organization (WHO) classification of myeloid neoplasms and acute leukemia: rationale and important changes. *Blood*, Vol. 114, No. 5, (July), pp. 937-951, ISSN 0006-4971

Vaughn, C.P. & Elenitoba-Johnson, K.S. (2004) High-resolution melting analysis for detection of internal tandem duplications. *Journal of Molecular Diagnostics*, Vol. 6, No. 3, (August), pp. 211-216, ISSN 1525-1578

Verhaak, R.G.; Goudswaard, C.S.; van Putten, W.; Bijl, M.A.; Sanders, M.A.; Hugens, W.; Uitterlinden, A.G.; Erpelinck, C.A.; Delwel, R.; Löwenberg, B. & Valk, P.J. (2005) Mutations in nucleophosmin (NPM1) in acute myeloid leukemia (AML): association with other gene abnormalities and previously established gene expression signatures and their favorable prognostic significance. *Blood*, Vol. 106, No. 12, (December), pp. 3747-3754, ISSN 0006-4971

Verhaak, R.G.; Wouters, B.J.; Erpelinck, C.A.; Abbas, S.; Beverloo, H.B.; Lugthart, S.; Löwenberg, B.; Delwel, R. & Valk, P.J. (2009) Prediction of molecular subtypes in acute myeloid leukemia based on gene expression profiling. *Haematologica*, Vol. 94, No. 1, (January), pp. 131-134, ISSN 0390-6078

Virappane, P.; Gale, R.; Hills, R.; Kakkas, I.; Summers, K.; Stevens, J.; Allen, C.; Green.; C, Quentmeier, H.; Drexler, H.; Burnett, A.; Linch, D.; Bonnet, D.; Lister, T.A. & Fitzgibbon J. (2008) Mutation of the Wilms' tumor 1 gene is a poor prognostic factor associated with chemotherapy resistance in normal karyotype acute myeloid leukemia: the United Kingdom Medical Research Council Adult Leukaemia Working Party. Mutation of the Wilms' tumor 1 gene is a poor prognostic factor associated with chemotherapy resistance in normal karyotype acute myeloid leukemia: the United Kingdom Medical Research Council Adult Leukaemia Working Party. *Journal of Clinical Oncology*, Vol. 26, No. 33, (November), pp. 5429-5435, ISSN 0732-183X

Wagner, K.; Damm, F.; Göhring, G.; Görlich, K.; Heuser, M.; Schäfer, I.; Ottmann, O.; Lübbert, M.; Heit, W.; Kanz, L.; Schlimok, G.; Raghavachar, A.A.; Fiedler, W.; Kirchner, H.H.; Brugger, W.; Zucknick, M.; Schlegelberger, B.; Heil, G.; Ganser, A. & Krauter, J. (2010) Impact of IDH1 R132 mutations and an IDH1 single nucleotide polymorphism in cytogenetically normal acute myeloid leukemia: SNP rs11554137 is an adverse prognostic factor. *Journal of Clinical Oncology*, Vol. 28, No. 14, (May), pp. 5078-5087, ISSN 0732-183X

Wang, N.D.; Finegold, M.J.; Bradley, A.; Ou, C.N.; Abdelsayed, S.V.; Wilde, M.D.; Taylor, L.R.; Wilson, D.R. & Darlington, G. (1995) Impaired energy homeostasis in C/EBP alpha knockout mice. *Science*, Vol. 269, No. 5227, (August) pp. 1108-1112, ISSN 0036-8075

Ward, P.S,; Patel, J.; Wise, D.R.; Abdel-Wahab, O.; Bennett, B.D.; Coller, H.A.; Cross, J.R.; Fantin, V.R.; Hedvat, C.V.; Perl, A.E.; Rabinowitz, J.D.; Carroll, M.; Su, S.M.; Sharp, K.A.; Levine, R.L. & Thompson, C.B. (2010) The common feature of leukemia-associated IDH1 and IDH2 mutations is a neomorphic enzyme activity converting alpha-ketoglutarate to 2-hydroxyglutarate. *Cancer Cell*, Vol. 17, No. 3, (March), pp. 225-234, ISSN 1535-6108

Watanabe, Y. & Maekawa, M. (2010) Methylation of DNA in cancer. *Advances in Clinical Chemistry*, Vol. 52, pp. 145-167. ISSN 0065-2423

Weisberg, E.; Barrett, R.; Liu, Q.; Stone, R.; Gray, N. & Griffin, J.D. (2009) FLT3 inhibition and mechanisms of drug resistance in mutant FLT3-positive AML. *Drug Resistance Updates*, Vol. 12, No. 3, (June), pp. 81-89, ISSN 1368-7646

Whitman, S.P.; Hackanson, B.; Liyanarachchi, S.; Liu, S.; Rush, L.J.; Maharry, K.; Margeson, D.; Davuluri, R.; Wen, J.; Witte, T.; Yu, L.; Liu, C.; Bloomfield, C.D.; Marcucci, G.; Plass, C. & Caligiuri, M.A. (2008a) DNA hypermethylation and epigenetic silencing of the tumor suppressor gene, SLC5A8, in acute myeloid leukemia with the MLL partial tandem duplication. *Blood*, Vol. 112, No. 5, (September), pp. 2013-2016, ISSN 0006-4971

Whitman, S.P.; Liu, S.; Vukosavljevic, T.; Rush, L.J.; Yu, L.; Liu, C.; Klisovic, M.I.; Maharry, K.; Guimond; M.; Strout, M.P.; Becknell, B.; Dorrance, A.; Klisovic, R.B.; Plass, C.; Bloomfield, C.D.; Marcucci, G. & Caligiuri, M.A. (2005) The MLL partial tandem duplication: evidence for recessive gain-of-function in acute myeloid leukemia identifies a novel patient subgroup for molecular-targeted therapy. *Blood*, Vol. 106, No. 1, (July), pp. 345-352, ISSN 0006-4971

Whitman, S.P.; Maharry, K.; Radmacher, M.D.; Becker, H.; Mrózek, K.; Margeson, D.; Holland, K.B.; Wu, Y.Z.; Schwind, S.; Metzeler, K.H.; Wen, J.; Baer, M.R.; Powell, B.L.; Carter, T.H.; Kolitz, J.E.; Wetzler, M.; Moore, J.O.; Stone, R.M.; Carroll, A.J.; Larson, R.A.; Caligiuri, M.A.; Marcucci, G. & Bloomfield, C.D. (2010) FLT3 internal tandem duplication associates with adverse outcome and gene- and microRNA-expression signatures in patients 60 years of age or older with primary cytogenetically normal acute myeloid leukemia: a Cancer and Leukemia Group B study. *Blood*, Vol. 116, No. 18, (November), pp. 3622-3626, ISSN 0006-4971

Whitman, S.P.; Ruppert, A.S.; Radmacher, M.D.; Mrózek, K.; Paschka, P.; Langer, C.; Baldus, C.D.; Wen, J.; Racke, F.; Powell, B.L.; Kolitz, J.E.; Larson, R.A.; Caligiuri, M.A.; Marcucci, G. & Bloomfield, C.D. (2008b) FLT3 D835/I836 mutations are associated with poor disease-free survival and a distinct gene-expression signature among younger adults with de novo cytogenetically normal acute myeloid leukemia lacking FLT3 internal tandem duplications. *Blood*, Vol. 111, No. 3, (February), pp. 1529-1559, ISSN 0006-4971

Wiernik, P. H. (2010) FLT3 Inhibitors for the Treatment of Acute Myeloid Leukemia. *Clinical Advances in Hematology and Oncoogy*, Vol. 8, No. 6, (June), pp. 429-444, ISSN 1543-0790

Wittwer, C.T. (2009) High-resolution DNA melting analysis: advancements and limitations. *Human Mutation*, Vol. 30, No. 6, (June), pp. 857-859, ISSN 1059-7794

Wouters, B.J.; Löwenberg, B. & Delwel, R. (2009a) A decade of genome-wide gene expression profiling in acute myeloid leukemia: flashback and prospects. *Blood*, Vol. 113, No. 2, (January), pp. 291-298, ISSN 0006-4971

Wouters, B.J.; Löwenberg, B.; Erpelinck-Verschueren, C.A.; van Putten, W.L.; Valk, P.J. & Delwel, R. (2009b) Double CEBPA mutations, but not single CEBPA mutations, define a subgroup of acute myeloid leukemia with a distinctive gene expression profile that is uniquely associated with a favorable outcome. *Blood*, Vol. 113, No. 13, (March), pp. 3088-3091, ISSN 0006-4971

Xiao, J.; Zhang, Z.; Chen, G.G.; Zhang, M.; Ding, Y.; Fu, J.; Li, M. & Yun J.P. (2009) Nucleophosmin/B23 interacts with p21WAF1/CIP1 and contributes to its stability. *Cell Cycle*, Vol. 8, No. 6, (March), pp. 889-895, ISSN 1551-4005

Xu, X.; Zhao, Y.; Xu, M.; Dai, Q.; Meng, W.; Yang, J. & Qin, R. (2010) Activation of Notch signal pathway is associated with a poorer prognosis in acute myeloid leukemia. *Medical Oncology*, [Epub ahead of print] PMID:20812035, ISSN 1357-0560

Yamamoto, Y.; Kiyoi, H.; Nakano, Y.; Suzuki, R.; Kodera, Y.; Miyawaki, S.; Asou, N.; Kuriyama, K.; Yagasaki, F.; Shimazaki, C.; Akiyama, H.; Saito, K.; Nishimura, M.; Motoji, T.; Shinagawa, K.; Takeshita, A.; Saito, H.; Ueda, R.; Ohno, R. & Naoe, T. (2001) Activating mutation of D835 within the activation loop of FLT3 in human hematologic malignancies. *Blood*, Vol. 97, No. 8, (April), pp. 2434-2439, ISSN 0006-4971

Yang, L.; Han, Y.; Suarez Saiz, F. & Minden, M.D. (2007) A tumor suppressor and oncogene: the WT1 story. *Leukemia*, Vol. 21, No. 5, (May), pp. 868-876, ISSN 0887-6924

Ysebaert, L.; Chicanne, G.; Demur, C.; De Toni, F.; Prade-Houdellier N; Ruidavets, J.B.; Mansat-De Mas, V.; Rigal-Huguet, F.; Laurent, G.; Payrastre, B.; Manenti, S. & Racaud-Sultan, C. (2006) Expression of beta-catenin by acute myeloid leukemia cells predicts enhanced clonogenic capacities and poor prognosis. *Leukemia*, Vol. 20, No. 7, (July), pp. 1211-1216, ISSN 0887-6924

Yu, Y.; Maggi Jr., L.B.; Brady, S.N.; Apicelli, A.J.; Dai, M.S.; Lu, H. & Weber, J.D. (2006) Nucleophosmin is essential for ribosomal protein L5 nuclear export. *Molecular and Cellular Biology*, Vol. 26, No. 10, (May), pp. 3798–3809, ISSN 0270- 7306

Zhang, D.E.; Zhang, P.; Wang, N.D.; Hetherington, C.J.; Darlington, G.J. & Tenen, D.G. (1997) Absence of granulocyte colony-stimulating factor signaling and neutrophil development in CCAAT enhancer binding protein alpha-deficient mice. *The Proceedings of the National Academy of Siences of the USA*, Vol. 94, No. 2, (January), pp. 569-574, ISSN 0027-8424

5

Epigenetics and Targeted Therapy in Acute Leukemia

Xudong Ma, Shaohong Jiang, Yiqun Huang,
Yong Zou, Ruiji Zheng and Liyun Xiao
Zhangzhou Affiliated Hospital of Fujian Medical University
China

1. Introduction

Chromatin is a highly ordered structure consisting of repeats of nucleosomes connected by linker DNA. It consists of DNA, histone, and nonhistone proteins condensed into nucleoprotein complexes and it functions as the physiological template of all eukaryotic genetic information. Histones are small basic proteins containing a globular domain and a flexible charged NH_2 terminus known as the histone tail, which protrudes from the nucleosome. Epigenetic codes are set up by modifications on the DNA (methylation) or on the histones (acetylation, methylation, phosphorylation, ubiquitination, and ADP ribosylation, etc.), by different classes of enzymes in a precise and targeted manner. Posttranslational modification to histones affects chromatin structure and function resulting in altered gene expression and changes in cell behavior. These modifications do not alter the primary sequence of DNA but have an impact on gene expression regulation, most frequently gene suppression. They lead to pathological states in hematopoietic system resulting in acute leukemia.

DNA methylation is catalyzed by DNA methyltransferases (DNMTs), of which three active enzymes have been identified in mammals, namely DNMT1, DNMT3A and DNMT3B. DNMT1 is responsible for maintaining pre-existing methylation patterns during DNA replication, while DNMT3A and DNMT3B are required for initiation of de novo methylation. Acetylation is a reversible process. The balance between acetylation (transcriptional activation) and deacetylation (transcriptional repression) is regulated by histone acetyltransferase (HATs) and histone deacetylases (HDACs) in specific lysine residues in the N-termini of histone tails and/or in transcription factors (eg, p53, E2F1, GATA1, RelA, YY1, and Mad/Max) without directly binding to the DNA (Minucci et al., 2006, Gallinare et al., 2007), and is critical in regulating gene expression. Mammalian HDACs are classified into three classes based on their homology to yeast HDACs. Class I HDACs (HDAC1, 2, 3, 8, and 11) are homologues of *Sacharomyces cerevisiae* histone deacetylase Rpd 3 (reduced potassium dependency 3) and those with greater similarity to yeast Hda1, are class II HDACs (Gray & Ekstrom, 2001; Gao et al., 2002; Kao et al., 2002). Class III HDACs are called Sirtuins, which are homologoues of yeast sir2 (silence information regulator). Histones can be mono-, di-, or tri-methylated at lysine and arginine residues by HMTs, and the recent identification of histone lysine demethylases such as KDM1/LSD1 and the Jumonji-domain (JMJD)-containing protein family shows that histone methylation is an enzymatically dynamic process (Lan et al., 2008). In general, methylation at H3K4, H3K36, and H3K79 is associated with transcriptional activation, whereas H3K9, H3K27, and H3K20 methylation is associated with transcriptional repression (Kouzarides et al., 2007). The involvement of HMTases, more so of DNMTs (DNA methyltransferase) is observed in cancer (Zhang et al., 2005). Several chromosomal translocations in acute myeloid leukemia (AML) that produce chimerical fusion oncoproteins have been shown to repress genes involved in cell-cycle growth inhibition, differentiation, and apoptosis (Bhalla et al., 2005; Hormaeche, 2007) . The reversal of aberrant epigenetic changes has therefore emerged as a potential strategy for the treatment of cancer. DNA methylation and histone deacetylation inhibitors and a number of compounds targeting enzymes that regulate DNA methylation, histone acetylation and histone methylation have been developed as epigenetic therapies, with some demonstrating efficacy in hematological malignancies and solid tumors. The aberrance of DNA methylation, histone acetylation and methylation has been found in acute leukemia. We found that PHI (Phenylhexyl isothiocyanate), synthetic phenylhexyl isothiocyanates, could correct the aberrance (Ma et al., 2006; Xiao et al., 2010 ; Jiang et al., 2010) .

2. Epigenetic event in acute leukemia

Epigenetic mechanisms controlling transcription of genes involved in cell differentiation, proliferation, and survival are often targets for deregulation in malignant development. Misregulation of epigenetic modification may be as significant as genetic mutation in driving cancer development and growth. There are some acute leukemias with cytogenetic translocations in WHO classification, which involved in epigenetic modification change. DNA methylation is established during early embryogenesis and continues through different generations of cell cycle and development. Abnormal patterns in DNA methylation are one of epigenetic deregulation to be characterized in human cancers, either as a result of DNMT over expression or aberrant recruitment. Acetylation and methylation are the two histone modification that has been clinically associated with pathological epigenetic disruption in cancer cells. Specific recurring chromosomal abnormalities are commonly associated with acute myeloid leukemia. These chromosomal anomalies influence the molecular and cellular phenotype of the leukemia blasts and may be responsible for their malignant potential (Caligiuri et al., 1997; Thandla et al., 1997). The aberrations often lead to the formation of one or more fusion genes resulting in the over expression or untimely expression of a normal gene, eg, the MYC/Ig gene enhancer fusion produced by the t (8;14) in Burkitt's lymphoma (Crosce et al., 1986; Thandla et al., 1997) , or the creation of a new gene product by fusing genes as in the PML-RAR fusion produced by the t(15;17) characteristic of acute promyelocytic leukemia (Zelent et al., 2001). Some regions are common partners in fusion events, and 11q23 is involved in at least 40 different translocations in acute leukemia.

2.1 DNA methylation and acute leukemia

The maintenance of appropriate DNA methylation within CpG nucleotide islands plays a significant role in regulation of a wide variety of molecular processes including stability of chromosomal structure and control of gene expression (Das, 2004). DNA methylation can also result in the recruitment of proteins that bind methylated CpG sequences (methyl-CpG-binding domain [MBD] proteins) complexes with histone deacetylases (HDACs) and histone methyltransferase (HMTase) prompting coordinated epigenetic modifications of the surrounding chromatin (Esteller, 2005). Tumor cell-specific promoter hypermethylation in genes that play important roles in regulating cell cycle, apoptosis, DNA repair, differentiation, and cell adhesion is often a hallmark of disease (Esteller, 2008). In addition, hypomethylation of repetitive sequences may result in chromosomal and genetic instability, leading to further oncogenic events. Transcriptional silencing via DNA hypermethylation can often be associated with poor clinical outcome in several malignancies (Bhalla et al., 2005; Das, 2004; Herranz, 2007). Abnormal gain in DNA methylation with aberrant silencing of transcription may occur at specific gene promoter regions and represents a mechanism for inactivation of tumor-suppressor genes. In a clinical experiment, the methylation profiles of 344 patients with acute myeloid leukemia (AML) were examined. A common aberrant DNA methylation signature consisting of 45 genes in most of them hypermethylated was identified, that was consistently detected in at least 10 of the 16 clusters' methylation signatures and affecting at least 70% of the cases studied. Genes in this signature are likely to be part of a common epigenetic pathway involved in leukemic transformation of hematopoietic cells. They are the tumor suppressor PDZD2, transcriptional regulators (ZNF667, ZNF582, PIAS2, CDK8), nuclear import receptors (TNPO3, IPO8), and CSDA, a repressor of GM-CSF. They could predict the clinical outcome (Maria et al., 2010). Silencing of CDKN2A and CDKN1A has been associated with poor clinical outcome in acute leukemias (Herman, 2003; Bernstein et al., 2007). Aberrant p15CDKN2B has been widely reported in leukemias and other myeloid neoplasms (Cameron et al., 1999; Christiansen et al., 2003; Shimamoto et al., 2005; Toyota et al., 2001). Roman-Gomez et al. reported an incidence of *p21CIP1* methylation of 41% in 124 patients with acute lymphocytic leukemia (ALL). Most importantly, they observed that *p21CIP1* methylation was an independent predictor of poor prognosis both in adults and children with this disease (Roman-Gomez et al., 2002). Zheng et al. reported that there are 35.29%, 48.65% hypermethylation of the p15 INK4, p16 INK4 gene exon 1 in acute leukemia respectively, 25%, 37.5% hypermethylation of the p15 INK4, p16 INK4 gene exon 1 in acute myeloid leukemia respectively, 60%, 69.23% hypermethylation of the p15 INK4, p16 INK4 gene exon 1 in acute lymphoid leukemia respectively (Zheng et al., 2004a, 2004b).

2.2 Histone acetylation and acute leukemia

Histone acetylation is associated with transcriptionally active chromatin, which has been established over 40 years ago (Littau et al., 1964). The acetylation of the histone tails was surmised to result in a decreased affinity of the histone for the DNA, on account of the decreasing positive charge, establishing an 'open' chromatin state. The transcriptionally active state may be mediated via the transient formation of $(H3\text{-}H4)_2$ tetrameric particle that could adopt an open structure only when H3 and H4 tails are acetylated (Morales et al., 2000). Mistargeting and mutations in HATs and HDACs are major factors leading to diseases and disorders. A classic example of one such disorder is the Rubinstein-Taybi syndrome (RSTS), which is a consequence of a single mutation in the gene encoding the HAT CREB binding protein (CBP) located on chromosome 16p13.3. In addition to functioning as a bridge between transcription factors and the basal transcription machinery, CBP has histone acetyltransferase activity (Bannister et al., 1996; Ogryzko et al., 1996). CBP causes an acetylation of core histone proteins, such as H2A, H2B, H3 and H4, and interacts with histone acetyltransferases, such as PCAF (P300/CBP associated factor), SRC-1 (steroid receptor coactivator-1) and ACTR (coactivator for nuclear hormone receptors). It is generally accepted that CBP is involved in the remodeling of nucleosomes via these factors. Altered HAT (histone acetylase) activity has been reported in both hematological and solid cancers, by inactivation of HAT activity through gene mutation or through deregulation of HAT activity by viral oncoproteins. Chromosomal translocations involving HATs and their consequent fusion proteins have been implicated in the onset and progression of acute leukemia. Such translocations have been identified in acute myeloid leukemia (AML) and acute lymphoblastic leukemia (ALL) cases in which the translocation t (11;16) (q23;p13) results in a fusion protein (MLL-CBP) consisting of the CBP and the mixed lineage leukemia (MLL) protein. The underlying mechanisms of effects of this fusion protein in the formation of AML may involve deregulation of MLL target genes by CBP-mediated chromatin remodeling and increased chromatin accessibility (Ayton et al., 2001). The fusion protein has A/T hooks and cysteine-rich DNA recognition domain of MLL fused to intact CBP and fails to recruit SWI/SNF to its target as it lacks the SET domain, which is important for interacting with hSNF5 (Taki et al., 1997). MLL can also be aberrantly fused to p300 in AML via the t (11;22)(q23;p13) translocation (Ida et al., 1997). In addition to p300 and CBP fusion proteins involving the HATs, TIF2, MOZ (monocytic zinc finger protein) and MORF that arise as a result of chromosomal translocations have also been identified in hematological malignancies (Cairns, 2001; Cairns et al., 2001; Panagopoulos et al., 2001; Liang J et al., 1998). The MOZ-CBP fusion proteins is expressed due to a translocation t (8;16)(p11;p13), associated with a subtype of acute monocytic leukemia (AML M5). The resulting fusion protein has been recently shown to increase expression of genes regulated by NF-κB (Chan et al., 2007). MORF gene fusions are expressed in t (10;16) (q22;p13) in childhood AML and myelodysplastic syndrome, in which the MORF gene is fused with the CBP gene (Champagne et al., 1999). The MOZ-TIF2 fusion is one of a new family of chromosomal rearrangements that associate HAT activity, transcriptional coactivation, and acute leukemia (Jian et al., 1998). The CBP gene has been shown to fuse with MOZ in AML patients with t (8;16)(p11;p13) (Borrow et al., 1996; Giles et al., 1997), and in MLL patients with therapy-related acute leukemia with t(11;16)(q23;p13) (Rowley et al., 1997; Satake et al., 1997; Sobulo et al., 1997; Taki et al., 1997).

Deregulation of HDAC activity by chromosomal translocations has been strongly implicated in aberrant gene silencing and the promotion of tumorigenesis, especially in leukemia. A well-understood link between tumorigenesis and aberrant HDAC activity occurs in acute promyelocytic leukemia (APL). In APL, the chromosomal translocations t (15;17) and t (11;17) results in fusion proteins RARα-PML (promyelocytic leukemia protein) and RARα-PLZF (promyelocytic zinc finger), respectively. These aberrant proteins retain the ability to bind RAREs and HDACs with high affinity and are no responsive to retinoids, resulting in the deregulated transcriptional silencing of RAR-targeted genes and prevention of cell differentiation (Zelent et al., 2001). The retinoic acid receptor (RAR) is important for myeloid differentiation and acts as a transcriptional regulator by binding its heterodimerization partner RXR, which in turn bind to retinoic acid response elements (RAREs) within the promoters of target genes (Bolden et al., 2006). Both PML-RARalpha and PLZF-RARalpha fusion proteins recruit the nuclear co-repressor (N-CoR)-histone deacetylase complex through the RARalpha CoR box (Iris & Luciano, 2011). AML1-ETO is a fusion protein that results from t (8;21) and CBFβ-MYH11 caused by the chromatin inversion 16(p13;q22) in cases of AML. It is of translocations in leukemogenesis that is capable of altering protein acetylation. Fusion proteins from these translocations result in the recruitment of HDACs to target gene promoters and consequent gene silencing (Wang et al., 2007; Bhalla et al., 2005).

We have studied on the state of histone acetylation in acute leukemia. The levels of acetylated H3 and H4 were examined in patients with or without complete remission response. The deficient histone acetylation existed in all 15 cases of acute leukemias, including both myeloid and lymphoid lineages. The results showed that both levels of histone H3 and H4 acetylation in 15 AL patients were significantly lower, as compared with 4 individuals without leukemia(H3 0.128±0.013 *vs* 0.386±0.104, H4 0.096± 0.008 *vs* 0.341±0.096 respectively, both $p<0.01$). This deficiency was revealed in all the acute leukemia cases investigated in all age groups from 2.5 to 69 years, including both myeloid and lymphoid lineages (Xiao et al., 2010).

2.3 Histone methylation and acute leukemia

Histone methylation is brought about by histone methyltransferases (HMTases), which catalyze the transfer of methyl group from the donor SAM (S-adenosyl methionine) predominantly to the lysine or arginine residues on the N-terminal histone tails. Based on the basis of amino acids that get modified, they are classified into the lysine methyltransferases (Martin & Zhang, 2005) and arginine methyltransferases (Bedford et al., 2005). The residues can be mono-, di- or tri-methylated, which further increase the scope and range of methylation-mediated regulation. Arginine methyltransferase have an additional level of regulation in catalyzing the formation of asymmetricdimethylarginine (aDMA) or symmetricdimethylarginine (sDMA). HMTases are versatile enzymes with their modifications being involved in both activation and repression. The exact residue on the histone tails that gets modification determines transcriptional activation or repression. The lysineme methyltransferases are involved in transcriptional activation (methylation on H3K4, H3K36 and H3K79) as well as transcription repression (methylation of H3K9, H3K27 and H4K20), while the arginine methyltransferases so far have been shown to be involved in transcriptional activation (Kourzarides et al., 2007). There are a form of chromosomal translocations involving HMTs (e.g., MLL1, NSD1, NSD3), gene over expression or amplification (e.g., EZH2, MLL2, NSD3, BMI1, GASC1), gene silencing (e.g., RIZ1), and gene deletion (e.g., MLL3).

Chromosomal rearrangements, affecting chromosome 11q23 and involving the human MLL gene, is a histone methyltransferase. It recurrently associated with the disease phenotype of acute leukemias (Pui et al., 2002, 2003). There are a total of 87 different MLL rearrangements of which 51 TPGs are now characterized at the molecular level. The four most frequently found TPGs (AF4, AF9, ENL and AF10) encode nuclear proteins that are part of a protein network involved in histone H3K79 methylation (Meyer et al., 2006). Because H3K79 methylation is important for transcriptional elongation (Krogan et al., 2003), global hypomethylation could also lead to a reduced expression of a great number of genes (Dik et al., 2005).

The key transcriptional pathways that are subordinate to both wild-type and oncogenic MLL proteins include Hox genes, which are master regulators of cell fate, proliferation, and morphogenesis (Owens & Hawley, 2002). Hematopoietic cells transformed by MLL oncoproteins consistently hyperexpress several Hoxa cluster genes, some of which have been shown to be direct targets of MLL and key contributors to the pathologic features of MLL associated leukemia (Ayton & Cleary, 2003; Kumar et al., 2004; Wang et al., 2005). This subtype of acute leukemia has a particularly aggressive with a very dismal prognosis. Thus, an interesting scenario about the contribution of CALM-AF10 in leukemogenesis can be envisioned whereby the CALM-AF10 fusion, in addition to up-regulating specific oncogenes (eg, HOXA5 genes) via local hypermethylation, might promote leukemogenesis by interfering with multiple cellular pathways through global hypomethylation of H3K79.

Lin et al. suggested that the increased chromosomal instability associated with H3K79 hypomethylation caused by the CALM-AF10 fusion might accelerate the acquisition of additional genetic abnormalities required for leukemogenesis. AF10 fusion proteins seem to use at least 2 mechanisms that promote leukemogenesis: (1) deregulation of target genes resulting from local epigenetic changes, and (2) increasing genomic instability due to global epigenetic changes (Lin et al., 2009).

ALL-1 is a member of the human trithorax/Polycomb gene family and is also involved in acute leukemia. ALL-1 is associated in a stable complex with at least 27 proteins (Tatsuya et al., 2002), most ALL-1-associated proteins can be classified into well-known complexes involved in transcription. The ALL-1 protein was found to be posttranslationally processed into two polypeptides, p300 and p180. The two ALL-1 polypeptides are present within a single supercomplex, which is physical association between segments spanning residues 1979–2130 and 3613–3876. p180 contains the SET domain which methylates H3-K4, as well as a domain (TAD) with transcriptional activation capacity. p300 comprises the HAT hooks which bind DNA, a bromodomain which binds acetylated lysines within histone H4 (Dhalluin et al., 1999; Jacobson et al., 2000), the PHD zinc fingers domain, and a region with homology to DNA methyltransferase. The cleavage might enable the formation of a spatial configuration accommodating the many interactions of ALL-1 with proteins and DNA. ALL-1-associated leukemias show some unusual and intriguing features (DiMartino et al., 1999). A study showed 16/22 (68%) infant's acute leukemia with ALL-1 gene rearrangements. It demonstrated that ALL-1, a highly intricate chromatin modifier, in acute leukemia is abnormal in its function (Cimino et al., 1997).

The t (8;21) is found in 10–15% of myeloid leukemia and gives rise to a fusion protein that contains the N-terminal portion of RUNX1 fused to nearly all of myeloid translocation gene on chromosome 8 (MTG8, also known as eight-twenty-one (ETO)) (Miyoshi et al., 1991, 1993; Erickson et al., 1994). The fusion protein appears to function as a transcriptional repressor of RUNX1-regulated genes (Peterson et al., 2004). The t (12;21) is found in up to 25% of pediatric B-cell acute leukemia and creates a chimerical gene encoding the TEL-RUNX1 fusion protein (Golub et al., 1995; Nucifora et al., 1995). RUNX1 function is also impaired by the inv (16), which fuses the RUNX1 associating factor, core binding factor b (CBFb or polyoma enhancer binding protein 2 betas) to the smooth muscle myosin heavy-chain gene MYH11, in approximately 8% of acute myeloid leukemia (Liu et al., 1993). Two SUV39H1 contact points within repression domain 2 of RUNX1, with one of these RUNX1 domains also contacting HDAC1 and HDAC3, begins to provide a mechanistic basis for gene silencing mediated by RUNX1. Both Runt and RUNX1 are required for gene silencing during development and a central domain of RUNX1, termed repression domain 2 (RD2). RD2 contacts SUV39H1, a histone methyltransferase, via two motifs and that endogenous SUV39H1 associates with a Runx1-regulated repression element in murine erythroleukemia

cells. In addition, one of these SUV39H1-binding motifs is also sufficient forbidding to histone deacetylases 1 and 3, and both of these domains are required for full RUNX1-mediated transcriptional repression. The association between RUNX1, histone deacetylases and SUV39H1 provides a molecular mechanism for repressor (E et al., 2006).
The state of histone methylation in acute leukemia has been studied. Aberrant histone methylations showed downregulation of H3K4 methylation and upregulation of H3K9 methylation in all acute leukemia. The methylation status of histone H3 at lysines 4 and 9 of mononuclear cells from 19 patients with acute leukemia, aged from 6 to 78, including AML and ALL and that from 9 individuals without leukemia were compared. The results showed that the level of H3K4 methylation was significantly lower in 19 AL patients than that in non leukemia (0.220±0.096 *vs* 0.447±0.186, P<0. 01), while the level of H3K9 methylation was significantly higher (0.409 4±0.106 *vs* 0.168±0.015, P<0.01). These results clearly demonstrated that the patients with acute leukemias are hypomethylated at H3K4, and hypermethylated at H3K9. (Ma et al., 2010).

3. Epigenetic therapy in acute leukemia

The cause of most epigenetic diseases can be traced to the enzymes that establish them. A great deal of research has gone into the discovery of the modulators of these enzymes, which not only leads to a better understanding of the mechanism, but also to therapeutic possibilities. Fusion protein, such as MLL-MOZ, PML-RARA results mutations in HATs, HDACs and HMTas, and misregulating gene expression. Inactivation of tumor suppressor genes is central to the development of cancer. Silencing of these genes occurs by epigenetic means and inhibition of these factors lead to reversal of tumor suppressor gene silencing and inhibition of tumorigenesis (Gibbons et al., 2005).
Chemical compound acting on epigenetic control of gene expression mainly fall into two broad categories: inhibitors of DNA methyltransferases and inhibitors of histone deacetylase (HDACi). Recently, compounds regulating histone methylations have been studied. These drugs have been used in phase I and II trials in patients with hematological and solid tumor. Some of them have been approved by FDA (U.S. Food and Drug Administration) to treat hematological disorders and solid tumor.
Pharmacologic inhibition of DNA methylation causes the trapping of DNMTs and their targeted degradation results in re-expression of genes that have been aberrantly silenced by hypermethylation, concomitant with inhibition of clonal expansion and tumor cell growth, induction of cell differentiation, and cancer cell death (Issa, 2007). A number of DNA methylation inhibitors are currently under investigation, including the pyrimidine nucleoside analogs Decitabine (Dacogen, SuperGen, Inc., Dublin, CA) and Azacitidine (Vidaza, Celgene, Summit, NJ), and the nonucleoside inhibitor Hydralazine. Azacitidine and Decitabine are both approved by FDA for the treatment of a number of myelodysplastic syndrome subtypes, including refractory anemia and chronic myelogenous leukemia (CML) (Gal-Yam et al., 2008; Issa. 2007; Wong et al., 2007).
Most current DNA-demethylating agents block the action of DNA methyltransferases (DNMTs), whose expression levels are usually moderately elevated in human tumors. The genetic inactivation of two DNMTs, DNMT1 and DNMT3B, induces demethylation of all known hypermethylated tumor-suppressor genes and remarkably slow growth. DNMTs have two binding sites: one for the cytosine residue and another for S-adenosyl- methionine.

It is expected that chemicals tightly binding any of these pockets will reduce the methylation rate because of competitive inhibition. The cytidine and 2-deoxycytidine analogs are the most extensively studied members of this class. The first analog tested to determine whether it was an inhibitor of DNA methylation was 5-azacytidine (5-aza-CR), which was first synthesized almost 50 years ago. 5-azacytidine could incorporate into DNA forming covalent adducts with cellular DNMT1, thereby depleting cells from enzyme activity and causing demethylation of genomic DNA as a secondary consequence. Schneider-Stock reported that 5-aza-CR caused a marked down-regulation of DNMT1 and DNMT3A mRNA levels, in contrast to a null effect on DNMT3B (Schneider-Stock, et al., 2005). In various in vitro experiments, 5-aza-CR treatment leads to re-expression of former silenced genes. The resulting DNA hypomethylation has been linked to the induction of cellular differentiation and altered expression of genes involved in tumor suppression. It was demonstrated to have a wide range of anti-metabolic activities when tested against cultured cancer cells and to be an effective chemotherapeutic agent for acute myelogenous leukemia. Their clinical efficacy in hematological malignancies has been demonstrated in vitro and in a series of phase I and II trials. Azacitidine was first approved by FDA in 2004 for the treatment of myelodyspalstic syndrome (MDS). The phase II trials recorded complete remission (CR), partial remission (PR) and hematological improvement (HI) rates of 15%, 2% and 27%, and of 17%, 0% and 23% in the CALGB 8421 and CALGB 8921, respectively. A subsequent phase III randomized trial in 191 MDS patients reported an overall response rate of 60% on the Azacitidine arm (CR, 7%) compared with 5% of patients receiving supportive care (Silverman et al., 1993). A recent re-analysis of three CALGB trials by applying WHO classification and International Working Group (IWG) responds criteria confirmed those response figures, with 90% of patients achieving a response by six cycles; however, whereas quality of life significantly ameliorated, there was no improvement in overall survival in the whole patient population or in the separate classes of risk (Silverman et al,. 2006). Because of 5-azacytidine's general toxicity, other nucleoside analogs were favored as therapeutics. There is now a revived interest in the use of Decitabine (5-aza-2 -deoxycytidine) as a therapeutic agent for cancers in which epigenetic silencing of critical regulatory genes has occurred (Christman, 2006).

Decitabine was approved by FDA in 2006 for the treatment of MDS. It is an analog of deoxycytidine that incorporates into DNA and forms irreversible covalent bonding with DNA-methyltransferases (Mtase) at cytosine sites targeted for methylation. That leads to DNA synthesis stalling and eventual degradation of DNA-Mtase. Resumption of DNA replication in the absence of Mtase results in gene hypomethylation and reactivation of gene expression, as has been demonstrated for multiple epigenetically inactivated loci (Karpf et al., 2002; Li et al., 1999; Toyota et al., 2002). At high doses, treated cells die via apoptosis triggered by the DNA adducts and DNA synthesis arrest. By contrast, at low doses, cells survive but change their gene expression profile to favor differentiation, reduced proliferation, and/or increased apoptosis. Thus, Decitabine has potentially dual effects on treated cells. Clinical development of Decitabine was initiated more than 2 decades ago, with classical phase I studies that defined 1500 to 2250 mg/m^2 per course as the maximum tolerated dose (MTD), and demonstrated a short half-life for the drug (Santini et al., 2001). In a multicenter, phase II study, patients older than 60 years who had AML (i.e., >20% bone marrow blasts) and no prior therapy for AML were treated with Decitabine 20 mg/m^2 intravenously for 5 consecutive days of a 4-week cycle. Response was assessed by weekly CBC and bone marrow biopsy after cycle 2nd and after each subsequent cycle. Patients continued to receive Decitabine until disease progression or an unacceptable adverse event occurred. Fifty-five patients (mean age, 74 years) were enrolled and were treated with a median of three cycles (range, 1 to 25 cycles) of Decitabine. The expert-reviewed overall response rate was 25% (complete response rate, 24%). The response rate was consistent across subgroups, including in patients with poor-risk cytogenetics and in those with a history of myelodysplastic syndrome. The overall median survival was 7.7 months, and the 30-day mortality rate was 7%. The most common toxicities were myelosuppression, febrile neutropenia, and fatigue (Amanda et al., 2010). Decitabine has been used also in Imatinib-resistant CML (Issa, et al., 2005) or in combination with Imatinib in patients with accelerated or leukaemic-phase CML (Oki et al., 2007).

Several classes of HDACIs have been identified, including: (a) short-chain fatty acids (e.g., butyrates); (b) organic hydroxamic acids (e.g., TSA and hybrid polar compounds [HPCs]); (c) cyclic tetrapeptides containing a 2-amino-8-oxo 9,10-epoxy-decanoyl (AOE) moiety (e.g., trapoxin); and (d) cyclic peptides not containing the AOE moiety (e.g., FR901228, apicidin).

HDAC inhibitors (HDACIs) also impact epigenetic expression. They display ability to affect several cellular processes which are dysregulated in neoplastic cells. One of the mechanism is that HDACIs could upregulate acetylation of histones, activate tumor suppressor genes and repress oncogenes. They are potent inducers of differentiation with arrest of cells in the G1 but sometimes also in the G2 phase. They activate transcription of the cyclin-dependent kinase (CDK) inhibitor WAF1 which are responsible for cell cycle arrest and subsequent cell differentiation (Rocchi et al., 2005). Another mechanism is that they can induce apoptosis in vitro and in vivo by activating both the death-receptor and intrinsic apoptotic pathway (Nebbioso et al., 2005; Peart et al., 2005) and increase p53 acetylation diminishes Mdm2-mediated ubiquitination and the subsequent proteasome-facilitated degradation (Luo et al., 2000). In addition, HDAC inhibitors might lead to activation of the host immune response and inhibition of tumor angiogenesis by multifactorial processes.

Drugs belonging to several classes of HDACIs are in clinical trials. TSA is a fermentation product of Streptomycin with anti-fungal properties and was found to be a reversible inhibitor of HDACs in vitro, as well as in vivo. It is a highly potent HDAC inhibitor. Because of its known pharmacology, it has come to be a "reference" substance in research aimed at changing the acetylation-deacetylation state of proteins for clinical as well as research applications. Januchowski R et al. found that TSA down-regulate DNMT1 mRNA and protein expression in Jurkat T leukemia cells clone E6-1. They also observed that TSA decreased DNMT1 mRNA stability and reduced this transcript half-life from approximately 7 to 2 h. The finding suggests that TSA not only alters histone acetylation, but also may affect DNA methylation (Januchowski et al, 2007).

Vorinostat, suberoylanilide hydroxamic acid (SAHA), is an inhibitor of class I and II HDAC enzymes, promoting cell-cycle arrest and apoptosis of cancer cells (Marks et al., 2007). Relevant target genes have been characterized through gene expression analysis (Peart et al., 2005). SAHA has been shown to have clinical activity in a transgenic animal model of therapy resistant acute promyelocytic leukemia, restoring sensitivity to retinoic acid, and to induce differentiation of human breast cancer cells (He et al., 2001). It has been approved by FDA for the treatment of CTCL in 2006. In phase I clinical trials, it was demonstrated that the maximum tolerated dose was 400 mg qd and 200 mg bid for continuous daily dosing and 300 mg bid for 3 consecutive days per week dosing. Histones isolated from peripheral-blood mononuclear cells showed consistent accumulation of acetylated histones post-therapy, and enzyme-linked immunosorbent assay demonstrated a trend towards a dose-dependent accumulation of acetylated histones from 200 to 600 mg of oral SAHA. There was one complete response, three partial responses, two unconfirmed partial responses, and 22 (30%) patients remained on study for 4 to 37+ months (William et al., 2005). Phase I studies with vorinostat (SAHA) have also resulted in complete and partial responses (CRs and PRs, respectively) in both refractory solid and hematological malignancies. The major adverse events (AEs) observed with vorinostat differ by route of administration, i.v. or oral, possibly due to differences in pharmacokinetics. Oral vorinostat produced fatigue, diarrhea, anorexia and dehydration as major AEs, whereas i.v. vorinostat produced myelosuppression and thrombocytopenia as major AEs (O'Connor et al., 2006). In another phase I/II study, vorinostat was used to treat 41 patients with leukaemia or MDS who were relapsed or refractory to previous therapy or who were not candidate to chemotherapy. Hematological improvement was observed in 17% of cases including two complete responses in AML. Evidence of histone H3 acetylation was found in peripheral blood and bone marrow cells, and down-regulation of proliferation-associated genes was associated with hematological improvement (Garcia-Manero et al., 2008).

Phenylbutyrate is a fatty acid with HDACi activity that has been studied extensively in patients with solid tumors, leukemia, and myelodysplastic syndromes (MDS). Depsipetide (FK-228) is a cyclic tetrapeptide with potent HDACi activity especially of Class I HDACs. Depsipeptide also has been studied in several clinical trials.

Valproic Acid is a short chain fatty acid that is clinically used as an anticonvulsant. It has excellent bioavailability and can be given orally. Its elimination half-life is 6–17 hours. And overall, it has a good toxicity profile (Garcia-Manero G &Issa, 2005). Clinical activity has been demonstrated in studies in MDS patients who received VPA orally on a continuous schedule to maintain a serum concentration of 50–100 mg/ml. The first pilot study reported a 44% overall response rate in MDS with a median response duration of 4 months (Kuendgen et al., 2004). In a follow-up study on 122 patients with MSD and AML, an overall response rate of 20% was reported, including one CR. A higher percentage of response was observed in low-risk MDS, according to morphological subtype (Kuendgen et al., 2007). VPA has been used in combination with all-trans retinoic acid in patients with acute leukaemia, eventually in association with cytotoxic therapy, without appreciable or with only minor improvements (Raffoux et al.,2005; Pilatrino et al., 2005; Bug et al., 2005).

The field of HMTase is relatively unexplored with just a few examples of which majority are substrate analogues. The only specific inhibitor is Chaetocin, a SU(VAR)3–9 inhibitor (Greiner et al., 2005) and the documented analogue inhibitors are AMI-1, analogue inhibitor of PRMT (Cheng et al., 2004). Chaetocin killed human tumor cell lines and primary myeloma cells in vitro whereas normal human B cells were insensitive to the compound (Isham et al., 2007). We have designed siRNA segments targeting JARID1B and SU (VAR) 3–9 gene and transfected them into tumor cells. The result showed that JARID1B siRNA upregulated histone methylated H3K4 remarkbly and histone acetylation of H3 slightly. SU (VAR) 3–9 siRNA downregulated H3K9, upregulated histone acetyaltion H3. JARID1B and SU (VAR) 3–9 siRNA upregulated P27 and suppressed the proliferation in tumor cells. The expression of BCL-2, procaspase-9, procaspase-3, and C-myc decreased and cells apoptosis induced. (Cai, et al., unpublished; Ma et al., unpublished).

Sinefungin is another analogue inhibitor of Arginine methyltransferase (Amur et al., 1986). Since the role of HMTases in cancer manifestations is well established, these inhibitors will be of great use for cancer treatment. The small molecule inhibitor BIX-01294 inhibited methylation at H3K9 at several G9a-targeting genes. 3-Deazaneplanocin (DZNep) is a compound capable of depleting levels of the polycomb-recessive complex 2 (PRC2) components EZH2, SUZ12, and EED. Treatment of tumor cell lines with DZNep inhibited methylation at H3K27 but not H3K9 reactivated a series of genes that are transcriptionally repressed by PRC2 and induced potent tumor cell-selective apoptosis (Tan et al., 2007). An alternative way to reactivate epigenetically silencing genes is to inhibit the activity of histone demethylases. Recently, polyamine-based inhibitors of LSD1 have been developed that induce mono- and di-methylation at H3K4 and concomitant reactivation of previously silenced genes in treated tumor cell lines (Huang et al., 2007). The biological effects of these agents have not yet been evaluated but they represent an important step forward in the development of new agents to target the epigenetics.

Both HDAC inhibitors and DNA demethylating agents have shown clinical efficacy as single agents; yet combination of the two therapies has been shown to have strong synergistic effects on the reactivation of silenced genes and antiproliferative and cytotoxic effects on cancer cells (Bhalla et al., 2005; Glaser et al., 2007).

Combination therapies employing DNMT inhibitors and HDACIs together or with other agents are being pursued clinically. The combination of azacitidine with histone deacetylase inhibitors, such as sodium phenylbutyrate (Maslak et al., 2006), valproic acid and all-trans retinoic acid (Soriano et al., 2007), has been explored with little evidence of improvement in patients with leukaemia or high-risk MDS.

A phase I/II trial of vorinostat in combination with azacitidine (NCT00392353) are currently underway; preliminary results from phase I of the combination trial indicated that the therapy is safe and well tolerated and appears superior to azacitidine alone for time to response, overall response and CR rate (Silverman et al., 2008).

Isothiocyanates has been found potential anti-tumor agents. Natural isothiocyanates occur as thioglucoside conjugates, i.e. glucosinolate, in a wide variety of cruciferous vegetables including broccoli, cabbages, watercress, and Brussel's sprouts. The isothiocyanates (ITS) are released when the vegetables are cut or masticated. The research currently demonstrated that natural and synthetic isothiocyanates are potent cancer chemopreventive agents in a number of carcinogen-induced cancer models in rodents. The primary mechanism is the blocking of initiation of carcinogenesis via inhibiting cytochrome P450s, and inducing detoxifying enzymes to remove carcinogens (Chiao et al, 2002). We have demonstrated that Phenylhexyl isothiocyanate (PHI), one of ITC, a man-made isothiocyanate, may induce cell cycle blocking and apoptosis via altering epigenetic modification. PHI inhibited cell cycle CDK activity and up-regulated p21WAF1 (p21) in cancer cells. Exposure of HL-60 and Molt-4 leukemia cells to PHI induced G1 arrest and apoptosis. Additionally, PHI reduced the expression of HDAC and increased the level of acetyl transferase p300, in favor of accumulation of acetylated histones. Within hours, global acetylation of histones was enhanced. PHI further mediated selective alterations of histone methylation, with upregulated H3K4 and downregulated H3K9, a pattern consistent to the marks of transcription competent chromatins. ChIP assay showed that chromatins from cells exposed to PHI contained more p21 DNA in the precipitates of hyperacetylated histones, indicating more accessibility of transcription machinery to the p21 promoter after chromatin unfolding (Ma XD et al., 2006; Xiao et al., 2010). On the other hand, PHI could induce DNA demethylation in Molt-4 cells. Hypermethylation of gene p15 was reversed and activation transcription could be de novo by PHI. Hypermethylation of gene p15 was attenuated and p15 gene was activated de novo after 5 days exposure to PHI in a concentration-dependent manner(0-40μM). DNMT1 and DNMT3B were inhibited by PHI ($P<0.05$). Alteration of DNMT3A was not significant at those concentrations (Jiang et al., 2010). PHI has multi-target in epigenetic, it might represent a combination target for correcting aberrant histone acetylation, histone methylation and DNA methylation, and a promising potential epigenetic regulators for preventing the progression of leukemia.

4. Conclusion

Epigenetic disorder may be the mechanism in acute leukemia. It is now understood that deregulated epigenetic mechanisms can cause, as well as compound, the effects of oncogenic mutations to promote tumor development and growth. Epigenetic therapy is a promising approach for the prevention and treatment of malignancies. The discovery of modulators of HATs and HMTases which are highly specific may bring a new era of epigenetics based drugs.

5. References

Amour SG, Shaker G, & Cochran JM, et al. (1986). Correlation between inhibition of myelin basic protein (argentine) methyltransferase by sinefungin and lack of compact myelin formation in cultures of cerebral cells from embryonic mice. *J Neurosci Res*, vol.16, No.2, (February 1986), pp. 367–376, ISSN 0360-4012

Ayton PM, Cleary ML. (2001). Molecular mechanisms of leukemogenesis mediated by MLL fusion proteins. *Oncogene*, Vol.20, No.40, (September 2001), pp. 5695–707, ISSN 0950-9232

Ayton PM, Cleary ML. (2003). Transformation of myeloid progenitors by MLL oncoproteins is dependent on Hoxa7 and Hoxa9. *Genes Dev.* Vol.17, No.18, （September 2003）, pp. 2298–307, ISSN 0890-9369

Bannister AJ, Kouzarides T. (1996). The CBP co-activator is a histone acetyltransferase. *Nature.* Vol.19, No.384, (December 1996) , pp. 641-3, ISSN 0028-0836

Bedford MT, Richard S. (2005) . Arginine methylation an emerging regulator of protein function. *Mol Cel.* Vol.18, No.4, (April 2005), pp. 263–272, ISSN 1097-2765

Bernstein BE, Meissner A, Lander ES. (2007). The mammalian epigenome. *Cell.* Vol.128, No.4, (February 2007), pp. 263–72, ISSN 0092-8674

Bhalla KN. (2005). Epigenetic and chromatin modifiers as targeted therapy ofhematologic malignancies. *J Clin Oncol.* Vol 23, No 17, (June 2005), pp. 3971-93, ISSN 0732-183X

Biondi A., Cimino G & Pieters R, et al. (2000) Biological and therapeutic aspects of infant leukemia. *Blood.* Vol 96, No 1, (July 2000), pp. 24-33, ISSN 0006-4971

Bolden JE, Peart MJ & Johnstone RW. (2006). Anticancer activities of histone deacetylase inhibitors. *Nat Rev Drug Discov.* Vol 5, (September 2006), pp. 769–84, ISSN 1474-1776

Bug G, Ritter M & Wassmann B, et al. (2005). Clinical trial of valproic acid and alltrans retinoic acid in patients with poor risk acute myeloid leukemia. *Cancer,* Vol.104, No.12, (December 2005), pp.2717-2725. eISSN 1097-0142.

C Meyer, B Schneider & S Jakob, et al. (2006). The MLL recombinome of acute leukemias. *Leukemia.* Vol.20, No.5, (May 2006), pp. 777–784, ISSN 0887-6924

Cai LS, Ma XD & Huang YQ, et al. Study on the Effect of Suv39H1 Gene Targeting siRNA on Gastric Carcinoma. Unpublished.

Cairns BR. (2001). Emerging roles for chromatin remodeling in cancer biology.*Trends Cell Biol.* Vol.11, No.11, (November 2001), pp. S15-21, ISSN 0962-8924

Caligiuri MA, Strout MP & Gilliland DG. (1997). Molecular biology of acute myeloid leukemia. *Semin Oncol.* Vol.24, No.1, (February 1997), pp. 32-44, ISSN 0093-7754

Cameron E.E., Baylin, S.B & Herman J.G. (1999). p15(INK4B) CpG island methylation in primary acute leukemia is heterogeneous and suggests density as a critical factor for transcriptional silencing. *Blood.* Vol.94, No.7, (October 1999), pp. 2445-2451, ISSN 0006-4971

Champagne N, Bertos NR & Pelletier N, et al.(1999). Identification of a human histone acetyltransferase related to monocytic leukemia zinc finger protein. *J Biol Chem.* Vol.274, No.40, (October 1999), pp. 28528-36, ISSN 0021-9258

Chan EM, Chan RJ & Comer EM, et al.(2007). MOZ and MOZ-CBP cooperate with NF-κB to activate transcription from NF-κB-dependent promoters. *Exp Hematol* . Vol.35, No.12 , (December 2007), pp. 1782-92, ISSN 0301-472X

Cheng D, Yadav N & King RW, et al. (2004). Small molecule regulators of protein arginine methyltransferases. *J Biol Chem.*Vol.279, No.23, (Jun 2004),pp.23892-23899. ISSN 0021-9258

Chiao JW, Chung FL & Kancherla R, et al.(2002). Sulforaphane and its metabolite growth arrest and apoptosis in human prostate cancer cells. *Int J Oncol.* Vol.20, No.3, (March 2002), pp.631-636. ISSN 1019-6439

Christiansen D.H., Andersen M.K. & Pedersen-Bjergaard J. (2003). Methylation of p15INK4B is common, is associated with deletion of genes on chromosome arm 7q and predicts a poor prognosis in therapy-related myelodysplasia and acute myeloid leukemia. *Leukemia.* Vol.17, No.9 , (September 2003), pp. 1813-1819, ISSN 0887-6924

Cimino G, Lanza C & Elia L, et al. (1997). Multigenetic lesions in infant acute leukaemias: correlations with ALL-1 gene status. *Br J Haematol.* Vol.17, No.9, (February 1997), pp. 308-13, ISSN 0007-1048

Croce CM, Nowell PC. Molecular genetics of human B cell neoplasia. (1986).*Adv Immunol.* Vol.38, (1986), pp. 245-74, ISSN 0065-2776

Das PM, Singal R.(2004). DNA methylation and cancer. *J Clin Oncol.* Vol.22, No.22, (November 2004), pp. 4632-42, ISSN 0732-183X

Dhalluin C, Carlson J.E. & Zeng L, et al. (1999). Structure and ligand of a histone acetyltransferase bromodomain. *Nature,* Vol.399, (June 1999), pp. 491-496, ISSN 0028-0836

Dik WA, Brahim W, Braun C, et al.(2005). CALM-AF10+ T-ALL expression profiles are characterized by overexpression of HOXA and BMI1 oncogenes. *Leukemia.* Vol.19, No.11, (November 2005), pp. 1948-1957, ISSN 0887-6924

DiMartino JF & Cleary M L. (1999). Mll rearrangements in haematological malignancies: lessons from clinical and biological studies. *Br J Haematol.* Vol.106, No.3, (September 1999), pp.614-626, ISSN 0007-1048

E Reed-Inderbitzin, I Moreno-Miralles & SK Vanden-Eynden, et al.(2006). RUNX1 associates with histone deacetylases and SUV39H1 to repress transcription. *Oncogene*.Vol.25, No.5, (May 2006), pp. 5777–5786, ISSN 0950-9232

Esteller M.(2007) .Cancer epigenomics: DNA methylomes and histonemodification maps. Nat Rev Genet.Vol.8,No.4, (April 2007), pp. 286–98, ISSN 1471-0056

Esteller M. (2008). Epigenetics in cancer. *N Engl J Med*. Vol.358, No.3, (March 2008), pp. 1148–59, ISSN 0028-4793

Gal-Yam EN, Saito Y & Egger G, et al.(2006). Cancer epigenetics: modifications, screening, and therapy. *Annu Rev Med*. Vol.59, (February 2008), pp.267-80, ISSN 0066-4219.

Gallinari P, Di Marco S & Jones P, et al.(2007). HDACs, histone deacetylation and gene transcription: from molecular biology to cancertherapeutics. *Cell Res*.Vol.17,No.2,(Febrary 2007),pp. :195-211,ISSN 1001-0602

Gao L, Cueto MA & Asselbergs F, et al.(2002). Cloning and functional characterization of HDAC11: A novel member of the human histone deacetylase family. *J Biol Chem*.Vol.277, No.28,(July 2002),pp. 25748–25755, ISSN 0021-9258

Garcia-Manero G, Yang H & Bueso-Ramos C, et al. (2008). Phase 1 study of the histone deacetylase inhibitor vorinostat (suberoylanilide hydroxamic acid [SAHA]) in patients with advanced leukemias and myelodysplastic syndromes. *Blood*. Vol.111, No.3, (February 2008), pp.1060–1066, ISSN 0006-4971

Garcia-Manero G, Issa JP (2005). Histone deacetylase inhibitors: A review of their clinical status as antineoplastic agents. *Cancer Invest*. Vol.23, No.7, (2005), pp.635–642, ISSN 0006-4971

Glaser KB. (2007). HDAC inhibitors: clinical update and mechanism-based potential. *Biochem Pharmacol*. Vol.74, No.5, (September 2007), pp.659–671, ISSN 0006-2952.

Gibbons RJ. (2005). Histone modifying and chromatin remodeling enzymes in cancer and dysplastic syndromes. *Hum Mol Genet*. Vol.14,spec No.1, (April 2005), pp.R85–R92, ISSN 0964-6906.

Golub TR, Barker GF & Bohlander SK, et al. (1995). Fusion of the TEL gene on 12pl3 to the AML1 gene on 21q22 in acute lymphoblastic leukemia. *Proc Natl Acad Sci USA*. Vol.92, No.5, (May 1995), pp. 4917–4921, ISSN 0027-8424

Gray SG, Ekstrom TJ. (2001).The human histone deacetylase family. *Exp Cell Res*. Vol.262, No.2, (January 2001), pp. 75–83, ISSN 0014-4827

Greiner D, Bonaldi T & Eskeland R, et al.(2005). Identification of a specific inhibitor of the histone methyltransferase SU(VAR)3–9. *Nat Chem Biol*. Vol.1,No.3, (August 2005), pp.143-5, ISSN 1552-4450.

He LZ, Tolentino T & Grayson P, et al. (2001). Histone deacetylase inhibitors induce remission in transgenic models of therapy-resistant acute promyelocytic leukemia. *J Clin Invest*. Vol.108, No.9, (November 2001), pp.1321-30, ISSN 1064-3745.

Herranz M, Esteller M. (2007). DNA methylation and histone modifications in patients with cancer: potential prognostic and therapeutic targets. *Methods Mol Biol*. Vol.361, (2007), pp. 25–62, ISSN 1064-3745

Hormaeche I, Licht JD. (2007). Chromatin modulation by oncogenic transcription factors: new complexity, new therapeutic targets. Cancer Cell. Vol.11, No.6, (June 2007),pp. 474-8, ISSN 1535-6108

Huang Y, Greene E & Murray Stewart T, et al.(2007). Inhibition of lysinespecific demethylase 1 by polyamine analogues results in reexpression of aberrantly silenced genes. *Proc Natl Acad Sci USA*. Vol.104, No.19, (May 2007), pp.8023–8, ISSN 0027-8424

Ida K, Kitabayashi I & Taki T, et al. Adenoviral E1A-associated protein p300 is involved in acute myeloid leukemia with t(11;22)(q23;q13). *Blood.* Vol.90, No.12, (December 1997), pp. 4699–704, ISSN 0006-4971

Iris U, Luciano DC. (2001). Dynamics of epigenetic modifications in leukemia. *Brief Funct Genomics.* Vol.10, No.1, (January 2001), pp. 18-29, ISSN 1473-9550

Isham CR, Tibodeau & JD, et al. (2007). Chaetocin: a promising new antimyeloma agent with in vitro and in vivo activity mediated via imposition of oxidative stress. *Blood.* Vol.109, No.6, (March 2007), pp.2579–88, ISSN 0006-4971

Issa JP. (2007). DNA methylation as a therapeutic target in cancer. *Clin Cancer Res.* Vol.13, No.6, (March 2007), pp.1634–7, ISSN 1078-0432.

Issa JP, Gharibyan V & Cortes J, et al. (2005) .Phase II study of low-dose decitabine in patients with chronic myelogenous leukemia resistant to imatinib mesylate. *J Clin Oncol.* Vol.23, No.17, (June 2005), pp. 3948–56, ISSN 0732-183X

Jacobson R.H., Ladurner A.G. & King D.S., et al. (2000). Structure and function of a human TAFII250 double bromodomain module. *Science.* Vol.288, No.5470, (May 2000), pp. 1422–25, ISSN 0036-8075

Januchowski R, Jagodzinski PP. (2007). Trichostatin A down-regulates ZAP-70, LAT and SLP-76 content in Jurkat T cells. *Int Immunopharmacol.* Vol.7, No.2, (February 2007), pp.198-204, ISSN 0732-183X.

Jian Liang, Leonard Prouty & B. Jill Williams, et al. (1998), Blanchard Acute Mixed Lineage Leukemia With an inv(8)(p11q13) Resulting in Fusion of the Genes for MOZ and TIF2. *Blood.* Vol.92, No.6, (September 1998), pp. 2118-22, ISSN 0006-4971

Jiang SH, Ma XD & Huang YQ, et al. (2010). Reactivating aberrantly hypermethylated p15 gene in leukemic T cells by a phenylhexylisothiocyanate mediated inter-active mechanism on DNA and chromatin. *Journal of Hematology & Oncology*, Vol.3, (November 2010), pp.48-53, ISSN 1756-8722.

Judith K Christman.(2002). 5-Azacytidine and 5-aza-2'-deoxycytidine as inhibitors of DNA methylation: mechanistic studies and their implications for cancer therapy. *Oncogene.* Vol.21, No.35, (August 2002), pp. 5483-95, ISSN 0950-9232.

Kao H-Y, Lee C-H & Komarov A.(2002). Isolation and characterization of mammalian HDAC10: A novel histone deacetylase. *J Biol Chem* .Vol.277, No.1, (January 2002), pp.187–93, ISSN 0021-9258

Karpf AR, Jones DA. (2002). Reactivating the expression of methylation silenced genes in human cancer. *Oncogene.* Vol.21, No.35, (August 2002), pp.5496-503, ISSN 0950-9232.

Kouzarides T. (2007). Chromatin modifications and their function. *Cell.* Vol.128, No.4, (February 2007), pp. 693–705, ISSN 0092-8764

Krogan NJ, Dover J & Wood A, et al. (2003). The Paf1 complex is required for histone H3 methylation by COMPASS and Dot1p: linking transcriptional elongation to histone methylation. *Mol Cell.* Vol.11, No.3, (March 2003), pp. 721-729, ISSN 1097-2765

Kuendgen A, Strupp C & Aivado M, et al.(2004). Treatment of myelodysplastic syndromes with valproic acid alone or in combination with all-trans retinoic acid. *Blood.* Vol.104, No.5, (September 2004), pp.1266-9, ISSN 0027-8424

Kuendgen A, Gattermann N.(2007). Valproic acid for the treatment of myeloid malignancies. *Cancer.* Vol.110 ,No.5, (September 2007), pp.943-54, ISSN 1097-0142

Kumar AR, Hudson WA & Chen W, et al. (2004). Hoxa9 influences the phenotype but not the incidence of Mll-AF9 fusion gene leukemia. *Blood.* Vol.103, No.5, (March 2004), pp. 1823–8, ISSN 0006-4971

Lan F, Nottke AC & Shi Y. (2008). Mechanisms involved in the regulation of histone lysine demethylases. *Curr Opin Cell Biol* . Vol.20, No.3, (June 2008), pp. 316–25, ISSN 0955-0674

Li Q, Ahuja N & Burger PC, et al. (1999). Methylation and silencing of the Thrombospondin-1 promoter in human cancer. *Oncogene.* Vol.18, No.21, (May 1999), pp. 3284-9, ISSN 0950-9232.

Liang J, Prouty L & Williams BJ, et al. (1998). Acute mixed lineage leukemia with an inv(8)(p11q13) resulting in fusion of the genes for MOZ and TIF2. *Blood.*Vol.92, No.6, (September 1998), pp. 2118–22, ISSN 0006-4971

Lin YH, Purvi M. Kakadia & Ying Chen. (2009). Global reduction of the epigenetic H3K79 methylation mark and increased chromosomal instability in CALM-AF10-positive leukemias ，*Blood.* Vol.114, No.3, (July 2009) , pp. 651-8, ISSN 0006-4971

Littau VC, Allfrey VG & Frenster JH, et al. (1964). Active and inactive regions of nuclear chromatin as revealed by electron microscope autoradiography. *Proc Natl Acad Sci USA.* Vol.52, No.1, (July 1964), pp. 93–100, ISSN 0027-8424

Liu P, Tarle SA & Hajra A, et al. (1993). Fusion between transcription factor CBF beta/PEBP2 beta and a myosin heavy chain in acute myeloid leukemia. *Science.* Vol. 261, No.24, (September,1993), pp. 1041–4, ISSN 0036-8075

Luo J, Su F, Chen D & Shiloh A, et al. (2000). Deacetylation of p53 modulates its effect on cell growth and apoptosis. *Nature.* Vol.408, (November 2000), pp.377–81, ISSN 0028-0836

Ma XD, Han HD & HuangYQ. Study on the Effect of JARID5 Gene Targeting siRNA on HL60 cells. Unpublished.

Ma XD, Huang YQ & Xiao LY, et al. (2010). Study on aberration in histone methylation and acetylation in acute leukemia. *Chin J Hematol,* Vol.31, No.8,(August 2010), pp. 523-6, ISSN 1009-4237

Ma XD, Fang YQ & Beklemisheva A, et al. (2006) . Phenylhexyl isothiocyanate inhibits histone deacetylases and remodels chromatins to induce growth arrest in human leukemia cells. *Int J Oncol* . Vol.28, No.5, (May 2006), pp.1287-93, ISSN 1019-6439

Marks PA, Breslow R. (2007). Dimethyl sulfoxide to vorinostat: development of this histone deacetylase inhibitor as an anticancer drug. *Nat Biotechnol.* Vol.25, (January 2007), pp. 84–90, ISSN 1087-1056

Maria E. Figueroa, Sanne Lugthart & Yushan Li, et al.(2010). DNA Methylation Signatures Identify Biologically Distinct Subtypes in Acute Myeloid Leukemia, *Cancer Cell.* Vol.17, No.1, (January 2010), pp. 13–27. ISSN 1535-6108

Martin C, Zhang Y .(2005) . The diverse functions of histone lysine methylation. *Nat Rev Mol Cell Biol.*Vol.6, (November 2005), pp. 838–49, ISSN 1471-0072

Maslak P, Chanel S & Camacho LH, et al.(2006). Pilot study of combination transcriptional modulation therapy with sodium phenylbutyrate and 5-azacytidine in patients with acute myeloid leukemia or myelodysplastic syndrome. *Leukemia.* Vol.20, No.2, (February 2006), pp. 212-7, ISSN 0887-6924

Minucci S, Pelicci PG.(2006).Histone deacetylase inhibitorsand the promise of epigenetic (and more) treatments for cancer. *Nat Rev Cancer.* Vol.6, No.1, (January 2006), pp.38-51, ISSN 1474-175X

Miyoshi H, Kozu T & Shimizu K, et al. (1993). The t(8;21) translocation in acute myeloid leukemia results in production of an AML 1- MTG8 fusion transcript. *EMBO J.* Vol.12, No.7, (1993), pp. 2715-21, ISSN 0291-4189

Morales V, Richard-Foy H. (2000). Role of Histone N-Terminal Tails and Their Acetylation in Nucleosome Dynamics. *Mol Cell Biol.* Vol.20, No.19, (October 2000), pp. 7230-7, ISSN 0270-1306

Nebbioso A, Clarke N & Voltz E, et al. (2005). Tumor-selective action of HDAC inhibitors involves TRAIL induction in acute myeloid leukemia cells. *Nature Med.* Vol.11, (2005), pp. 77-84, ISSN 1078-8956

Nucifora G, Begy CR & Erickson P, et al. (1995). Fusion of the TEL gene on 12pl3 to the AML1 gene on 21q22 in acute lymphoblastic leukemia . *PROC NATL ACAD SCI USA.* . Vol.92, (May 1995), pp. 4917-21, ISSN 0027-8424

O'Connor OA, Heaney ML & Schwartz L, et al.(2006). Clinical experience with intravenous intravenous and oral formulations of the novel histone deacetylase inhibitor suberoylanilide hydroxamic acid in patients with advanced hematologic malignancies. *J Clin Oncol,* Vol.24, No.1, (January 2006), pp. 166-73, ISSN 0732-183X

Ogryzko VV, Schiltz RL & Russanova V, et al. (1996). The transcriptional coactivators p300 and CBP are histone acetyltransferases. *Cell.* Vol.87, No.5, (November 1996),pp. 953-9. ISSN 0092-8674

Oki Y, Kantarjian HM & Gharibyan V, et al. (2007).Phase II study of low-dose decitabine in combination with imatinib mesylate in patients with accelerated or myeloid blastic phase of chronic myelogenous leukemia. *Cancer.* Vol.109, No.5, (March 2007), pp.899-906, ISSN 1097-0142

Owens BM, Hawley RG.(2002). HOX and non-HOX homeobox genes in leukemic hematopoiesis. *Stem Cells.* Vol.20, No.5, (2002) ,pp. 364-79, ISSN 1066-5099

Panagopoulos I, Fioretos T & Isaksson M, et al. (2001). Fusion of the MORF and CBP genes in acute myeloid leukemia with the t(10;16)(q22;p13). *Hum Mol Genet.* Vol.10, No.4, (February 2001), pp. 395-404, ISSN 0964-6906

Peterson LF, Zhang DE. (2004). The 8;21 translocation in leukemogenesis. *Oncogene.* Vol.23, (May 2004), pp.4255-62, ISSN 0950-9232

Peart MJ, Smyth GK & van Laar RK, et al. (2005). Identification and functional significance of genes regulated by structurally different histone deacetylase inhibitors. *PROC NATL ACAD SCI USA.* Vol.102, No.10, (January 2005), pp.3697-702, ISSN 0027-8424.

Pilatrino C, Cilloni D & Messa E, et al.(2005).Increase in platelet count in older, poorrisk patients with acute myeloid leukemia or myelodysplastic syndrome treated with valproic acid and all-trans retinoic acid. *Cancer.* Vol.104, No.1, (January 2005),pp.101-9,ISSN 1097-0142

Pui CH, Chessells JM & Camitta B, et al. (2003). Clinical heterogeneity in childhood acute lymphoblastic leukemia with 11q23 rearrangements. *Leukemia.* Vol.17, (2003), pp. 700–706, ISSN 0887-6924

Pui CH, Gaynon PS & Boyett JM, et al.(2002). Outcome of treatment in childhood acute lymphoblasticleukaemia with rearrangements of the 11q23 chromosomal region. *Lancet.* Vol.359, No.9321, (June 2002), pp. 1909–1915, ISSN 0140-6736

Roman-Gomez, Roman-Gomez J & Castillejo JA, et al. (2002). 5' CpG island hypermethylation is associated with transcriptional silencing of the p21(CIP1/WAF1/SDI1) gene and confers poor prognosis in acute lymphoblastic leukemia. *Blood.* Vol.99, No.7, (April 2002), ISSN 0006-4971

Raffoux E, Chaibi P & Dombret H, et al.(2005). Valproic acid and all-trans retinoic acid for the treatment of elderly patients with acute myeloid leukemia. *Haematologica.* Vol.90, No.7, (2005); pp.986-8,ISSN 0390-8721

Regine Schneider-Stock, Mona Diab-Assef &Astrid Rohrbeck, et al. (2005). 5-aza-Cytidine Is a Potent Inhibitor of DNA Methyltransferase3a and Induces Apoptosis in HCT-116 Colon Cancer Cells via Gadd45- and p53-Dependent Mechanisms. *JPET.* Vol.312, No.2, (February 2005),pp. 525-36, ISSN 0022-3565

Rocchi P, Tonelli R & Camerin C, et al. (2005). p21Waf1/Cip1 is a common target induced by short-chain fatty acid HDAC inhibitors (valproic acid, tributyrin and sodium butyrate) in neuroblastoma cells. *Oncol Rep,* Vol.13, No.6, (June 2005),pp.1139–44,ISSN 1021-335X

Rowley JD, Reshmi S & Sobulo O, et al.(1997). AlIl patients with the T(11;16)(q23;p13.3) that involves MLL and CBP have treatment-related hematologic disorders. *Blood.* Vol.90, No.2, (July 1997), pp. 535-41, ISSN 0006-4971

Shimamoto T, Ohyashiki JH & Ohyashiki K. (2005). Methylation of p15(INK4b) and E-cadherin genes is independently correlated with poor prognosis in acute myeloid leukemia. *Leuk. Res.* Vol.29, No.6, (June 2005), pp. 653–9. ISSN 0145-2126

Silverman LR, Holland JF & Weinberg RS, et al. (1993). Effects of treatment with 5-azacytidine on the in vivo and in vitro hematopoiesis in patients with myelodysplastic syndromes. *Leukemia.* Vol.7, Suppl 1, (May 1993), pp. 21–9, ISSN:0887-6924

Silverman LR, McKenzie DR & Peterson BL, et al. (2006). Further analysis of trials with azacitidine in patients with myelodysplastic syndrome: studies 8421, 8921, and 9221 by the Cancer and Leukemia Group B. *J Clin Oncol.* Vol.24, No.24, (August 2006), pp.3895–903, ISSN 0732-183X

Silverman LR, Verma A & Odchimar-Reissig R, et al. (2008). A phase I/II study of vorinostat, an oral histone deacethylase inhibitor, in combination with azacitidine in patients with the myelodysplastic syndromes and acute myeloid leukemia(AML). Initial results of the phase I trial: a New York Cancer Consortium. J Clin Oncol. Suppl, (May 2008), 7000A, ISSN 0732-183X

Soriano AO, Yang H & Faderl S, et al. (2007). Safety and clinical activity of the combination of 5-azacytidine, valproic acid, and alltrans retinoic acid in acute myeloid leukemia and myelodysplastic syndrome. *Blood.* Vol.110, No.7, (October 2007), pp. 2302–8, ISSN 0006-4971

Taki T, Sako M & Tsuchida M, et al. (1997) .The t(11;16)(q23;p13) translocation in Myelodysplastic syndrome fuses the MLL gene to the CBP gene. *Blood.* Vol.89, No.11, (June 1997), pp. 3945–50, ISSN 0006-4971

Tan J, Yang X & Zhuang L, et al.(2007). Pharmacologic disruption of Polycombrepressive complex 2-mediated gene repression selectively induces apoptosis in cancer cells. *Genes Dev.* Vol.21, No.9, (May 2007), pp.1050–63, ISSN:0890-9369

Tatsuya Nakamura, Toshiki Mori & Shinichiro Tada, et al.(2002). ALL-1 Is a Histone Methyltransferase that Assembles a Supercomplex of Proteins Involved in Transcriptional Regulation. *Mol Cell,* Vol.10, No.5, (2002), pp. 1119–28, ISSN1097-2765

Thandla S, Aplan PD. (1997). Molecular biology of acute lymphocytic leukemia. *Semin Oncol.* Vol.24, No.1, (February 1997), pp. 45-56, ISSN 0093-7754

Toyota M, Kopecky KJ, Toyota MO, et al. (2001). Methylation profiling in acute myeloid leukemia. *Blood.* Vol.97, No.9, (May 2001), pp. 2823–2829, ISSN 0006-4971

Toyota M, Issa JP.(2002). Methylated CpG island amplifi- cation for methylation analysis and cloning differentially methylated sequences. Methods Mol Biol. Vol.200, (2002), pp.101-10, ISSN 1064-3745.

Wang GG, Allis CD & Chi P.(2007). Chromatin remodeling and cancer, Part I: Covalent histone modifications. *Trends Mol Med.* Vol.13, No.9, (September 2007), pp. 363–72, ISSN 1471-4914

Wang, J., Iwasaki & H., Krivtsov, et al.(2005). Conditional MLL-CBP targets GMP and models therapyrelated myeloproliferative disease. *EMBO J.* Vol.24, (January 2005), pp. 368–81, ISSN 0261-4189

William Kk，Owen O C & Lee Km . (2005). Phase I Study of an Oral Histone Deacetylase Inhibitor，Suberoylanilide Hydroxamic Acid，in Patients With Advanced Cancer. *J Clin Oncol.* Vol.23, No.14, (June 2005)，pp.3923–31, ISSN 0732-183X

Wong S, Weber JD. (2007).Deacetylation of the retinoblastoma tumour suppressor protein by SIRT1. *Biochem J.* Vol.407, No.3, (November 2007), pp.451–60, ISSN 0264-6021

Xiao LY, Huang YQ & Zhen RJ, et al. (2010). Deficient Histone Acetylation in Acute Leukemia and the Correction by an Isothiocyanate. *Acta Haematol.* Vol.123, No.2, (2010), pp.71–6, ISSN 0001-5792

Yi-Hui Lin, Purvi M. Kakadia & ing Chen.(2009). Global reduction of the epigenetic H3K79 methylation mark and increased chromosomal instability in CALM-AF10–positive leukemias，*Blood.* Vol.114, No.3, (July 2009), pp. 651-8, ISSN 0006-4971

Zelent A, Guidez F & Melnick A,et al. (2001). Translocations of the RARalpha gene in acute promyelocytic leukemia. *Oncogene.* Vol.20, No.49, (Octber 2001), pp. 7186-203, ISSN 0950-9232

Zhang K, Dent SY. (2005) . Histone modifying enzymes and cancer: Going beyond histones. *J Cell Biochem.* Vol.96, No.6, (December 2005), pp. 1137–48, ISSN 0730-2312

Zheng RJ, Ma XD.(2010). Study on p16, p15 p18, p19 homozygous deletion and methylation in leukemia. *Joural of Leukemia and lymphoma* .Vol.19, No.4, (April 2010), pp. 230-3, ISSN 1672-4194

Zheng RJ, Sheng SF & Shen JZ, et al. (2004). Study on p15, p16 p18, p19 methylation of INK4 series cancer inhibitive gene in leukemia. *Jornal of Fujian Medical university*. Vol.38, No.3, (March 2004), pp. 257-9, ISSN 1672-4194

Zheng RJ, Sheng SF& Shen JZ, et al.(2004). Study on p16, p15 p18, p19 homozygous deletion in leukemia. *Joural of Leukemia and lymphoma*. Vol.18, No.5, (May 2004), pp. 280-2. ISSN 1009-9921

6

The PI3K/PKB Signaling Module in Normal and Malignant Hematopoiesis

Roel Polak[1] and Miranda Buitenhuis[1,2]
[1]*Department of Hematology, Erasmus MC, Rotterdam,*
[2]*Erasmus MC Stem Cell Institute for Regenerative Medicine, Erasmus MC, Rotterdam, The Netherlands*

1. Introduction

Hematopoiesis is a complex series of events resulting in the formation of mature blood cells. This process is regulated by cytokines at various levels, including self-renewal, proliferation, and differentiation. Upon binding of cytokines to their cognate receptors, the activity of intracellular signal transduction pathways is regulated, leading to modulation of gene expression. Although our appreciation of the transcriptional regulators of hematopoiesis has developed considerably, until recently, the roles of specific intracellular signal transduction pathways were largely unknown. An important mediator of cytokine signaling implicated in regulation of hematopoiesis is the Phosphatidylinositol-3-Kinase (PI3K) / Protein Kinase B (PKB/c-Akt) signaling module (Figure 1).

The PI3K family consists of three distinct subclasses of which, to date, only the class I isoforms have been implicated in regulation of hematopoiesis. Four distinct catalytic class I isoforms have been identified; p110α, p110β, p110δ and p110γ (reviewed by Vanhaesebroeck et al., 2001). These isoforms are predominantly activated by protein tyrosine kinases and form heterodimers with a group a regulatory adapter molecules, including p85α, p85β, p50α p55α, p55γ and p101γ (reviewed by Vanhaesebroeck et al., 2001). The most important substrate for these Class I PI3Ks is phosphatidylinositol 4,5 bisphosphate (PI(4,5)P_2) which can be phosphorylated at the D3 position of the inositol ring upon extracellular stimulation, resulting in the formation of phosphatidylinositol 3,4,5 trisphosphate (PI(3,4,5)P_3) (reviewed by Hawkins et al., 2006). PI(3,4,5)P_3 subsequently serves as an anchor for pleckstrin homology (PH) domain-containing proteins, such as Protein Kinase B (PKB/ c-akt) (Burgering & Coffer, 1995). Activation of PKB requires phosphorylation on both Thr^{308}, in the activation loop, by phosphoinositide-dependent kinase 1 (PDK1) and Ser^{473}, within the carboxyl-terminal hydrophobic motif, by the MTORC2 complex that consists of multiple proteins, including Mammalian Target of Rapamycin (mTOR) and Rictor (Sarbassov et al., 2005).

PKB itself subsequently regulates the activity of multiple downstream effectors, including the serine/threonine kinase Glycogen Synthase Kinase-3 (GSK-3) (Cross et al., 1995), members of the FoxO subfamily of forkhead transcription factors FoxO1, FoxO3, and FoxO4 (Brunet et al., 1999; Kops et al., 1999) and the serine/threonine kinase mammalian target of rapamycin (mTOR) as part of the MTORC1 complex, which also includes the regulatory associated protein of mTOR (Raptor). In contrast to GSK-3 and the FoxO transcription factors that are inhibitory phosphorylated by PKB, activation of mTOR is positively regulated (Nave et al., 1999; Inoki et al., 2002). It has been demonstrated that PKB can inhibit the GTPase activating protein Tuberous sclerosis protein 2 (TSC2)/TSC1 complex, resulting in accumulation of GTP-bound Rheb and subsequent activation of mTOR (Inoki et al., 2002).

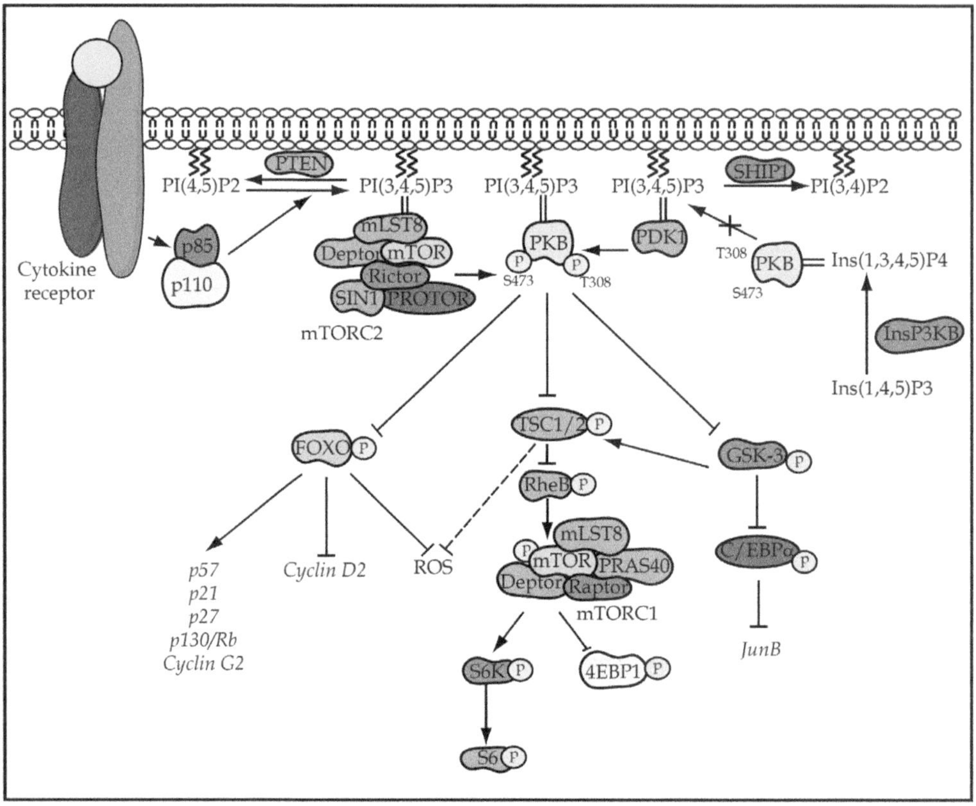

Fig. 1. *Schematic representation of the PI3K/PKB signaling module.* Activation of PI3K by receptor stimulation results in the production of PtdIns(3,4,5)P_3 at the plasma membrane. PKB subsequently translocates to the plasma membrane where it is phopshorylated by PDK1 and the mTORC2 complex. Upon phosphorylation, PKB is released into the cytoplasm where it can both inhibitory phosphorylate multiple substrates, including FoxO transcription factors and GSK-3 and induce the activity of other substrates such as mTOR as part of the mTORC1 complex. Negative regulators of the PI3K/PKB signaling module include PTEN, SHIP1 and Ins(1,3,4,5)P4.

While cytokines and growth factors positively induce PI3K activity, its activity can also be inhibited by SH2-containing inositol-5'-phosphatase 1 (SHIP1) (Damen et al., 1996), a protein predominantly expressed in hematopoietic cells (Liu et al., 1998), that hydrolyzes PIP_3 to generate PI(3,4)P_2 (Damen et al., 1996). Similarly, Phosphate and Tensin Homologue (PTEN) (Maehama & Dixon, 1998), a ubiquitously expressed tumor suppressor protein, can dephosphorylate PIP_3 resulting in the formation of $PI(4,5)P_2$ (Maehama & Dixon, 1998). Although both PTEN and SHIP1 act on the main product of PI3K activity, PIP_3, the products generated are distinct. $PI(3,4)P_2$ and $PI(4,5)P_2$ both act as discrete second messengers activating distinct downstream events (Dowler et al., 2000; Golub & Caroni, 2005) indicating that the activation of SHIP1 and PTEN not only inhibit PI3K activity, but also can re-route the signal transduction pathways activated by PI-lipid second messengers.

2. PI3K/PKB signaling and normal hematopoiesis

2.1 PI3K

The role of PI3K class I isoforms was initially examined utilizing knockout mice deficient for one or multiple regulatory or catalytic subunits. Combined deletion of p85α, p55α and p50α resulted in a complete block in B cell development (Fruman et al., 2000). Similarly, introduction of a mutated, catalytically inactive p110δ ($p110\delta^{D910A}$) in the normal p110δ locus also resulted in a block in early B cell development while T cell development was unaffected (Jou et al., 2002; Okkenhaug et al., 2002). These results indicate that PI3K activity is essential for normal B lymphocyte development. Pharmacological inhibition of PI3K activity in human umbilical cord blood derived CD34+ hematopoietic stem and progenitor cells revealed that inhibition of the activity of PI3K is sufficient to completely abrogate both proliferation and differentiation during *ex vivo* eosinophil and neutrophil development eventually leading to cell death (Buitenhuis et al., 2008). Conditional deletion of either PTEN or SHIP1 in adult HSCs resulting in activation of the PI3K pathway not only reduced the level of B-lymphocytes but also enhanced the level of myeloid cells (Helgason et al., 1998; Liu et al., 1999; Zhang et al., 2006). In addition, these mice developed a myeloproliferative disorder that progressed to leukemia (Helgason et al., 1998; Liu et al., 1999; Zhang et al., 2006). Furthermore, enhanced levels of megakaryocyte progenitors have been observed in SHIP1 deficient mice (Perez et al., 2008). In PTEN heterozygote (+/-) SHIP null (-/-) mice, a more severe myeloproliferative phenotype, displayed by reduced erythrocyte and platelet numbers and enhanced white blood cell counts including elevated levels of neutrophils and monocytes in the peripheral blood, could be observed (Moody et al., 2004). Interestingly, PI3K appears not only to be involved in lineage development, but is also required for stem cell maintenance. In PTEN and SHIP1 deficient mice, an initial expansion of HSCs could be observed which was followed by a depletion of long-term repopulating HSCs (Damen et al., 1996; Helgason et al., 2003). Recently, a shorter SHIP1 isoform (s-SHIP1), which is transcribed from an internal promoter in the SHIP1 gene, has also been implicated in positive regulation of lymphocyte development during hematopoiesis. (Nguyen et al., 2011). Its role in regulation of HSCs and long-term hematopoiesis remains to be investigated (Nguyen et al., 2011). A third negative regulator of the PI3K/PKB signaling module is Inositol 1,3,4,5-tetrakiphosphate (Ins(1,3,4,5)P4), which is generated from Inositol 1,4,5-triphosphate (Ins(1,4,5)P3) by Inositol triphosphate 3-kinase B (InsP3KB). It has been shown that Ins(1,3,4,5)P4 can bind to the PIP3-specific PH domains and competes for binding to those PH domains with PIP3 (Jia et al., 2007). In the bone marrow of mice deficient for InsP3KB, an acceleration of proliferation of the granulocyte macrophage progenitor has been observed resulting in higher levels of GMPs and mature neutrophils (Jia et al., 2008). In addition, although B lymphocytes could still be observed in InsP3KB deficient mice, mature CD4+ and CD8+ T lymphocytes were almost completely absent (Pouillon et al., 2003). Although InsP3KB is also involved in regulation of other pathways, the enhanced PKB phosphorylation in these mice (Jia et al., 2008) suggest that the observed phenotype is at least partially due to activation of the PI3K/PKB signaling module. Taken together, these studies suggest that correct temporal regulation of PI3K activity is critical for both HSC maintenance and regulation of lineage development.

2.2 PKB

PKB, an important effector of PI3K signaling, has been demonstrated to play an important role in regulation of cell survival and proliferation in a variety of systems (reviewed by Manning & Cantley, 2007). Three highly homologous PKB isoforms have been described to be expressed in mammalian cells; PKBα, PKBβ, and PKBγ. Analysis of HSCs derived from PKBα/PKBβ double-knockout mice revealed that PKB plays an important role in maintenance of long-term repopulating HSCs. These PKBα/PKBβ double-deficient HSCs were found to persist in the G_0 phase of the cell cycle, suggesting that the long-term functional defects observed in these mice were caused by enhanced quiescence (Juntilla et al., 2010). In contrast, loss of only one of the isoforms only minimally affected HSCs (Juntilla et al., 2010). In addition, analysis of mice deficient for both PKBα and PKBβ revealed that the generation of marginal zone and B1 B cells and the survival of mature follicular B cells highly depend on the combined expression of PKBα and PKBβ. Again no significant differences could be observed in mice deficient for the single isoforms (Calamito et al., 2010). In addition, ectopic expression of constitutively active PKB in mouse HSCs conversely resulted in transient expansion and increased cycling of HSCs, followed by apoptosis and expansion of immature progenitors in BM and spleen, which was also associated with impaired engraftment (Kharas et al., 2010), again demonstrating the importance of PKB in HSC maintenance. Utilizing an *ex vivo* human granulocyte differentiation system and a mouse transplantation model, it has recently been demonstrated that PKB not only plays a role in expansion of hematopoietic progenitors, but also has an important function in regulation of cell fate decisions during hematopoietic lineage commitment (Buitenhuis et al., 2008). High PKB activity was found to promote neutrophil and monocyte development and to inhibit B lymphocyte development, while conversely reduction of PKB activity is required to induce optimal eosinophil differentiation (Buitenhuis et al., 2008). In addition, PKB plays an important role in regulation of proliferation and survival of dendritic cell (DC) progenitors, but not maturation (van de Laar et al., 2010). Transplantion of mouse bone marrow cells ectopically expressing constitutively active PKB was sufficient to induce a myeloproliferative disease in most mice, characterized by extramedullary hematopoiesis in liver and spleen. In the majority of those mice, lymphoblastic thymic T cell lymphoma could also be observed. In addition, an undifferentiated AML developed in those mice that did not develop a myeloproliferative disease (Kharas et al., 2010).

2.3 Downstream effectors of PKB

To understand the molecular mechanisms underlying PKB mediated regulation of hematopoiesis, the roles of its downstream effectors in hematopoiesis have been investigated. FoxO transcription factors are known to play an important role in regulation of proliferation and survival of various cell types (reviewed by Birkenkamp & Coffer, 2003). Although proliferation and differentiation of hematopoietic progenitors appears not to be affected in FoxO3 deficient mice, competitive repopulation experiments revealed that deletion of FoxO3 is sufficient to impair long-term reconstitution (Miyamoto et al., 2007). In addition, in aging mice, the frequency of HSCs was increased compared to wild type littermate controls

(Miyamoto et al., 2007) and neutrophilia developed upon myelosuppressive stress conditions (Miyamoto et al., 2007). In contrast to FoxO3 deficient mice in which neutrophilia only occurred after myelosuppression while aging, conditional deletion of FoxO1, 3, and 4 in the adult hematopoietic system, was sufficient to increase the levels of myeloid cells and decrease the number of peripheral blood lymphocytes under normal conditions. In time, these mice developed leukocytosis characterized by a relative neutrophilia and lymphopenia (Tothova et al., 2007). In addition, an initial expansion of HSCs has been observed in these mice which correlated with an HSC-specific up-regulation of Cyclin D2 and down-regulation of Cyclin G2, p130/Rb, p27, and p21 (Tothova et al., 2007). Furthermore, a defective long-term repopulating capacity of bone marrow cells was observed, which could be explained by the reduction in HSC numbers that followed the initial expansion (Tothova et al., 2007). Although deletion of FoxO3 alone was not sufficient to improve myeloid development, ectopic expression of a constitutively active, non-phosphorylatable, FoxO3 mutant in mouse hematopoietic progenitors did result in a decrease in the formation of both myeloid and erythroid colonies (Engstrom et al., 2003), suggesting that FoxO3 does plays an important role in lineage development.

Modulation of the activity of the PI3K signaling pathway has been observed to alter the level of reactive oxygen species (ROS). While ROS levels are reduced in PKBα/β deficient mice (Juntilla et al., 2010), increased levels have been observed in mice deficient for FoxO (Miyamoto et al., 2007). Increasing ROS levels in PKBα/β deficient mice was sufficient to rescue differentiation defects, but not impaired long-term hematopoiesis (Juntilla et al., 2010). Restoring the ROS levels in FoxO deficient mice by *in vivo* treatment with an antioxidative agent N-acetyl-L-cysteine was sufficient to abrogate the enhanced levels of proliferation and apoptosis in FoxO deficient HSCs and to restore the reduced colony forming ability of these cells (Tothova et al., 2007). These studies demonstrate that correct regulation of ROS by FoxO transcription factors is essential for normal hematopoiesis.

Recent findings have demonstrated that correct regulation of the activity of GSK-3, another downstream effector of PKB, is also essential for maintenance of hematopoietic stem cell homeostasis. A reduction in long-term, but not short-term repopulating HSCs has, for example, been observed in GSK3 deficient mice (Huang et al., 2009). In addition, disruption of GSK-3 activity in mice with a pharmacological inhibitor or shRNAs has been shown to transiently induce expansion of both hematopoietic stem and progenitor cells followed by exhaustion of long-term repopulation HSCs (Trowbridge et al., 2006; Huang et al., 2009). In addition, since GSK-3 has been demonstrated to inhibit mTOR activity by phosphorylation and activation of TSC1/2 (Inoki et al., 2006) and the level of phosphorylated S6 was enhanced in cells with reduced GSK-3 levels, mice were treated with rapamycin. Rapamycin induced the number of LSK cells when GSK3 was depleted, but not in un-manipulated cells, suggesting that mTOR is an important effector of GSK-3 in regulation of HSC numbers (Huang et al., 2009) In addition to the observed expansion of HSCs in mice treated with a GSK-3 inhibitor, the recovery of neutrophil and megakaryocyte numbers after transplantation was accelerated in these mice, resulting in improved survival of the recipients (Trowbridge et al., 2006). In addition, *ex vivo* experiments revealed that GSK-3 can enhance eosinophil differentiation and inhibit neutrophil development (Buitenhuis et al., 2008). C/EBPα, a key regulator of hematopoiesis, has been demonstrated to be an important mediator of PKB/GSK-3 signaling in regulation of granulocyte development (Buitenhuis et al., 2008).

A third, important mediator of PI3K/PKB signaling is mTOR. Conditional deletion of TSC1 in mice, resulting in activation of mTOR, has been demonstrated to enhance the percentage of cycling HSCs and to reduce the self-renewal capacity of HSCs in serial transplantation assays (Chen et al., 2008). In addition, a reduction in the number of granulocytes and lymphocytes has been observed in those mice (Chen et al., 2008). As described above, activation of the PI3K signaling pathway by conditional deletion of PTEN in adult murine HSCs resulted in an initial expansion followed by exhaustion of LT-HSCs. Inhibition of mTOR in murine HSCs deficient for PTEN with Rapamycin was sufficient to revert this phenotype, again suggesting that mTORC1 signaling plays an important role in proliferation of HSCs (Yilmaz et al., 2006). A role for mTOR in progenitor expansion has been demonstrated utilizing an *ex vivo* human granulocyte differentiation system (Geest et al., 2009). In contrast to inhibition of PKB activity which not only affects progenitor expansion but also alters lineage development (Buitenhuis et al., 2008), inhibition of mTOR activity with Rapamycin only reduced the expansion of hematopoietic progenitors, during both eosinophil and neutrophil differentiation, without altering levels of apoptosis or maturation (Geest et al., 2009). Similarly, inhibition of mTOR reduced the number of interstitial DCs and Langerhans cells in *in vitro* experiments (van de Laar et al., 2010). In contrast to granulocyte development, treatment with rapamycin appears not only to affect proliferation during megakaryocyte (MK) development, but also appears to delay the generation of pro-platelet MKs (Raslova et al., 2006). Similar to FOXO transcription factors, TSC1 also appears to be involved in regulation of ROS levels in HSCs. Elevated levels of ROS have been observed in TSC1 deficient mice. *In vivo* treatment of those mice with a ROS antagonist restored HSC numbers and function (Chen et al., 2008), suggesting that TSC1 regulates HSC numbers at least in part via ROS. In addition to GSK3, the activity of C/EBPα also appears to be regulated by mTOR, albeit in a different manner. It has recently been shown that the ratio of wild type C/EBPα (C/EBPαp42) and truncated C/EBPαp30, which is generated by alternative translation initiation, is decreased by mTOR, resulting in high levels of the smaller p30 C/EBPα isoform (Fu et al., 2010) that inhibits trans-activation of C/EBPα target genes in a dominant-negative manner (Pabst et al., 2001) and binds to the promoters of a unique set of target genes to suppress their transcription (Wang et al., 2007).

3. PI3K/PKB signaling and malignant hematopoiesis

3.1 Deregulated PI3K/PKB signaling in malignant hematopoiesis

The above described studies clearly demonstrate that the PI3K/PKB signaling module plays a critical role in regulation of hematopoiesis. Since constitutive activation of PI3K and/or its downstream effectors has been observed in a high percentage of patients with hematological malignancies, it is likely that the development of leukemia may at least in part depend on aberrant regulation of this signaling module.

3.1.1 PI3K

Constitutive activation of class I PI3K isoforms has been observed in a high percentage of patients with acute leukemia (Kubota et al., 2004; Silva et al., 2008; Billottet et al., 2009; Zhao, 2010). In contrast to the expression of p110α, β and γ which is only up-regulated in leukemic blasts of some patients, p110δ expression appears to be consistently up-regulated in cells from patients with either AML or APL (Sujobert et al., 2005; Billottet et al., 2009). Activating mutations in p110α, have been detected in a wide variety of human solid tumors (Ligresti et al., 2009). The most common mutations in p110α are located in the kinase domain (H1047R) and in the helical domain (E545A) (Lee et al., 2005). The E545A mutation has also been detected in acute, but not further specified, leukemia, albeit in a very low percentage (1/88) (Lee et al., 2005). In a series of 44 pediatric T-ALL patients, activating mutations in the catalytic subunit of PI3K (PIK3CA) have been observed in 2 patients, while in frame insertions/deletions have been detected in the PI3K regulatory subunit PIK3R1 in two other patients (Gutierrez et al., 2009). Transplantation of mice with bone marrow cells ectopically expressing mutated p110α resulted in the development of a leukemia-like disease within 5 weeks after transplantation (Horn et al., 2008), suggesting that mutations in p110α would be sufficient to induce leukemia. However, since mutations in PI3K appear to be very rare, it is unlikely that these mutations would be a major cause of leukemic development. Alternatively, the constitutive activation of PI3K observed in many patients with leukemia could also be caused by either aberrant expression or activation of modulators of PI3K activity, including PTEN and SHIP1.

Reduced expression of PTEN has, for example, been observed in different types of leukemia (Xu et al., 2003; Nyakern et al., 2006). Both homozygous and heterozygous deletion of PTEN as well as non-synonymous sequence alterations in exon 7 have been detected in approximately 15% and 25% of T-ALL patients, respectively (Gutierrez et al., 2009). In contrast, analysis of both leukemic cell lines and primary AML blasts indicate that PTEN mutations are rare in AML (Aggerholm et al., 2000; Liu et al., 2000). In addition to mutations in PTEN itself, aberrant PTEN expression may also be caused by mutations in its upstream regulators. Both enhanced casein kinase 2 (CK2) expression/activity and enhanced ROS levels appear, for example, to correlate with decreased PTEN phosphatase activity in T-ALL cells (Silva et al., 2008). Both CK2 inhibitors and ROS scavengers were sufficient to restore PTEN activity and impaired PI3K/PKB signaling in those T-ALL cells, demonstrating that aberrant CK2 and ROS levels may affect PI3K signaling in leukemia (Silva et al., 2008). Another important, negative regulator of PI3K activity that has been demonstrated to play a critical role in hematopoiesis is SHIP1. Analysis of primary T-ALL cells revealed that full length SHIP1 expression is often low or undetectable. However, when using an antibody against the C terminal domain of SHIP1, low molecular weight proteins can frequently be observed. These low molecular weight proteins are thought to be the result of mutation induced alternative splicing (Lo et al., 2009). In addition, in leukemic cells from an AML patient, a mutation in the phosphatase domain of SHIP1 has also been detected which results in reduced catalytic activity and enhanced PKB phosphorylation (Luo et al., 2003). For an overview of all known mutations affecting PI3K/PKB signaling, see table 1.

3.1.2 PKB

Constitutive activation of PKB has been demonstrated in a significant fraction of AML patients (Min et al., 2003; Xu et al., 2003; Zhao et al., 2004; Grandage et al., 2005; Gallay et al., 2009). Until recently, no PKB mutations were found in patients with leukemia. However, an activating mutation in the pleckstrin homology domain of PKB (E17K) has recently been detected in solid tumors (Carpten et al., 2007). Transplantation of mice with bone marrow cells ectopically expressing this E17K mutation was sufficient to induce leukemia, ten weeks after transplantation (Carpten et al., 2007). Although this particular mutation has been observed in different types of cancer, it appears to be rare in leukemic patients. Thus far, this mutation has only been detected in one pediatric T-ALL patient (Gutierrez et al., 2009). To date, no other mutations in PKB have been described.

	Mutation	Activation/ loss	Detected in:	Location	References
Pathway					
PI3K	E545A	Activation	AML & ALL	Helical domain p110α	Lee , 2005; Horn , 2008
	E542K	Activation	#	Helical domain p110α	Horn , 2008
	H1047R	Activation	#	Kinase domain p110α	Horn , 2008
	PIK3CA	Activation	T-ALL	Catalytic subunit PI3K	Gutierrez , 2009
	PIK3R1	Deletion	T-ALL	Regulatory subunit PI3K	Gutierrez , 2009
PTEN	PTEN	Deletion	T-ALL	Homozygous and heterozygous	Gutierrez , 2009
		Dysruption	T-ALL	Sequence alterations in exon 7	Gutierrez , 2009
		Deletion	ALL cell line	Exons 2 through 5	Sakai , 1998
		Deletion	AMl cell line	Exons 2 through 5	Aggerholm , 2000
SHIP1	SHIP1	Deactivation	AML	Phosphatase domain	Luo , 2003
PKB	E17K	Activation	T-ALL	Pleckstrin homology domain	Carpten , 2007; Gutierrez , 2009
PP2A	Deletion	Deletion/Loss	AML		Cristobal , 2011
Upstream					
Flt3	Flt3-ITD	Activation	AML & ALL	Juxtamembrane (JM) domain	Reviewed by Parcells , 2006
	JM-point mutation	Less autoinhibition	AML	Juxtamembrane (JM) domain	
	AL-point mutation	Activation	AML & ALL	Activation loop (AL) of the kinase domain	
	K663Q	Activation	AML	First mutation outside JM and AL domain	
c-Kit	EC-point mutation	Activation	AML	Extracellular (EC) domain of the kinase	Yuzawa, 2007
	AL-point mutation	Activation	AML	Activation loop (AL) of the kinase domain	Reviewed by Scholl , 2008
Ras	Mutations	Activation	AML & ALL		Gutierrez , 2009; Dicker , 2010
Bcr-Abl	Translocati on	Activation	ALL	t(9;22) (q34;q11)	Clark , 1988; Varticovski , 1991

Mutation induces leukemia in mouse model.

Table 1. Mutations in the PI3K/PKB pathway.

3.1.3 Activating mutations upstream of PI3K/PKB signaling pathway

The PI3K/PKB signaling module is an important mediator of cytokine signals. In hematological malignancies, mutations in cytokine receptors have been described to affect

PI3K signaling. Constitutive activation of FMS-like tyrosine kinase 3 (FLT3), by internal tandem duplication (Flt3-ITD) (Brandts et al., 2005) and mutation in c-Kit (Ning et al., 2001) have, for example, been demonstrated to induce PKB activity. This induction of PKB activity appears to be essential for the survival and proliferation of cells expressing FLT3-ITD (Brandts et al., 2005) or mutated c-Kit (Hashimoto et al., 2003; Cammenga et al., 2005; Horn et al., 2008). In addition to these tyrosine kinase receptors, the activity of the PI3K/PKB pathway can also be enhanced by several fusion proteins, including Bcr-Abl, which can be detected in virtually all patients with CML (Ben-Neriah et al., 1986) and in patients with ALL (Clark et al., 1988). It has been demonstrated that the PI3K/PKB signal transduction pathway plays an important role in Bcr-abl mediated leukemic transformation (Varticovski et al., 1991; Skorski et al., 1997; Hirano et al., 2009). Other potential regulators of PI3K often mutated in leukemia include Ras (Rodriguez-Viciana et al., 1994; reviewed by Schubbert et al., 2007; Gutierrez et al., 2009) Evi1 (Yoshimi et al., 2011) and PP2A. In AML patients, decreased PP2A activity has, for example, been reported to correlate with enhanced levels of PKB phosphorylation on Thr308 (Gallay et al., 2009). In addition, restoration of PP2A activity also resulted in a reduction of PKB phosphorylation (Cristobal et al., 2011).

3.2 Prognosis of acute leukemia with activated PI3K/PKB signaling

As described above, the PI3K/PKB signaling module appears to be aberrantly regulated in a large fraction of patients with leukemia. Recent evidence suggests that the level of PI3K/PKB activation in leukemic blasts could be used to predict the survival rate of patients. Comparison of pediatric T-ALL patients with either no mutations in PTEN, mono-allelic mutations or bi-allelic mutations revealed that the survival rate of patients positively correlates with the level of PTEN (Jotta et al., 2010). Similar observations were made in a different cohort of pediatric T-ALL patients, in which PTEN deletions correlated with early treatment failure in T-ALL (Gutierrez et al., 2009). These studies suggest that constitutive activation of PI3K and its downstream effectors reduces the survival rate of ALL patients. To determine whether the level of mTOR activity similarly correlates with reduced survival of ALL patients, mice were transplanted with blasts from pediatric de novo B cell progenitor ALL patients. In those experiments, a rapid induction of leukemia correlated with enhanced mTOR activity in the leukemic blasts (Meyer et al., 2011). In addition to ALL, constitutive activation of PI3K, as measured by enhanced FoxO3 expression or phosphorylation, is also considered to be an independent adverse prognostic factor in AML patients (Santamaria et al., 2009; Kornblau et al., 2010). In addition, a reduced survival rate has also been observed in AML patients displaying enhanced levels of phosphorylated, and therefore inactive, PTEN (Cheong et al., 2003) and phosphorylated PKB on Serine 473 (Kornblau et al., 2006) and Threonine 308 (Gallay et al., 2009). In contrast, Tamburini *et al.* suggest that PI3K activity, as was determined by analysis of the level of phosphorylation of PKB on Ser^{473}, positively correlates with the survival of AML patients (Tamburini et al., 2007). Although the short-term survival rate (within 12 months) appeared to be slightly lower in the group displaying high PKB phosphorylation compared to the group with low levels of phosphorylated PKB, both the long-term survival and relapse free survival were significantly enhanced (Tamburini et al., 2007). Except for this last study, all other studies suggest that enhanced PI3K/PKB activity correlates with reduced survival rate in both ALL and AML patients. The molecular mechanisms underlying this reduced prognosis are, thus far, incompletely understood. However, it has been demonstrated that AML blasts

displaying enhanced PI3K/PKB activation exhibit a reduced apoptotic response (Rosen et al., 2010) which might be due to positive regulation of the anti-apoptotic NF-kB pathway and negative regulation of the P53 pathway (Grandage et al., 2005).
In addition, since PI3K has been demonstrated to induce expression of the multidrug resistance-associated protein 1 (MRP1), a member of the ATP-binding cassette (ABC) membrane transporters that functions as a drug efflux pump (Tazzari, Cappellini et al. 2007), it could also be hypothesized that constitutive activation of this signaling module results in drug-resistance. The observation that high levels of MRP1 correlates with enhanced drug resistance of AML cells and poor prognosis supports this hypothesis (Legrand et al., 1999; Mahadevan & List, 2004).

3.3 PI3K/PKB signaling as therapeutic target in acute leukemia

3.3.1 PI3K inhibitors

Since aberrant regulation of PI3K and its downstream effectors has frequently been observed in leukemic cells and are known to play a critical role in normal hematopoiesis, these molecules are considered to be promising targets for therapy (Table 2). Wortmannin and LY294002 are two well characterized inhibitors of PI3K activity that prevent ATP to bind to and activate PI3K by association with its catalytic subunit (Vlahos et al., 1994; Wymann et al., 1996). Although pre-clinical experiments indicate that both LY294002 and Wortmannin are potent inhibitors of PI3K activity, induce apoptosis in leukemic cells (Xu et al., 2003; Zhao et al., 2004) and rescue drug sensitivity (Neri et al., 2003), it has been demonstrated that both inhibitors exhibit little specificity within the PI3K family and can also inhibit other kinases, including CK2 and smMLCK, respectively (Davies et al., 2000; Gharbi et al., 2007). Since both inhibitors are also insoluble in an aqueous solution (Garlich et al., 2008; Zask et al., 2008) and are detrimental for normal cells (Gunther et al., 1989; Buitenhuis et al., 2008), different PI3K inhibitors are currently developed. Recently, while screening for inhibitors of Cyclin D expression, a novel inhibitor of PI3K activity (S14161) has been discovered that appears to be able to delay tumor growth in mice transplanted with human leukemic cell lines (Mao et al., 2011). In addition, novel inhibitors have been developed that efficiently block the activity of individual p110 isoforms. The p110δ-selective inhibitor IC87114, for example, significantly reduced proliferation and survival of AML blasts (Sujobert et al., 2005) and APL cells (Billottet et al., 2009) without affecting the proliferation of normal hematopoietic progenitors (Sujobert et al., 2005). Similar results were obtained in APL cells treated with an inhibitor directed against p110β (TGX-115) (Billottet et al., 2009).

3.3.2 PKB inhibitors

In addition to PI3K inhibitors, research has also focused on the development of pharmacological compounds that inhibit its downstream effector PKB. Perifosine, a synthetic alkylphosphocholine with oral bioavailability inhibits PKB phosphorylation by competitive interaction with its PH domalin (Kondapaka et al., 2003) and promotes degradation of PKB, mTOR, Raptor, Rictor, p70S6K and 4E-BP1 (Fu et al., 2009). *In vitro* experiments with multidrug-resistant human T-ALL cells and primary AML cells revealed that treatment with Perisofine is sufficient to induce apoptosis (Chiarini et al., 2008; Papa et al., 2008). Moreover, Perifosine reduced the clonogenic activity of AML blasts, but not normal $CD34^+$ hematopoietic progenitor cells (Papa et al., 2008). The efficacy of Perifosine in treatment of different types of leukemia is currently examined in several phase II clinical trials (NCT00391560, NCT00873457). Phosphatidylinositol ether lipid analogues (PIA) inhibit PKB activity in a similar manner compared to Perifosine. Treatment of HL60 cells with PIA resulted in inhibition of proliferation and sensitization to chemotherapeutic agents in concentrations which did not affect proliferation of normal hematopoietic progenitors (Tabellini et al., 2004). Another specific PKB inhibitor (AKT-I-1/2 inhibitor) (Bain et al., 2007), has been demonstrated to efficiently reduce colony formation in high-risk AML samples (Gallay et al., 2009). The PKB inhibitor Triciribine (API-2), a purine analog that has initially been identified as an inhibitor of DNA synthesis, inhibits PKB phosphorylation by interacting with the PH domain of PKB, thus preventing PKB membrane localization and phosphorylation (Berndt et al., 2010). Experiments in T-ALL cell lines revealed that API-2 induces cell cycle arrest and caspase-dependent apoptosis (Evangelisti et al., 2011a). The safety of this inhibitor is currently under investigation in a phase I clinical trial in patients with advanced hematologic malignancies (NCT00363454).

3.3.3 mTOR inhibitors

Rapamycin and its analogues RAD001 (everolimus), CCI-779 (temsirolimus) and AP23573 (deforolimus) inhibit the mTORC1 complex by association with FKBP-12 which prohibits association of Raptor with mTOR. (Choi et al., 1996; Oshiro et al., 2004). The efficacy of these compounds as therapeutic drugs has been examined in various preclinical and clinical studies for a wide range of malignancies (reviewed by Yuan et al., 2009; reviewed by Chapuis et al., 2010a). The anti-tumor properties of Rapamycin have also been examined in both AML derived cell lines and primary AML blasts, revealing a strong anti-tumor effect of this agent in short-term cultures (Recher et al., 2005). Furthermore, Rapamycin and its analog CCI-779 showed promising effects in preclinical models of T-ALL (Teachey et al., 2008; Meyer et al., 2011) and pre-B ALL (Teachey et al., 2006), respectively. Clinical trials initiated to examine the efficacy of Rapamycin (Recher et al., 2005) and its analog AP23573 in hematological malignancies only resulted in a partial response (Rizzieri et al., 2008). The limited therapeutic effects of Rapamycin and AP23573 may be explained by the induction of PKB activity in AML blasts treated with these compounds (Easton & Houghton, 2006; Tamburini et al., 2008; Yap et al., 2008). Furthermore, experiments with PTEN deficient mice revealed that, due to failure to eliminate the leukemic stem cell population, withdrawal of rapamycin results in a rapid re-induction of leukemia and death in the majority of mice (Guo et al., 2011). This suggests that rapamycin primarily has cytostatic, but not cytotoxic, effects on hematopoietic stem cells.

To circumvent the observed up-regulation of PKB phosphorylation by Rapamycin and its analogs, ATP-competitive mTOR inhibitors have been generated that inhibit both the activity of mTORC1 and mTORC2 (Garcia-Martinez et al., 2009; Bhagwat & Crew, 2010; Janes et al., 2010). Treatment of mice transplanted with primary ALL blasts or pre-leukemic thymocytes over-expressing PKB with the mTORC 1/2 inhibitor PP242, but not Rapamycin, significantly reduced the development of leukemia (Hsieh et al., 2010; Janes et al., 2010). Importantly, PP242 appears to induce less adverse effects on proliferation and function of normal lymphocytes in comparison to Rapamycin (Janes et al., 2010; Evangelisti et al., 2011b). In addition to PP-242, another mTORC1/2 inhibitor, OSI-027, has recently been described. (Evangelisti et al., 2011). It has been demonstrated that this inhibitor exhibits anti-leukemic effects in both Ph+ ALL and CML cells (Carayol et al., 2010). Furthermore, proliferation experiments indicate that, in comparison to Rapamycin, OSI-027 is a more efficient suppressor of proliferation of AML cell lines (Altman et al., 2011).

3.3.4 Dual inhibition of the PI3K/PKB pathway

In addition to the recently developed mTORC1/2 inhibitors, dual specificity inhibitors have been generated to further optimize inhibition of the PI3K signaling module. PI-103, a synthetic small molecule of the pyridofuropyrimidine class is, for example, a potent inhibitor for both class I PI3K isoforms and mTORC1 (Raynaud et al., 2007). PI-103 has been demonstrated to reduce proliferation and survival of cells from T-ALL (Chiarini et al., 2009) and AML patients (Kojima et al., 2008; Park et al., 2008) and appears to exhibit a stronger anti-leukemic activity compared to both Rapamycin (Chiarini et al., 2009) and the combination of RAD001 and IC87114 (Park et al., 2008). Importantly, although PI-103 reduces proliferation of normal hematopoietic progenitors, survival is not affected (Park et al., 2008). Recently, NVP-BEZ235, another dual PI3K/mTOR inhibitor has been identified. This orally bioavailable imidazoquinoline derivative, has been demonstrated to inhibit the activity of both PI3K and mTOR by binding to their ATP-binding pocket (Maira et al., 2008). In both primary T-ALL (Chiarini et al., 2010) and AML cells (Chapuis, Tamburini et al. 2010b) as well as leukemic cell lines, NVP-BEZ235 significantly reduced proliferation and survival (Chapuis et al., 2010b; Chiarini et al., 2010). Furthermore, this compound did not affect the clonogenic capacity of normal hematopoietic progenitors (Chapuis et al., 2010b). A dual PI3K/PDK1 inhibitor called BAG956 has also recently been described to inhibit proliferation of BCR-ABL and FLT3-ITD expressing cells. However, in contrast to RAD001 which efficiently reduced the tumor load in mice transplanted with BCR-ABL expressing cells, treatment with BAG956 alone was not sufficient to reduce the tumor load (Weisberg et al., 2008). In addition to these dual inhibitors, KP372-1, a multiple kinase inhibitor capable of inhibiting PKB, PDK1, and FLT3 has been described (Zeng et al., 2006). It has been demonstrated that KP372-1 can induce apoptosis in primary AML cells and leukemic cell lines, as was visualized by mitochondrial depolarization and phosphatidylserine externalization (Zeng et al., 2006). Although the survival of normal hematopoietic progenitors was not impaired by this compound, their clonogenic capacity was, albeit with a low efficiency (Zeng et al., 2006).

In addition to the above described dual inhibitors, the efficacy of combination therapy utilizing multiple inhibitors, which are directed against different intermediates of the PI3K signaling module, is also under investigation. To abrogate the RAD001 mediated up-regulation of PKB phosphorylation, the p110δ inhibitor IC87114 has, for example, been added to leukemic cells simultaneously with RAD001. Combined inhibition of mTOR and p110δ not only resulted in a block in PKB phosphorylation in primary AML blasts, but a synergistic reduction in proliferation could also be observed (Tamburini et al., 2008). Similarly, combining the PI3K/PDK1 inhibitor BAG956 with RAD001 also resulted in a synergistic reduction in tumor volume in a mouse model transplanted with BCR-ABL expressing cells (Weisberg et al., 2008). Recently, a phase I trial focusing on development of a combination regimen including both perifosine and UCN-01 (NCT00301938), a PDK1 inhibitor which is known to induce apoptosis in AML cells *in vitro* (Hahn et al., 2005), has been initiated.

3.3.5 Combination of PI3K/PKB pathway inhibitors with other pathway inhibitors

Leukemogenesis involves aberrant regulation of various signal transduction pathways, including, but not limited to, the PI3K signaling module. Simultaneous targeting of multiple

Target	Compound	Effect		Clinical Trials (phase)	Leukemia	References
		In vitro	*In vivo*			
PI3K	Wortmannin	+	-	-		Wymann , 1996
	LY294002	+	-	-		Xu , 2003; Zhao , 2004
	S14161	+	+	-		Mao , 2011
p110β	TGX-115	+	-	-		Billottet , 2009
p110δ	IC87114	+	-	-		Sujobert , 2005; Billottet , 2006, 2009
	AMG 319	-	-	NCT01300026 (I)	ALL	
PDK1	UCN-01	+	-	-		Hahn , 2005
PKB	Perifosine	+	-	NCT00391560 (II)	AML&ALL	Chiarini , 2008; Fu , 2009; Papa , 2008
				NCT00873457 (II)	CLL	
	PIA	+	-	-		Tabellini , 2004
	AKT-I-1/2	+	-	-		Gallay , 2009
	Triciribine (API-2)	+	-	NCT00363454 (I)	-	Evangelisti , 2011a
	GSK690693	+	-	NCT00666081 (I)	AML&ALL	Levy , 2009
	MK2206	-	-	NCT01231919 (I)	AML&ALL	
				NCT01253447 (II)	AML	
	SR13668	-	-	NCT00896207 (I)	-	
	GSK2141795	-	-	NCT00920257 (I)	-	
	GSK2111018 3	-	-	NCT00881946 (I/II)	AML&ALL	
mTOR	Rapamycin	+	+	NCT00795886 (I)	ALL	Recher 2005; Meyer , 2011;
						Teachey , 2008; Gu , 2010; Guo , 2011
	RAD001	+	+	Yee, 2006 (I/II)	AML	Yee , 2006
	CCI-779	+	+	Recher, 2005 (II)	AML	Teachey , 2006; Recher, 2005
	AP23573	-	-	Rizzieri, 2008 (II)	AML	Rizzieri, 2008
				NCT00086125 (II)	AML&ALL	
	PP242	+	+	-		Hsieh , 2010; Janes , 2010; Evangelisti , 2011b
	OSI-027	+	-	-		Evangelisti, 2011b ; Carayol, 2010; Altman, 2011
	AZD-8050	+	-	-	-	Evangelisti , 2011b
PI3K/mTOR	PI-103	+	+	-	-	Chiarini , 2009; Kojima , 2008; Park , 2008
PI3K/mTOR	NVP-BEZ235	+	+	-	-	Maira , 2008; Chiarini , 2010; Chapuis , 2010b
PI3K/PDK1	BAG956	+	+	-	-	Weisberg , 2008
PKB/PDK1/Flt3	KP372-1	+	-	-	-	Zeng , 2006

Table 2. Inhibitors of PI3K/PKB signaling pathway

aberrantly regulated signal transduction pathways is considered to be a promising therapeutic strategy (Table 3). Proteosome inhibitors are considered to be a new class of therapeutic agents. However, treatment of both pediatric and adult B-ALL patients with such an inhibitor (Bortezomib) alone was not sufficient to induce a robust anti-tumor response (Cortes et al., 2004; Horton et al., 2007). Experiments in leukemic cell lines and primary cells from B-ALL patients revealed that while MG132, a proteosome inhibitor, and RAD001 alone only modestly reduce cell viability, combined inhibition of proteosomes and mTOR significantly enhanced cell death (Saunders et al., 2011), suggesting a synergistic effect of both inhibitors. In addition to proteosome inhibitors, HDAC inhibitors have also emerged as a promising class of anti-tumor agents (reviewed by Minucci & Pelicci, 2006). Although the HDAC inhibitor MS-275 appears to induce growth arrest, apoptosis and differentiation of leukemic cell lines, in mouse models only a partial reduction in tumor volume could be observed (Nishioka et al., 2008). Combined administration of MS-275 and RAD001, however, potentiated the effect of both inhibitors individually both *in vitro* and *in vivo* (Nishioka et al., 2008). Synergistic effects on proliferation and survival of leukemic cell lines have also been observed after co-administration of HDAC inhibitors and the PKB inhibitor Perisofine (Rahmani et al., 2005). Additionally, the efficacy of specific inhibitors targeting constitutively activated tyrosine kinases in leukemia, including inhibitors of Flt3, Abl, and c-Kit, has been investigated in preclinical and clinical models. Although anti-leukemia effects were observed *in vivo* and *in vitro*, combined inhibition of tyrosine kinases and the PI3K/PKB pathway resulted in a synergistically enhanced anti-leukemia effect in ALL (Kharas et al., 2008; Weisberg et al., 2008) and AML (Weisberg et al., 2008) compared to the individual inhibitors. Phase I/II clinical trials have already been initiated to investigate the synergistic effects of combined inhibition of PI3K/PKB and Flt3 (NCT00819546) or c-Kit (NCT00762632).

3.3.6 Combination of PI3K/PKB pathway inhibitors with chemotherapeutical agents

Despite the effectiveness of chemotherapy in a subset of patients, incomplete remission and the development of a refractory disease have been observed in many patients with acute leukemia (Thomas, 2009; Burnett et al., 2011). To optimize treatment of those patients, chemotherapy could potentially be combined with leukemia-specific inhibitors or chemosensitizing drugs (Table 3). Co-administration of mTOR inhibitors with different types of chemotherapeutic drugs, including Etoposide, Ara-C, Cytarabine and Dexamethason has, for example, been demonstrated to induce synergistic anti-leukemia effects in cells from AML patients (Xu et al., 2003; Xu et al., 2005) and ALL patients (Avellino et al., 2005; Teachey et al., 2008; Bonapace et al., 2010; Gu et al., 2010; Saunders et al., 2011). Several phase I/II clinical trials have been initiated to investigate and optimize the synergistic effect of mTOR inhibitors and chemotherapeutic drugs in patients with acute leukemia (NCT00544999, NCT01184898, NCT00780104, NCT01162551 and NCT00776373). In addition, co-administration of chemotherapeutic agents with IC87114 (Billottet et al., 2006), UCN-01 (Sampath et al., 2006) or Triciribine (Evangelisti et al., 2011a) showed similar synergistic effects in AML cells. Strong synergistic, cytotoxic, activity was also observed in T-ALL cells when combining the dual specificity inhibitors PI-103 and NVP-BEZ235 with chemotherapy (Chiarini et al., 2009; Chiarini et al., 2010).

Target	Compound	Combination regimens	Effects *in vitro*/	*in vivo*	Clinical trials (phase)	Leukemia	References
PI3K	Wortmannin	ATRA (DA)	+	-	-		Neri , 2003
	LY294002	Apigenin (CK2 I)	+	-	-		Cheong , 2010
		ATRA (DA)	+	-	-		Neri , 2003
p110δ	IC87114	VP16 (CT)	+	-	-		Billottet , 2006
PDK1	UCN-01	Ara-c (CT)	+	-	Sampath, 2006 (II)	AML	Sampath , 2006
		Cytarabine (CT)	-	-	NCT00004263 (I)	AML	
		Fludarabine (CT)	-	-	NCT00019838 (I)	AML&ALL	
PP2A	Forskolin	Idarubicine/Ara-C	+	-	-		Cristobal , 2011
PKB	Perifosine	UCN-01	-	-	NCT00301938 (I)	AML&ALL	
		HDAC I	+	-	-		Rahmani , 2005
		TRAIL (AI)	+	-	-		Tazzari , 2008
		Etoposide (CT	+	-	-		Papa , 2008
	PIA	CT	+	-	-		Tabellini , 2004
	Triciribine	Cytarabine (CT)	+	-	-		Evangelisti , 2011a
mTOR	Rapamycin	UCN-01	+	-	-		Hahn , 2005
		3-BrOP (glycolysis I)	+	-	-		Akers , 2011
		Notch I	+	-	-		Chan , 2007
		Dexamethason	+	-	-		Gu, 2010; Bonapace , 2010
		Etoposide (CT)	+	+	-		Xu , 2005
		Methotrexate (CT)	+	+	NCT01162551 (II)	ALL	Teachey , 2008
		Anthracyclin (CT)	+	-	-		Avellino , 2005
		CT	+	-	NCT00776373 (I/II)	ALL	
			+	-	NCT01184898 (I/II)	AML	
					NCT00780104 (I/II)	AML	
	RAD001	IC87114	+	-	-		Tamburini , 2008
		BAG956	+	+	-		Weisberg , 2008
		Bortezomib (PI)	+	-	-		Saunders , 2011
		MS-275 (HDAC I)	+	+	-		Nishioka , 2008
		PKC412 (Flt3 TKI)	-	-	NCT00819546 (I)	AML	
		Nilotinib (c-Kit-TKI)	-	-	NCT00762632 (I/II)	AML	
		ATRA (DA)	+	+	-		Nishioko , 2009
		Ara-c (CT)	+	-	-		Xu , 2003; Saunders , 2011
		Vincristine (CT)	+	-	-	ALL	Crazzolara, 2009
		CT	+	-	NCT00544999 (I)	AML&ALL	
	CCI-779	Methotrexate (CT)	+	+	-		Teachey , 2008
	PP242	Vincristine (CT)	+	-			Evangelisti , 2011b
PI3K/mTOR	PI-103	Nutlin-3 (MDM2-I)	+	-			Kojima , 2008
		Vincristine (CT)	+	-			Chiarini , 2009
		Imatinib (Bcr-Abl-TKI)	+	-			Kharas , 2008
PI3K/mTOR	NVP-BEZ235	CT	+	-			Chiarini , 2010
PI3K/PDK1	BAG956	Imatinib (Bcr-Abl-TKI)	+	+			Weisberg , 2008
		PKC412 (Flt3 TKI)	+	+			Weisberg , 2008

DA: Differentiating agents; I: Inhibitor; CT: Chemotherapy; AI: Apoptosis inducer; PI: Proteasome inhibitor; TKI: Tyrosine kinase inhibitor.

Table 3. Combination regimens.

4. Conclusion

During the last two decades, it has become clear that intracellular signal transduction pathways play an important role in both normal and malignant hematopoiesis. One such module implicated in playing a critical role in regulation of various hematopoietic processes includes PI3K and PKB. Aberrant regulation of these molecules appears to be sufficient to induce hematological malignancies. As discussed in this chapter, constitutive activation of this signaling module has been observed in a large group of acute leukemia's. Although activating mutations in PI3K and PKB have been detected in cells from patients with leukemia, these mutations appear to be very rare. In patients, mutations have also been observed in PTEN and SHIP1 resulting in activation of PI3K and its downstream effectors. These mutations, however, cannot account for the large incidence of constitutive activation of PI3K in patients with leukemia. Alternatively, constitutive activation of PI3K and PKB can also be induced by mutations in, for example, tyrosine kinase receptors and by translocation induced formation of fusion proteins. Since PI3K is frequently activated in leukemia and activation of this molecule is thought to correlate with poor prognosis and drug resistance, it is considered to be a promising target for therapy. A high number of pharmacological inhibitors directed against both individual and multiple components of this pathway has already been developed in order to improve therapy. Especially the dual specificity inhibitors seem to possess promising anti-leukemic activities. In addition, research currently focuses on combining inhibitors of the PI3K signaling module with either inhibitors directed against other signal transduction molecules or classic chemotherapy. Mouse models and in vitro experiments indicate that both strategies could be used to improve current therapeutic regimes in specific patient groups. To confirm the pre-clinical data and to examine the safety and efficacy of the individual inhibitors and combination regimes in patients with leukemia, several phase I and II clinical trials have already been initiated.

5. Acknowledgements

R. Polak was supported by a grant from KiKa (Children Cancer free).

6. References

Aggerholm, A.,K. Gronbaek, et al. (2000). Mutational analysis of the tumour suppressor gene MMAC1/PTEN in malignant myeloid disorders. *European Journal of Haematology*, Vol.65, No.2, pp. 109-113, ISSN 0902-4441

Akers, L. J.,W. Fang, et al. (2011). Targeting glycolysis in leukemia: A novel inhibitor 3-BrOP in combination with rapamycin. *Leukemia Research*, pp. ISSN 1873-5835

Altman, J. K.,A. Sassano, et al. (2011). Dual mTORC2/mTORC1 targeting results in potent suppressive effects on acute myeloid leukemia (AML) progenitors. *Clinical Cancer Research*, pp. ISSN 1078-0432

Avellino, R.,S. Romano, et al. (2005). Rapamycin stimulates apoptosis of childhood acute lymphoblastic leukemia cells. *Blood*, Vol.106, No.4, pp. 1400-1406, ISSN 0006-4971

Bain, J.,L. Plater, et al. (2007). The selectivity of protein kinase inhibitors: a further update. *The Biochemical Journal*, Vol.408, No.3, pp. 297-315, ISSN 1470-8728

Ben-Neriah, Y.,G. Q. Daley, et al. (1986). The chronic myelogenous leukemia-specific P210 protein is the product of the bcr/abl hybrid gene. *Science*, Vol.233, No.4760, pp. 212-214, ISSN 0036-8075

Berndt, N.,H. Yang, et al. (2010). The Akt activation inhibitor TCN-P inhibits Akt phosphorylation by binding to the PH domain of Akt and blocking its recruitment to the plasma membrane. *Cell Death and Differentiation*, Vol.17, No.11, pp. 1795-1804, ISSN 1476-5403

Bhagwat, S. V. and A. P. Crew. (2010). Novel inhibitors of mTORC1 and mTORC2. *Current Opinion in Investigational Drugs*, Vol.11, No.6, pp. 638-645, ISSN 2040-3429

Billottet, C.,L. Banerjee, et al. (2009). Inhibition of class I phosphoinositide 3-kinase activity impairs proliferation and triggers apoptosis in acute promyelocytic leukemia without affecting atra-induced differentiation. *Cancer Research*, Vol.69, No.3, pp. 1027-1036, ISSN 1538-7445

Billottet, C.,V. L. Grandage, et al. (2006). A selective inhibitor of the p110delta isoform of PI 3-kinase inhibits AML cell proliferation and survival and increases the cytotoxic effects of VP16. *Oncogene*, Vol.25, No.50, pp. 6648-6659, ISSN 0950-9232

Birkenkamp, K. U. and P. J. Coffer. (2003). FOXO transcription factors as regulators of immune homeostasis: molecules to die for? *Journal of Immunology*, Vol.171, No.4, pp. 1623-1629, ISSN 0022-1767

Bonapace, L.,B. C. Bornhauser, et al. (2010). Induction of autophagy-dependent necroptosis is required for childhood acute lymphoblastic leukemia cells to overcome glucocorticoid resistance. *Journal of Clinical Investigation*, Vol.120, No.4, pp. 1310-1323, ISSN 1558-8238

Brandts, C. H.,B. Sargin, et al. (2005). Constitutive activation of Akt by Flt3 internal tandem duplications is necessary for increased survival, proliferation, and myeloid transformation. *Cancer Research*, Vol.65, No.21, pp. 9643-9650, ISSN 0008-5472

Brunet, A.,A. Bonni, et al. (1999). Akt promotes cell survival by phosphorylating and inhibiting a Forkhead transcription factor. *Cell*, Vol.96, No.6, pp. 857-868, ISSN 0092-8674

Buitenhuis, M.,L. P. Verhagen, et al. (2008). Protein kinase B (c-akt) regulates hematopoietic lineage choice decisions during myelopoiesis. *Blood*, Vol.111, No.1, pp. 112-121, ISSN 0006-4971

Burgering, B. M. and P. J. Coffer. (1995). Protein kinase B (c-Akt) in phosphatidylinositol-3-OH kinase signal transduction. *Nature*, Vol.376, No.6541, pp. 599-602, ISSN 0028-0836

Burnett, A.,M. Wetzler, et al. (2011). Therapeutic advances in acute myeloid leukemia. *Journal of Clinical Oncology*, Vol.29, No.5, pp. 487-494, ISSN 1527-7755

Calamito, M.,M. M. Juntilla, et al. (2010). Akt1 and Akt2 promote peripheral B-cell maturation and survival. *Blood*, Vol.115, No.20, pp. 4043-4050, ISSN 1528-0020

Cammenga, J.,S. Horn, et al. (2005). Extracellular KIT receptor mutants, commonly found in core binding factor AML, are constitutively active and respond to imatinib mesylate. *Blood*, Vol.106, No.12, pp. 3958-3961, ISSN 0006-4971

Carayol, N.,E. Vakana, et al. (2010). Critical roles for mTORC2- and rapamycin-insensitive mTORC1-complexes in growth and survival of BCR-ABL-expressing leukemic cells. *Proceedings of the National Academy of Sciences of the United States of America*, Vol.107, No.28, pp. 12469-12474, ISSN 1091-6490

Carpten, J. D.,A. L. Faber, et al. (2007). A transforming mutation in the pleckstrin homology domain of AKT1 in cancer. *Nature*, Vol.448, No.7152, pp. 439-444, ISSN 1476-4687

Chan, S. M.,A. P. Weng, et al. (2007). Notch signals positively regulate activity of the mTOR pathway in T-cell acute lymphoblastic leukemia. *Blood*, Vol.110, No.1, pp. 278-286, ISSN 0006-4971

Chapuis, N.,J. Tamburini, et al. (2010)a. Perspectives on inhibiting mTOR as a future treatment strategy for hematological malignancies. *Leukemia*, Vol.24, No.10, pp. 1686-1699, ISSN 1476-5551

Chapuis, N.,J. Tamburini, et al. (2010)b. Dual inhibition of PI3K and mTORC1/2 signaling by NVP-BEZ235 as a new therapeutic strategy for acute myeloid leukemia. *Clinical Cancer Research*, Vol.16, No.22, pp. 5424-5435, ISSN 1078-0432

Chen, C.,Y. Liu, et al. (2008). TSC-mTOR maintains quiescence and function of hematopoietic stem cells by repressing mitochondrial biogenesis and reactive oxygen species. *The Journal of Experimental Medicine*, Vol.205, No.10, pp. 2397-2408, ISSN 1540-9538

Cheong, J. W.,J. I. Eom, et al. (2003). Phosphatase and tensin homologue phosphorylation in the C-terminal regulatory domain is frequently observed in acute myeloid leukaemia and associated with poor clinical outcome. *British Journal of Haematology*, Vol.122, No.3, pp. 454-456, ISSN 0007-1048

Cheong, J. W.,Y. H. Min, et al. (2010). Inhibition of CK2{alpha} and PI3K/Akt synergistically induces apoptosis of CD34+CD38- leukaemia cells while sparing haematopoietic stem cells. *Anticancer Research*, Vol.30, No.11, pp. 4625-4634, ISSN 1791-7530

Chiarini, F.,M. Del Sole, et al. (2008). The novel Akt inhibitor, perifosine, induces caspase-dependent apoptosis and downregulates P-glycoprotein expression in multidrug-resistant human T-acute leukemia cells by a JNK-dependent mechanism. *Leukemia*, Vol.22, No.6, pp. 1106-1116, ISSN 1476-5551

Chiarini, F.,F. Fala, et al. (2009). Dual inhibition of class IA phosphatidylinositol 3-kinase and mammalian target of rapamycin as a new therapeutic option for T-cell acute lymphoblastic leukemia. *Cancer Research*, Vol.69, No.8, pp. 3520-3528, ISSN 1538-7445

Chiarini, F.,C. Grimaldi, et al. (2010). Activity of the novel dual phosphatidylinositol 3-kinase/mammalian target of rapamycin inhibitor NVP-BEZ235 against T-cell acute lymphoblastic leukemia. *Cancer Research*, Vol.70, No.20, pp. 8097-8107, ISSN 1538-7445

Choi, J.,J. Chen, et al. (1996). Structure of the FKBP12-rapamycin complex interacting with the binding domain of human FRAP. *Science*, Vol.273, No.5272, pp. 239-242, ISSN 0036-8075

Clark, S. S.,J. McLaughlin, et al. (1988). Expression of a distinctive BCR-ABL oncogene in Ph1-positive acute lymphocytic leukemia (ALL). *Science*, Vol.239, No.4841 Pt 1, pp. 775-777, ISSN 0036-8075

Cortes, J.,D. Thomas, et al. (2004). Phase I study of bortezomib in refractory or relapsed acute leukemias. *Clinical Cancer Research*, Vol.10, No.10, pp. 3371-3376, ISSN 1078-0432

Crazzolara, R.,A. Cisterne, et al. (2009). Potentiating effects of RAD001 (Everolimus) on vincristine therapy in childhood acute lymphoblastic leukemia. *Blood*, Vol.113, No.14, pp. 3297-3306, ISSN 1528-0020

Cristobal, I.,L. Garcia-Orti, et al. (2011). PP2A impaired activity is a common event in acute myeloid leukemia and its activation by forskolin has a potent anti-leukemic effect. *Leukemia*, pp. ISSN 1476-5551

Cross, D. A.,D. R. Alessi, et al. (1995). Inhibition of glycogen synthase kinase-3 by insulin mediated by protein kinase B. *Nature*, Vol.378, No.6559, pp. 785-789, ISSN 0028-0836

Damen, J. E.,L. Liu, et al. (1996). The 145-kDa protein induced to associate with Shc by multiple cytokines is an inositol tetraphosphate and phosphatidylinositol 3,4,5-triphosphate 5-phosphatase. *Proceedings of the National Academy of Sciences of the United States of America*, Vol.93, No.4, pp. 1689-1693, ISSN 0027-8424

Davies, S. P.,H. Reddy, et al. (2000). Specificity and mechanism of action of some commonly used protein kinase inhibitors. *The Biochemical Journal*, Vol.351, No.Pt 1, pp. 95-105, ISSN 0264-6021

Dowler, S.,R. A. Currie, et al. (2000). Identification of pleckstrin-homology-domain-containing proteins with novel phosphoinositide-binding specificities. *The Biochemical Journal*, Vol.351, No.Pt 1, pp. 19-31, ISSN 0264-6021

Easton, J. B. and P. J. Houghton. (2006). mTOR and cancer therapy. *Oncogene*, Vol.25, No.48, pp. 6436-6446, ISSN 0950-9232

Engstrom, M.,R. Karlsson, et al. (2003). Inactivation of the forkhead transcription factor FoxO3 is essential for PKB-mediated survival of hematopoietic progenitor cells by kit ligand. *Experimental Hematology*, Vol.31, No.4, pp. 316-323, ISSN 0301-472X

Evangelisti, C.,F. Ricci, et al. (2011)a. Preclinical testing of the Akt inhibitor triciribine in T-cell acute lymphoblastic leukemia. *Journal of Cellular Physiology*, Vol.226, No.3, pp. 822-831, ISSN 1097-4652

Evangelisti, C.,F. Ricci, et al. (2011)b. Targeted inhibition of mTORC1 and mTORC2 by active-site mTOR inhibitors has cytotoxic effects in T-cell acute lymphoblastic leukemia. *Leukemia*, pp. ISSN 1476-5551

Fruman, D. A.,F. Mauvais-Jarvis, et al. (2000). Hypoglycaemia, liver necrosis and perinatal death in mice lacking all isoforms of phosphoinositide 3-kinase p85 alpha. *Nature Genetics*, Vol.26, No.3, pp. 379-382, ISSN 1061-4036

Fu, C. T.,K. Y. Zhu, et al. (2010). An evolutionarily conserved PTEN-C/EBPalpha-CTNNA1 axis controls myeloid development and transformation. *Blood*, Vol.115, No.23, pp. 4715-4724, ISSN 1528-0020

Fu, L.,Y. A. Kim, et al. (2009). Perifosine inhibits mammalian target of rapamycin signaling through facilitating degradation of major components in the mTOR axis and induces autophagy. *Cancer Research*, Vol.69, No.23, pp. 8967-8976, ISSN 1538-7445

Gallay, N.,C. Dos Santos, et al. (2009). The level of AKT phosphorylation on threonine 308 but not on serine 473 is associated with high-risk cytogenetics and predicts poor overall survival in acute myeloid leukaemia. *Leukemia*, Vol.23, No.6, pp. 1029-1038, ISSN 1476-5551

Garcia-Martinez, J. M.,J. Moran, et al. (2009). Ku-0063794 is a specific inhibitor of the mammalian target of rapamycin (mTOR). *The Biochemical Journal*, Vol.421, No.1, pp. 29-42, ISSN 1470-8728

Garlich, J. R.,P. De, et al. (2008). A vascular targeted pan phosphoinositide 3-kinase inhibitor prodrug, SF1126, with antitumor and antiangiogenic activity. *Cancer Research*, Vol.68, No.1, pp. 206-215, ISSN 1538-7445

Geest, C. R.,F. J. Zwartkruis, et al. (2009). Mammalian target of rapamycin activity is required for expansion of CD34+ hematopoietic progenitor cells. *Haematologica*, Vol.94, No.7, pp. 901-910, ISSN 1592-8721

Gharbi, S. I.,M. J. Zvelebil, et al. (2007). Exploring the specificity of the PI3K family inhibitor LY294002. *The Biochemical Journal*, Vol.404, No.1, pp. 15-21, ISSN 1470-8728

Golub, T. and P. Caroni. (2005). PI(4,5)P2-dependent microdomain assemblies capture microtubules to promote and control leading edge motility. *Journal of Cell Biology*, Vol.169, No.1, pp. 151-165, ISSN 0021-9525

Grandage, V. L.,R. E. Gale, et al. (2005). PI3-kinase/Akt is constitutively active in primary acute myeloid leukaemia cells and regulates survival and chemoresistance via NF-kappaB, Mapkinase and p53 pathways. *Leukemia*, Vol.19, No.4, pp. 586-594, ISSN 0887-6924

Gu, L.,C. Zhou, et al. (2010). Rapamycin sensitizes T-ALL cells to dexamethasone-induced apoptosis. *Journal of Experimental & Clinical Cancer Research*, Vol.29, pp. 150, ISSN 1756-9966

Gunther, R.,H. K. Abbas, et al. (1989). Acute pathological effects on rats of orally administered wortmannin-containing preparations and purified wortmannin from Fusarium oxysporum. *Food and Chemical Toxicology*, Vol.27, No.3, pp. 173-179, ISSN 0278-6915

Guo, W.,S. Schubbert, et al. (2011). Suppression of leukemia development caused by PTEN loss. *Proceedings of the National Academy of Sciences of the United States of America*, Vol.108, No.4, pp. 1409-1414, ISSN 1091-6490

Gutierrez, A.,T. Sanda, et al. (2009). High frequency of PTEN, PI3K, and AKT abnormalities in T-cell acute lymphoblastic leukemia. *Blood*, Vol.114, No.3, pp. 647-650, ISSN 1528-0020

Hahn, M.,W. Li, et al. (2005). Rapamycin and UCN-01 synergistically induce apoptosis in human leukemia cells through a process that is regulated by the Raf-1/MEK/ERK, Akt, and JNK signal transduction pathways. *Molecular Cancer Therapeutics*, Vol.4, No.3, pp. 457-470, ISSN 1535-7163

Hashimoto, K.,I. Matsumura, et al. (2003). Necessity of tyrosine 719 and phosphatidylinositol 3'-kinase-mediated signal pathway in constitutive activation and oncogenic potential of c-kit receptor tyrosine kinase with the Asp814Val mutation. *Blood*, Vol.101, No.3, pp. 1094-1102, ISSN 0006-4971

Hawkins, P. T.,K. E. Anderson, et al. (2006). Signalling through Class I PI3Ks in mammalian cells. *Biochemical Society Transactions*, Vol.34, No.Pt 5, pp. 647-662, ISSN 0300-5127

Helgason, C. D.,J. Antonchuk, et al. (2003). Homeostasis and regeneration of the hematopoietic stem cell pool are altered in SHIP-deficient mice. *Blood*, Vol.102, No.10, pp. 3541-3547, ISSN 0006-4971

Helgason, C. D.,J. E. Damen, et al. (1998). Targeted disruption of SHIP leads to hemopoietic perturbations, lung pathology, and a shortened life span. *Genes and Development*, Vol.12, No.11, pp. 1610-1620, ISSN 0890-9369

Hirano, I.,S. Nakamura, et al. (2009). Depletion of Pleckstrin homology domain leucine-rich repeat protein phosphatases 1 and 2 by Bcr-Abl promotes chronic myelogenous leukemia cell proliferation through continuous phosphorylation of Akt isoforms. *Journal of Biological Chemistry*, Vol.284, No.33, pp. 22155-22165, ISSN 0021-9258

Horn, S.,U. Bergholz, et al. (2008). Mutations in the catalytic subunit of class IA PI3K confer leukemogenic potential to hematopoietic cells. *Oncogene*, Vol.27, No.29, pp. 4096-4106, ISSN 1476-5594

Horton, T. M.,D. Pati, et al. (2007). A phase 1 study of the proteasome inhibitor bortezomib in pediatric patients with refractory leukemia: a Children's Oncology Group study. *Clinical Cancer Research*, Vol.13, No.5, pp. 1516-1522, ISSN 1078-0432

Hsieh, A. C.,M. Costa, et al. (2010). Genetic dissection of the oncogenic mTOR pathway reveals druggable addiction to translational control via 4EBP-eIF4E. *Cancer Cell*, Vol.17, No.3, pp. 249-261, ISSN 1878-3686

Huang, J.,Y. Zhang, et al. (2009). Pivotal role for glycogen synthase kinase-3 in hematopoietic stem cell homeostasis in mice. *The Journal of Clinical Investigation*, Vol.119, No.12, pp. 3519-3529, ISSN 1558-8238

Inoki, K.,Y. Li, et al. (2002). TSC2 is phosphorylated and inhibited by Akt and suppresses mTOR signalling. *Nature Cell Biology*, Vol.4, No.9, pp. 648-657, ISSN 1465-7392

Inoki, K.,H. Ouyang, et al. (2006). TSC2 integrates Wnt and energy signals via a coordinated phosphorylation by AMPK and GSK3 to regulate cell growth. *Cell*, Vol.126, No.5, pp. 955-968, ISSN 0092-8674

Janes, M. R.,J. J. Limon, et al. (2010). Effective and selective targeting of leukemia cells using a TORC1/2 kinase inhibitor. *Nature Medicine*, Vol.16, No.2, pp. 205-213, ISSN 1546-170X

Jia, Y.,F. Loison, et al. (2008). Inositol trisphosphate 3-kinase B (InsP3KB) as a physiological modulator of myelopoiesis. *Proceedings of the National Academy of Sciences of the United States of America*, Vol.105, No.12, pp. 4739-4744, ISSN 1091-6490

Jia, Y.,K. K. Subramanian, et al. (2007). Inositol 1,3,4,5-tetrakisphosphate negatively regulates phosphatidylinositol-3,4,5- trisphosphate signaling in neutrophils. *Immunity*, Vol.27, No.3, pp. 453-467, ISSN 1074-7613

Jotta, P. Y.,M. A. Ganazza, et al. (2010). Negative prognostic impact of PTEN mutation in pediatric T-cell acute lymphoblastic leukemia. *Leukemia*, Vol.24, No.1, pp. 239-242, ISSN 1476-5551

Jou, S. T.,N. Carpino, et al. (2002). Essential, nonredundant role for the phosphoinositide 3-kinase p110delta in signaling by the B-cell receptor complex. *Molecular and Cellular Biology*, Vol.22, No.24, pp. 8580-8591, ISSN 0270-7306

Juntilla, M. M.,V. D. Patil, et al. (2010). AKT1 and AKT2 maintain hematopoietic stem cell function by regulating reactive oxygen species. *Blood*, Vol.115, No.20, pp. 4030-4038, ISSN 1528-0020

Kharas, M. G.,M. R. Janes, et al. (2008). Ablation of PI3K blocks BCR-ABL leukemogenesis in mice, and a dual PI3K/mTOR inhibitor prevents expansion of human BCR-ABL+ leukemia cells. *The Journal of Clinical Investigation*, Vol.118, No.9, pp. 3038-3050, ISSN 0021-9738

Kharas, M. G.,R. Okabe, et al. (2010). Constitutively active AKT depletes hematopoietic stem cells and induces leukemia in mice. *Blood*, Vol.115, No.7, pp. 1406-1415, ISSN 1528-0020

Kojima, K.,M. Shimanuki, et al. (2008). The dual PI3 kinase/mTOR inhibitor PI-103 prevents p53 induction by Mdm2 inhibition but enhances p53-mediated mitochondrial apoptosis in p53 wild-type AML. *Leukemia*, Vol.22, No.9, pp. 1728-1736, ISSN 1476-5551

Kondapaka, S. B.,S. S. Singh, et al. (2003). Perifosine, a novel alkylphospholipid, inhibits protein kinase B activation. *Molecular Cancer Therapeutics*, Vol.2, No.11, pp. 1093-1103, ISSN 1535-7163

Kops, G. J.,N. D. de Ruiter, et al. (1999). Direct control of the Forkhead transcription factor AFX by protein kinase B. *Nature*, Vol.398, No.6728, pp. 630-634, ISSN 0028-0836

Kornblau, S. M.,N. Singh, et al. (2010). Highly phosphorylated FOXO3A is an adverse prognostic factor in acute myeloid leukemia. *Clinical Cancer Research*, Vol.16, No.6, pp. 1865-1874, ISSN 1078-0432

Kornblau, S. M.,M. Womble, et al. (2006). Simultaneous activation of multiple signal transduction pathways confers poor prognosis in acute myelogenous leukemia. *Blood*, Vol.108, No.7, pp. 2358-2365, ISSN 0006-4971

Kubota, Y.,H. Ohnishi, et al. (2004). Constitutive activation of PI3K is involved in the spontaneous proliferation of primary acute myeloid leukemia cells: direct evidence of PI3K activation. *Leukemia*, Vol.18, No.8, pp. 1438-1440, ISSN 0887-6924

Lee, J. W.,Y. H. Soung, et al. (2005). PIK3CA gene is frequently mutated in breast carcinomas and hepatocellular carcinomas. *Oncogene*, Vol.24, No.8, pp. 1477-1480, ISSN 0950-9232

Legrand, O.,G. Simonin, et al. (1999). Simultaneous activity of MRP1 and Pgp is correlated with in vitro resistance to daunorubicin and with in vivo resistance in adult acute myeloid leukemia. *Blood*, Vol.94, No.3, pp. 1046-1056, ISSN 0006-4971

Levy, D. S.,J. A. Kahana, et al. (2009). AKT inhibitor, GSK690693, induces growth inhibition and apoptosis in acute lymphoblastic leukemia cell lines. *Blood*, Vol.113, No.8, pp. 1723-1729, ISSN 1528-0020

Ligresti, G.,L. Militello, et al. (2009). PIK3CA mutations in human solid tumors: role in sensitivity to various therapeutic approaches. *Cell Cycle*, Vol.8, No.9, pp. 1352-1358, ISSN 1551-4005

Liu, Q.,G. Nozari, et al. (1998). Single-tube polymerase chain reaction for rapid diagnosis of the inversion hotspot of mutation in hemophilia A. *Blood*, Vol.92, No.4, pp. 1458-1459, ISSN 0006-4971

Liu, Q.,T. Sasaki, et al. (1999). SHIP is a negative regulator of growth factor receptor-mediated PKB/Akt activation and myeloid cell survival. *Genes and Development*, Vol.13, No.7, pp. 786-791, ISSN 0890-9369

Liu, T. C.,P. M. Lin, et al. (2000). Mutation analysis of PTEN/MMAC1 in acute myeloid leukemia. *Am J Hematol*, Vol.63, No.4, pp. 170-175, ISSN 0361-8609

Lo, T. C.,L. M. Barnhill, et al. (2009). Inactivation of SHIP1 in T-cell acute lymphoblastic leukemia due to mutation and extensive alternative splicing. *Leukemia Research*, Vol.33, No.11, pp. 1562-1566, ISSN 1873-5835

Luo, J. M.,H. Yoshida, et al. (2003). Possible dominant-negative mutation of the SHIP gene in acute myeloid leukemia. *Leukemia*, Vol.17, No.1, pp. 1-8, ISSN 0887-6924

Maehama, T. and J. E. Dixon. (1998). The tumor suppressor, PTEN/MMAC1, dephosphorylates the lipid second messenger, phosphatidylinositol 3,4,5-trisphosphate. *Journal of Biological Chemistry*, Vol.273, No.22, pp. 13375-13378, ISSN 0021-9258

Mahadevan, D. and A. F. List. (2004). Targeting the multidrug resistance-1 transporter in AML: molecular regulation and therapeutic strategies. *Blood*, Vol.104, No.7, pp. 1940-1951, ISSN 0006-4971

Maira, S. M.,F. Stauffer, et al. (2008). Identification and characterization of NVP-BEZ235, a new orally available dual phosphatidylinositol 3-kinase/mammalian target of rapamycin inhibitor with potent in vivo antitumor activity. *Molecular Cancer Therapy*, Vol.7, No.7, pp. 1851-1863, ISSN 1535-7163

Manning, B. D. and L. C. Cantley. (2007). AKT/PKB signaling: navigating downstream. *Cell*, Vol.129, No.7, pp. 1261-1274, ISSN 0092-8674

Mao, X.,B. Cao, et al. (2011). A small-molecule inhibitor of D-cyclin transactivation displays preclinical efficacy in myeloma and leukemia via phosphoinositide 3-kinase pathway. *Blood*, Vol.117, No.6, pp. 1986-1997, ISSN 1528-0020

Meyer, L. H.,S. M. Eckhoff, et al. (2011). Early Relapse in ALL Is Identified by Time to Leukemia in NOD/SCID Mice and Is Characterized by a Gene Signature Involving Survival Pathways. *Cancer Cell*, Vol.19, No.2, pp. 206-217, ISSN 1878-3686

Min, Y. H.,J. I. Eom, et al. (2003). Constitutive phosphorylation of Akt/PKB protein in acute myeloid leukemia: its significance as a prognostic variable. *Leukemia*, Vol.17, No.5, pp. 995-997, ISSN 0887-6924

Minucci, S. and P. G. Pelicci. (2006). Histone deacetylase inhibitors and the promise of epigenetic (and more) treatments for cancer. *Nature Reviews Cancer*, Vol.6, No.1, pp. 38-51, ISSN 1474-175X

Miyamoto, K.,K. Y. Araki, et al. (2007). Foxo3a is essential for maintenance of the hematopoietic stem cell pool. *Cell Stem Cell*, Vol.1, No.1, pp. 101-112, ISSN 1875-9777

Miyamoto, K.,T. Miyamoto, et al. (2008). FoxO3a regulates hematopoietic homeostasis through a negative feedback pathway in conditions of stress or aging. *Blood*, Vol.112, No.12, pp. 4485-4493, ISSN 1528-0020

Moody, J. L.,L. Xu, et al. (2004). Anemia, thrombocytopenia, leukocytosis, extramedullary hematopoiesis, and impaired progenitor function in Pten+/-SHIP-/- mice: a novel model of myelodysplasia. *Blood*, Vol.103, No.12, pp. 4503-4510, ISSN 0006-4971

Nave, B. T.,M. Ouwens, et al. (1999). Mammalian target of rapamycin is a direct target for protein kinase B: identification of a convergence point for opposing effects of insulin and amino-acid deficiency on protein translation. *The Biochemical Journal*, Vol.344 Pt 2, pp. 427-431, ISSN 0264-6021

Neri, L. M.,P. Borgatti, et al. (2003). The phosphoinositide 3-kinase/AKT1 pathway involvement in drug and all-trans-retinoic acid resistance of leukemia cells. *Molecular Cancer Research*, Vol.1, No.3, pp. 234-246, ISSN 1541-7786

Nguyen, N. Y.,M. J. Maxwell, et al. (2011). An ENU-induced mouse mutant of SHIP1 reveals a critical role of the stem cell isoform for suppression of macrophage activation. *Blood*, pp. ISSN 1528-0020

Ning, Z. Q.,J. Li, et al. (2001). Signal transducer and activator of transcription 3 activation is required for Asp(816) mutant c-Kit-mediated cytokine-independent survival and proliferation in human leukemia cells. *Blood*, Vol.97, No.11, pp. 3559-3567, ISSN 0006-4971

Nishioka, C.,T. Ikezoe, et al. (2008). Blockade of mTOR signaling potentiates the ability of histone deacetylase inhibitor to induce growth arrest and differentiation of acute myelogenous leukemia cells. *Leukemia*, Vol.22, No.12, pp. 2159-2168, ISSN 1476-5551

Nyakern, M.,P. L. Tazzari, et al. (2006). Frequent elevation of Akt kinase phosphorylation in blood marrow and peripheral blood mononuclear cells from high-risk myelodysplastic syndrome patients. *Leukemia*, Vol.20, No.2, pp. 230-238, ISSN 0887-6924

Okkenhaug, K.,A. Bilancio, et al. (2002). Impaired B and T cell antigen receptor signaling in p110delta PI 3-kinase mutant mice. *Science*, Vol.297, No.5583, pp. 1031-1034, ISSN 1095-9203

Oshiro, N.,K. Yoshino, et al. (2004). Dissociation of raptor from mTOR is a mechanism of rapamycin-induced inhibition of mTOR function. *Genes to Cells*, Vol.9, No.4, pp. 359-366, ISSN 1356-9597

Pabst, T.,B. U. Mueller, et al. (2001). Dominant-negative mutations of CEBPA, encoding CCAAT/enhancer binding protein-alpha (C/EBPalpha), in acute myeloid leukemia. *Nature Genetics*, Vol.27, No.3, pp. 263-270, ISSN 1061-4036

Papa, V.,P. L. Tazzari, et al. (2008). Proapoptotic activity and chemosensitizing effect of the novel Akt inhibitor perifosine in acute myelogenous leukemia cells. *Leukemia*, Vol.22, No.1, pp. 147-160, ISSN 1476-5551

Park, S.,N. Chapuis, et al. (2008). PI-103, a dual inhibitor of Class IA phosphatidylinositide 3-kinase and mTOR, has antileukemic activity in AML. *Leukemia*, Vol.22, No.9, pp. 1698-1706, ISSN 1476-5551

Perez, L. E.,C. Desponts, et al. (2008). SH2-inositol phosphatase 1 negatively influences early megakaryocyte progenitors. *PLoS One*, Vol.3, No.10, pp. e3565, ISSN 1932-6203

Pouillon, V.,R. Hascakova-Bartova, et al. (2003). Inositol 1,3,4,5-tetrakisphosphate is essential for T lymphocyte development. *Nature Immunology*, Vol.4, No.11, pp. 1136-1143, ISSN 1529-2908

Rahmani, M.,E. Reese, et al. (2005). Coadministration of histone deacetylase inhibitors and perifosine synergistically induces apoptosis in human leukemia cells through Akt and ERK1/2 inactivation and the generation of ceramide and reactive oxygen species. *Cancer Research*, Vol.65, No.6, pp. 2422-2432, ISSN 0008-5472

Raslova, H.,V. Baccini, et al. (2006). Mammalian target of rapamycin (mTOR) regulates both proliferation of megakaryocyte progenitors and late stages of megakaryocyte differentiation. *Blood*, Vol.107, No.6, pp. 2303-2310, ISSN 0006-4971

Raynaud, F. I.,S. Eccles, et al. (2007). Pharmacologic characterization of a potent inhibitor of class I phosphatidylinositide 3-kinases. *Cancer Research*, Vol.67, No.12, pp. 5840-5850, ISSN 0008-5472

Recher, C.,O. Beyne-Rauzy, et al. (2005). Antileukemic activity of rapamycin in acute myeloid leukemia. *Blood*, Vol.105, No.6, pp. 2527-2534, ISSN 0006-4971

Rizzieri, D. A.,E. Feldman, et al. (2008). A phase 2 clinical trial of deforolimus (AP23573, MK-8669), a novel mammalian target of rapamycin inhibitor, in patients with relapsed or refractory hematologic malignancies. *Clinical Cancer Research*, Vol.14, No.9, pp. 2756-2762, ISSN 1078-0432

Rodriguez-Viciana, P.,P. H. Warne, et al. (1994). Phosphatidylinositol-3-OH kinase as a direct target of Ras. *Nature*, Vol.370, No.6490, pp. 527-532, ISSN 0028-0836

Sampath, D.,J. Cortes, et al. (2006). Pharmacodynamics of cytarabine alone and in combination with 7-hydroxystaurosporine (UCN-01) in AML blasts in vitro and during a clinical trial. *Blood*, Vol.107, No.6, pp. 2517-2524, ISSN 0006-4971

Santamaria, C. M.,M. C. Chillon, et al. (2009). High FOXO3a expression is associated with a poorer prognosis in AML with normal cytogenetics. *Leukemia Research*, Vol.33, No.12, pp. 1706-1709, ISSN 1873-5835

Sarbassov, D. D.,D. A. Guertin, et al. (2005). Phosphorylation and regulation of Akt/PKB by the rictor-mTOR complex. *Science*, Vol.307, No.5712, pp. 1098-1101, ISSN 1095-9203

Saunders, P.,A. Cisterne, et al. (2011). The mammalian target of rapamycin inhibitor RAD001 (everolimus) synergizes with chemotherapeutic agents, ionizing radiation and proteasome inhibitors in pre-B acute lymphocytic leukemia. *Haematologica*, Vol.96, No.1, pp. 69-77, ISSN 1592-8721

Schubbert, S.,K. Shannon, et al. (2007). Hyperactive Ras in developmental disorders and cancer. *Nature Reviews Cancer*, Vol.7, No.4, pp. 295-308, ISSN 1474-175X

Silva, A.,J. A. Yunes, et al. (2008). PTEN posttranslational inactivation and hyperactivation of the PI3K/Akt pathway sustain primary T cell leukemia viability. *The Journal of Clinical Investigation*, Vol.118, No.11, pp. 3762-3774, ISSN 0021-9738

Skorski, T.,A. Bellacosa, et al. (1997). Transformation of hematopoietic cells by BCR/ABL requires activation of a PI-3k/Akt-dependent pathway. *EMBO Journal*, Vol.16, No.20, pp. 6151-6161, ISSN 0261-4189

Sujobert, P.,V. Bardet, et al. (2005). Essential role for the p110delta isoform in phosphoinositide 3-kinase activation and cell proliferation in acute myeloid leukemia. *Blood*, Vol.106, No.3, pp. 1063-1066, ISSN 0006-4971

Tabellini, G.,P. L. Tazzari, et al. (2004). Novel 2'-substituted, 3'-deoxy-phosphatidyl-myo-inositol analogues reduce drug resistance in human leukaemia cell lines with an activated phosphoinositide 3-kinase/Akt pathway. *British Journal of Haematology*, Vol.126, No.4, pp. 574-582, ISSN 0007-1048

Tamburini, J.,N. Chapuis, et al. (2008). Mammalian target of rapamycin (mTOR) inhibition activates phosphatidylinositol 3-kinase/Akt by up-regulating insulin-like growth factor-1 receptor signaling in acute myeloid leukemia: rationale for therapeutic inhibition of both pathways. *Blood*, Vol.111, No.1, pp. 379-382, ISSN 0006-4971

Tamburini, J.,C. Elie, et al. (2007). Constitutive phosphoinositide 3-kinase/Akt activation represents a favorable prognostic factor in de novo acute myelogenous leukemia patients. *Blood*, Vol.110, No.3, pp. 1025-1028, ISSN 0006-4971

Tazzari, P. L.,G. Tabellini, et al. (2008). Synergistic proapoptotic activity of recombinant TRAIL plus the Akt inhibitor Perifosine in acute myelogenous leukemia cells. *Cancer Research*, Vol.68, No.22, pp. 9394-9403, ISSN 1538-7445

Teachey, D. T.,D. A. Obzut, et al. (2006). The mTOR inhibitor CCI-779 induces apoptosis and inhibits growth in preclinical models of primary adult human ALL. *Blood*, Vol.107, No.3, pp. 1149-1155, ISSN 0006-4971

Teachey, D. T.,C. Sheen, et al. (2008). mTOR inhibitors are synergistic with methotrexate: an effective combination to treat acute lymphoblastic leukemia. *Blood*, Vol.112, No.5, pp. 2020-2023, ISSN 1528-0020

Thomas, X. (2009). Chemotherapy of acute leukemia in adults. *Expert Opinion on Pharmacotherapy*, Vol.10, No.2, pp. 221-237, ISSN 1744-7666

Tothova, Z.,R. Kollipara, et al. (2007). FoxOs are critical mediators of hematopoietic stem cell resistance to physiologic oxidative stress. *Cell*, Vol.128, No.2, pp. 325-339, ISSN 0092-8674

Trowbridge, J. J.,A. Xenocostas, et al. (2006). Glycogen synthase kinase-3 is an in vivo regulator of hematopoietic stem cell repopulation. *Nature Medicine*, Vol.12, No.1, pp. 89-98, ISSN 1078-8956

van de Laar, L.,M. Buitenhuis, et al. (2010). Human CD34-derived myeloid dendritic cell development requires intact phosphatidylinositol 3-kinase-protein kinase B-mammalian target of rapamycin signaling. *Journal of Immunology*, Vol.184, No.12, pp. 6600-6611, ISSN 1550-6606

Vanhaesebroeck, B.,S. J. Leevers, et al. (2001). Synthesis and function of 3-phosphorylated inositol lipids. *Annu Rev Biochem*, Vol.70, pp. 535-602, ISSN 0066-4154

Varticovski, L.,G. Q. Daley, et al. (1991). Activation of phosphatidylinositol 3-kinase in cells expressing abl oncogene variants. *Molecular and Cellular Biology*, Vol.11, No.2, pp. 1107-1113, ISSN 0270-7306

Vlahos, C. J.,W. F. Matter, et al. (1994). A specific inhibitor of phosphatidylinositol 3-kinase, 2-(4-morpholinyl)-8-phenyl-4H-1-benzopyran-4-one (LY294002). *Journal of Biological Chemistry*, Vol.269, No.7, pp. 5241-5248, ISSN 0021-9258

Wang, C.,X. Chen, et al. (2007). C/EBPalphap30 plays transcriptional regulatory roles distinct from C/EBPalphap42. *Cell Res*, Vol.17, No.4, pp. 374-383, ISSN 1748-7838

Weisberg, E.,L. Banerji, et al. (2008). Potentiation of antileukemic therapies by the dual PI3K/PDK-1 inhibitor, BAG956: effects on BCR-ABL- and mutant FLT3-expressing cells. *Blood*, Vol.111, No.7, pp. 3723-3734, ISSN 0006-4971

Wymann, M. P.,G. Bulgarelli-Leva, et al. (1996). Wortmannin inactivates phosphoinositide 3-kinase by covalent modification of Lys-802, a residue involved in the phosphate transfer reaction. *Molecular and Cellular Biology*, Vol.16, No.4, pp. 1722-1733, ISSN 0270-7306

Xu, Q.,S. E. Simpson, et al. (2003). Survival of acute myeloid leukemia cells requires PI3 kinase activation. *Blood*, Vol.102, No.3, pp. 972-980, ISSN 0006-4971

Xu, Q.,J. E. Thompson, et al. (2005). mTOR regulates cell survival after etoposide treatment in primary AML cells. *Blood*, Vol.106, No.13, pp. 4261-4268, ISSN 0006-4971

Yap, T. A.,M. D. Garrett, et al. (2008). Targeting the PI3K-AKT-mTOR pathway: progress, pitfalls, and promises. *Current Opinion in Pharmacology*, Vol.8, No.4, pp. 393-412, ISSN 1471-4892

Yilmaz, O. H.,R. Valdez, et al. (2006). Pten dependence distinguishes haematopoietic stem cells from leukaemia-initiating cells. *Nature*, Vol.441, No.7092, pp. 475-482, ISSN 1476-4687

Yoshimi, A.,S. Goyama, et al. (2011). Evi1 represses PTEN expression by interacting with polycomb complexes and activates PI3K/AKT/mTOR signaling. *Blood*, pp. ISSN 1528-0020

Yuan, R.,A. Kay, et al. (2009). Targeting tumorigenesis: development and use of mTOR inhibitors in cancer therapy. *Journal of Hematology and Oncology*, Vol.2, pp. 45, ISSN 1756-8722

Zask, A.,J. Kaplan, et al. (2008). Synthesis and structure-activity relationships of ring-opened 17-hydroxywortmannins: potent phosphoinositide 3-kinase inhibitors with improved properties and anticancer efficacy. *Journal of Medicinal Chemistry*, Vol.51, No.5, pp. 1319-1323, ISSN 0022-2623

Zeng, Z.,I. J. Samudio, et al. (2006). Simultaneous inhibition of PDK1/AKT and Fms-like tyrosine kinase 3 signaling by a small-molecule KP372-1 induces mitochondrial dysfunction and apoptosis in acute myelogenous leukemia. *Cancer Research*, Vol.66, No.7, pp. 3737-3746, ISSN 0008-5472

Zhang, J.,J. C. Grindley, et al. (2006). PTEN maintains haematopoietic stem cells and acts in lineage choice and leukaemia prevention. *Nature*, Vol.441, No.7092, pp. 518-522, ISSN 1476-4687

Zhao, S.,M. Konopleva, et al. (2004). Inhibition of phosphatidylinositol 3-kinase dephosphorylates BAD and promotes apoptosis in myeloid leukemias. *Leukemia*, Vol.18, No.2, pp. 267-275, ISSN 0887-6924

Zhao, W. L. (2010). Targeted therapy in T-cell malignancies: dysregulation of the cellular signaling pathways. *Leukemia*, Vol.24, No.1, pp. 13-21, ISSN 1476-5551

7

Biochemistry of the Mixed Lineage Leukemia 1 (MLL1) Protein and Targeted Therapies for Associated Leukemia

Venkatasubramanian Dharmarajan and Michael S. Cosgrove
Department of Biology, Syracuse University, Syracuse, New York
USA

1. Introduction

Mixed Lineage Leukemia constitutes a heterogeneous category of rare acute leukemias that are characterized by a mixed population of poorly differentiated lymphoid and myeloid progenitor cells. The mixed lineage leukemia (MLL1) gene, also known as HRX or ALL-1, is a frequent site of genetic rearrangements in infant acute leukemias and therapy-related malignancies (Daser and Rabbitts, 2005) and since its discovery (Djabali et al., 1992; Tkachuk et al., 1992; Ziemin-van der Poel et al., 1991), significant progress has been made in understanding its role in human biology and leukemogenesis (Liu et al., 2009; Slany, 2009). Chromosomal abnormalities involving the MLL1 gene include reciprocal chromosomal translocations, internal partial tandem duplications (PTD), and amplifications of un-rearranged MLL1 (Dou and Hess, 2008). These chromosomal aberrations are associated with mechanistically distinct gain-of-function phenotypes that may be amenable to targeted therapeutic approaches. However, progress in this area has been impeded by a lack of understanding of the molecular details by which MLL1 translocations, amplifications and PTDs contribute to leukemogenesis. To date, more than 60 MLL1 fusion partners have been described (Krivtsov and Armstrong, 2007), and detailed genetic/biochemical studies have identified several functional domains within chimeric MLL1-fusion proteins that are essential for leukemic transformation (Daser and Rabbitts, 2005; Debernardi et al., 2002; Eguchi et al., 2004; Ernst et al., 2002; Krivtsov and Armstrong, 2007; Lavau et al., 2000; Liu et al., 2009; Luo et al., 2001; Mitterbauer-Hohendanner and Mannhalter, 2004; Mueller et al., 2009; Prasad et al., 1995). Although our understanding of the molecular pathology of MLL1-associated leukemias remains incomplete, recent biochemical and structural information is contributing to an evolution of potential treatment strategies from a broadly-based chemotherapeutics approach towards therapies targeted to the underlying molecular pathogenesis of leukemia (Liedtke and Cleary, 2009). This chapter reviews recent advances in our efforts to develop novel MLL1-targeted therapies.

2. MLL1- a master epigenetic regulator with multiple roles in transcription

2.1 MLL1 in embryonic development and hematopoiesis

The MLL1 protein is a histone H3 lysine 4 (H3K4) methyltransferase that functions to maintain gene expression during development and hematopoiesis (Hess et al., 1997; Milne et al., 2002;

Yagi et al., 1998). The best studied target genes of MLL1 include the homeobox transcription factors or HOX genes, which are important for segment identity and cell fate during metazoan development (Abramovich and Humphries, 2005; Ernst et al., 2004b). Genetic studies in mice have demonstrated that the homozygous knock out of MLL1 is embryonic lethal and is associated with multiple developmental defects including neural crest patterning and hematopoietic abnormalities (Ernst et al., 2004a; Hess et al., 1997; Yagi et al., 1998; Yu et al., 1995). Notably, the expression levels of several HOX genes including HOXa4, HOXa7, HOXa9, and HOXa10 are decreased in MLL1$^{-/-}$ mice and are associated with defects in fetal liver hematopoiesis (Hanson et al., 1999; Yagi et al., 1998). MLL1$^{+/-}$ mice are not embryonic lethal but are anemic and exhibit homeotic developmental defects that are related to posterior shifts in HOX gene expression patterns (Yagi et al., 1998; Yu et al., 1995). Likewise, MLL1 is also required for adult hematopoiesis and stem cell self-renewal. In MLL1 conditional knockout mice fetal hematopoiesis is unaltered; however, adult mice exhibit anemia, a significant reduction in the number of bone marrow hematopoietic stem cell progenitors, and poor survival rates (Gan et al., 2010). In addition, it has been demonstrated that MLL1 plays a crucial role in self-renewal in cultured fetal liver and adult bone marrow stem cells (Jude et al., 2007; McMahon et al., 2007). These studies suggest that MLL1 orchestrates its biological functions at least in part through the regulation of HOX genes. Indeed, HOX dysregulation is a common phenotype that underlies the pathogenesis of acute leukemias associated with alterations in the MLL1 gene (Armstrong et al., 2002; Ayton and Cleary, 2003; Dorrance et al., 2006; Ferrando et al., 2003; Liu et al., 2009). However, MLL1 is also required for the regulation of cell cycle dependent genes such as: cyclins A, B, and E (Takeda et al., 2006) and CDK inhibitors p16^{Ink4a}, p18, p27 (Milne et al., 2005; Takeda et al., 2006); E2F family of transcription factors (E2F2, E2F4 and E2F6) (Takeda et al., 2006) as well as the transcription factor GATA3, which plays an essential role in specifying lymphoid subtype (Yamashita et al., 2006). In addition, MLL1 regulates expression of several genes involved in organogenesis and differentiation (Ansari and Mandal, 2010; Scharf et al., 2007) . Therefore, MLL1 is a master regulator that is critical for many gene expression programs required for normal development, hematopoiesis and the cell cycle.

2.2 MLL1 regulates the degree of H3K4 methylation and transcription

In eukaryotes, DNA is condensed into highly ordered structures known as chromatin- the structure of which is dynamically altered according to the needs of the cell. The basic repeating unit of chromatin is the nucleosome, which is composed of ~146 base pairs of DNA wrapped around an octameric disc of histone proteins containing two copies each of histones H2A, H2B, H3 and H4 (Luger and Hansen, 2005). Cellular processes that require access to DNA often use enzymes that dynamically regulate the structure of chromatin either through recruitment of adaptor proteins or additional enzymatic machineries that alter the positioning of nucleosomes on DNA (Cosgrove and Wolberger, 2005). One such enzymatic activity is the methylation of lysine 4 of histone H3 (H3K4), an evolutionarily conserved epigenetic mark predominantly associated with transcriptional activation in eukaryotes (Bernstein et al., 2002; Boggs et al., 2002; Litt et al., 2001; Noma and Grewal, 2002; Strahl et al., 1999). The epsilon amino group of lysine 4 can be mono-, di-, or trimethylated, with each modification correlating with distinct transcriptional outcomes (Bernstein et al., 2005; Ng et al., 2003; Pokholok et al., 2005; Santos-Rosa et al., 2002; Schneider et al., 2004; Schubeler et al., 2004). For example, genome-wide chromatin immunoprecipitation studies have demonstrated that high levels of H3K4 trimethylation are present within the 5′ regions of actively transcribed genes (Pokholok et al., 2005; Santos-Rosa et al., 2002; Schneider et al., 2004; Schubeler et al., 2004). It has been demonstrated that H3K4 trimethylation functions to recruit ATP dependent nucleosome remodeling enzymes that increase promoter DNA accessibility by sliding or displacing nucleosomes (Pray-Grant et al., 2005; Santos-Rosa et al., 2003; Wysocka et al., 2006). H3K4 dimethylation is spread more evenly across the coding regions of genes and is thought to be associated with a transcriptionally "poised" state of chromatin (Bernstein et al., 2002; Schneider et al., 2004; Schubeler et al., 2004). In contrast, H3K4 monomethylation is enriched at the 3′ ends of the genes and distal enhancer sequences, and is associated with ribosomal DNA (rDNA) and telomeric silencing (Bernstein et al., 2002; Heintzman et al., 2007; Pokholok et al., 2005; Santos-Rosa et al., 2002; Schneider et al., 2004; Schubeler et al., 2004)(Nislow, Ray et al. 1997; Briggs, Bryk et al. 2001; Schneider, Wood et al. 2005; van Dijk, Marley et al. 2005). These studies suggest that the degree of H3K4 methylation is a highly regulated process. Indeed eukaryotes have evolved a number of highly conserved enzymes whose function appears to precisely regulate the degree of H3K4 methylation.

H3K4 methylation is mainly deposited by a group of enzymes that share an evolutionarily conserved SET (SuVar, E(z), Trithorax) domain (Dillon et al., 2005) , although a new H3K4 methyltransferase lacking a SET domain has recently been reported (Patel et al., 2009; Patel et al., 2011). While there are several SET domains enzymes that differ with regard to their substrate specificity (Dillon et al., 2005; Qian and Zhou, 2006), members of the SET1 family share the properties that they all methylate H3K4, and all interact with an evolutionarily conserved core group of proteins that function to regulate the degree of H3K4 methylation. MLL1 belongs to the SET1 family of histone methyltransferases and evidence suggests that its transcriptional co-activator function is mediated in part by the enzymatic activity of its SET domain (Dillon et al., 2005; Milne et al., 2002). For example, homozygous deletion of the MLL1 SET domain in mice, while not embryonic lethal, exhibits skeletal defects and altered expression of several HOX genes that partially phenocopy the heterozygous knockout of the whole MLL1 gene (Terranova et al., 2006). These changes are correlated with decreased levels of mono- and dimethylation of H3K4 and deregulated DNA methylation patterns at several HOX gene promoters (Terranova et al., 2006).

MLL1 functions within a large macromolecular complex with more than 30 subunits that regulate the degree of H3K4 methylation and MLL1's target gene specificity (Cosgrove and Patel, 2010). While subunit composition of different SET1 family members varies to some degree, each SET1 family member interacts with a conserved core group of proteins that include WD-40 repeat protein-5 (WDR5), Retinoblastoma binding protein-5 (RbBP5), Absent small homeotic 2-like protein (Ash2L) and Dumpy30 (Dpy-30) (Cho et al., 2007; Dou et al., 2006; Lee et al., 2007). WRD5, RbBP5, Ash2L and DPY-30 form an indepedent complex called WRAD that possesses an intrisic histone methyltransferase activity on its own (Patel et al., 2009; Patel et al., 2011). When WRAD interacts with MLL1, it forms what is known as the MLL1 core complex, which is required for mono- and dimethylation of H3K4 (Dou et al., 2006; Patel et al., 2009). These studies have led to a model in which H3K4 methylation is sequentially catalyzed by a complex that contains multiple distinct active sites for the addition of each methyl group (Patel et al., 2009).

2.3 Mechanism of multiple lysine methylation catalyzed by MLL1 core complex

Previously it was thought that mono-, di-, and trimethylation of H3K4 could be attributed to the SET domain dependent methyltransferase activity of MLL1 alone and that the WRAD complex functions merely as an allosteric regulator of MLL1 (Cheng et al., 2005; Collins et al., 2005; Dou et al., 2006; Han et al., 2006; Ruthenburg et al., 2006; Southall et al., 2009; Steward et al., 2006; Takahashi et al., 2009). However, since it has more recently been demonstrated that the WRAD complex dimethylates H3K4 in a manner that is independent of the enzymatic activity of the MLL1 SET domain (Patel et al., 2009), the allosteric model needs to be revised. Indeed, in vitro methylation assays demonstrate that the isolated MLL1 SET domain is predominantly a monomethyltranferse, which can be attributed to the presence of a conserved tyrosine residue in the SET domain active site (Patel et al., 2009). Furthermore, loss of the WDR5, RbBP5 or Ash2L subunits of WRAD results in the loss of di- and trimethylation of H3K4 both in vivo and in vitro without significant changes in H3K4 monomethylation (Dou et al., 2006; Patel et al., 2009; Patel et al., 2008b; Wysocka et al., 2005). These results are consistent with a sequential mechanism whereby the MLL1 SET domain catalyzes H3K4 monomethylation and the WRAD enzyme catalyzes H3K4 dimethylation within the MLL1 core complex. However, WRAD lacks the ability to dimethylate H3K4 without MLL1, suggesting that MLL1 amino acid sequences, distinct from the MLL1 SET domain active site, contributes to the WRAD active site within the MLL1 core complex. That a complex between WRAD and MLL1 is required for H3K4 dimethylation is supported by the demonstration that amino acid substitutions that disrupt the interaction between MLL1 and WRAD also disrupt the H3K4 dimethylation activity of the MLL1 core complex (Patel et al., 2008b). Therefore, the completely assembled MLL1 core complex is required for efficient H3K4 dimethylation and for nucleosome methylation (Patel et al., 2011). The existence of a sequential mechanism utilizing several active sites for multiple lysine methylation suggests that the degree of H3K4 methylation is more highly regulated than previously appreciated.

2.4 WRAD components are associated with development and oncogenesis

One of the common features of the greater than 60-MLL fusion proteins associated with leukemias is that in most cases they lose the amino acid sequences required for interaction with WRAD. This raises questions about WRAD's role in MLL1 associated oncogenesis. WRAD subunits are conserved within SET1 family complexes ranging from yeast to humans (Cho et al., 2007; Dou et al., 2006; Lee and Skalnik, 2005; Lee et al., 2007; Steward et al., 2006) and have been shown to play essential roles in cellular differentiation (Gori and Demay, 2005; Gori et al., 2005; Zhu et al., 2008), development (Adamson and Shearn, 1996; Wysocka et al., 2005), dosage compensation (Hsu et al., 1995; Hsu and Meyer, 1994), embryogenesis (Stoller et al.), and transcription (Tan et al., 2008). However, the WRAD enzyme lacks sequence homology to known methyltransferase folds and as a result relatively little is understood about its methyltransferase activity and the role it might play in oncogenesis. WRAD's potential role in oncogenesis is supported by the observation that the Ash2L component of WRAD is overexpressed at the protein level in many human tumors, and that knockdown of Ash2L inhibits tumor cell proliferation (Luscher-Firzlaff et al., 2008). In addition, the RbBP5 component of WRAD has been shown to be amplified in several glioblastomas, suggesting that it may be a novel oncogene (Bralten et al., 2010). Further studies will be required to better understand WRAD's role in MLL1 associated leukemogenesis and other cancers.

In contrast, the MLL1 component of the MLL1 core complex is more extensively characterized and several functional domains implicated in transcriptional regulation have been identified (for recent reviews refer to Ansari and Mandal, 2010; Cosgrove and Patel, 2010). Furthermore, MLL1 is a frequent site of chromosomal alterations that sometimes disrupt the functions of these domains. The next subsection summarizes recent genetic, biochemical and structural studies of the functional domains that regulate MLL1's gene targeting and H3K4 methyltransferase activity.

2.5 MLL1 functional domains implicated in transcriptional regulation

The MLL1 gene encodes a large protein of 3,969 amino acid residues and contains several functional domains including: menin binding motif (MBM), Lens epithelium derived growth factor (LEDGF) binding domain (LBD), DNA-binding AT hooks, a cysteine-rich CXXC DNA binding motif, plant homeodomain (PHD) fingers, a bromo domain (BD), a transactivation domain (TAD), a WDR5 interaction (Win) motif, and a C-terminal histone methyltransferase SET domain (Figure 1) (Cosgrove and Patel, 2010). The full-length MLL1 protein, synthesized as a single transcript, is cleaved by taspase I into MLL1-N (320 kDa) and MLL1-C (180 kDa) fragments, which then re-associate through the FYRN and FYRC motifs to form the functional MLL1 complex in vivo (Figure 1) (Hsieh et al., 2003a; Hsieh et al., 2003b; Yokoyama et al., 2002). The mature MLL1 protein assembles into macromolecular complexes with several regulatory proteins that are essential for MLL1's transcriptional co-activator properties. Biochemical and genetic studies have identified several direct and

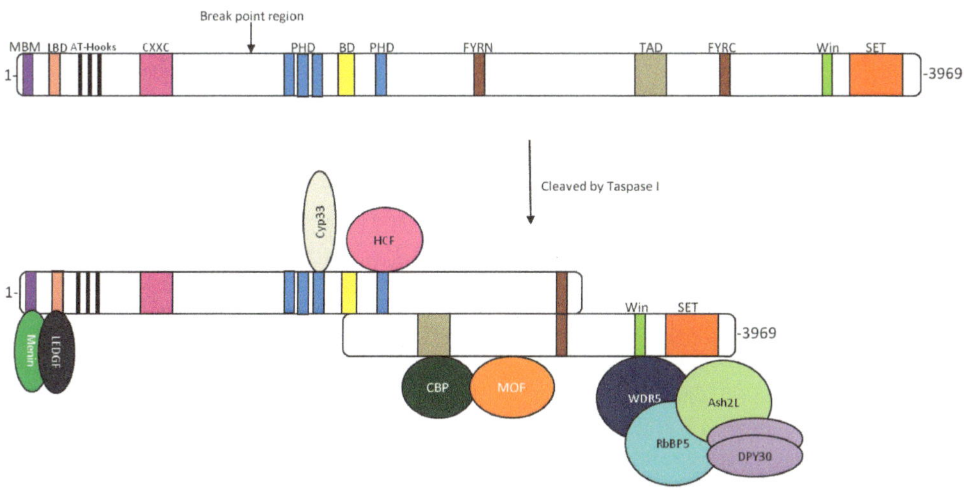

Schematic representation showing the functional domains present in the MLL1 protein. Menin binding motif MBM (purple), LEDGF binding domain or LBD (light red), DNA binding AT-hooks (black), zinc finger containing CXXC motifs (pink), plant homeodomain (PHD) fingers (blue), bromodomain (BD) (yellow), phenylalanine-tyrosine rich regions (FYR) (brown), WDR5 interaction (*Win)* motif (light green), and the histone methyltransferase SET domain (red) are highlighted. a) The full-length MLL1 protein (3969 amino acids) is cleaved by Taspase 1 into MLL-N (300 kDa) and MLL-C (180 kDa) fragments that then re-associate through FYRN and FYRC motifs to form a stable complex. This mature MLL1 protein then assembles into a macromolecular complex with a number of proteins including- menin (green); lens epithelium derived growth factor or LEDGF (dark grey); nuclear cyclophilin (Cyp33) (light grey); host cell factor (HCF) (light pink); CREB binding protein (CBP) (dark green); histone acetyltransferase MOF (orange); WD-40 repeat containing protein-5 (WDR5) (dark blue); retinoblastoma binding protein-5 (RbBP5) (cyan); absent, small, homeotic disc-2 like (Ash2L) (olive green); and DPY-30 (light purple).

Fig. 1. Domain architecture of human MLL1.

indirect interaction partners for MLL1 that include; the menin tumor suppressor protein (Hughes et al., 2004; Yokoyama et al., 2004); cell cycle regulators such as E2Fs and HCF-1 (Tyagi et al., 2007; Yokoyama et al., 2004); polycomb group proteins, BMI-1 and HPC-2 (Xia et al., 2003); histone deacetylases (Nakamura et al., 2002; Xia et al., 2003); nuclear cyclophilin, Cyp33 (Xia et al., 2003); acetyltransferases such as p300, CBP and MOF (Dou et al., 2005; Ernst et al., 2001); chromatin remodeling factors, INI1/SNF5 (Rozenblatt-Rosen et al., 1998); and WDR5/RbBP5/Ash2L and DPY30, which are core components of SET1 family methyltransferases (Dou et al., 2006). In addition, a recent paper describes the identification of a gene internal promoter that transcribes the C-terminal half of MLL1 (Scharf et al., 2007), the function of which is not known. Interestingly, the gene internal promoter coincides with an MLL1 breakpoint region, suggesting that the pathogenesis of MLL1 translocation induced leukemia could be due in part to the loss of this N-terminally truncated form of MLL1 when the breakpoint is 5′ to the gene internal promoter. However, in cases where the MLL1 breakpoint is 3′ to the gene internal promoter, it could result in aberrant expression of the fusion protein (Scharf et al., 2007). Indeed, it has been noted that the common MLL1 translocation partners AF4, AF6, and ENL have potential AUG start codons in positions where they could be transcribed within the context of the translocated MLL1 gene (Scharf et al., 2007).

These studies suggest that the transcriptional activator properties of MLL1 are mediated through multiple functional domains through protein-protein and protein-DNA interactions. Many of these interactions are retained in leukemogenic MLL1s, some participating in gain-of function phenotypes, making them candidates for molecular targeted therapy. We review progress in this area in sections 3-5. In section 2, we describe in more detail our current understanding of the role of MLL1 alterations in hematopoietic malignancies.

3. MLL1-A key player in hematologic malignancies

3.1 Acute myeloid and lymphoblastic leukemia with 11q23 abnormalities

3.1.1 Incidence and clinical significance of 11q23 chromosomal translocations

The MLL1 gene located at chromosome 11, band q23, is frequently involved in reciprocal translocations found in several cases of acute myeloid (AML) and acute lymphoblastic leukemia (ALL) (Djabali et al., 1992; Gu et al., 1992; Ziemin-van der Poel et al., 1991) and identify a patient sub-population with a poor prognosis (Daser and Rabbitts, 2005). Recurrent MLL1 translocations account for >70% of infant acute leukemias (both ALL and AML) and are also observed in approximately 10% of de novo AML in adults (Krivtsov and Armstrong, 2007), and in therapy-related leukemias that develop in patients treated with topoisomerase II inhibitors (Bigoni et al., 1999; Felix et al., 1995; Krivtsov and Armstrong, 2007). Chromosomal translocations fuse the N-terminal part (~1400 amino acids) of the MLL1 protein in-frame to one of more than 60 partner proteins that range from nuclear factors to cytoplasmic proteins (Daser and Rabbitts, 2005; Huret et al., 2001; Schoch et al., 2003).

The five most common MLL1 translocations include: MLL1-AF4 or t(4;11)(q21;q23); MLL1-ENL or t(11;19)(q23;p13.3); MLL1-AF9 or t(9;11)(p23;q23), MLL1-AF10 or t(10;11)(p12;q23), and MLL1-AF6 or t(6;11)(q27;q23) and account for greater than 80% of MLL1-rearranged leukemias (Burmeister et al., 2009; Meyer et al., 2009; Meyer et al., 2006; Slany, 2009). In addition, chimeric MLL1-fusions involving ELL, EEN, GAS7, AF1p, AFx, Septins, and histone acetyltransferases CBP/p300 have also been reported (Bernard et al., 1994; Dobson et al., 2000; Hall and Russell, 2004; Ida et al., 1997; Krivtsov and Armstrong,

2007; Meyer et al., 2009; Schichman et al., 1995; So et al., 2003; Taki et al., 1997; Tkachuk et al., 1992; Wang et al., 2005). The translocation partners identified to date are diverse and do not share any biochemical function or structural motifs. However, all known MLL1 fusion proteins share the property that the N-terminal portion containing the AT hooks and CxxC domains of MLL1 are retained, suggesting the preservation of DNA binding activity (Ayton et al., 2004; Macrini et al., 2003). In contrast, the taspase cleavage site, gene internal promoter, TAD domain, PHD fingers, *Win* motif and the SET domain are lost (Figure 2) (Liu et al., 2009).

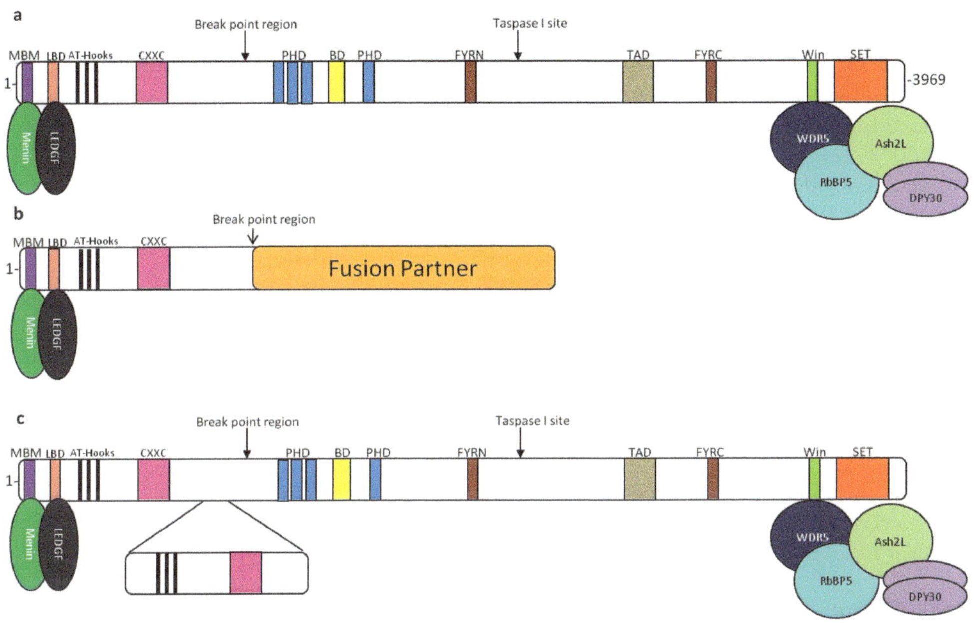

The putative protein products generated by the two most common chromosomal alterations associated with the MLL1 gene are indicated along with wild-type MLL1: a) wild-type MLL1, b) reciprocal chromosomal translocations involving MLL1, and c) partial tandem duplications (PTDs) in MLL1. The various functional domains are color coded as in Figure 1. Chromosomal translocations fuse the N-terminal ~1400 amino acids of MLL1 in-frame to one of over 60 different fusion partners (indicated in orange in b). PTDs have a duplicated N-terminus (AT-hooks and CXXC motifs) in addition to all the functional domains present in wild-type MLL1.

Fig. 2. Schematic representation of the most common genetic alterations associated with the MLL1 gene.

3.1.2 Pathogenesis of acute leukemias with MLL1-translocations

While it is expected that the loss of SET domain in MLL1 translocations would result in decreased H3K4 methylation and Hox gene expression, genetic studies have revealed that the individual fusion partners possess transcriptional activator properties and are indispensable for leukemogenesis (Chen et al., 2006a; Dobson et al., 1999; Dobson et al., 2000; Wang et al., 2005). Given the complexity of different translocation partners, MLL1-fusions may activate a common leukemia-associated gene expression program through multiple mechanisms. Indeed, AF4, AF5, AF9, ENL, ELL and AF10 proteins are all implicated in transcriptional elongation via association with the EAF complex, pTEFb kinase, and hDOT1 mediated methylation of H3K79 (Bitoun et al., 2007; Luo et al., 2001; Mueller et al., 2007; Mueller et al., 2009; Okada et al., 2005; Simone et al., 2001). Another mechanism could involve transcriptional activation via increased or aberrant histone acetylation (MLL-CBP/p300) (Lavau et al., 2000; Sobulo et al., 1997), protein arginine methyltransferase-1 (PRMT1) association (MLL-EEN) (Cheung et al., 2007), SWI-SNF chromatin-remodeling complex recruitment (MLL-ENL, -AF9, -AF10) (Debernardi et al., 2002; Nie et al., 2003; Schreiner et al., 1999), and self-association or dimerization of the N-terminal part of MLL1 (MLL-GAS7, -AF1p, -beta-galactosidase, -gephyrin, -SEPT6) (Dobson et al., 2000; Eguchi et al., 2004; Martin et al., 2003; So et al., 2003).

Regardless of the mechanism, aberrant expression of MLL1 target genes are a common feature of MLL1-rearrangements examined to date. For example, HOXa7, HOXa9, and the HOX cofactor MEIS1 are consistently over expressed in human leukemias with MLL1-translocations (Armstrong et al., 2002; Ayton and Cleary, 2003; Rozovskaia et al., 2001; Yeoh et al., 2002; Zeisig et al., 2004) and act, at least partially, through the activation of the proto-oncogene c-Myb (Hess et al., 2006). Furthermore, retroviral co-transduction studies in mice have demonstrated that HOXa9 and MEIS1 expression immortalizes hematopoietic progenitors in vitro and rapidly accelerates leukemia development (Kroon et al., 1998). In addition, MLL1-fusion proteins fail to transform bone marrow cells in which HOXa7 and HOXa9 expression are genetically ablated (Ayton and Cleary, 2003). Similarly, it has been demonstrated that expression of HOXa9 and MEIS1 can replace the leukemogenic activity of MLL1-ENL (Zeisig et al., 2004). Collectively, these results suggest that HOXa9 dysregulation is an important factor in some MLL1-fusion induced leukemias (Ayton and Cleary, 2003). However, not all leukemogenic fusions result in HOXa9 dysregulation. For example, MLL1-GAS7 and MLL1-AF9 fusions were shown to transform bone marrow cells or mice that do not express HOXa9 (Kumar et al., 2004; So et al., 2004).

However, in addition to disregulation of HOX genes, other signaling pathways are perturbed by MLL-translocations and may contribute to leukemogeneis. For example, transcriptional deregulation of FMS-like tyrosine kinase 3(FLT3), glycogen synthase kinase 3 (GSK3), heat shock protein-90 (HSP-90), myeloid cell leukemia sequence-1 (MCL-1), and components of the RAS pathway have been implicated in MLL1-induced leukemogenesis (Armstrong et al., 2003; Brown et al., 2005; Carnicer et al., 2004; Liang et al., 2006; Stubbs et al., 2008; Wang et al., 2008; Yao et al., 2005; Yasui et al., 2005; Yocum et al., 2006). MLL1's role as a master regulator of gene expression significantly complicates understanding its role in MLL1 associated leukemogenesis.

The master regulatory role of MLL1 in transcriptional control has implications that affect our normal understanding of malignancy. For example, it has been suggested that second-hit mutations are required to initiate the full leukemia phenotype (Dobson et al., 2000). Indeed, recent studies have identified mutations in p53, ATM, Ras, and FLT3 genes in MLL1 leukemia patients (Felix et al., 1998; Mahgoub et al., 1998; Oguchi et al., 2003; Taketani et al., 2004). However, because of MLL1's role in epigenetic gene control, second hit mutations could also arise in the form of epigenetic mutations that result in silencing of tumor suppressors genes without changes in their DNA sequence. For example, it has been demonstrated that the FHIT tumor suppressor gene is epigenetically silenced in human primary tumor cells and tumor cell lines with MLL1-translocations (Stam et al., 2006). These data suggest that epigenetic alterations may be just as important as genetic mutations in sources of so called "2nd hit" mutations that underlie the pathogenesis of leukemia. Recent advances in deep sequencing technologies such as RNA-SEQ and CHIP-SEq will likely allow us to better distinguish genetic versus epigenetic aberrations in future studies.

3.2 Partial tandem duplications: A cytogenetically normal rearrangement in MLL1

3.2.1 Clinical significance of MLL1 partial tandem duplications (MLL1-PTDs)

The second common MLL1-rearrangement, internal partial tandem duplication (MLL1-PTD) was first observed in de novo AML patients with a normal karyotype or trisomy 11 (Caligiuri et al., 1994). MLL1-PTDs are found in 4-7% of the cases of AML and present a cytogenetically normal rearrangement that is associated with poor prognosis (Caligiuri et al., 1998; Dohner et al., 2002; Schichman et al., 1994; Schichman et al., 1995). MLL1-PTDs result from an in frame fusion of exons 11-5 or 12-5 upstream of exon 5, partially duplicating sequences in the 5′ end of MLL1 (Caligiuri et al., 1994; Quentmeier et al., 2003; Schichman et al., 1994). The protein product of MLL1-PTDs has a duplicated N-terminus that contains an additional AT-hook and CXXC domain while essentially retaining all the conserved domains in wild-type MLL1 (Quentmeier et al., 2003; Schichman et al., 1994). In contrast to the variety of MLL1-fusions that delete the MLL1 C-terminus, MLL1-PTDs retain the 3′-portion of the gene that encodes the SET domain methyltransferase motif (Figure 2). Recent data suggests that the enzymatic activity of the MLL-PTD SET domain participates in a gain-of function phenotype in AML.

3.2.2 Mechanism of leukemic transformation by MLL1-PTDs

The molecular mechanisms that underlie MLL1-PTD transformation in AML are currently unknown. The crucial alteration is the duplication of AT hooks and CXXC DNA binding motifs, which may alter target gene specificity. It has been suggested that duplication of these segments may also mimic dimerization observed in several MLL1 chimeric fusion proteins (Martin et al., 2003). Indeed, it has been demonstrated that a synthetic MLL1 N-terminal construct containing duplicated AT-hook and CXXC domains possesses potent transactivation activity in luciferase reporter assays (Martin et al., 2003). However, comparison of genome-wide gene expression data shows that MLL1-PTD primary cells have gene expression patterns that are distinct from that of cells bearing MLL1 chimeric fusions suggesting that the mechanism underlying transformation is distinct (Ross et al., 2004). Alternatively, it has been suggested that the additional amino acid sequences in MLL1-PTD might adopt a conformation that potentially interferes with the normal function of MLL1 by distancing the regulatory domains from its target site (Dou and Hess, 2008).

There is a growing body of evidence that suggests that epigenetic alterations underlie the pathogenesis of MLL1-PTDs. For example, it has been demonstrated that knock-in mice bearing $MLL1^{PTD/WT}$ exhibit increased expression of HOXa7, HOXa9, and HOXa10 that is associated with increased H3K4 methylation and H3/H4 acetylation within these promoters (Dorrance et al., 2006). Similar gene expression and H3K4 dimethylation changes were seen in the presence and absence of the wild type MLL1 allele in primary MLL1-PTD mouse fetal liver cells, suggesting that MLL1-PTD behaves as a dominant gain-of-function mutation (Dorrance et al., 2008). This phenotype may also be due to other epigenetic alterations. For example, Whitman and colleagues (2005) have demonstrated that the wild type MLL1 allele in $MLL1^{PTD/WT}$ AML cells is silenced in a manner that is associated with hypoacetylation of histones H3 and H4 (Whitman et al., 2005). Treatment of MLL1-PTD cells with histone deacetylase inhibitors partially reactivates wild type MLL1 expression and reduces AML blast colony forming units (Whitman et al., 2008). In addition, it has been demonstrated that the SLC5A8 tumor suppressor gene is silenced in MLL-PTD cells in a manner that is associated with increased DNA methylation in its promoter, a phenotype that is partially reversed with DNA methyltransferase inhibitors (Whitman et al., 2008). SLC5A8 encodes a membrane monocarboxylate transporter that regulates intracellular concentrations of histone deacetylase inhibitors, such as butyrate and pyruvate (Ganapathy et al., 2005; Gupta et al., 2006). Together, these observations suggest that targeting MLL1-PTD may have therapeutic value in the treatment of AML (Whitman et al., 2005). Indeed, it has been demonstrated that down regulation of MLL1-PTD using antisense oligodeoxynucleotides (aODNs) in primary human MLL-PTD AMLs results in reactivation of the wild type MLL1 gene, reduced AML blast-derived colony forming units, and increased sensitivity to cell death (Whitman et al., 2008).

3.3 Acute myeloid leukemia with amplifications in MLL1

Amplifications of the MLL1 gene, including trisomy 11 and intrachromosomal amplifications, are found with less frequency in AML and other myelodysplastic syndromes and are associated with a complex karyotype and poor prognosis (Allen et al., 1998; Ariyama et al., 1998; Avet-Loiseau et al., 1999; Cuthbert et al., 1999; Herry et al., 2006; Poppe et al., 2004; Streubel et al., 2000). Amplifications involving MLL1 result in up-regulation of several HOX genes including, HOXa7, HOXa9, and MEIS1 (Herry et al., 2006; Poppe et al., 2004). These studies suggest that MLL1-amplifications contribute to leukemogenesis through mechanisms that share some features with that of MLL1-fusions and MLL1-PTDs. In addition, gene expression analyses have identified other proteins that are up-regulated in AML with 11q23 amplifications including cell surface receptors PROML1, ADAM10, and NKG2D, and the inosine triphosphatase (ITPA) (Poppe et al., 2004). These data suggest that MLL1 amplifications are associated with a gain-of-function phenotype that may be responsive to targeted therapy (Poppe et al., 2004).

In spite of these advances in our understanding of the pathogenesis of MLL1-linked leukemias, identification of inhibitors that specifically target MLL1 or MLL1-chimeric fusion proteins has so far proven elusive. Although in recent years the introduction of broadly based chemotherapeutic interventions such as all-trans retinoic acid, cytosine arabinoside, histone deacetylase and DNA methyltransferase inhibitors has increased the survival rates in some leukemia patients (Altucci et al., 2005; Downing, 2008; Liedtke and Cleary, 2009), molecular therapies that target MLL1 are still lacking. Recent advances in our understanding of the protein-protein interactions involving MLL1 suggest several novel therapeutic strategies for targeted inhibition of MLL1 or MLL1 chimeric fusion activity in leukemic cells. These advances are reviewed in sections 3-6 (and are summarized in Figure 8).

4. Targeting MLL1-Menin interaction as a therapeutic strategy to treat Mixed Lineage Leukemia

4.1 Menin is a common component of wild-type and mutant MLL1 complexes

Despite the growing evidence demonstrating a role for HOX genes in hematopoiesis, it is unclear how the array of mutations involving the MLL1 gene all contribute to altered HOX gene expression in acute leukemias. While there is little that is common among the different types of MLL1 aberrations, all types of MLL1 gene mutations including: chromosomal translocations, internal partial tandem duplications, and gene amplifications, retain the N-terminus of MLL1 (Daser and Rabbitts, 2005; Hess, 2004; Mitterbauer-Hohendanner and Mannhalter, 2004). These ~1400 N-terminal amino acids contain the DNA binding AT-hooks and CXXC domains as well as the binding site for nuclear proteins menin (called the Menin Binding Motif or MBM) and the LEDGF binding domain (LBD) (Figures 1 and 2). Menin, which directly binds wild-type MLL1 and MLL1-oncogenic fusion proteins, is an essential co-factor for the maintenance of normal hematopoiesis and the leukemogenic activity of MLL1-associated translocations (Chen et al., 2006b; Hughes et al., 2004; Yokoyama et al., 2005; Yokoyama et al., 2004). The importance of menin in the pathogenesis of MLL1-related leukemia and progress on the development of inhibitors that target the MLL1-menin interaction is reviewed in this section.

4.2 MEN1 tumorigenesis

Menin is the product of MEN1 gene located at chromosome band 11q13. Menin functions as a tumor suppressor protein that is mutated in patients with an inherited syndrome called Multiple Endocrine Neoplasia 1 (MEN1) (Chandrasekharappa et al., 1997; Chandrasekharappa and Teh, 2001; Larsson et al., 1988). To date, more than 400 nonsense and frame-shift mutations have been reported in MEN1 patients often developing parathyroid, pancreatic or pituitary tumors after the loss of the wild-type MEN1 allele (Dong et al., 1997; Larsson et al., 1988; Lemmens et al., 1997; Thakker, 2001). Homozygous knockout of MEN1 (-/-) is embryonic lethal in mice, which die at the mid-gestation period with profound defects in liver, heart and the neural tube (Bertolino et al., 2003a; Crabtree et al., 2001; Stewart et al., 1998). Heterozygous knockout mice are viable until the adult stages, but develop tumors similar to human MEN1 syndrome in pancreatic islets, parathyroid, anterior pituitary, adrenal cortex and adrenal medulla (Bertolino et al., 2003b; Crabtree et al., 2001). Although the loss of menin results in tumors of the endocrine lineage, the MEN1 gene is ubiquitously expressed in most adult tissues and at all developmental stages (Chandrasekharappa and Teh, 2001, 2003). In spite of the increasing evidence that highlights a role for menin in MEN1 tumors, the basic biology of menin dependent tumor suppression is unclear.

4.3 Menin homology and conserved domain architecture

Menin is highly conserved among vertebrates including, humans, mouse, rat, and zebrafish. However, menin orthologs have not been identified in budding yeast *Saccharomyces cerevisiae* or in the nematode *Caenorhabditis elegans* (Stewart et al., 1998) (Guru et al., 1999; Guru et al., 2001; Khodaei et al., 1999; Manickam et al., 2000). Strikingly, several of the disease-associated MEN1 mutations occur at conserved amino acid positions, highlighting a crucial role for menin in regulating cell proliferation in higher eukaryotes (Chandrasekharappa and Teh, 2003; Poisson et al., 2003). Menin is a novel nuclear protein of ~610 amino acids and does not share significant sequence homology to any other known proteins (Chandrasekharappa et al., 1997; Guru et al., 1998; Poisson et al., 2003). However, extensive analysis of sequence alignments among menin homologues has revealed several domains with putative roles in nuclear targeting and transcriptional regulation. Conserved domain search using the human menin amino acid sequence identified putative domains such as: consensus GTPase-like motifs (G1-G5), two leucine-zipper motifs, a proline-rich region and two nuclear localization signals (NLS) (Balogh et al., 2006; Chandrasekharappa and Teh, 2003; Poisson et al., 2003) (Figure 3). However, it is unclear as to how these conserved motifs contribute to the tumor suppressor function of menin.

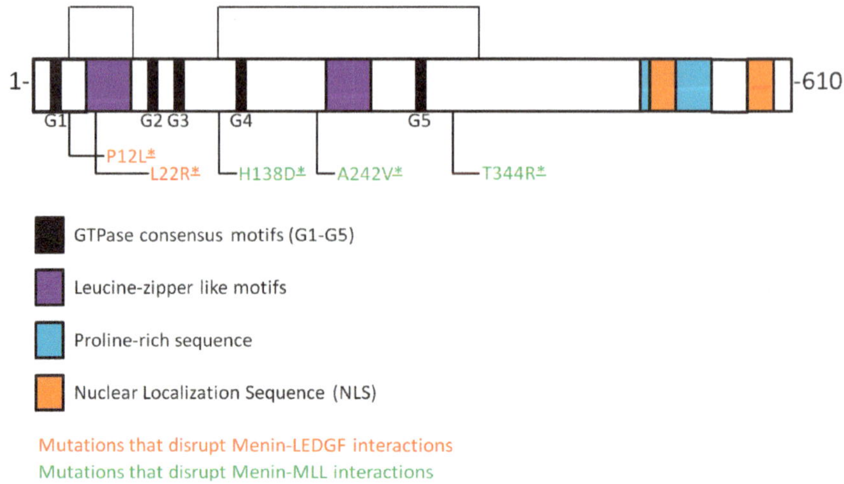

Schematic representation of the conserved regions in human menin with the various functional domains indicated in different colors: GTPase consensus-motifs G1-G5 (black), leucine-zipper-like motifs (purple), proline-rich sequence (blue), and nuclear localization signal (NLS) (orange). Naturally occurring MEN1 mutations that disrupt its interaction with MLL1 (green) and LEDGF (red) are indicated below.

Fig. 3. Domain architecture of human menin showing conserved domains

4.4 Menin molecular interaction network

The precise biochemical function of menin has so far proven elusive due to the lack of any known functional domains in menin. However, it has been suggested that the transcriptional regulatory properties of menin are regulated by protein-protein interactions (Balogh et al., 2006; Jin et al.; Poisson et al., 2003; Yokoyama and Cleary, 2008; Yokoyama et al., 2004). Recent biochemical efforts have been undertaken to elucidate the molecular pathways that underlie menin-dependent transcriptional regulation (Balogh et al., 2006). Using yeast two-hybrid, GST pull-down and co-immunoprecipitation assays, menin was shown to interact with a cohort of proteins that are involved in cell cycle regulation, DNA replication and repair, genome stability, endocrine metabolism, bone morphogenesis and hematopoiesis (Balogh et al., 2006; Chandrasekharappa and Teh, 2003; Hughes et al., 2004; Wu and Hua, 2008). These studies uncovered a wide variety of proteins that may or may not interact directly with menin. These proteins (menin interacting proteins or MIPs) can be grouped into four major functional classes: Class I, which includes transcription factors like JunD (Agarwal et al., 1999; Gobl et al., 1999; Heppner et al., 2001), NFkB (p50, p52 and p65) (Heppner et al., 2001), Smad3 (Kaji et al., 2001), BMP2 (bone morphogenic protein 2) (Sowa et al., 2004), IGFBP-2 (Insulin-like growth factor binding protein 2) (La et al., 2004), FANCD2 (fanconi anemia complementation group D2 protein) (Jin et al., 2003), Pem (a homeobox containing transcription factor) (Lemmens et al., 2001), cMyb (Jin et al.); Class II, which includes DNA damage and replication proteins such as RPA (replication protein A 1 and 2) (Sukhodolets et al., 2003); Class III, which includes cell cycle regulatory proteins such as CDK inhibitors (p18 and p27) (Milne et al., 2005), ASK (activator s-phase kinase)

(Schnepp et al., 2004), type III intermediate filaments (glial fibrillary acidic protein or GFAP and Vimentin) (Lopez-Egido et al., 2002); and Class IV, which includes transcriptional activators such as MLL1/2 (mixed lineage leukemia proteins) (Hughes et al., 2004; Yokoyama et al., 2004), RNA polymerase II phosphorylated carboxy terminal domain (Hughes et al., 2004), LEDGF (Yokoyama and Cleary, 2008), and CHD1 (chromo domain helicase I) (Chen et al., 2006b). Based on these studies it has been suggested that MIPs modulate the transcriptional activator/repressor functions of menin (Agarwal et al., 1999; Agarwal et al., 2003; Heppner et al., 2001; Kaji et al., 2001). While a direct role for the interaction of menin with all MIPs has yet to be validated in vivo, it is possible that MIPs regulate transcription by binding directly or indirectly to menin (Balogh et al., 2006; Chandrasekharappa and Teh, 2003; Wu and Hua, 2008). In addition, menin also binds to a putative tumor metastasis suppressor/nucleoside diphosphate kinase (Nm23), which stimulates the GTP hydrolyzing activity of menin (Ohkura et al., 2001). Moreover, menin also functions as a transcriptional co-activator of the nuclear receptor pathway by binding with estrogen receptor-alpha (ERalpha) in a hormone-dependent manner (Dreijerink et al., 2006). A non-specific DNA binding activity through the C-terminal NLS has also been reported for menin (La et al., 2004). Of the multitude of interactions reported for menin, it is the association with the SET1 family methyltransferases MLL1/2 that has generated a lot of interest due to their roles in hematopoiesis and leukemia.

4.5 Role of menin in Hematopoiesis

Menin is an essential component of MLL1/2 family complexes with specific roles in the maintenance of HOX gene expression patterns during hematopoiesis (Hughes et al., 2004; Yokoyama et al., 2004). Conditional knockouts of the MEN1 gene in mice decreases peripheral white blood cell counts as well as colony forming potential of bone marrow hematopoietic progenitors (Chen et al., 2006b). Recent work by Maillard et al., (2009a), suggests that while conditional menin knockouts have modest effects on hematopoiesis under steady-state conditions, more severe defects are observed in competitive transplantation assays and during drug-mediated chemoablation (Maillard et al., 2009). These studies suggest that menin functions as an essential regulator of hematopoietic stem cell (HSC) homeostasis specifically in situations of hematopoietic stress (Maillard and Hess, 2009). These phenotypes may be due, at least in part, to menin's role in regulating *HOX* gene expression. For example, small-interfering RNA (siRNA) mediated knockdown of menin or conditional MEN1 (-/-) knockout embryos show significant decreases in the expression levels of several HOX genes including HOXa9, HOXc6, and HOXc8 (Chen et al., 2006b; Hughes et al., 2004; Wu and Hua, 2008; Yokoyama et al., 2004). Interestingly, these hematopoietic defects are rescued by the ectopic expression of menin or its downstream targets HOXa9/MEIS1 (Chen et al., 2006b; Hughes et al., 2004). Evidence indicates that menin's interaction with MLL1/2 complexes is required for its role in transcription. For example, chromatin immunoprecipitation studies using antibodies specific to menin, MLL1, trimethylated H3K4 or CHD1 (which binds trimethylated H3K4) (Flanagan et al., 2005; Pray-Grant et al., 2005; Sims et al., 2005) have further established that menin co-localizes with these components at HOXa9 promoters and is required for transcriptional activation (Chen et al., 2006b; Wu and Hua, 2008). Furthermore, it has been shown that a subset of naturally occurring mutations in menin (H139D, A242V, and T344R) disrupts its association with MLL1 and fails to associate with MLL1-dependent H3K4 methyltransferase activity

(Hughes et al., 2004) (Refer to figure 3 for MEN1 mutations). These findings underscore the importance of the menin-MLL1 interaction in regulating HOX gene expression in hematopoiesis.

4.6 Role of menin in leukemogenesis

The first evidence for the involvement of menin in MLL1-associated leukemogenesis came from the initial biochemical studies carried out by Yokoyama et al., (2005) who identified a menin binding motif (MBM) located within the first 330 amino acids of MLL1, a region that is also retained in all types of MLL1 aberrations (Figures 1 and 2) (Yokoyama et al., 2005). Using leukemia cells that carry specific MLL1-translocations (MLL1-AF6, MLL1-ENL, MLL1-AF9, MLL1-AF10, and MLL1-GAS7) it was demonstrated that menin specifically associates with these MLL1-fusion proteins at the promoter of HOX genes such as: HOXa7, HOXa9 and HOXa10, which are constitutively expressed in several cases of acute leukemia (Chen et al., 2006b; Yokoyama et al., 2005; Yokoyama et al., 2004). Acute loss of menin reduces the aberrant HOX gene expression and abrogates the differentiation arrest associated with these MLL1-fusions (Yokoyama et al., 2005). Furthermore, conditional knockouts of the MEN1 gene suggests that menin is essential for the initiation and maintenance of MLL1-associated, but not other oncogene induced, myeloid transformations (Caslini et al., 2007; Chen et al., 2006b; Yokoyama et al., 2005). Together, these results demonstrate that MLL1-fusion proteins are dependent on menin for their oncogenic properties and raise the possibility that molecular therapies that target the menin-MLL1 interaction might be an effective strategy to treat leukemias.

While it is unclear how menin modulates the activities of wild-type and MLL1-fusion proteins, recent studies suggest that menin functions to recruit other proteins that are required for targeting MLL1 to downstream genes. For example, a recent study by Yokoyama and Cleary (2008) suggests that menin promotes LEDGF binding to MLL1. LEDGF contains a highly conserved PWWP motif that is required for MLL1's association with downstream target genes (Yokoyama and Cleary, 2008). In addition, menin amino acid substitutions that disrupt its interaction with LEDGF without affecting menin's interaction with MLL1 also display decreased Hoxa9 gene expression (Roudaia and Speck, 2008; Yokoyama and Cleary, 2008). These data indicate that part of menin's function is to stabilize the interaction between MLL1 and LEDGF. More recently, it has been shown that menin recruits the transcription factor cMyb to the MLL1 complex, which is required for recruitment of MLL1 to the Hoxa9 promoter (Jin et al., 2010). It has been shown that depletion of cMyb decreases the transforming potential of the MLL1-ENL fusion protein (Jin et al., 2010), suggesting that molecules that inhibit the menin-cMyb interaction may also be useful therapeutic agents.

4.7 Menin interacts with the N-terminus of MLL1 through an evolutionarily conserved Menin Binding Motif (MBM)

The interaction of menin with N-terminal sequences of wild-type MLL1 and MLL1-chimeric fusion proteins have been demonstrated by three independent reports (Caslini et al., 2007; Grembecka et al., 2010; Yokoyama et al., 2005). While the conclusions of these studies differ with respect to the exact length of the MLL1 fragment predicted to be involved in the interaction with menin, they have collectively identified a highly conserved "menin binding motif" (MBM) localized within the first 46 residues of MLL1. For example, Yokoyama et al.,

(2005) demonstrated that a consensus sequence (RXRFP), called the high-affinity MBM, is present between MLL1 amino acids 6-10. Sequence analysis reveals that the MBM is highly conserved among MLL1 orthologs and in MLL2 (residues 17-21) (Figure 3). Deletions of the MBM in the MLL1-ENL and MLL1-GAS7 fusion proteins abrogates the interaction with menin in 293T cells (Yokoyama et al., 2005). Furthermore, MLL1-ENL fusions that lack the MBM fails to induce acute myeloid leukemia in syngeneic recipient mice (Yokoyama et al., 2005). This failure is associated with impaired expression of HOXa7 and HOXa9 genes in the MBM-deleted MLL1-ENL transduced murine myeloid progenitors (Yokoyama et al., 2005). Moreover, MBM deletion mutants of MLL1-ENL lose their clonogenic potential and induce differentiation in leukemia blasts, a phenotype similar to the conditional knock out of menin or MLL1-ENL itself (Ayton and Cleary, 2003; Yokoyama et al., 2005; Zeisig et al., 2004). These studies demonstrate the importance of menin-MLL1 interaction in the pathogenesis of MLL1-associated leukemias.

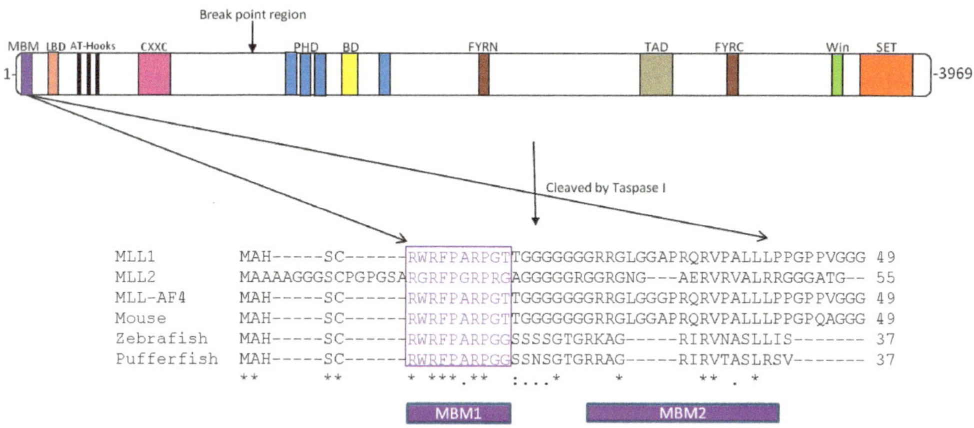

The different functional domains in MLL1 are indicated and color coded as in Figure 1. The menin binding motif encompassing residues 5-44 (purple) along with LEDGF binding domain (LBD)(light red), AT-hooks (black), and the CXXC motif (pink) are retained by both MLL1-translocations and PTD mutations. The blow up region shows a ClustalW multiple sequence alignment of the high affinity menin binding motifs, MBM1 and MBM2, present in human (Q03164), mouse (NP_001074518), zebrafish (ACN88688), and pufferfish (AAC41377) MLL1s; and human MLL2 (O14686), and MLL1-AF4 (AAC37520) fusions (indicated in purple). MBM1 and 2 were identified based on three independent studies (Yokoyama et al., 2005; Caslini et al., 2007; Grembecka et al., 2010).

Fig. 4. Menin Binding Motifs (MBMs) are present in the wild-type MLL1, MLL1 chimeric fusions and partial tandem duplications

In an attempt to further characterize the physiological significance of the MLL1-menin interaction in acute leukemias, Caslini et al., (Caslini et al., 2007) demonstrated that MLL1 residues 5-44 are required for high affinity binding with menin. This MBM region spans the RWRFP motif (residues 6-10) and also includes a second region between MLL1 residues 35 and 44 that is necessary, but not sufficient, for high-affinity interaction with menin (Caslini et al., 2007). Internal deletions in the MLL1-AF9 fusion protein that lacked amino acids 5-15 (high affinity MBM) or 35-44 (low affinity MBM) failed to co-immunoprecipitate with menin from 293T cells (Caslini et al., 2007). Furthermore, Caslini et al., (2007) also demonstrated that MLL1-AF9 MBM sequences were essential for the transformation of hematopoietic progenitors by the MLL1-AF9 fusion protein. Interestingly, the MLL1 constructs MLL1(2-167), MLL1(2-62), and MLL1(2-44) function as dominant negative inhibitors of the MLL1-menin interaction by titrating menin from the endogenous MLL1-AF9 protein resulting in reduced HOXa9 and MEIS1 expression and inhibition of the growth of transformed bone marrow progenitors (Caslini et al., 2007). Together, these results suggest that expression of dominant negative MLL1 constructs or peptide inhibitors that mimic the MLL1-menin interaction can inhibit the transforming potential of MLL1-fusion proteins by specifically down regulating the expression of target HOX genes. Unexpectedly, dominant negative constructs of MLL1 also inhibited the colony-forming ability of wild-type hematopoietic progenitors since these constructs also mimic the interaction surface between wild-type MLL1 and menin (Caslini et al., 2007). Collectively, these findings suggest that small molecule inhibitors that target menin-MLL1 interaction have a therapeutic potential to treat MLL1-associated leukemias, but with the caveat that normal hematopoiesis might also be impaired (Caslini et al., 2007).

4.8 MBM based peptides as novel therapeutic agents for acute leukemias with MLL1-rearrangements

Structural and biochemical studies that characterize the menin-MLL1 interaction in detail is an important step in the development of MBM-based small molecule inhibitors that can specifically help treat MLL1-mediated cancers. Grembecka et al., (2010) carried out a detailed biophysical characterization of the interaction between menin and MLL1 using a combination of NMR, Isothermal Titration Calorimetry (ITC) and Fluorescence Anisotropy (FP). They found that MLL1 binds menin with high affinity (K_d=~10nM) utilizing two menin binding motifs (MBM1 and 2) located within the first 43 amino acids of MLL1 as previously suggested (Caslini et al., 2007; Yokoyama et al., 2005). Furthermore, peptides derived from the MBM1 (amino acids 5-14) and MBM2 (23-40) in MLL1 bind menin with interaction affinities of 53nM and 1400nM, respectively (Grembecka et al., 2010). Using a series of peptide competition experiments, MBM1 and MBM2 peptides were shown to displace a construct of MLL1 (amino acids 2-43) from bound menin in vitro with IC_{50} values of 0.5 μM and 37 μM, respectively (Grembecka et al., 2010). Moreover, based on transfer-nuclear overhauser effects (Tr-NOEs) based NMR experiments, it was further suggested that MBM1 interacts with menin in an extended conformation and that the binding is facilitated by hydrophobic residues Phe9, Pro10 and Pro13 (Grembecka et al., 2010). Substitution to alanine of these amino acid residues significantly impaired the binding of MLL1 constructs to menin (Grembecka et al., 2010). Together, these studies have identified MBM1 (which encompasses the consensus RWRFP) as a potential drug target for leukemias with MLL1 translocations.

5. Molecular targeting of MLL1-rearranged leukemias - Peptide inhibitors that target the activity of MLL1-AF4 and MLL1-AF9 fusion proteins

5.1 Clinical significance of t(4;11) and t(9;11) translocations

MLL1 translocations do not share a common structural motif or biochemical function. However, based on sequence similarities, the most commonly occurring MLL1 fusions can be grouped into three major gene families: AF10/AF17, ENL/AF9, and the largest family,

AF4/LAF4/AF5q31/FMR2 (Nilson et al., 1997). The most common translocation is t(4;11)(q21;q23) and is associated with more than 50% of acute leukemia cases in infants, and for 3-6% of cases in older children (Behm et al., 1996; Faderl et al., 1998; Heerema et al., 1999). The t(4;11) translocations results in leukemic blasts expressing phenotypic markers for ALL in 95% of the cases (Chen et al., 1993; Pui et al., 2003)). t4:11 translocations result in cancers that often spread beyond the hematopoietic lineage and have a poor prognosis (Armstrong et al., 2002; Chen et al., 1993; Rubnitz et al., 1994a). The t(4:11) translocation retains the 5′ portion of MLL1 gene containing the menin binding motif (MBM), AT hooks and the CXXC DNA binding motifs, which are fused in-frame to the 3′ portion of the gene at the 4q21 locus called AF4 (Gu et al., 1992). The high occurrence rates of t(4;11) translocation in infants along with the poor prognosis and absence of chemotherapeutics to treat these leukemias highlight an urgent need for the development of inhibitors that specifically target the gain-of-function phenotypes associated with the MLL1-AF4 fusion. In this regard, inhibitors that target the interaction between AF4 and its partner protein AF9 have been developed recently and show promising results in inhibiting the transforming potential of leukemia cell lines bearing MLL1-AF4 or MLL1-AF9 translocations (Bennett et al., 2009; Palermo et al., 2008; Srinivasan et al., 2004). The biochemical studies that form the basis for these conclusions are summarized in this section.

5.2 Domain architecture and the functional roles of AF4 family

AF4, also known as AFF1/FEL, is a serine/proline-rich nuclear protein with crucial roles in B and T lymphocyte development. AF4 has several putative functional domains including the ALF (AF4/LAF4/FMR2 homology) domain, which mediates the interaction with a family of ubiquitin ligases called SIAH (seven in absentia homolog), a serine/proline-rich transcriptional activation domain (TAD), nuclear localization signals (NLS), a guanosine triphosphate (GTP) binding motif (GBM), and a C-terminal homology domain involved in intra-nuclear localization and binding to pre-mRNA splicing factors (Bensaid et al., 2009; Chen et al., 1993; Isnard et al., 2000; Melko et al.; Morrissey et al., 1993; Oliver et al., 2004) (Figure 5). AF4 is located at a fragile break-point region on chromosome 4 and is associated with a wide variety of chromosomal translocations. AF4 is a member of AF4/LAF4/AF5q31/FMR2 family of nuclear transcription factors (Gu et al., 1996; von Bergh et al., 2001; von Bergh et al., 2002) and also shows significant homology to the Drosophila melanogaster pair-rule gene *Lilliputian* (Su et al., 2001). Surprisingly, three of these family members (AF4/LAF4/AF5q31) are associated with infant leukemias involving reciprocal translocations with the MLL1 gene (Domer et al., 1993; Ma and Staudt, 1996; Taki et al., 1999). The second family member LAF4, isolated from Burkitt's lymphoma, is a lymphoid-specific transcription factor and has transcriptional activation domains and nuclear localization signals that are highly similar to AF4 (Ma and Staudt, 1996). Indeed, the MLL1-LAF4 fusion proteins also retain the TAD in LAF4, which can functionally substitute for the activation domain in MLL1, thereby the contributing to the leukemogenic potential of these chimeric fusion proteins (Ma and Staudt, 1996). The third AF4 homologue AF5q31 was originally identified from infant acute leukemias with a (5;11)(q31;q13q23) translocation (Taki et al., 1999). Strikingly, each of these MLL1-AF4 gene family fusions manifest very similar clinical characteristics- that is, early onset, poor prognosis, and a mixed immunophenotype. However, the fourth AF4 family member, FMR2, is associated with mental retardation and is located in the folate-sensitive break-point region at chromosome X band q28 (Gecz, Gedeon et al. 1996; Gu, Shen et al. 1996). FMR2 has not been reported to be a part of any MLL1 fusions.

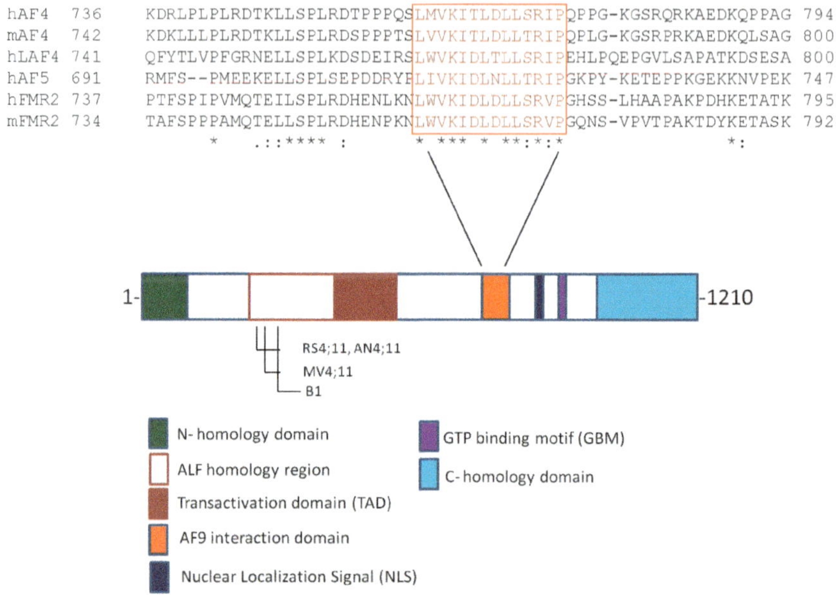

Overview of the protein domain structure of human AF4 adapted from (Li et al., 1998; Srinivasan et al., 2004 and Melko et al., 2011). The different domains are highlighted: N-homology region with an unknown function (green), ALF (AF4/LAF4/FMR2 homology) region which includes the transcription activation domain (dark red), AF9 interaction region (orange), nuclear localization signals (dark blue), a putative consensus guanosine triphosphate (GTP) binding motif (purple), and C-terminal homology domain (light blue). The domains are not drawn to scale. The ClustalW multiple protein sequence alignment of the AF9 binding regions of AF4 family members: human AF4 (hAF4, Pubmed ID: P51825), mouse AF4 (mAF4, Pubmed: AAU93698), human LAF4 (hLAF4, PubMed ID: NP002276), human AF5 (hAF5, PubMed ID: Q9UHB7), human FMR2 (hFMR2, PubMed ID: BAC81113) and mouse FMR2 (mFMR2, PubMed ID: CAA04821) are shown with the AF9 interaction region boxed. Chromosomal break points are also indicated for cell lines carrying t(4;11) translocations.

Fig. 5. Domain representation of human AF4 highlighting the AF9 interaction region.

Despite the growing amount of clinical evidence suggesting the involvement of MLL1-AF4 family translocations in human acute leukemias, the molecular mechanisms by which the MLL1-AF4 fusion proteins induce neoplasia are not fully understood. One possibility is that the resulting MLL1-AF4 fusion protein has a gain-of function phenotype wherein the transcriptional activation domain of AF4 is fused to the DNA binding domains of MLL1 and alters the regulation of MLL1 dependent genes (Prasad et al., 1995). However, genetic studies using mouse knock-in models suggest that the two fusion proteins MLL1-AF4 and AF4-MLL1 resulting from the balanced reciprocal translocation between MLL1 and AF4 could independently contribute to the pathogenesis of t(4;11) mediated acute leukemias (Bursen et al.; Chen et al., 2006a; Isnard et al., 2000). Importantly, the AF4-MLL1 fusion protein retains the C-terminal portion of MLL1 including its SET domain, and is sufficient to induce leukemia in the absence of MLL1-AF4 (Bursen et al., 2010).

5.3 Molecular interaction network for AF4 fusion proteins

These studies raise the possibility that MLL1-AF4 and AF4-MLL1 participate in different sets of interaction networks as compared to the native full-length proteins (MLL1 and AF4) and result in gene expression signatures that are a representative of the physiological function of the fusion partners. This hypothesis is supported by the studies of Benedikt et al., (2011), who used affinity purified AF4 and AF4-MLL1 complexes from 293T cells to elucidate the subunit composition of the two complexes (Benedikt et al., 2011). Wild-type AF4 was purified in a complex containing the CDK9/Cyclin T heterodimer, which resembles the positive transcription elongation factor b (p-TEFb) (Benedikt et al., 2011; Estable et al., 2002) and also co-purifies with the wild type versions of two other known MLL1 fusion partners, AF9 and ENL, both of which bind to the C-terminus of AF4 family members (Benedikt et al., 2011; Erfurth et al., 2004; Mueller et al., 2009). Furthermore, ENL binding to AF4 creates a binding site for AF10, DOT1 methyltransferase and histone H3 (Benedikt et al., 2011; Mueller et al., 2007). Both the DOT1 mediated H3K79 methylation and the p-TEFb mediated phosphorylation of RNA Pol II C-terminal domain could lead to transcriptional elongation and is facilitated by the interaction of wild-type AF4 with these proteins (Benedikt et al., 2011; Bitoun et al., 2007). In contrast, the subunit composition of the AF4-MLL1 complex is different from the wild-type AF4 protein alone due to additional proteins that interact with the fused MLL1 C-terminal fragment. These proteins likely modulate the transcriptional activating properties of AF4-MLL1 fusion protein (Benedikt et al., 2011). MLL1-AF4 chimeric fusions on the other hand have an intact C-terminus of AF4 and therefore retain the transcriptional activation domains and its ability to interact with AF9 and ENL.

5.4 Functional significance of AF9/ENL family

Reciprocal translocations involving the AF9 (t(9;11)(p22;q23)) and ENL (t(11;19)(q23;p13)) genes are also associated with several cases of ALL and AML (Mitelman and Heim, 1992). Similar to AF4, AF9 also belongs to a family of serine/proline-rich transcription factors (Hemenway et al., 2001; Nakamura et al., 1993; Prasad et al., 1995) and shares significant similarity to ENL and the yeast protein ANC1 (Rubnitz et al., 1994b; Welch and Drubin, 1994). Interestingly, ANC1 has been demonstrated to be a part of the yeast RNA polymerase II complex, as well as the SWI/SNF nucleosome-remodeling complex, a macromolecular complex which functions as ATP-dependent chromatin remodeler (Cairns et al., 1996; Carlson and Laurent, 1994; Cote et al., 1994). The high degree of sequence similarity between human AF9/ENL and the yeast ANC1 protein has led to the hypothesis that AF9 and ENL may also interact with a human SWI/SNF remodeling complex similar to yeast ANC1, and the MLL1-AF9/ENL fusion proteins may retain these features. The biological functions of AF4, AF9 and ENL are not clearly understood, however, gene deletion studies in mice have demonstrated important roles for these proteins during development (Collins et al., 2002; Doty et al., 2002; Isnard et al., 2000). Furthermore, the endogenous ENL protein was purified as a part of a macromolecular complex (ENL associated protein complex or EAP) that also contains p-TEFb, DOT1 and AF4 and plays a putative role in transcriptional elongation (Bitoun et al., 2007; Mueller et al., 2007). Despite the fact that MLL1-AF4 translocations and MLL1-AF9/ENL fusions account for more than 50% of MLL1 11q23 associated leukemias (Burmeister et al., 2009; Meyer et al., 2009; Meyer et al., 2006), there exists no functional similarity between these MLL1 fusion partners. It is tempting to hypothesize that MLL1 fusion proteins might hijack the p-TEFb/DOT1 mediated transcriptional elongation activity or the SWI/SNF dependent nucleosome remodeling activity through the fusion partner and result in constitutive target gene expression leading to leukemia. These studies suggest that pTEFb, DOT1 and the MLL1 fusion partners AF4/AF9/ENL are all molecular targets in the development of therapeutics that target MLL1-fusion mediated leukemias.

5.5 Domain mapping of the interaction region between AF4 and AF9

Co-localization studies carried out by (Erfurth et al., 2004) have established that the two most common MLL1 fusion partners AF4 and AF9 form a stable complex within the nucleus and are restricted to discrete nuclear foci called "AF4 bodies". AF4 bodies are nuclear speckle-like in appearance and are distinct from the nucleolus, cajal bodies, PML body or regions associated with DNA replication and repair (Erfurth et al., 2004). Using yeast two-hybrid screens it was demonstrated that the minimum motif in human AF4 required for binding AF9 encompasses 14 residues (761-774) that are proximal to the bipartite nuclear localization signal (NLS) in AF4 (refer to figure 5 for domain representation). Deletion of these residues completely abolishes the interaction between AF4 and AF9 and also results in diffuse AF4 bodies (Erfurth et al., 2004; Srinivasan et al., 2004). Site-directed mutagenesis studies reveals that bulky hydrophobic residues within the conserved AF9 binding region in mouse AF4 (mAF4) dictate its binding affinity to AF9 (Srinivasan et al., 2004). Using fluorescent tagged AF4 and AF9 constructs it was further demonstrated that both the 14 residue AF9 binding motif and the bipartite NLS was required for the punctate nuclear speckle distribution of AF4-AF9 complexes (Erfurth et al., 2004). Likewise, the terminal 93 residues in AF9 (and the terminal 84 in the case of ENL) were identified as the minimal region required for binding AF4 (Erfurth et al., 2004). Interestingly, the mutual interaction domains between AF4 and AF9 are highly conserved in the AF4 and AF9 homologues (refer to figure 5 for sequence alignment) (Erfurth et al., 2004; Srinivasan et al., 2004) and the AF4-AF9 interaction region is retained by the MLL1 fusion proteins (MLL1-AF4 and MLL1-AF9) (Dobson et al., 1999; Domer et al., 1993; Erfurth et al., 2004), suggesting that AF4-AF9 interaction might be an important step in the pathogenesis associated with these MLL1 fusions. The functional significance of the interaction between AF4 and AF9 is unclear; however, the co-localization of these two proteins to specific sub-nuclear foci suggests that AF4-AF9 interaction might be required for normal cellular functions as well as in the pathogenesis of MLL1-AF4 or MLL1-AF9 associated leukemias (Erfurth et al., 2004). Furthermore, the presence of this interaction region in MLL1-AF4 and MLL1-AF9 fusion proteins, and the ability of MLL1-AF4 fusions to alter the localization of endogenous AF9 also suggest that AF4-AF9 protein complex is a pharmacological target for leukemia therapy (Erfurth et al., 2004; Srinivasan et al., 2004).

5.6 A synthetic peptide PFWT disrupts the interaction between AF4 and AF9

Based on the initial mapping studies of the AF9 binding region in AF4, a synthetic peptide, designated "PFWT" that mimics the interaction region was developed and tested for its ability to disrupt the AF4-AF9 interaction both in vitro and in vivo (Erfurth et al., 2004; Srinivasan et al., 2004). The initial PFWT peptide developed in this study was based on the highly conserved AF4-AF9 interaction sequence in the mouse FMR2 protein and encompasses residues (759-771) (see Figure 5 for the sequence alignment of the AF9 interaction region in AF4 family members). To enable nuclear uptake, the PFWT peptide was conjugated to a penetratin transporter sequence at its N-terminus (Srinivasan et al., 2004). Using pull-down assays with GST-tagged AF4 and biotinylated AF9, it was shown that this PFWT peptide disrupts the interaction between human AF4 and AF9 in a concentration dependent manner (Srinivasan et al., 2004). However, a control peptide (containing amino acid substitutions at V763E and I765S) did not interfere with the binding of AF4-AF9 complex (Srinivasan et al., 2004). The specificity of PFWT peptide against AF4-AF9 complexes was further demonstrated by its inability to disrupt the interaction between AF9 and two other proteins, the Polycomb protein (MPC3) and the mouse homolog of BCL-6 co-repressor (mBCoR), both of which interact through the C-terminus of AF9 (Hemenway et al., 2001; Srinivasan et al., 2003; Srinivasan et al., 2004). Furthermore, the PFWT peptide was shown to be readily taken up by NIH3T3 cells and disrupts the co-localization of AF4-AF9 in vivo (Srinivasan et al., 2004). These results corroborated the in vitro findings that the PFWT peptide has the ability to specifically disrupt the interaction between AF4 and AF9 protein complexes.

5.7 PFWT peptide inhibits the cell proliferation of leukemia cell lines with t(4;11) and t(9;11) translocations

Based on these observations it was further predicted that the PFWT peptide will have the ability to inhibit the proliferation of leukemia cell lines that carry a t(4;11)(q21;q23) or t(9;11)(p22;q23) translocations (Bennett et al., 2009; Palermo et al., 2008; Srinivasan et al., 2004). As expected, PFWT peptide specifically inhibits the proliferation of leukemia cell lines B1, MV4-11 and RS4;11 (Cohen et al., 1991; Lange et al., 1987; Stong et al., 1985) that harbor the MLL1-AF4 translocation (Bennett et al., 2009; Palermo et al., 2008; Srinivasan et al., 2004). Interestingly, the PFWT peptide also inhibits the survival capacity of KP-L-RY cell lines (Cohen et al., 1991) that are characterized by a t(5;11) translocation associated with MLL1-AF5q31 fusions (Srinivasan et al., 2004). In contrast to cell lines that carry either the MLL1-AF4 or MLL1-AF5q31 translocations, the PFWT peptide shows mixed effects in the inhibition of the proliferative capacity of leukemia cell lines that carry MLL1-AF9 translocations (Palermo et al., 2008; Srinivasan et al., 2004).). For instance, based on the study by (Srinivasan et al., 2004), the PFWT peptide failed to inhibit the growth of THP-1 cells (Tsuchiya et al., 1980) that are associated with MLL1-AF9 translocations. However, a more recent study demonstrated that Molm13 leukemia cells that are also associated with MLL1-AF9 translocations are sensitive to treatments with PFWT peptide in a dose dependent manner (Palermo et al., 2008). While these findings suggest that there are differences in the inhibitory properties of the PFWT peptide towards cell lines that carry a similar translocation, it highlights the fact that these leukemias might operate through additional pathways that lead to misregulated gene expression profiles (Palermo et al., 2008; Srinivasan et al., 2004). Furthermore, the specificity of PFWT peptide in inhibiting leukemia cells with MLL1-AF4 and MLL1-AF9 mutations is corroborated by the findings that the MOLT-4 (T-ALL) cell line (Minowada et al., 1972) that does not contain a MLL1-AF4 translocation is not affected by the PFWT peptide even at higher doses (Srinivasan et al., 2004). However, the Reh (B-precursor) cell lines (Koziner et al., 1985) that do not carry a MLL1-AF4 chimeric fusion are susceptible to the PFWT peptide (Srinivasan et al., 2004). These results suggest that some cell lines might require the function of normal AF4-AF9 complexes for its carcinogenesis and these native complexes are also targeted by the PFWT peptides

(Srinivasan et al., 2004). Nevertheless, these findings demonstrate the wide range of specificity for the PFWT peptide and suggest that PFWT-like peptides are promising lead compounds in the development of treatment regimens for the most frequent 11q23 translocations. The pharmacological importance of PFWT based peptides is further enhanced by the fact that these peptides have little effect on the number and colony forming potential of hematopoietic progenitor cells (Srinivasan et al., 2004), suggesting that PFWT-like peptides may have fewer side effects .

5.8 PFWT peptide as a lead compound in the treatment of MLL1-rearranged leukemias

While initial studies suggest that the growth inhibitory properties of the PFWT peptide is mediated through apoptosis (Srinivasan et al., 2004), recent work by (Palermo et al., 2008) demonstrates that PFWT peptide induces cell death by necrosis in MV4-11 and Molm13 cell lines. Necrotic cell death was further demonstrated by the changes in plasma membrane integrity in the absence of traditional apoptotic markers: nuclear disintegration, caspase activation, DNA fragmentation or mitochondrial membrane depolarization (Palermo et al., 2008). Given the resistance of t(4;11) translocations to conventional pro-apoptotic chemotherapeutic drugs, PFWT mediated necrotic cell death is an attractive alternative strategy to treat these acute leukemias. More recently, Bennett et al., (Bennett et al., 2009) demonstrated that the PFWT peptide in combination with standard chemotherapeutic agents such as etoposide, 17AAG (17-(allylamino)-17-demthoxygeldamycin), cytarabine, and Flt-3 kinase inhibitor results in synergistic cytotoxicity in MV4-11 cells that harbor t(4;11) translocations. Furthermore, cell death was mediated through both apoptotic and necrotic pathways suggesting that PFWT peptides could be useful in combinatorial therapy to treat leukemia cell lines that are relatively resistant to current apoptotic drugs (Bennett et al., 2009; Campo Dell'Orto et al., 2007; Nakanishi et al., 2007; Wiederschain et al., 2005). Together, these findings emphasize that PFWT peptides inhibit the proliferation of t(4;11), t(5;11) and t(9;11) leukemia cell lines by specifically disrupting the association of AF4 or AF5q31 with AF9 and serves as a starting point for the development of more effective therapeutic strategies. In the absence of a crystal structure that clearly demonstrates the interaction mode between AF4 and AF9 proteins, systematic site-directed mutagenesis experiments can help identify amino acid positions that are more important for the overall binding affinity. Such an approach has the potential to help identify additional PFWT-based peptido-mimetic compounds that have better inhibitory properties than the initial PFWT peptide and prevent the potential toxic side effects that could occur at high doses of the PFWT peptide.

6. Win motif-based inhibitors that target the assembly and enzymatic activity of the MLL1 core complex

6.1 Novel strategies that target the histone methyltransferase activity of MLL1 amplifications and MLL1-PTDs

Growing evidence suggests that increased HOXa gene expression associated with MLL1 amplifications and MLL1-PTDs underlie the pathogenesis of these leukemias (Basecke et al., 2006; Dorrance et al., 2006). HOXa gene expression is dependent on the histone methyltransferase activity of MLL1 ((Milne et al., 2002), and given the increased H3K4 methylation observed in MLL1-PTDs (Dorrance et al., 2008; Dorrance et al., 2006), inhibitors that down-regulate the histone methyltransferase activity of MLL1-PTD have the potential to reverse this aberrant epigenetic program. Until recently, inhibitors that specifically target MLL1's H3K4 methyltransferase activity have been difficult to develop due to lack of a clear understanding of MLL1's structure and function. However, recent findings have established that H3K4 methylation levels are precisely regulated by the function of two independent methyltransferases: the MLL1 SET domain and a novel multi-subunit enzyme, WDR5-RbBP5-Ash2L-DPY30 (WRAD), that lacks sequence homology to known methyltransferases (Patel et al., 2009; Patel et al., 2011). Because multiple methylation on H3K4 is catalyzed by two different enzymes, it is interesting to speculate that inhibitors that prevent the association of two methyltransferases will have clinical significance in the treatment of acute leukemias that are characterized by aberrant H3K4 methylation (Dorrance et al., 2008; Dorrance et al., 2006).

6.2 WDR5 is central for the assembly and H3K4 methylation activity of MLL1 core complex

The WD-40 repeat protein WDR5 is a conserved component of MLL1 family complexes ranging from yeast to humans and has been shown to be crucial for the assembly and H3K4 dimethylation activity of MLL1 core complex HOX (Dou et al., 2006; Patel et al., 2008a; Patel et al., 2008b). Consistent with the role of WDR5 in the regulation of degree of H3K4 methylation, siRNA mediated knock-down of WDR5 in mammalian cells results in a global decrease in the levels of H3K4 di- and trimethylation, down-regulation of HOXa9 and HOXc8 genes, and defects in hematopoiesis and development (Dou et al., 2006; Wysocka et al., 2005). WDR5 knock down and MLL1ΔSET mice show similar phenotypes suggesting that MLL1 and WDR5 function together to regulate H3K4 di/trimethylation and HOX gene expression in vivo (Terranova et al., 2006; Wysocka et al., 2005). Furthermore, growing evidence suggest that WDR5 interacts directly with MLL1 or other SET1 family members and functions as a scaffold to bridge the interactions between MLL1 and rest of the components of MLL1 core complex (Dou et al., 2006; Patel et al., 2008b; Trievel and Shilatifard, 2009; Wysocka et al., 2005). Indeed, MLL1 and WRAD enzymatic complexes fail to associate in the absence of WDR5 (Dou et al., 2006; Patel et al., 2008b), suggesting a crucial role for WDR5 in the assembly and H3K4 methylation activity of MLL1 core complex.

6.3 WDR5 recognizes a conserved arginine containing sequence in the N-SET region of MLL1

Previous studies have suggested that WDR5 functions within the MLL1 core complex as a histone "effector" or "presenter" domain, a domain that specifically recognizes methylated histones (Couture et al., 2006; Han et al., 2006; Ruthenburg et al., 2006; Schuetz et al., 2006; Trievel and Shilatifard, 2009; Wysocka et al., 2005). However, recent studies by Patel et al., (2008a and b) and Song and Kingston., (2008) demonstrate that WDR5 recognizes a conserved arginine containing motif in the N-SET region of MLL1 called the WDR5 interaction (Win) motif (Patel et al., 2008b), thereby promoting the assembly and the H3K4 dimethylation activity of the MLL1 core complex (Patel et al., 2008a; Patel et al., 2008b; Song and Kingston, 2008) (Figure 6). Based on sedimentation velocity analytical ultracentrifugation experiments, Patel et al., (2008b) demonstrated that an MLL1 construct (encompassing residues 3745-3969) containing the highly conserved *Win* motif binds to WDR5 as a 1:1 complex with a dissociation constant of 120nM. Whereas, a shorter construct in MLL1 (encompassing residues 3811-3969) that lacks the *Win* motif sequence fails to associate with WDR5 (Patel et al., 2008b). In their efforts to further map the interaction region between MLL1 and WDR5, the two groups showed that the conserved *Win* motif closely resembles the sequence surrounding arginine 2 of histone H3 and is highly conserved among metazoan MLL1 orthologs and other SET1 family members (Patel et al., 2008b; Song and Kingston, 2008) (Figure 6). Using a combination of analytical ultracentrifugation and MALDI-TOF mass spectrometry, it was demonstrated that the conserved arginine (R3765) of the MLL1 *Win* motif is crucial for the interaction with WDR5 and that substitution of R3765 with alanine in MLL1 abolishes the interaction between MLL1 and the WRAD sub-complex, which also results in the loss of the H3K4 dimethylation activity of the MLL1 core complex (Patel et al., 2008b). However, replacement of other residues such as serine 3763 and glutamate 3767 in the conserved *Win* motif sequence only modestly weakens MLL1's interaction with the WRAD sub-complex (Patel et al., 2008b). Furthermore, the MLL1 R3765A mutant fails to co-immunoprecipitate the rest of the core complex components RbBP5 and Ash2L from HeLa cells, consistent with a central role for the MLL1 *Win* motif in the assembly of MLL1 core complex in vivo (unpublished results from Lee and Skalnik). These results have led to a model in which the conserved *Win* motif of MLL1 and other metazoan SET1 family members functions to bind the WDR5 component of the WDR5-RbBP5-Ash2L sub-complex, which is required for the assembly and H3K4 dimethylation activity of the MLL1 core complex (Cosgrove and Patel, 2010; Trievel and Shilatifard, 2009). These observations suggest that targeting MLL1-WDR5 interaction might be an effective strategy to down-regulate H3K4 dimethylation and HOX gene expression mediated by the MLL1 core complex.

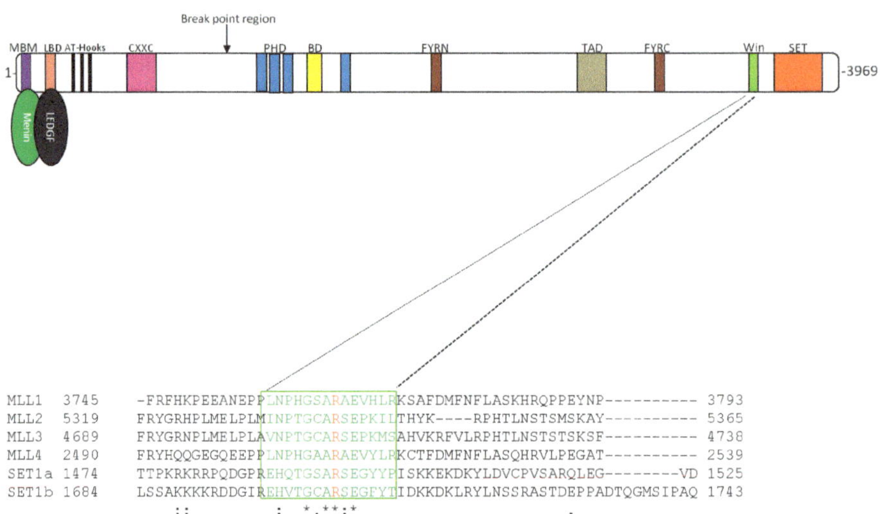

Schematic representation of the *Win* motif present in SET1 family members. At the top the domain architecture of wild-type MLL1 is shown and color coded as in Figure 1. The six-residue *Win* motif is present within the N-SET region of MLL1 (amino acid residues 3762-3767). The lower inset (green) shows the ClustalW multiple sequence alignment of the *Win* motif present in human SET1 family members: MLL1 (Q03164), MLL2 (O14686), MLL3 (AAK00583), MLL4 (Q9UMN6), SET1a (O15047), and SET1b (Q9UPS6). The conserved arginine of the *Win* motif is highlighted in red.

Fig. 6. WDR5 Interaction (*Win*) motif is highly conserved among human SET1 family members

6.4 Peptides derived from the MLL1 *Win* motif specifically inhibit the H3K4 dimethylation activity of MLL1 core complex

Based on mapping studies of the WDR5 binding region in MLL1, Patel et al., (2008b) developed a peptide, designated the MLL1 *Win* motif peptide (3762-3773) that can bind WDR5 with high affinity (K_d=1700nM) and disrupt the assembly of the MLL1 core complex in vitro (Patel et al., 2008a; Patel et al., 2008b). Consequently, this 12-residue MLL1 *Win* motif peptide inhibits the in vitro H3K4 dimethylation activity of the MLL1 core complex in a dose dependent manner by competing with wild-type MLL1 for the arginine binding pocket in WDR5 (Patel et al., 2008b). However, a control p53 peptide that has an arginine in a different sequence context failed to inhibit the H3K4 dimethylation activity even with a 60-fold excess, suggesting that *Win* motif peptides are highly specific inhibitors of MLL1 family complexes (Patel et al., 2008b). Furthermore, recent unpublished results from our lab demonstrate that peptides derived from other human SET1 family members bind WDR5 with dissociation constants ranging from 50nM-1700nM (in preparation). In accordance with the binding studies, MALDI-TOF mass spectrometry based methylation assays further demonstrate that other human SET1 family *Win* motif peptides are significantly more potent inhibitors of the H3K4 dimethylation activity of the MLL1 core complex as compared to the MLL1 *Win* motif peptide (Dharmarajan and Cosgrove, unpublished results). These studies suggest that the MLL1 *Win* motif based peptide represents an excellent starting point for the design of lead compounds that would specifically disrupt the interaction between MLL1 and WDR5 and inhibit the H3K4 dimethylation activity of MLL1 core complex in vivo.

6.5 MLL1 *Win* motif peptide binds to WDR5 by adopting a 3_{10}–helical conformation

Design of *Win* motif based inhibitors with better efficiency could be greatly enhanced by determining the protein structural features within the *Win* motif that are required for the high affinity binding to WDR5. To facilitate the process of structure-based drug design and to understand the molecular basis for MLL1-WDR5 interaction, two independent groups determined the three-dimensional structure of WDR5 bound to a peptide derived from the MLL1 *Win* motif (Patel et al., 2008a; Song and Kingston, 2008). The structures reveal that MLL1 *Win* motif peptide binds WDR5 by adopting a partial 3_{10}-helical conformation (Figure 7) (Patel et al., 2008a; Song and Kingston, 2008). The conserved *Win* motif residues (3762-3767) all participate in the formation of 3_{10}–helix with two-intramolecular i->i+3 main-chain hydrogen bonds stabilizing this conformation (Figure 7). MLL1 *Win* peptide binding is further stabilized by the insertion of conserved R3765 of MLL1 into a central water filled tunnel of WDR5 (Patel et al., 2008a; Song and Kingston, 2008). The structures also demonstrate that the side chain guanidinium of R3765 is sandwiched between two aromatic rings from WDR5- residues Phe-133 and Phe-263. R3765 is also stabilized by an extensive network of hydrogen bond, pi-pi and cation-pi, and hydrophobic interactions (Patel et al., 2008a; Song and Kingston, 2008) (Figure 7). These structural studies further corroborate the role of R3765 in mediating the interaction with WDR5 and explain the high sequence conservation of this arginine within SET1 family *Win* motifs. Accordingly, structures of WDR5 bound to *Win* motif peptides derived from other human SET1 family members reveal that WDR5 recognizes the different SET1 family *Win* motifs using the same arginine binding pocket as previously described for MLL1 (Dharmarajan and Cosgrove, unpublished results). However, the different *Win* motif peptides also participate in additional sets of interactions that might contribute to their differential inhibitory properties and suggest a framework for the use of *Win* motif peptides as lead compounds for drug development (Dharmarajan and Cosgrove, unpublished results). While the *Win* peptide binding mode is similar to the previously determined structures of WDR5 bound to histone peptides, which bind by inserting R2 of histone H3 into the central tunnel in WDR5 (Couture et al., 2006; Han et al., 2006; Schuetz et al., 2006), the SET1 family *Win* motif peptides participate in more favorable interactions with WDR5 (Patel et al., 2008a; Song and Kingston, 2008). These findings suggest that peptidomimetics based on the *Win* motif sequence can specifically bind WDR5 and down-regulate the activity of MLL1 core complex.

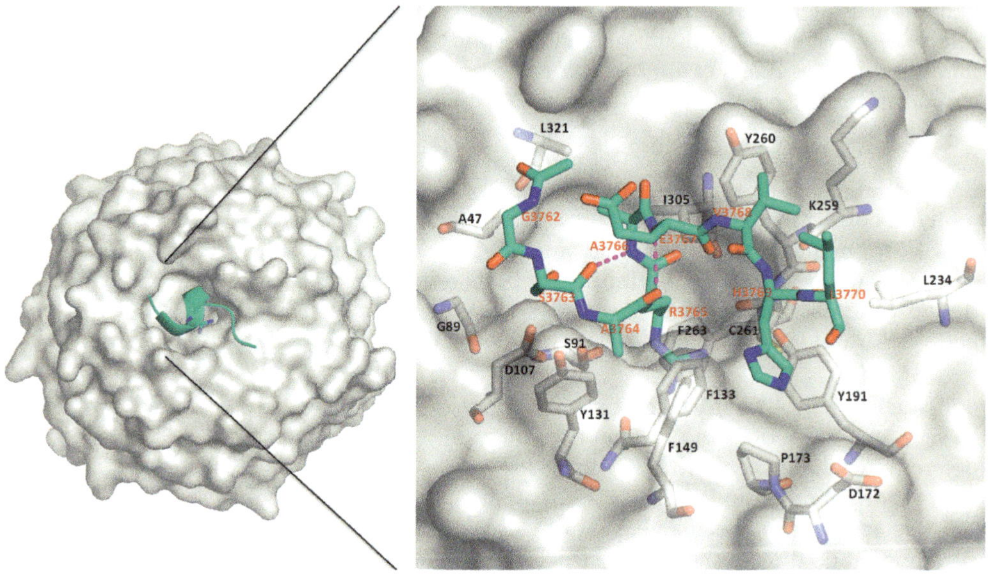

Three-dimensional structure of WDR5 (PDB code 3EG6) in complex with MLL1 *Win* motif peptide (3762-3773). a) On the left, the MLL1 *Win* motif peptide (cyan) is shown bound to the central tunnel in WDR5 (white). MLL1 *Win* motif peptide binds WDR5 by adopting a 3_{10}-helical conformation. On the right, blow up of the peptide binding site with MLL1 residues indicated in red and WDR5 residues indicated in black. Atom coloring: oxygen (red), nitrogen (blue), carbon (cyan for Win motif residues and grey for WDR5 residues).

Fig. 7. Crystal structure of MLL1 *Win* motif peptide bound to WDR5

6.6 Analysis of the binding of MLL1 *Win* motif and histone H3 peptides to WDR5: identification of key structural elements required for binding WDR5

To facilitate the design of small-molecule inhibitors of MLL1-WDR5 interaction, Karatas et al (2010) performed a systematic deletion analysis on the original 12-residue MLL1 *Win* motif peptide (3762-3773) and showed that a three residue sequence composed of $_{\text{Acetyl}}$-ARA- $_{\text{NH2}}$ is the minimal motif that is required for its interaction with WDR5 (Karatas et al., 2010). The acetyl group on the N-terminus is essential as its removal results in the loss of binding.

The $_{\text{Acetyl}}$-ARA-$_{\text{NH2}}$ peptide binds WDR5 in peptide competition experiments with similar affinity to that of the original 12 residue MLL1 *Win* motif peptide (~120 nM) (Karatas et al., 2010; Patel et al., 2008b). Moreover, systematic mutagenesis and molecular dynamics simulations further suggest that $_{Acetyl}$-ARA-$_{NH2}$ peptide could recapitulate the two intramolecular i-> i+3 main chain hydrogen bonds that are present in the original 12-residue MLL1 *Win* motif peptide. Absence of one or both of these hydrogen bonds significantly weakens the interaction affinity between the 3-residue peptide and WDR5 (Karatas et al., 2010). These results suggest that $_{Acetyl}$-ARA-$_{NH2}$ peptide binds WDR5 by adopting a partial 3_{10}-helical conformation similar to that of the 12-residue MLL1 *Win* motif peptide and participates in similar sets of interactions (Karatas et al., 2010; Patel et al., 2008b). However, the most potent inhibitor derived from the MLL1 *Win* motif peptide sequence is the acetyl-10mer ($_{acetyl}$-ARAEVHLRKS-$_{NH2}$) encompassing residues 3764-3773, which binds WDR5 with a K_i = 3nM (Karatas et al., 2010). These results suggest that sequences outside of the ARA sequence contribute to the affinity and would likely increase specificity. In addition, replacement of alanine at the +1 position (1 residue C-terminal to R3765) with a threonine in the acetyl-10mer ($_{acetyl}$-ARTEVHLRKS-$_{NH2}$) or 3-mer ($_{Acetyl}$-ART-$_{NH2}$) results in a 3-to-6-fold increase in binding affinity to WDR5, respectively (Karatas et al., 2010). In summary, these experiments suggest that the $_{Acetyl}$-ARA-$_{NH2}$ motif anchors the peptide to the arginine binding pocket of WDR5 and that the 3_{10} -helical conformation is crucial for interaction. In addition, sequences N- and C-terminal to the ARA motif are important for increasing binding specificity. It remains to be determined if the $_{Acetyl}$-ARA-$_{NH2}$ peptide actually inhibits the WDR5-MLL1 interaction within the context of the assembled MLL1 core complex.

6.7 *Win* motif based inhibitors - a novel class of compounds with potential to treat Acute Myeloid Leukemia

The extensive biochemical characterization of the peptide derived from the MLL1 Win motif have demonstrated that these peptidomimetic compounds have the potential to inhibit the H3K4 methyltransferase activity of the MLL1 core complex by specifically disrupting the association of MLL1 with the WRAD sub-complex (Patel et al., 2008b). Furthermore, the crystal structures of WDR5 bound to human SET1 family *Win* motif peptides provides a rationale for the design of new peptides and non-peptide mimetics with better inhibitory properties. The structures also reveal that conserved residues from the MLL1 Win motif (GSARAE) form a cyclical shaped 3_{10}-helix that fits snugly into the outer opening in WDR5 and raises the possibility that other cyclic peptidomimetic compounds might also bind WDR5 with similar or better inhibitory properties. The efficacy of *Win* motif based inhibitors in down regulating the H3K4 methylation activity of MLL1 core complex *in vitro* has yet to be demonstrated *in vivo*. However, based on the in vitro studies it is expected that the *Win* motif based peptides will have the ability to down regulate the increased H3K4 dimethylation, and aberrant HOX gene expression associated with MLL1-PTDs and gene amplification mutations in MLL1. Hence, the MLL1 *Win* motif peptide is a novel "first in class" inhibitor that is expected to have the ability to specifically regulate H3K4 dimethylation levels in cells without perturbing K3K4 monomethylation, or the methylation activities of other H3K4 methyltransferases.

7. Conclusions and future perspectives - are there other molecular targets for leukemia therapy?

Over the past decade, we have witnessed remarkable strides towards understanding the fundamental mechanisms of MLL1-mediated transcription and leukemogenesis, and many targets that are likely to be biomedically important are beginning to be characterized (Dou and Hess, 2008; Liedtke and Cleary, 2009; Marschalek, 2010). Genetic, biochemical and structural studies have demonstrated that several MLL1 partner proteins (AF4, AF9, AF10, ENL, and EEN) are either directly or indirectly associated with macromolecular complexes involved in transcriptional initiation and elongation (Bitoun et al., 2007; Cheung et al., 2007; Marschalek; Mueller et al., 2007; Mueller et al., 2009; Okada et al., 2005; Okada et al., 2006). Based on these studies, it was also suggested that leukemogenic properties of these MLL1-fusions are mediated in part through their association with the histone methyltransferases:

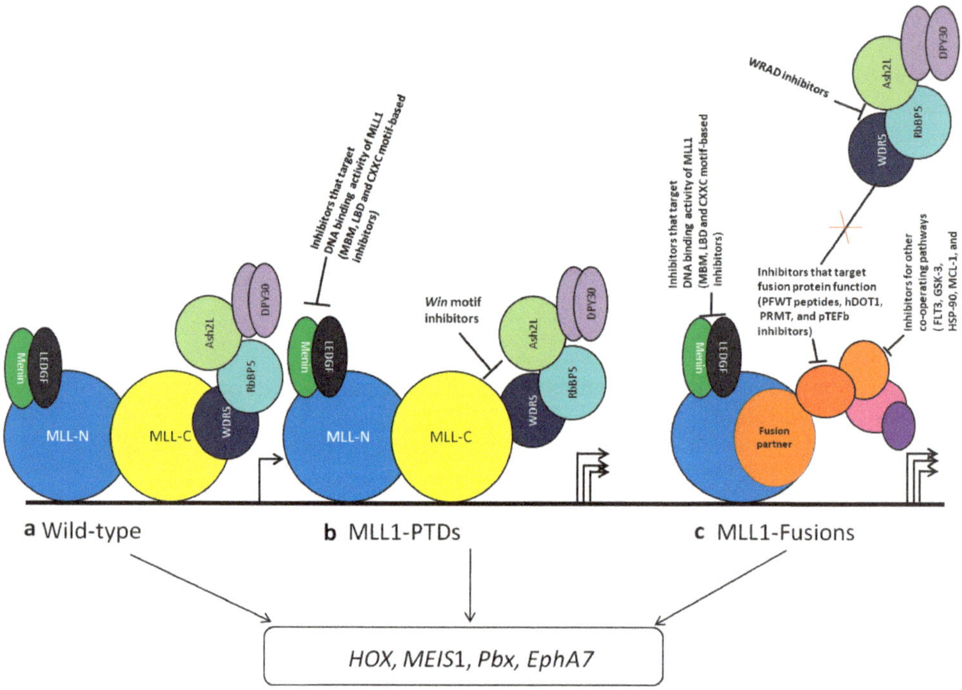

Cartoon representation of the different forms of MLL1 (a. wild-type, b. PTDs, and c. chromosomal translocations) and a summary of emerging potential molecular targeted therapies for mixed lineage leukemia. Key molecular targets include: i) inhibitors that disrupt the association of MLL1 with its target genes (MBM-based or CXXC motif-based inhibitors), ii) inhibitors that target the assembly of MLL1 core complex (*Win* motif-based inhibitors), iii) inhibitors that target the functions of fusion proteins (PFWT-like peptides, hDOT1L inhibitors, pTEFb kinase inhibitors), iv) WRAD sub-complex inhibitors and v) Inhibitors that target other co-operating pathways in leukemia (GSK-3, FLT3, MCL-1, and Ras). MLL-N (blue) and MLL-C (yellow) fragments are shown as localized to a hypothetical MLL1 target gene. In a). menin (green), LEDGF (dark grey) and WRAD sub-complex associate with wild-type MLL1 to regulate the normal expression (indicated by a single arrow) of MLL1 target genes. Target gene expression is dysregulated in MLL1-PTDs and MLL1-fusions (b and c) as indicated by multiple arrows. b) MLL1-PTDs retain all the functional interactions as seen in wild-type MLL1 and c) MLL1-fusions do not retain the MLL-C fragment and many interacting proteins.. Figure 8 was adapted from Liedtke and Cleary (2009).

Fig. 8. Potential protein:protein interaction targets for the development of novel therapies for MLL1-associated leukemias

hDOT1 (Bitoun et al., 2007; Okada et al., 2005; Okada et al., 2006) and protein arginine methyltransferase-1 or PRMT1 (Cheung et al., 2007). These studies have led to the proposal of the "MLL1 web hypothesis", which states that MLL1 fusion partners are components of larger macromolecular complexes that are involved in transcriptional activation and/or elongation (Erfurth et al., 2004). Molecular therapies directed at the interactions of these proteins within the "MLL1 web hypothesis" or inhibiting the activity of associated histone modifying enzymes are emerging as promising targets (Dou and Hess, 2008; Liedtke and Cleary, 2009; Marschalek, 2010). In addition to targeting the function of MLL1-fusion proteins, inhibitors that target the association of MLL1-fusion proteins to target DNA might also have potential therapeutic implications. In this regard, inhibitors that disrupt the interaction between MLL1's CXXC motif and unmethylated CpG containing target DNA are being investigated as molecular drug targets in MLL1-related leukemias (Allen et al., 2006; Cierpicki et al., 2010). In addition to these molecular targets, recent studies have also identified other cooperating pathways such as positive transcription elongation factor-b (pTEFb) recruitment (Marschalek, 2010; Mueller et al., 2007; Mueller et al., 2009; Shapiro, 2006), activation of FMS-like tyrosine kinase 3 (FLT3) (Armstrong et al., 2003; Brown et al., 2005; Stubbs et al., 2008; Yao et al., 2005), glycogen synthase kinase 3 (GSK3) (Wang et al., 2008), heat shock protein-90 (HSP-90) (Yao et al., 2005; Yocum et al., 2006), myeloid cell leukemia sequence-1 (MCL-1) expression (Chen et al., 2009), and RAS pathways (Liang et al., 2006) that are implicated in MLL1-induced leukemogenesis. The therapeutic significance of these molecular targets in MLL1-therapy were reviewed recently (Dou and Hess, 2008; Liedtke and Cleary, 2009; Marschalek, 2010) and since then, additional potential pharmacological targets such as the multi-subunit complex WRAD, which regulates the degree of H3K4 methylation by the MLL1 core complex, have emerged (Patel et al., 2009; Patel et al., 2011) (Figure 8).

In conclusion, this chapter summarizes recent biochemical studies that have contributed significantly to our understanding of how MLL1 works and have led to the identification of promising therapeutic targets for MLL1-related leukemias. In particular, inhibitors that target molecular interactions between menin and MLL1, AF4 and AF9, and MLL1 and WRAD have emerged as novel candidate small molecule targets. These MLL1-targeted therapies have enhanced pharmacological potential as compared to the existing broadly-based chemotherapeutics for MLL1-associated leukemias and will hopefully result in better treatment outcomes. In the future, similar biochemical, structural and genetic studies will be instrumental in identifying additional molecular targets that will form the basis for novel treatment strategies.

8. References

Abramovich, C., and Humphries, R.K. (2005). Hox regulation of normal and leukemic hematopoietic stem cells. Curr Opin Hematol *12*, 210-216.

Adamson, A.L., and Shearn, A. (1996). Molecular genetic analysis of Drosophila ash2, a member of the trithorax group required for imaginal disc pattern formation. Genetics *144*, 621-633.

Agarwal, S.K., Guru, S.C., Heppner, C., Erdos, M.R., Collins, R.M., Park, S.Y., Saggar, S., Chandrasekharappa, S.C., Collins, F.S., Spiegel, A.M., *et al.* (1999). Menin interacts with the AP1 transcription factor JunD and represses JunD-activated transcription. Cell *96*, 143-152.

Agarwal, S.K., Novotny, E.A., Crabtree, J.S., Weitzman, J.B., Yaniv, M., Burns, A.L., Chandrasekharappa, S.C., Collins, F.S., Spiegel, A.M., and Marx, S.J. (2003). Transcription factor JunD, deprived of menin, switches from growth suppressor to growth promoter. Proc Natl Acad Sci U S A *100*, 10770-10775.

Allen, M.D., Grummitt, C.G., Hilcenko, C., Min, S.Y., Tonkin, L.M., Johnson, C.M., Freund, S.M., Bycroft, M., and Warren, A.J. (2006). Solution structure of the nonmethyl-CpG-binding CXXC domain of the leukaemia-associated MLL histone methyltransferase. Embo J *25*, 4503-4512.

Allen, R.J., Smith, S.D., Moldwin, R.L., Lu, M.M., Giordano, L., Vignon, C., Suto, Y., Harden, A., Tomek, R., Veldman, T., *et al.* (1998). Establishment and characterization of a megakaryoblast cell line with amplification of MLL. Leukemia *12*, 1119-1127.

Altucci, L., Clarke, N., Nebbioso, A., Scognamiglio, A., and Gronemeyer, H. (2005). Acute myeloid leukemia: therapeutic impact of epigenetic drugs. Int J Biochem Cell Biol *37*, 1752-1762.

Ansari, K.I., and Mandal, S.S. (2010). Mixed lineage leukemia: roles in gene expression, hormone signaling and mRNA processing. Febs J *277*, 1790-1804.

Ariyama, Y., Fukuda, Y., Okuno, Y., Seto, M., Date, K., Abe, T., Nakamura, Y., and Inazawa, J. (1998). Amplification on double-minute chromosomes and partial-tandem duplication of the MLL gene in leukemic cells of a patient with acute myelogenous leukemia. Genes Chromosomes Cancer *23*, 267-272.

Armstrong, S.A., Kung, A.L., Mabon, M.E., Silverman, L.B., Stam, R.W., Den Boer, M.L., Pieters, R., Kersey, J.H., Sallan, S.E., Fletcher, J.A., *et al.* (2003). Inhibition of FLT3 in MLL. Validation of a therapeutic target identified by gene expression based classification. Cancer Cell *3*, 173-183.

Armstrong, S.A., Staunton, J.E., Silverman, L.B., Pieters, R., den Boer, M.L., Minden, M.D., Sallan, S.E., Lander, E.S., Golub, T.R., and Korsmeyer, S.J. (2002). MLL translocations specify a distinct gene expression profile that distinguishes a unique leukemia. Nat Genet *30*, 41-47.

Avet-Loiseau, H., Godon, C., Li, J.Y., Daviet, A., Mellerin, M.P., Talmant, P., Harousseau, J.L., and Bataille, R. (1999). Amplification of the 11q23 region in acute myeloid leukemia. Genes Chromosomes Cancer *26*, 166-170.

Ayton, P.M., Chen, E.H., and Cleary, M.L. (2004). Binding to nonmethylated CpG DNA is essential for target recognition, transactivation, and myeloid transformation by an MLL oncoprotein. Mol Cell Biol *24*, 10470-10478.

Ayton, P.M., and Cleary, M.L. (2003). Transformation of myeloid progenitors by MLL oncoproteins is dependent on Hoxa7 and Hoxa9. Genes Dev *17*, 2298-2307.

Balogh, K., Racz, K., Patocs, A., and Hunyady, L. (2006). Menin and its interacting proteins: elucidation of menin function. Trends Endocrinol Metab *17*, 357-364.

Basecke, J., Whelan, J.T., Griesinger, F., and Bertrand, F.E. (2006). The MLL partial tandem duplication in acute myeloid leukaemia. Br J Haematol *135*, 438-449.

Behm, F.G., Raimondi, S.C., Frestedt, J.L., Liu, Q., Crist, W.M., Downing, J.R., Rivera, G.K., Kersey, J.H., and Pui, C.H. (1996). Rearrangement of the MLL gene confers a poor prognosis in childhood acute lymphoblastic leukemia, regardless of presenting age. Blood *87*, 2870-2877.

Benedikt, A., Baltruschat, S., Scholz, B., Bursen, A., Arrey, T.N., Meyer, B., Varagnolo, L., Muller, A.M., Karas, M., Dingermann, T., *et al.* (2011). The leukemogenic AF4-MLL fusion protein causes P-TEFb kinase activation and altered epigenetic signatures. Leukemia *25*, 135-144.

Bennett, C.A., Winters, A.C., Barretto, N.N., and Hemenway, C.S. (2009). Molecular targeting of MLL-rearranged leukemia cell lines with the synthetic peptide PFWT synergistically enhances the cytotoxic effect of established chemotherapeutic agents. Leuk Res *33*, 937-947.

Bensaid, M., Melko, M., Bechara, E.G., Davidovic, L., Berretta, A., Catania, M.V., Gecz, J., Lalli, E., and Bardoni, B. (2009). FRAXE-associated mental retardation protein (FMR2) is an RNA-binding protein with high affinity for G-quartet RNA forming structure. Nucleic Acids Res *37*, 1269-1279.

Bernard, O.A., Mauchauffe, M., Mecucci, C., Van den Berghe, H., and Berger, R. (1994). A novel gene, AF-1p, fused to HRX in t(1;11)(p32;q23), is not related to AF-4, AF-9 nor ENL. Oncogene *9*, 1039-1045.

Bernstein, B.E., Humphrey, E.L., Erlich, R.L., Schneider, R., Bouman, P., Liu, J.S., Kouzarides, T., and Schreiber, S.L. (2002). Methylation of histone H3 Lys 4 in coding regions of active genes. Proc Natl Acad Sci U S A *99*, 8695-8700.

Bernstein, B.E., Kamal, M., Lindblad-Toh, K., Bekiranov, S., Bailey, D.K., Huebert, D.J., McMahon, S., Karlsson, E.K., Kulbokas, E.J., 3rd, Gingeras, T.R., *et al.* (2005). Genomic maps and comparative analysis of histone modifications in human and mouse. Cell *120*, 169-181.

Bertolino, P., Radovanovic, I., Casse, H., Aguzzi, A., Wang, Z.Q., and Zhang, C.X. (2003a). Genetic ablation of the tumor suppressor menin causes lethality at mid-gestation with defects in multiple organs. Mech Dev *120*, 549-560.

Bertolino, P., Tong, W.M., Galendo, D., Wang, Z.Q., and Zhang, C.X. (2003b). Heterozygous Men1 mutant mice develop a range of endocrine tumors mimicking multiple endocrine neoplasia type 1. Mol Endocrinol *17*, 1880-1892.

Bigoni, R., Cuneo, A., Roberti, M.G., Moretti, S., De Angeli, C., Dabusti, M., Campioni, D., del Senno, L., Biondi, A., Chaplin, T., *et al.* (1999). Therapy-related adult acute lymphoblastic leukemia with t(4;11)(q21; q23): MLL rearrangement, p53 mutation and multilineage involvement. Leukemia *13*, 704-707.

Bitoun, E., Oliver, P.L., and Davies, K.E. (2007). The mixed-lineage leukemia fusion partner AF4 stimulates RNA polymerase II transcriptional elongation and mediates coordinated chromatin remodeling. Hum Mol Genet *16*, 92-106.

Boggs, B.A., Cheung, P., Heard, E., Spector, D.L., Chinault, A.C., and Allis, C.D. (2002). Differentially methylated forms of histone H3 show unique association patterns with inactive human X chromosomes. Nat Genet *30*, 73-76.

Bralten, L.B., Kloosterhof, N.K., Gravendeel, L.A., Sacchetti, A., Duijm, E.J., Kros, J.M., van den Bent, M.J., Hoogenraad, C.C., Sillevis Smitt, P.A., and French, P.J. (2010). Integrated genomic profiling identifies candidate genes implicated in glioma-genesis and a novel LEO1-SLC12A1 fusion gene. Genes Chromosomes Cancer *49*, 509-517.

Brown, P., Levis, M., Shurtleff, S., Campana, D., Downing, J., and Small, D. (2005). FLT3 inhibition selectively kills childhood acute lymphoblastic leukemia cells with high levels of FLT3 expression. Blood *105*, 812-820.

Burmeister, T., Meyer, C., Schwartz, S., Hofmann, J., Molkentin, M., Kowarz, E., Schneider, B., Raff, T., Reinhardt, R., Gokbuget, N., *et al.* (2009). The MLL recombinome of adult CD10-negative B-cell precursor acute lymphoblastic leukemia: results from the GMALL study group. Blood *113*, 4011-4015.

Bursen, A., Schwabe, K., Ruster, B., Henschler, R., Ruthardt, M., Dingermann, T., and Marschalek, R. (2010). The AF4.MLL fusion protein is capable of inducing ALL in mice without requirement of MLL.AF4. Blood *115*, 3570-3579.

Cairns, B.R., Henry, N.L., and Kornberg, R.D. (1996). TFG/TAF30/ANC1, a component of the yeast SWI/SNF complex that is similar to the leukemogenic proteins ENL and AF-9. Mol Cell Biol *16*, 3308-3316.

Caligiuri, M.A., Schichman, S.A., Strout, M.P., Mrozek, K., Baer, M.R., Frankel, S.R., Barcos, M., Herzig, G.P., Croce, C.M., and Bloomfield, C.D. (1994). Molecular rearrangement of the ALL-1 gene in acute myeloid leukemia without cytogenetic evidence of 11q23 chromosomal translocations. Cancer Res *54*, 370-373.

Caligiuri, M.A., Strout, M.P., Lawrence, D., Arthur, D.C., Baer, M.R., Yu, F., Knuutila, S., Mrozek, K., Oberkircher, A.R., Marcucci, G., *et al.* (1998). Rearrangement of ALL1 (MLL) in acute myeloid leukemia with normal cytogenetics. Cancer Res *58*, 55-59.

Campo Dell'Orto, M., Banelli, B., Giarin, E., Accordi, B., Trentin, L., Romani, M., te Kronnie, G., and Basso, G. (2007). Down-regulation of DLX3 expression in MLL-AF4 childhood lymphoblastic leukemias is mediated by promoter region hypermethylation. Oncol Rep *18*, 417-423.

Carlson, M., and Laurent, B.C. (1994). The SNF/SWI family of global transcriptional activators. Curr Opin Cell Biol *6*, 396-402.

Carnicer, M.J., Nomdedeu, J.F., Lasa, A., Estivill, C., Brunet, S., Aventin, A., and Sierra, J. (2004). FLT3 mutations are associated with other molecular lesions in AML. Leuk Res *28*, 19-23.

Caslini, C., Yang, Z., El-Osta, M., Milne, T.A., Slany, R.K., and Hess, J.L. (2007). Interaction of MLL amino terminal sequences with menin is required for transformation. Cancer Res *67*, 7275-7283.

Chandrasekharappa, S.C., Guru, S.C., Manickam, P., Olufemi, S.E., Collins, F.S., Emmert-Buck, M.R., Debelenko, L.V., Zhuang, Z., Lubensky, I.A., Liotta, L.A., *et al.* (1997). Positional cloning of the gene for multiple endocrine neoplasia-type 1. Science *276*, 404-407.

Chandrasekharappa, S.C., and Teh, B.T. (2001). Clinical and molecular aspects of multiple endocrine neoplasia type 1. Front Horm Res *28*, 50-80.

Chandrasekharappa, S.C., and Teh, B.T. (2003). Functional studies of the MEN1 gene. J Intern Med *253*, 606-615.

Chen, C.S., Hilden, J.M., Frestedt, J., Domer, P.H., Moore, R., Korsmeyer, S.J., and Kersey, J.H. (1993). The chromosome 4q21 gene (AF-4/FEL) is widely expressed in normal tissues and shows breakpoint diversity in t(4;11)(q21;q23) acute leukemia. Blood *82*, 1080-1085.

Chen, R., Wierda, W.G., Chubb, S., Hawtin, R.E., Fox, J.A., Keating, M.J., Gandhi, V., and Plunkett, W. (2009). Mechanism of action of SNS-032, a novel cyclin-dependent kinase inhibitor, in chronic lymphocytic leukemia. Blood *113*, 4637-4645.

Chen, W., Li, Q., Hudson, W.A., Kumar, A., Kirchhof, N., and Kersey, J.H. (2006a). A murine Mll-AF4 knock-in model results in lymphoid and myeloid deregulation and hematologic malignancy. Blood *108*, 669-677.

Chen, Y.X., Yan, J., Keeshan, K., Tubbs, A.T., Wang, H., Silva, A., Brown, E.J., Hess, J.L., Pear, W.S., and Hua, X. (2006b). The tumor suppressor menin regulates hematopoiesis and myeloid transformation by influencing Hox gene expression. Proc Natl Acad Sci U S A *103*, 1018-1023.

Cheng, X., Collins, R.E., and Zhang, X. (2005). Structural and sequence motifs of protein (histone) methylation enzymes. Annu Rev Biophys Biomol Struct *34*, 267-294.

Cheung, N., Chan, L.C., Thompson, A., Cleary, M.L., and So, C.W. (2007). Protein arginine-methyltransferase-dependent oncogenesis. Nat Cell Biol *9*, 1208-1215.

Cho, Y.W., Hong, T., Hong, S., Guo, H., Yu, H., Kim, D., Guszczynski, T., Dressler, G.R., Copeland, T.D., Kalkum, M., *et al.* (2007). PTIP associates with MLL3- and MLL4-containing histone H3 lysine 4 methyltransferase complex. J Biol Chem *282*, 20395-20406.

Cierpicki, T., Risner, L.E., Grembecka, J., Lukasik, S.M., Popovic, R., Omonkowska, M., Shultis, D.D., Zeleznik-Le, N.J., and Bushweller, J.H. (2010). Structure of the MLL CXXC domain-DNA complex and its functional role in MLL-AF9 leukemia. Nat Struct Mol Biol *17*, 62-68.

Cohen, A., Grunberger, T., Vanek, W., Dube, I.D., Doherty, P.J., Letarte, M., Roifman, C., and Freedman, M.H. (1991). Constitutive expression and role in growth regulation of interleukin-1 and multiple cytokine receptors in a biphenotypic leukemic cell line. Blood *78*, 94-102.

Collins, E.C., Appert, A., Ariza-McNaughton, L., Pannell, R., Yamada, Y., and Rabbitts, T.H. (2002). Mouse Af9 is a controller of embryo patterning, like Mll, whose human homologue fuses with Af9 after chromosomal translocation in leukemia. Mol Cell Biol *22*, 7313-7324.

Collins, R.E., Tachibana, M., Tamaru, H., Smith, K.M., Jia, D., Zhang, X., Selker, E.U., Shinkai, Y., and Cheng, X. (2005). In vitro and in vivo analyses of a Phe/Tyr switch controlling product specificity of histone lysine methyltransferases. J Biol Chem *280*, 5563-5570.

Cosgrove, M.S., and Patel, A. (2010). Mixed lineage leukemia: a structure-function perspective of the MLL1 protein. Febs Journal *277*, 1832-1842.

Cosgrove, M.S., and Wolberger, C. (2005). How does the histone code work? Biochem Cell Biol *83*, 468-476.

Cote, J., Quinn, J., Workman, J.L., and Peterson, C.L. (1994). Stimulation of GAL4 derivative binding to nucleosomal DNA by the yeast SWI/SNF complex. Science *265*, 53-60.

Couture, J.F., Collazo, E., and Trievel, R.C. (2006). Molecular recognition of histone H3 by the WD40 protein WDR5. Nat Struct Mol Biol *13*, 698-703.

Crabtree, J.S., Scacheri, P.C., Ward, J.M., Garrett-Beal, L., Emmert-Buck, M.R., Edgemon, K.A., Lorang, D., Libutti, S.K., Chandrasekharappa, S.C., Marx, S.J., *et al.* (2001). A mouse model of multiple endocrine neoplasia, type 1, develops multiple endocrine tumors. Proc Natl Acad Sci U S A *98*, 1118-1123.

Cuthbert, G., McCullough, S., Finney, R., Breese, G., and Bown, N. (1999). Jumping translocation at 11q23 with MLL gene rearrangement and interstitial telomeric sequences. Genes Chromosomes Cancer *24*, 295-298.

Daser, A., and Rabbitts, T.H. (2005). The versatile mixed lineage leukaemia gene MLL and its many associations in leukaemogenesis. Semin Cancer Biol *15*, 175-188.

Debernardi, S., Bassini, A., Jones, L.K., Chaplin, T., Linder, B., de Bruijn, D.R., Meese, E., and Young, B.D. (2002). The MLL fusion partner AF10 binds GAS41, a protein that interacts with the human SWI/SNF complex. Blood *99*, 275-281.

Dillon, S.C., Zhang, X., Trievel, R.C., and Cheng, X. (2005). The SET-domain protein superfamily: protein lysine methyltransferases. Genome Biol *6*, 227.

Djabali, M., Selleri, L., Parry, P., Bower, M., Young, B.D., and Evans, G.A. (1992). A trithorax-like gene is interrupted by chromosome 11q23 translocations in acute leukaemias. Nat Genet *2*, 113-118.

Dobson, C.L., Warren, A.J., Pannell, R., Forster, A., Lavenir, I., Corral, J., Smith, A.J., and Rabbitts, T.H. (1999). The mll-AF9 gene fusion in mice controls myeloproliferation and specifies acute myeloid leukaemogenesis. Embo J *18*, 3564-3574.

Dobson, C.L., Warren, A.J., Pannell, R., Forster, A., and Rabbitts, T.H. (2000). Tumorigenesis in mice with a fusion of the leukaemia oncogene Mll and the bacterial lacZ gene. Embo J *19*, 843-851.

Dohner, K., Tobis, K., Ulrich, R., Frohling, S., Benner, A., Schlenk, R.F., and Dohner, H. (2002). Prognostic significance of partial tandem duplications of the MLL gene in adult patients 16 to 60 years old with acute myeloid leukemia and normal cytogenetics: a study of the Acute Myeloid Leukemia Study Group Ulm. J Clin Oncol *20*, 3254-3261.

Domer, P.H., Fakharzadeh, S.S., Chen, C.S., Jockel, J., Johansen, L., Silverman, G.A., Kersey, J.H., and Korsmeyer, S.J. (1993). Acute mixed-lineage leukemia t(4;11)(q21;q23) generates an MLL-AF4 fusion product. Proc Natl Acad Sci U S A *90*, 7884-7888.

Dong, Q., Debelenko, L.V., Chandrasekharappa, S.C., Emmert-Buck, M.R., Zhuang, Z., Guru, S.C., Manickam, P., Skarulis, M., Lubensky, I.A., Liotta, L.A., *et al.* (1997). Loss of heterozygosity at 11q13: analysis of pituitary tumors, lung carcinoids, lipomas, and other uncommon tumors in subjects with familial multiple endocrine neoplasia type 1. J Clin Endocrinol Metab *82*, 1416-1420.

Dorrance, A.M., Liu, S., Chong, A., Pulley, B., Nemer, D., Guimond, M., Yuan, W., Chang, D., Whitman, S.P., Marcucci, G., *et al.* (2008). The Mll partial tandem duplication: differential, tissue-specific activity in the presence or absence of the wild-type allele. Blood *112*, 2508-2511.

Dorrance, A.M., Liu, S., Yuan, W., Becknell, B., Arnoczky, K.J., Guimond, M., Strout, M.P., Feng, L., Nakamura, T., Yu, L., *et al.* (2006). Mll partial tandem duplication induces aberrant Hox expression in vivo via specific epigenetic alterations. J Clin Invest *116*, 2707-2716.

Doty, R.T., Vanasse, G.J., Disteche, C.M., and Willerford, D.M. (2002). The leukemia-associated gene Mllt1/ENL: characterization of a murine homolog and demonstration of an essential role in embryonic development. Blood Cells Mol Dis *28*, 407-417.

Dou, Y., and Hess, J.L. (2008). Mechanisms of transcriptional regulation by MLL and its disruption in acute leukemia. Int J Hematol *87*, 10-18.

Dou, Y., Milne, T.A., Ruthenburg, A.J., Lee, S., Lee, J.W., Verdine, G.L., Allis, C.D., and Roeder, R.G. (2006). Regulation of MLL1 H3K4 methyltransferase activity by its core components. Nat Struct Mol Biol *13*, 713-719.

Dou, Y., Milne, T.A., Tackett, A.J., Smith, E.R., Fukuda, A., Wysocka, J., Allis, C.D., Chait, B.T., Hess, J.L., and Roeder, R.G. (2005). Physical association and coordinate function of the H3 K4 methyltransferase MLL1 and the H4 K16 acetyltransferase MOF. Cell *121*, 873-885.

Downing, J.R. (2008). Targeted therapy in leukemia. Mod Pathol *21 Suppl 2*, S2-7.

Dreijerink, K.M., Mulder, K.W., Winkler, G.S., Hoppener, J.W., Lips, C.J., and Timmers, H.T. (2006). Menin links estrogen receptor activation to histone H3K4 trimethylation. Cancer Res *66*, 4929-4935.

Eguchi, M., Eguchi-Ishimae, M., and Greaves, M. (2004). The small oligomerization domain of gephyrin converts MLL to an oncogene. Blood *103*, 3876-3882.

Erfurth, F., Hemenway, C.S., de Erkenez, A.C., and Domer, P.H. (2004). MLL fusion partners AF4 and AF9 interact at subnuclear foci. Leukemia *18*, 92-102.

Ernst, P., Fisher, J.K., Avery, W., Wade, S., Foy, D., and Korsmeyer, S.J. (2004a). Definitive hematopoiesis requires the mixed-lineage leukemia gene. Dev Cell *6*, 437-443.

Ernst, P., Mabon, M., Davidson, A.J., Zon, L.I., and Korsmeyer, S.J. (2004b). An Mll-dependent Hox program drives hematopoietic progenitor expansion. Curr Biol *14*, 2063-2069.

Ernst, P., Wang, J., Huang, M., Goodman, R.H., and Korsmeyer, S.J. (2001). MLL and CREB bind cooperatively to the nuclear coactivator CREB-binding protein. Mol Cell Biol *21*, 2249-2258.

Ernst, P., Wang, J., and Korsmeyer, S.J. (2002). The role of MLL in hematopoiesis and leukemia. Curr Opin Hematol *9*, 282-287.

Estable, M.C., Naghavi, M.H., Kato, H., Xiao, H., Qin, J., Vahlne, A., and Roeder, R.G. (2002). MCEF, the newest member of the AF4 family of transcription factors involved in leukemia, is a positive transcription elongation factor-b-associated protein. J Biomed Sci *9*, 234-245.

Faderl, S., Kantarjian, H.M., Talpaz, M., and Estrov, Z. (1998). Clinical significance of cytogenetic abnormalities in adult acute lymphoblastic leukemia. Blood *91*, 3995-4019.

Felix, C.A., Lange, B.J., Hosler, M.R., Fertala, J., and Bjornsti, M.A. (1995). Chromosome band 11q23 translocation breakpoints are DNA topoisomerase II cleavage sites. Cancer Res *55*, 4287-4292.

Felix, C.A., Megonigal, M.D., Chervinsky, D.S., Leonard, D.G., Tsuchida, N., Kakati, S., Block, A.M., Fisher, J., Grossi, M., Salhany, K.I., *et al.* (1998). Association of germline p53 mutation with MLL segmental jumping translocation in treatment-related leukemia. Blood *91*, 4451-4456.

Ferrando, A.A., Armstrong, S.A., Neuberg, D.S., Sallan, S.E., Silverman, L.B., Korsmeyer, S.J., and Look, A.T. (2003). Gene expression signatures in MLL-rearranged T-lineage and B-precursor acute leukemias: dominance of HOX dysregulation. Blood *102*, 262-268.

Flanagan, J.F., Mi, L.Z., Chruszcz, M., Cymborowski, M., Clines, K.L., Kim, Y., Minor, W., Rastinejad, F., and Khorasanizadeh, S. (2005). Double chromodomains cooperate to recognize the methylated histone H3 tail. Nature *438*, 1181-1185.

Gan, T., Jude, C.D., Zaffuto, K., and Ernst, P. (2010). Developmentally induced Mll1 loss reveals defects in postnatal haematopoiesis. Leukemia *24*, 1732-1741.

Ganapathy, V., Gopal, E., Miyauchi, S., and Prasad, P.D. (2005). Biological functions of SLC5A8, a candidate tumour suppressor. Biochem Soc Trans *33*, 237-240.

Gobl, A.E., Berg, M., Lopez-Egido, J.R., Oberg, K., Skogseid, B., and Westin, G. (1999). Menin represses JunD-activated transcription by a histone deacetylase-dependent mechanism. Biochim Biophys Acta *1447*, 51-56.

Gori, F., and Demay, M.B. (2005). The effects of BIG-3 on osteoblast differentiation are not dependent upon endogenously produced BMPs. Exp Cell Res *304*, 287-292.

Gori, F., Friedman, L., and Demay, M.B. (2005). Wdr5, a novel WD repeat protein, regulates osteoblast and chondrocyte differentiation in vivo. J Musculoskelet Neuronal Interact *5*, 338-339.

Grembecka, J., Belcher, A.M., Hartley, T., and Cierpicki, T. (2010). Molecular basis of the mixed lineage leukemia-menin interaction: implications for targeting mixed lineage leukemias. J Biol Chem *285*, 40690-40698.

Gu, Y., Nakamura, T., Alder, H., Prasad, R., Canaani, O., Cimino, G., Croce, C.M., and Canaani, E. (1992). The t(4;11) chromosome translocation of human acute leukemias fuses the ALL-1 gene, related to Drosophila trithorax, to the AF-4 gene. Cell *71*, 701-708.

Gu, Y., Shen, Y., Gibbs, R.A., and Nelson, D.L. (1996). Identification of FMR2, a novel gene associated with the FRAXE CCG repeat and CpG island. Nat Genet *13*, 109-113.

Gupta, N., Martin, P.M., Prasad, P.D., and Ganapathy, V. (2006). SLC5A8 (SMCT1)-mediated transport of butyrate forms the basis for the tumor suppressive function of the transporter. Life Sci *78*, 2419-2425.

Guru, S.C., Crabtree, J.S., Brown, K.D., Dunn, K.J., Manickam, P., Prasad, N.B., Wangsa, D., Burns, A.L., Spiegel, A.M., Marx, S.J., *et al.* (1999). Isolation, genomic organization, and expression analysis of Men1, the murine homolog of the MEN1 gene. Mamm Genome *10*, 592-596.

Guru, S.C., Goldsmith, P.K., Burns, A.L., Marx, S.J., Spiegel, A.M., Collins, F.S., and Chandrasekharappa, S.C. (1998). Menin, the product of the MEN1 gene, is a nuclear protein. Proc Natl Acad Sci U S A *95*, 1630-1634.

Guru, S.C., Prasad, N.B., Shin, E.J., Hemavathy, K., Lu, J., Ip, Y.T., Agarwal, S.K., Marx, S.J., Spiegel, A.M., Collins, F.S., *et al.* (2001). Characterization of a MEN1 ortholog from Drosophila melanogaster. Gene *263*, 31-38.

Hall, P.A., and Russell, S.E. (2004). The pathobiology of the septin gene family. J Pathol *204*, 489-505.

Han, Z., Guo, L., Wang, H., Shen, Y., Deng, X.W., and Chai, J. (2006). Structural basis for the specific recognition of methylated histone H3 lysine 4 by the WD-40 protein WDR5. Mol Cell *22*, 137-144.

Hanson, R.D., Hess, J.L., Yu, B.D., Ernst, P., van Lohuizen, M., Berns, A., van der Lugt, N.M., Shashikant, C.S., Ruddle, F.H., Seto, M., *et al.* (1999). Mammalian Trithorax and polycomb-group homologues are antagonistic regulators of homeotic development. Proc Natl Acad Sci U S A *96*, 14372-14377.

Heerema, N.A., Sather, H.N., Ge, J., Arthur, D.C., Hilden, J.M., Trigg, M.E., and Reaman, G.H. (1999). Cytogenetic studies of infant acute lymphoblastic leukemia: poor prognosis of infants with t(4;11) - a report of the Children's Cancer Group. Leukemia *13*, 679-686.

Heintzman, N.D., Stuart, R.K., Hon, G., Fu, Y., Ching, C.W., Hawkins, R.D., Barrera, L.O., Van Calcar, S., Qu, C., Ching, K.A., *et al.* (2007). Distinct and predictive chromatin signatures of transcriptional promoters and enhancers in the human genome. Nat Genet *39*, 311-318.

Hemenway, C.S., de Erkenez, A.C., and Gould, G.C. (2001). The polycomb protein MPc3 interacts with AF9, an MLL fusion partner in t(9;11)(p22;q23) acute leukemias. Oncogene *20*, 3798-3805.

Heppner, C., Bilimoria, K.Y., Agarwal, S.K., Kester, M., Whitty, L.J., Guru, S.C., Chandrasekharappa, S.C., Collins, F.S., Spiegel, A.M., Marx, S.J., *et al.* (2001). The tumor suppressor protein menin interacts with NF-kappaB proteins and inhibits NF-kappaB-mediated transactivation. Oncogene *20*, 4917-4925.

Herry, A., Douet-Guilbert, N., Gueganic, N., Morel, F., Le Bris, M.J., Berthou, C., and De Braekeleer, M. (2006). Del(5q) and MLL amplification in homogeneously staining region in acute myeloblastic leukemia: a recurrent cytogenetic association. Ann Hematol *85*, 244-249.

Hess, J.L. (2004). MLL: a histone methyltransferase disrupted in leukemia. Trends Mol Med *10*, 500-507.

Hess, J.L., Bittner, C.B., Zeisig, D.T., Bach, C., Fuchs, U., Borkhardt, A., Frampton, J., and Slany, R.K. (2006). c-Myb is an essential downstream target for homeobox-mediated transformation of hematopoietic cells. Blood *108*, 297-304.

Hess, J.L., Yu, B.D., Li, B., Hanson, R., and Korsmeyer, S.J. (1997). Defects in yolk sac hematopoiesis in Mll-null embryos. Blood *90*, 1799-1806.

Hsieh, J.J., Cheng, E.H., and Korsmeyer, S.J. (2003a). Taspase1: a threonine aspartase required for cleavage of MLL and proper HOX gene expression. Cell *115*, 293-303.

Hsieh, J.J., Ernst, P., Erdjument-Bromage, H., Tempst, P., and Korsmeyer, S.J. (2003b). Proteolytic cleavage of MLL generates a complex of N- and C-terminal fragments that confers protein stability and subnuclear localization. Mol Cell Biol *23*, 186-194.

Hsu, D.R., Chuang, P.T., and Meyer, B.J. (1995). DPY-30, a nuclear protein essential early in embryogenesis for Caenorhabditis elegans dosage compensation. Development *121*, 3323-3334.

Hsu, D.R., and Meyer, B.J. (1994). The dpy-30 gene encodes an essential component of the Caenorhabditis elegans dosage compensation machinery. Genetics *137*, 999-1018.

Hughes, C.M., Rozenblatt-Rosen, O., Milne, T.A., Copeland, T.D., Levine, S.S., Lee, J.C., Hayes, D.N., Shanmugam, K.S., Bhattacharjee, A., Biondi, C.A., *et al.* (2004). Menin associates with a trithorax family histone methyltransferase complex and with the hoxc8 locus. Mol Cell *13*, 587-597.

Huret, J.L., Dessen, P., and Bernheim, A. (2001). An atlas of chromosomes in hematological malignancies. Example: 11q23 and MLL partners. Leukemia *15*, 987-989.

Ida, K., Kitabayashi, I., Taki, T., Taniwaki, M., Noro, K., Yamamoto, M., Ohki, M., and Hayashi, Y. (1997). Adenoviral E1A-associated protein p300 is involved in acute myeloid leukemia with t(11;22)(q23;q13). Blood *90*, 4699-4704.

Isnard, P., Core, N., Naquet, P., and Djabali, M. (2000). Altered lymphoid development in mice deficient for the mAF4 proto-oncogene. Blood *96*, 705-710.

Jin, S., Mao, H., Schnepp, R.W., Sykes, S.M., Silva, A.C., D'Andrea, A.D., and Hua, X. (2003). Menin associates with FANCD2, a protein involved in repair of DNA damage. Cancer Res *63*, 4204-4210.

Jin, S., Zhao, H., Yi, Y., Nakata, Y., Kalota, A., and Gewirtz, A.M. (2010). c-Myb binds MLL through menin in human leukemia cells and is an important driver of MLL-associated leukemogenesis. J Clin Invest *120*, 593-606.

Jude, C.D., Climer, L., Xu, D., Artinger, E., Fisher, J.K., and Ernst, P. (2007). Unique and independent roles for MLL in adult hematopoietic stem cells and progenitors. Cell Stem Cell *1*, 324-337.

Kaji, H., Canaff, L., Lebrun, J.J., Goltzman, D., and Hendy, G.N. (2001). Inactivation of menin, a Smad3-interacting protein, blocks transforming growth factor type beta signaling. Proc Natl Acad Sci U S A *98*, 3837-3842.

Karatas, H., Townsend, E.C., Bernard, D., Dou, Y., and Wang, S. (2010). Analysis of the binding of mixed lineage leukemia 1 (MLL1) and histone 3 peptides to WD repeat domain 5 (WDR5) for the design of inhibitors of the MLL1-WDR5 interaction. J Med Chem *53*, 5179-5185.

Khodaei, S., O'Brien, K.P., Dumanski, J., Wong, F.K., and Weber, G. (1999). Characterization of the MEN1 ortholog in zebrafish. Biochem Biophys Res Commun *264*, 404-408.

Koziner, B., Stavnezer, J., and Al-Katib, A. (1985). Surface immunoglobulin light-chain expression by the "common" all cell line REH. Clin Immunol Immunopathol *37*, 135-141.

Krivtsov, A.V., and Armstrong, S.A. (2007). MLL translocations, histone modifications and leukaemia stem-cell development. Nat Rev Cancer *7*, 823-833.

Kroon, E., Krosl, J., Thorsteinsdottir, U., Baban, S., Buchberg, A.M., and Sauvageau, G. (1998). Hoxa9 transforms primary bone marrow cells through specific collaboration with Meis1a but not Pbx1b. Embo J *17*, 3714-3725.

Kumar, A.R., Hudson, W.A., Chen, W., Nishiuchi, R., Yao, Q., and Kersey, J.H. (2004). Hoxa9 influences the phenotype but not the incidence of Mll-AF9 fusion gene leukemia. Blood *103*, 1823-1828.

La, P., Schnepp, R.W., C, D.P., A, C.S., and Hua, X. (2004). Tumor suppressor menin regulates expression of insulin-like growth factor binding protein 2. Endocrinology *145*, 3443-3450.

Lange, B., Valtieri, M., Santoli, D., Caracciolo, D., Mavilio, F., Gemperlein, I., Griffin, C., Emanuel, B., Finan, J., Nowell, P., *et al.* (1987). Growth factor requirements of childhood acute leukemia: establishment of GM-CSF-dependent cell lines. Blood *70*, 192-199.

Larsson, C., Skogseid, B., Oberg, K., Nakamura, Y., and Nordenskjold, M. (1988). Multiple endocrine neoplasia type 1 gene maps to chromosome 11 and is lost in insulinoma. Nature *332*, 85-87.

Lavau, C., Du, C., Thirman, M., and Zeleznik-Le, N. (2000). Chromatin-related properties of CBP fused to MLL generate a myelodysplastic-like syndrome that evolves into myeloid leukemia. Embo J *19*, 4655-4664.

Lee, J.H., and Skalnik, D.G. (2005). CpG-binding protein (CXXC finger protein 1) is a component of the mammalian Set1 histone H3-Lys4 methyltransferase complex, the analogue of the yeast Set1/COMPASS complex. J Biol Chem *280*, 41725-41731.

Lee, J.H., Tate, C.M., You, J.S., and Skalnik, D.G. (2007). Identification and characterization of the human Set1B histone H3-Lys4 methyltransferase complex. J Biol Chem *282*, 13419-13428.

Lemmens, I., Van de Ven, W.J., Kas, K., Zhang, C.X., Giraud, S., Wautot, V., Buisson, N., De Witte, K., Salandre, J., Lenoir, G., *et al.* (1997). Identification of the multiple endocrine neoplasia type 1 (MEN1) gene. The European Consortium on MEN1. Hum Mol Genet *6*, 1177-1183.

Lemmens, I.H., Forsberg, L., Pannett, A.A., Meyen, E., Piehl, F., Turner, J.J., Van de Ven, W.J., Thakker, R.V., Larsson, C., and Kas, K. (2001). Menin interacts directly with the homeobox-containing protein Pem. Biochem Biophys Res Commun *286*, 426-431.

Liang, D.C., Shih, L.Y., Fu, J.F., Li, H.Y., Wang, H.I., Hung, I.J., Yang, C.P., Jaing, T.H., Chen, S.H., and Liu, H.C. (2006). K-Ras mutations and N-Ras mutations in childhood acute leukemias with or without mixed-lineage leukemia gene rearrangements. Cancer *106*, 950-956.

Liedtke, M., and Cleary, M.L. (2009). Therapeutic targeting of MLL. Blood *113*, 6061-6068.

Litt, M.D., Simpson, M., Gaszner, M., Allis, C.D., and Felsenfeld, G. (2001). Correlation between histone lysine methylation and developmental changes at the chicken beta-globin locus. Science *293*, 2453-2455.

Liu, H., Cheng, E.H., and Hsieh, J.J. (2009). MLL fusions: pathways to leukemia. Cancer Biol Ther *8*, 1204-1211.

Lopez-Egido, J., Cunningham, J., Berg, M., Oberg, K., Bongcam-Rudloff, E., and Gobl, A. (2002). Menin's interaction with glial fibrillary acidic protein and vimentin suggests a role for the intermediate filament network in regulating menin activity. Exp Cell Res *278*, 175-183.

Luger, K., and Hansen, J.C. (2005). Nucleosome and chromatin fiber dynamics. Curr Opin Struct Biol *15*, 188-196.

Luo, R.T., Lavau, C., Du, C., Simone, F., Polak, P.E., Kawamata, S., and Thirman, M.J. (2001). The elongation domain of ELL is dispensable but its ELL-associated factor 1 interaction domain is essential for MLL-ELL-induced leukemogenesis. Mol Cell Biol *21*, 5678-5687.

Luscher-Firzlaff, J., Gawlista, I., Vervoorts, J., Kapelle, K., Braunschweig, T., Walsemann, G., Rodgarkia-Schamberger, C., Schuchlautz, H., Dreschers, S., Kremmer, E., *et al.* (2008). The human trithorax protein hASH2 functions as an oncoprotein. Cancer Res *68*, 749-758.

Ma, C., and Staudt, L.M. (1996). LAF-4 encodes a lymphoid nuclear protein with transactivation potential that is homologous to AF-4, the gene fused to MLL in t(4;11) leukemias. Blood *87*, 734-745.

Macrini, C.M., Pombo-de-Oliveira, M.S., Ford, A.M., and Alves, G. (2003). MLL AT-hook sequence is strongly conserved in infant acute leukemia with or without MLL gene rearrangement. Leukemia *17*, 1432-1433.

Mahgoub, N., Parker, R.I., Hosler, M.R., Close, P., Winick, N.J., Masterson, M., Shannon, K.M., and Felix, C.A. (1998). RAS mutations in pediatric leukemias with MLL gene rearrangements. Genes Chromosomes Cancer *21*, 270-275.

Maillard, I., Chen, Y.X., Friedman, A., Yang, Y., Tubbs, A.T., Shestova, O., Pear, W.S., and Hua, X. (2009). Menin regulates the function of hematopoietic stem cells and lymphoid progenitors. Blood *113*, 1661-1669.

Maillard, I., and Hess, J.L. (2009). The role of menin in hematopoiesis. Adv Exp Med Biol *668*, 51-57.

Manickam, P., Vogel, A.M., Agarwal, S.K., Oda, T., Spiegel, A.M., Marx, S.J., Collins, F.S., Weinstein, B.M., and Chandrasekharappa, S.C. (2000). Isolation, characterization, expression and functional analysis of the zebrafish ortholog of MEN1. Mamm Genome *11*, 448-454.

Marschalek, R. (2010). Mixed lineage leukemia: roles in human malignancies and potential therapy. Febs J *277*, 1822-1831.

Martin, M.E., Milne, T.A., Bloyer, S., Galoian, K., Shen, W., Gibbs, D., Brock, H.W., Slany, R., and Hess, J.L. (2003). Dimerization of MLL fusion proteins immortalizes hematopoietic cells. Cancer Cell *4*, 197-207.

McMahon, K.A., Hiew, S.Y., Hadjur, S., Veiga-Fernandes, H., Menzel, U., Price, A.J., Kioussis, D., Williams, O., and Brady, H.J. (2007). Mll has a critical role in fetal and adult hematopoietic stem cell self-renewal. Cell Stem Cell *1*, 338-345.

Melko, M., Douguet, D., Bensaid, M., Zongaro, S., Verheggen, C., Gecz, J., and Bardoni, B. Functional characterization of the AFF (AF4/FMR2) family of RNA-binding proteins: insights into the molecular pathology of FRAXE intellectual disability. Hum Mol Genet *20*, 1873-1885.

Meyer, C., Kowarz, E., Hofmann, J., Renneville, A., Zuna, J., Trka, J., Ben Abdelali, R., Macintyre, E., De Braekeleer, E., De Braekeleer, M., *et al.* (2009). New insights to the MLL recombinome of acute leukemias. Leukemia *23*, 1490-1499.

Meyer, C., Schneider, B., Jakob, S., Strehl, S., Attarbaschi, A., Schnittger, S., Schoch, C., Jansen, M.W., van Dongen, J.J., den Boer, M.L., *et al.* (2006). The MLL recombinome of acute leukemias. Leukemia *20*, 777-784.

Milne, T.A., Briggs, S.D., Brock, H.W., Martin, M.E., Gibbs, D., Allis, C.D., and Hess, J.L. (2002). MLL targets SET domain methyltransferase activity to Hox gene promoters. Mol Cell *10*, 1107-1117.

Milne, T.A., Hughes, C.M., Lloyd, R., Yang, Z., Rozenblatt-Rosen, O., Dou, Y., Schnepp, R.W., Krankel, C., Livolsi, V.A., Gibbs, D., *et al.* (2005). Menin and MLL cooperatively regulate expression of cyclin-dependent kinase inhibitors. Proc Natl Acad Sci U S A *102*, 749-754.

Minowada, J., Onuma, T., and Moore, G.E. (1972). Rosette-forming human lymphoid cell lines. I. Establishment and evidence for origin of thymus-derived lymphocytes. J Natl Cancer Inst *49*, 891-895.

Mitelman, F., and Heim, S. (1992). Quantitative acute leukemia cytogenetics. Genes Chromosomes Cancer *5*, 57-66.

Mitterbauer-Hohendanner, G., and Mannhalter, C. (2004). The biological and clinical significance of MLL abnormalities in haematological malignancies. Eur J Clin Invest *34 Suppl 2*, 12-24.

Morrissey, J., Tkachuk, D.C., Milatovich, A., Francke, U., Link, M., and Cleary, M.L. (1993). A serine/proline-rich protein is fused to HRX in t(4;11) acute leukemias. Blood *81*, 1124-1131.

Mueller, D., Bach, C., Zeisig, D., Garcia-Cuellar, M.P., Monroe, S., Sreekumar, A., Zhou, R., Nesvizhskii, A., Chinnaiyan, A., Hess, J.L., *et al.* (2007). A role for the MLL fusion partner ENL in transcriptional elongation and chromatin modification. Blood *110*, 4445-4454.

Mueller, D., Garcia-Cuellar, M.P., Bach, C., Buhl, S., Maethner, E., and Slany, R.K. (2009). Misguided transcriptional elongation causes mixed lineage leukemia. PLoS Biol *7*, e1000249.

Nakamura, T., Alder, H., Gu, Y., Prasad, R., Canaani, O., Kamada, N., Gale, R.P., Lange, B., Crist, W.M., Nowell, P.C., *et al.* (1993). Genes on chromosomes 4, 9, and 19 involved in 11q23 abnormalities in acute leukemia share sequence homology and/or common motifs. Proc Natl Acad Sci U S A *90*, 4631-4635.

Nakamura, T., Mori, T., Tada, S., Krajewski, W., Rozovskaia, T., Wassell, R., Dubois, G., Mazo, A., Croce, C.M., and Canaani, E. (2002). ALL-1 is a histone methyltransferase that assembles a supercomplex of proteins involved in transcriptional regulation. Mol Cell *10*, 1119-1128.

Nakanishi, H., Nakamura, T., Canaani, E., and Croce, C.M. (2007). ALL1 fusion proteins induce deregulation of EphA7 and ERK phosphorylation in human acute leukemias. Proc Natl Acad Sci U S A *104*, 14442-14447.

Ng, H.H., Robert, F., Young, R.A., and Struhl, K. (2003). Targeted recruitment of Set1 histone methylase by elongating Pol II provides a localized mark and memory of recent transcriptional activity. Mol Cell *11*, 709-719.

Nie, Z., Yan, Z., Chen, E.H., Sechi, S., Ling, C., Zhou, S., Xue, Y., Yang, D., Murray, D., Kanakubo, E., *et al.* (2003). Novel SWI/SNF chromatin-remodeling complexes contain a mixed-lineage leukemia chromosomal translocation partner. Mol Cell Biol *23*, 2942-2952.

Nilson, I., Reichel, M., Ennas, M.G., Greim, R., Knorr, C., Siegler, G., Greil, J., Fey, G.H., and Marschalek, R. (1997). Exon/intron structure of the human AF-4 gene, a member of the AF-4/LAF-4/FMR-2 gene family coding for a nuclear protein with structural alterations in acute leukaemia. Br J Haematol *98*, 157-169.

Noma, K., and Grewal, S.I. (2002). Histone H3 lysine 4 methylation is mediated by Set1 and promotes maintenance of active chromatin states in fission yeast. Proc Natl Acad Sci U S A *99 Suppl 4*, 16438-16445.

Oguchi, K., Takagi, M., Tsuchida, R., Taya, Y., Ito, E., Isoyama, K., Ishii, E., Zannini, L., Delia, D., and Mizutani, S. (2003). Missense mutation and defective function of ATM in a childhood acute leukemia patient with MLL gene rearrangement. Blood *101*, 3622-3627.

Ohkura, N., Kishi, M., Tsukada, T., and Yamaguchi, K. (2001). Menin, a gene product responsible for multiple endocrine neoplasia type 1, interacts with the putative tumor metastasis suppressor nm23. Biochem Biophys Res Commun *282*, 1206-1210.

Okada, Y., Feng, Q., Lin, Y., Jiang, Q., Li, Y., Coffield, V.M., Su, L., Xu, G., and Zhang, Y. (2005). hDOT1L links histone methylation to leukemogenesis. Cell *121*, 167-178.

Okada, Y., Jiang, Q., Lemieux, M., Jeannotte, L., Su, L., and Zhang, Y. (2006). Leukaemic transformation by CALM-AF10 involves upregulation of Hoxa5 by hDOT1L. Nat Cell Biol *8*, 1017-1024.

Oliver, P.L., Bitoun, E., Clark, J., Jones, E.L., and Davies, K.E. (2004). Mediation of Af4 protein function in the cerebellum by Siah proteins. Proc Natl Acad Sci U S A *101*, 14901-14906.

Palermo, C.M., Bennett, C.A., Winters, A.C., and Hemenway, C.S. (2008). The AF4-mimetic peptide, PFWT, induces necrotic cell death in MV4-11 leukemia cells. Leuk Res *32*, 633-642.

Patel, A., Dharmarajan, V., and Cosgrove, M.S. (2008a). Structure of WDR5 bound to mixed lineage leukemia protein-1 peptide. J Biol Chem *283*, 32158-32161.

Patel, A., Dharmarajan, V., Vought, V.E., and Cosgrove, M.S. (2009). On the mechanism of multiple lysine methylation by the human mixed lineage leukemia protein-1 (MLL1) core complex. J Biol Chem *284*, 24242-24256.

Patel, A., Vought, V.E., Dharmarajan, V., and Cosgrove, M.S. (2008b). A conserved arginine-containing motif crucial for the assembly and enzymatic activity of the mixed lineage leukemia protein-1 core complex. J Biol Chem *283*, 32162-32175.

Patel, A., Vought, V.E., Dharmarajan, V., and Cosgrove, M.S. (2011). A novel non-SET domain multi-subunit methyltransferase required for sequential nucleosomal histone H3 methylation by the mixed lineage leukemia protein-1 (MLL1) core complex. J Biol Chem *286*, 3359-3369.

Poisson, A., Zablewska, B., and Gaudray, P. (2003). Menin interacting proteins as clues toward the understanding of multiple endocrine neoplasia type 1. Cancer Lett *189*, 1-10.

Pokholok, D.K., Harbison, C.T., Levine, S., Cole, M., Hannett, N.M., Lee, T.I., Bell, G.W., Walker, K., Rolfe, P.A., Herbolsheimer, E., *et al.* (2005). Genome-wide map of nucleosome acetylation and methylation in yeast. Cell *122*, 517-527.

Poppe, B., Vandesompele, J., Schoch, C., Lindvall, C., Mrozek, K., Bloomfield, C.D., Beverloo, H.B., Michaux, L., Dastugue, N., Herens, C., *et al.* (2004). Expression analyses identify MLL as a prominent target of 11q23 amplification and support an etiologic role for MLL gain of function in myeloid malignancies. Blood *103*, 229-235.

Prasad, R., Yano, T., Sorio, C., Nakamura, T., Rallapalli, R., Gu, Y., Leshkowitz, D., Croce, C.M., and Canaani, E. (1995). Domains with transcriptional regulatory activity within the ALL1 and AF4 proteins involved in acute leukemia. Proc Natl Acad Sci U S A *92*, 12160-12164.

Pray-Grant, M.G., Daniel, J.A., Schieltz, D., Yates, J.R., 3rd, and Grant, P.A. (2005). Chd1 chromodomain links histone H3 methylation with SAGA- and SLIK-dependent acetylation. Nature *433*, 434-438.

Pui, C.H., Chessells, J.M., Camitta, B., Baruchel, A., Biondi, A., Boyett, J.M., Carroll, A., Eden, O.B., Evans, W.E., Gadner, H., *et al.* (2003). Clinical heterogeneity in childhood acute lymphoblastic leukemia with 11q23 rearrangements. Leukemia *17*, 700-706.

Qian, C., and Zhou, M.M. (2006). SET domain protein lysine methyltransferases: Structure, specificity and catalysis. Cell Mol Life Sci *63*, 2755-2763.

Quentmeier, H., Reinhardt, J., Zaborski, M., and Drexler, H.G. (2003). MLL partial tandem duplications in acute leukemia cell lines. Leukemia *17*, 980-981.

Ross, M.E., Mahfouz, R., Onciu, M., Liu, H.C., Zhou, X., Song, G., Shurtleff, S.A., Pounds, S., Cheng, C., Ma, J., *et al.* (2004). Gene expression profiling of pediatric acute myelogenous leukemia. Blood *104*, 3679-3687.

Roudaia, L., and Speck, N.A. (2008). A MENage a Trois in leukemia. Cancer Cell *14*, 3-5.

Rozenblatt-Rosen, O., Rozovskaia, T., Burakov, D., Sedkov, Y., Tillib, S., Blechman, J., Nakamura, T., Croce, C.M., Mazo, A., and Canaani, E. (1998). The C-terminal SET domains of ALL-1 and TRITHORAX interact with the INI1 and SNR1 proteins, components of the SWI/SNF complex. Proc Natl Acad Sci U S A *95*, 4152-4157.

Rozovskaia, T., Feinstein, E., Mor, O., Foa, R., Blechman, J., Nakamura, T., Croce, C.M., Cimino, G., and Canaani, E. (2001). Upregulation of Meis1 and HoxA9 in acute lymphocytic leukemias with the t(4 : 11) abnormality. Oncogene *20*, 874-878.

Rubnitz, J.E., Link, M.P., Shuster, J.J., Carroll, A.J., Hakami, N., Frankel, L.S., Pullen, D.J., and Cleary, M.L. (1994a). Frequency and prognostic significance of HRX rearrangements in infant acute lymphoblastic leukemia: a Pediatric Oncology Group study. Blood *84*, 570-573.

Rubnitz, J.E., Morrissey, J., Savage, P.A., and Cleary, M.L. (1994b). ENL, the gene fused with HRX in t(11;19) leukemias, encodes a nuclear protein with transcriptional activation potential in lymphoid and myeloid cells. Blood *84*, 1747-1752.

Ruthenburg, A.J., Wang, W., Graybosch, D.M., Li, H., Allis, C.D., Patel, D.J., and Verdine, G.L. (2006). Histone H3 recognition and presentation by the WDR5 module of the MLL1 complex. Nat Struct Mol Biol *13*, 704-712.

Santos-Rosa, H., Schneider, R., Bannister, A.J., Sherriff, J., Bernstein, B.E., Emre, N.C., Schreiber, S.L., Mellor, J., and Kouzarides, T. (2002). Active genes are tri-methylated at K4 of histone H3. Nature *419*, 407-411.

Santos-Rosa, H., Schneider, R., Bernstein, B.E., Karabetsou, N., Morillon, A., Weise, C., Schreiber, S.L., Mellor, J., and Kouzarides, T. (2003). Methylation of histone H3 K4 mediates association of the Isw1p ATPase with chromatin. Mol Cell *12*, 1325-1332.

Scharf, S., Zech, J., Bursen, A., Schraets, D., Oliver, P.L., Kliem, S., Pfitzner, E., Gillert, E., Dingermann, T., and Marschalek, R. (2007). Transcription linked to recombination: a gene-internal promoter coincides with the recombination hot spot II of the human MLL gene. Oncogene *26*, 1361-1371.

Schichman, S.A., Caligiuri, M.A., Strout, M.P., Carter, S.L., Gu, Y., Canaani, E., Bloomfield, C.D., and Croce, C.M. (1994). ALL-1 tandem duplication in acute myeloid leukemia with a normal karyotype involves homologous recombination between Alu elements. Cancer Res *54*, 4277-4280.

Schichman, S.A., Canaani, E., and Croce, C.M. (1995). Self-fusion of the ALL1 gene. A new genetic mechanism for acute leukemia. Jama *273*, 571-576.

Schneider, R., Bannister, A.J., Myers, F.A., Thorne, A.W., Crane-Robinson, C., and Kouzarides, T. (2004). Histone H3 lysine 4 methylation patterns in higher eukaryotic genes. Nat Cell Biol *6*, 73-77.

Schnepp, R.W., Hou, Z., Wang, H., Petersen, C., Silva, A., Masai, H., and Hua, X. (2004). Functional interaction between tumor suppressor menin and activator of S-phase kinase. Cancer Res *64*, 6791-6796.

Schoch, C., Schnittger, S., Klaus, M., Kern, W., Hiddemann, W., and Haferlach, T. (2003). AML with 11q23/MLL abnormalities as defined by the WHO classification: incidence, partner chromosomes, FAB subtype, age distribution, and prognostic impact in an unselected series of 1897 cytogenetically analyzed AML cases. Blood *102*, 2395-2402.

Schreiner, S.A., Garcia-Cuellar, M.P., Fey, G.H., and Slany, R.K. (1999). The leukemogenic fusion of MLL with ENL creates a novel transcriptional transactivator. Leukemia *13*, 1525-1533.

Schubeler, D., MacAlpine, D.M., Scalzo, D., Wirbelauer, C., Kooperberg, C., van Leeuwen, F., Gottschling, D.E., O'Neill, L.P., Turner, B.M., Delrow, J., *et al.* (2004). The histone modification pattern of active genes revealed through genome-wide chromatin analysis of a higher eukaryote. Genes Dev *18*, 1263-1271.

Schuetz, A., Allali-Hassani, A., Martin, F., Loppnau, P., Vedadi, M., Bochkarev, A., Plotnikov, A.N., Arrowsmith, C.H., and Min, J. (2006). Structural basis for molecular recognition and presentation of histone H3 by WDR5. Embo J *25*, 4245-4252.

Shapiro, G.I. (2006). Cyclin-dependent kinase pathways as targets for cancer treatment. J Clin Oncol *24*, 1770-1783.

Simone, F., Polak, P.E., Kaberlein, J.J., Luo, R.T., Levitan, D.A., and Thirman, M.J. (2001). EAF1, a novel ELL-associated factor that is delocalized by expression of the MLL-ELL fusion protein. Blood *98*, 201-209.

Sims, R.J., 3rd, Chen, C.F., Santos-Rosa, H., Kouzarides, T., Patel, S.S., and Reinberg, D. (2005). Human but not yeast CHD1 binds directly and selectively to histone H3 methylated at lysine 4 via its tandem chromodomains. J Biol Chem *280*, 41789-41792.

Slany, R.K. (2009). The molecular biology of mixed lineage leukemia. Haematologica *94*, 984-993.

So, C.W., Karsunky, H., Passegue, E., Cozzio, A., Weissman, I.L., and Cleary, M.L. (2003). MLL-GAS7 transforms multipotent hematopoietic progenitors and induces mixed lineage leukemias in mice. Cancer Cell *3*, 161-171.

So, C.W., Karsunky, H., Wong, P., Weissman, I.L., and Cleary, M.L. (2004). Leukemic transformation of hematopoietic progenitors by MLL-GAS7 in the absence of Hoxa7 or Hoxa9. Blood *103*, 3192-3199.

Sobulo, O.M., Borrow, J., Tomek, R., Reshmi, S., Harden, A., Schlegelberger, B., Housman, D., Doggett, N.A., Rowley, J.D., and Zeleznik-Le, N.J. (1997). MLL is fused to CBP, a histone acetyltransferase, in therapy-related acute myeloid leukemia with a t(11;16)(q23;p13.3). Proc Natl Acad Sci U S A *94*, 8732-8737.

Song, J.J., and Kingston, R.E. (2008). WDR5 interacts with mixed lineage leukemia (MLL) protein via the histone H3-binding pocket. J Biol Chem *283*, 35258-35264.

Southall, S.M., Wong, P.S., Odho, Z., Roe, S.M., and Wilson, J.R. (2009). Structural basis for the requirement of additional factors for MLL1 SET domain activity and recognition of epigenetic marks. Mol Cell *33*, 181-191.

Sowa, H., Kaji, H., Hendy, G.N., Canaff, L., Komori, T., Sugimoto, T., and Chihara, K. (2004). Menin is required for bone morphogenetic protein 2- and transforming growth factor beta-regulated osteoblastic differentiation through interaction with Smads and Runx2. J Biol Chem *279*, 40267-40275.

Srinivasan, R.S., de Erkenez, A.C., and Hemenway, C.S. (2003). The mixed lineage leukemia fusion partner AF9 binds specific isoforms of the BCL-6 corepressor. Oncogene *22*, 3395-3406.

Srinivasan, R.S., Nesbit, J.B., Marrero, L., Erfurth, F., LaRussa, V.F., and Hemenway, C.S. (2004). The synthetic peptide PFWT disrupts AF4-AF9 protein complexes and induces apoptosis in t(4;11) leukemia cells. Leukemia *18*, 1364-1372.

Stam, R.W., den Boer, M.L., Passier, M.M., Janka-Schaub, G.E., Sallan, S.E., Armstrong, S.A., and Pieters, R. (2006). Silencing of the tumor suppressor gene FHIT is highly characteristic for MLL gene rearranged infant acute lymphoblastic leukemia. Leukemia *20*, 264-271.

Steward, M.M., Lee, J.S., O'Donovan, A., Wyatt, M., Bernstein, B.E., and Shilatifard, A. (2006). Molecular regulation of H3K4 trimethylation by ASH2L, a shared subunit of MLL complexes. Nat Struct Mol Biol *13*, 852-854.

Stewart, C., Parente, F., Piehl, F., Farnebo, F., Quincey, D., Silins, G., Bergman, L., Carle, G.F., Lemmens, I., Grimmond, S., *et al.* (1998). Characterization of the mouse Men1 gene and its expression during development. Oncogene *17*, 2485-2493.

Stoller, J.Z., Huang, L., Tan, C.C., Huang, F., Zhou, D.D., Yang, J., Gelb, B.D., and Epstein, J.A. Ash2l interacts with Tbx1 and is required during early embryogenesis. Exp Biol Med (Maywood) *235*, 569-576.

Stong, R.C., Korsmeyer, S.J., Parkin, J.L., Arthur, D.C., and Kersey, J.H. (1985). Human acute leukemia cell line with the t(4;11) chromosomal rearrangement exhibits B lineage and monocytic characteristics. Blood *65*, 21-31.

Strahl, B.D., Ohba, R., Cook, R.G., and Allis, C.D. (1999). Methylation of histone H3 at lysine 4 is highly conserved and correlates with transcriptionally active nuclei in Tetrahymena. Proc Natl Acad Sci U S A *96*, 14967-14972.

Streubel, B., Valent, P., Jager, U., Edelhauser, M., Wandt, H., Wagner, T., Buchner, T., Lechner, K., and Fonatsch, C. (2000). Amplification of the MLL gene on double minutes, a homogeneously staining region, and ring chromosomes in five patients with acute myeloid leukemia or myelodysplastic syndrome. Genes Chromosomes Cancer *27*, 380-386.

Stubbs, M.C., Kim, Y.M., Krivtsov, A.V., Wright, R.D., Feng, Z., Agarwal, J., Kung, A.L., and Armstrong, S.A. (2008). MLL-AF9 and FLT3 cooperation in acute myelogenous leukemia: development of a model for rapid therapeutic assessment. Leukemia *22*, 66-77.

Su, M.A., Wisotzkey, R.G., and Newfeld, S.J. (2001). A screen for modifiers of decapentaplegic mutant phenotypes identifies lilliputian, the only member of the Fragile-X/Burkitt's Lymphoma family of transcription factors in Drosophila melanogaster. Genetics *157*, 717-725.

Sukhodolets, K.E., Hickman, A.B., Agarwal, S.K., Sukhodolets, M.V., Obungu, V.H., Novotny, E.A., Crabtree, J.S., Chandrasekharappa, S.C., Collins, F.S., Spiegel, A.M., *et al.* (2003). The 32-kilodalton subunit of replication protein A interacts with menin, the product of the MEN1 tumor suppressor gene. Mol Cell Biol *23*, 493-509.

Takahashi, Y.H., Lee, J.S., Swanson, S.K., Saraf, A., Florens, L., Washburn, M.P., Trievel, R.C., and Shilatifard, A. (2009). Regulation of H3K4 trimethylation via Cps40 (Spp1) of COMPASS is monoubiquitination independent: implication for a Phe/Tyr switch by the catalytic domain of Set1. Mol Cell Biol *29*, 3478-3486.

Takeda, S., Chen, D.Y., Westergard, T.D., Fisher, J.K., Rubens, J.A., Sasagawa, S., Kan, J.T., Korsmeyer, S.J., Cheng, E.H., and Hsieh, J.J. (2006). Proteolysis of MLL family proteins is essential for taspase1-orchestrated cell cycle progression. Genes Dev *20*, 2397-2409.

Taketani, T., Taki, T., Sugita, K., Furuichi, Y., Ishii, E., Hanada, R., Tsuchida, M., Sugita, K., Ida, K., and Hayashi, Y. (2004). FLT3 mutations in the activation loop of tyrosine kinase domain are frequently found in infant ALL with MLL rearrangements and pediatric ALL with hyperdiploidy. Blood *103*, 1085-1088.

Taki, T., Kano, H., Taniwaki, M., Sako, M., Yanagisawa, M., and Hayashi, Y. (1999). AF5q31, a newly identified AF4-related gene, is fused to MLL in infant acute lymphoblastic leukemia with ins(5;11)(q31;q13q23). Proc Natl Acad Sci U S A *96*, 14535-14540.

Taki, T., Sako, M., Tsuchida, M., and Hayashi, Y. (1997). The t(11;16)(q23;p13) translocation in myelodysplastic syndrome fuses the MLL gene to the CBP gene. Blood *89*, 3945-3950.

Tan, C.C., Sindhu, K.V., Li, S., Nishio, H., Stoller, J.Z., Oishi, K., Puttreddy, S., Lee, T.J., Epstein, J.A., Walsh, M.J., *et al.* (2008). Transcription factor Ap2delta associates with Ash2l and ALR, a trithorax family histone methyltransferase, to activate Hoxc8 transcription. Proc Natl Acad Sci U S A *105*, 7472-7477.

Terranova, R., Agherbi, H., Boned, A., Meresse, S., and Djabali, M. (2006). Histone and DNA methylation defects at Hox genes in mice expressing a SET domain-truncated form of Mll. Proc Natl Acad Sci U S A *103*, 6629-6634.

Thakker, R.V. (2001). Multiple endocrine neoplasia. Horm Res *56 Suppl 1*, 67-72.

Tkachuk, D.C., Kohler, S., and Cleary, M.L. (1992). Involvement of a homolog of Drosophila trithorax by 11q23 chromosomal translocations in acute leukemias. Cell *71*, 691-700.

Trievel, R.C., and Shilatifard, A. (2009). WDR5, a complexed protein. Nat Struct Mol Biol *16*, 678-680.

Tsuchiya, S., Yamabe, M., Yamaguchi, Y., Kobayashi, Y., Konno, T., and Tada, K. (1980). Establishment and characterization of a human acute monocytic leukemia cell line (THP-1). Int J Cancer *26*, 171-176.

Tyagi, S., Chabes, A.L., Wysocka, J., and Herr, W. (2007). E2F activation of S phase promoters via association with HCF-1 and the MLL family of histone H3K4 methyltransferases. Mol Cell *27*, 107-119.

von Bergh, A., Gargallo, P., De Prijck, B., Vranckx, H., Marschalek, R., Larripa, I., Kluin, P., Schuuring, E., and Hagemeijer, A. (2001). Cryptic t(4;11) encoding MLL-AF4 due to insertion of 5' MLL sequences in chromosome 4. Leukemia *15*, 595-600.

von Bergh, A.R., Beverloo, H.B., Rombout, P., van Wering, E.R., van Weel, M.H., Beverstock, G.C., Kluin, P.M., Slater, R.M., and Schuuring, E. (2002). LAF4, an AF4-related gene, is fused to MLL in infant acute lymphoblastic leukemia. Genes Chromosomes Cancer *35*, 92-96.

Wang, J., Iwasaki, H., Krivtsov, A., Febbo, P.G., Thorner, A.R., Ernst, P., Anastasiadou, E., Kutok, J.L., Kogan, S.C., Zinkel, S.S., *et al.* (2005). Conditional MLL-CBP targets GMP and models therapy-related myeloproliferative disease. Embo J *24*, 368-381.

Wang, Z., Smith, K.S., Murphy, M., Piloto, O., Somervaille, T.C., and Cleary, M.L. (2008). Glycogen synthase kinase 3 in MLL leukaemia maintenance and targeted therapy. Nature *455*, 1205-1209.

Welch, M.D., and Drubin, D.G. (1994). A nuclear protein with sequence similarity to proteins implicated in human acute leukemias is important for cellular morphogenesis and actin cytoskeletal function in Saccharomyces cerevisiae. Mol Biol Cell *5*, 617-632.

Whitman, S.P., Hackanson, B., Liyanarachchi, S., Liu, S., Rush, L.J., Maharry, K., Margeson, D., Davuluri, R., Wen, J., Witte, T., *et al.* (2008). DNA hypermethylation and epigenetic silencing of the tumor suppressor gene, SLC5A8, in acute myeloid leukemia with the MLL partial tandem duplication. Blood *112*, 2013-2016.

Whitman, S.P., Liu, S., Vukosavljevic, T., Rush, L.J., Yu, L., Liu, C., Klisovic, M.I., Maharry, K., Guimond, M., Strout, M.P., *et al.* (2005). The MLL partial tandem duplication: evidence for recessive gain-of-function in acute myeloid leukemia identifies a novel patient subgroup for molecular-targeted therapy. Blood *106*, 345-352.

Wiederschain, D., Kawai, H., Shilatifard, A., and Yuan, Z.M. (2005). Multiple mixed lineage leukemia (MLL) fusion proteins suppress p53-mediated response to DNA damage. J Biol Chem *280*, 24315-24321.

Wu, X., and Hua, X. (2008). Menin, histone h3 methyltransferases, and regulation of cell proliferation: current knowledge and perspective. Curr Mol Med *8*, 805-815.

Wysocka, J., Swigut, T., Milne, T.A., Dou, Y., Zhang, X., Burlingame, A.L., Roeder, R.G., Brivanlou, A.H., and Allis, C.D. (2005). WDR5 associates with histone H3 methylated at K4 and is essential for H3 K4 methylation and vertebrate development. Cell *121*, 859-872.

Wysocka, J., Swigut, T., Xiao, H., Milne, T.A., Kwon, S.Y., Landry, J., Kauer, M., Tackett, A.J., Chait, B.T., Badenhorst, P., *et al.* (2006). A PHD finger of NURF couples histone H3 lysine 4 trimethylation with chromatin remodelling. Nature *442*, 86-90.

Xia, Z.B., Anderson, M., Diaz, M.O., and Zeleznik-Le, N.J. (2003). MLL repression domain interacts with histone deacetylases, the polycomb group proteins HPC2 and BMI-1, and the corepressor C-terminal-binding protein. Proc Natl Acad Sci U S A *100*, 8342-8347.

Yagi, H., Deguchi, K., Aono, A., Tani, Y., Kishimoto, T., and Komori, T. (1998). Growth disturbance in fetal liver hematopoiesis of Mll-mutant mice. Blood *92*, 108-117.

Yamashita, M., Hirahara, K., Shinnakasu, R., Hosokawa, H., Norikane, S., Kimura, M.Y., Hasegawa, A., and Nakayama, T. (2006). Crucial role of MLL for the maintenance of memory T helper type 2 cell responses. Immunity *24*, 611-622.

Yao, Q., Nishiuchi, R., Kitamura, T., and Kersey, J.H. (2005). Human leukemias with mutated FLT3 kinase are synergistically sensitive to FLT3 and Hsp90 inhibitors: the key role of the STAT5 signal transduction pathway. Leukemia *19*, 1605-1612.

Yasui, H., Hideshima, T., Hamasaki, M., Roccaro, A.M., Shiraishi, N., Kumar, S., Tassone, P., Ishitsuka, K., Raje, N., Tai, Y.T., *et al.* (2005). SDX-101, the R-enantiomer of etodolac, induces cytotoxicity, overcomes drug resistance, and enhances the activity of dexamethasone in multiple myeloma. Blood *106*, 706-712.

Yeoh, E.J., Ross, M.E., Shurtleff, S.A., Williams, W.K., Patel, D., Mahfouz, R., Behm, F.G., Raimondi, S.C., Relling, M.V., Patel, A., *et al.* (2002). Classification, subtype discovery, and prediction of outcome in pediatric acute lymphoblastic leukemia by gene expression profiling. Cancer Cell *1*, 133-143.

Yocum, A.K., Busch, C.M., Felix, C.A., and Blair, I.A. (2006). Proteomics-based strategy to identify biomarkers and pharmacological targets in leukemias with t(4;11) translocations. J Proteome Res *5*, 2743-2753.

Yokoyama, A., and Cleary, M.L. (2008). Menin critically links MLL proteins with LEDGF on cancer-associated target genes. Cancer Cell *14*, 36-46.

Yokoyama, A., Kitabayashi, I., Ayton, P.M., Cleary, M.L., and Ohki, M. (2002). Leukemia proto-oncoprotein MLL is proteolytically processed into 2 fragments with opposite transcriptional properties. Blood *100*, 3710-3718.

Yokoyama, A., Somervaille, T.C., Smith, K.S., Rozenblatt-Rosen, O., Meyerson, M., and Cleary, M.L. (2005). The menin tumor suppressor protein is an essential oncogenic cofactor for MLL-associated leukemogenesis. Cell *123*, 207-218.

Yokoyama, A., Wang, Z., Wysocka, J., Sanyal, M., Aufiero, D.J., Kitabayashi, I., Herr, W., and Cleary, M.L. (2004). Leukemia proto-oncoprotein MLL forms a SET1-like histone methyltransferase complex with menin to regulate Hox gene expression. Mol Cell Biol *24*, 5639-5649.

Yu, B.D., Hess, J.L., Horning, S.E., Brown, G.A., and Korsmeyer, S.J. (1995). Altered Hox expression and segmental identity in Mll-mutant mice. Nature *378*, 505-508.

Zeisig, B.B., Milne, T., Garcia-Cuellar, M.P., Schreiner, S., Martin, M.E., Fuchs, U., Borkhardt, A., Chanda, S.K., Walker, J., Soden, R., *et al.* (2004). Hoxa9 and Meis1 are key targets for MLL-ENL-mediated cellular immortalization. Mol Cell Biol *24*, 617-628.

Zhu, E.D., Demay, M.B., and Gori, F. (2008). Wdr5 is essential for osteoblast differentiation. J Biol Chem *283*, 7361-7367.

Ziemin-van der Poel, S., McCabe, N.R., Gill, H.J., Espinosa, R., 3rd, Patel, Y., Harden, A., Rubinelli, P., Smith, S.D., LeBeau, M.M., Rowley, J.D., *et al.* (1991). Identification of a gene, MLL, that spans the breakpoint in 11q23 translocations associated with human leukemias. Proc Natl Acad Sci U S A *88*, 10735-10739.

8

Trafficking of Acute Leukemia Cells – Chemokine Receptor Pathways that Modulate Leukemia Cell Dissemination

Seiji Fukuda[1], Chie Onishi[2] and Louis M. Pelus[3]
[1]*Department of Pediatrics, Shimane University School of Medicine*
[2]*Department of Hematology, Shimane University School of Medicine*
[3]*Department of Microbiology and Immunology, Indiana University School of Medicine*
[1,2]*Japan*
[3]*United States*

1. Introduction

Recent advances in therapeutic regimens targeting aberrant proliferation of leukemia cells have led to a decline in the mortality of patients with acute leukemia. Nevertheless, a number of patients still suffer from refractory disease or relapse, indicating that more innovative and effective therapeutic strategies are required to achieve superior outcomes. One of the major indicators of poor prognosis in leukemia patients is extramedullary infiltration or dissemination of leukemia cells. In particular, leukemia cell infiltration into the central nervous system is one of the major complications negatively influencing prognosis. However, little is known about the mechanisms responsible for extramedullary dissemination of leukemia cells compared to those responsible for solid tumor metastasis.

The chemokine SDF1 (stromal derived factor-1) and its receptor CXCR4 regulate trafficking of normal hematopoietic stem cells (HSC) as well as metastasis of solid tumor cells. Similarly, the majority of acute myeloid leukemia (AML) cells express CXCR4 and migrate in response to SDF1, suggesting that the SDF1/CXCR4 axis may be involved in the dissemination of AML cells to various organs. A recent study also suggests that chemokine/chemokine receptor interactions orchestrate extramedullary dissemination in childhood AML. Moreover, signaling through the chemokine receptor CCR7 is crucial for infiltration of T-ALL cells in the central nervous system. Our recent studies indicate that internal tandem duplication mutations of the Flt3 gene (ITD-Flt3), found in patients with AML, significantly augments migration of hematopoietic cells by deregulating CXCR4 signaling that are qualitatively distinct from cells lacking ITD-Flt3 and facilitate their infiltration to visceral organs while decreasing their homing to the bone marrow. ITD-Flt3 regulates overlapping as well as functionally distinct signaling pathways down-stream of SDF1/CXCR4 compared to cells that do not harbor ITD-Flt3 mutations. The data suggest that ITD-Flt3 may facilitate dissemination of leukemia cells by modulating SDF1/CXCR4 signaling and that blocking this functional cross-talk between ITD-Flt3 and CXCR4 pathways may have therapeutic benefit. Therefore, genes differentially regulated by SDF1 specifically in ITD-Flt3 cells may represent key targets regulating aberrant migration by

ITD-Flt3 in response to SDF1 to prevent unnecessary dissemination and invasiveness of ITD-Flt3+ acute leukemia cells without affecting normal hematopoiesis. This chapter will describe gene and receptor signaling pathways responsible for aberrant trafficking of acute leukemia cells and discuss therapeutic implications of antagonizing chemokine receptor signaling to selectively block extramedullary dissemination of leukemia cells.

2. Dissemination of acute leukemia and the role of chemokines and chemokine receptors

Despite significant advances in treatments for patients with acute leukemia during the past decade, the prognosis of patients with minimal residual disease is generally poor and recurrence of the disease is common. One of the major complications that leads to poor outcomes of both adults and pediatric patients with acute leukemia is central nervous system (CNS) infiltration of leukemia cells. Intensified intrathecal chemotherapy and cranial irradiation for prophylaxis of CNS relapse can lead to serious adverse side effects, particularly secondary tumors, bone marrow suppression, growth impairment and endocrine complications (Pui CH & Howard SC, 2008). In order to minimize the treatment associated mortality, blocking leukemia cell invasion and migration may represent a rational alternative strategy. However, despite the clinical importance of CNS infiltration of leukemia cells, little is known about the underlying mechanism. In addition to CNS, leukemia cells are often found in other extramedullary sites, including skin and visceral organs, which is also an adverse prognostic factor (Byrd JC *et al.*, 1995, Kaneider NC *et al.*, 2002). It is conceivable that leukemia stem cells are derived from a single transformed clone in the bone marrow that subsequently peripheralize into the peripheral blood circulation and home to other organs or different sites within the marrow where they occupy normal hematopoietic niches and impair production of functionally normal blood cells. Similar processes can take place in simultaneously or successive manner, which in turn causes serious hematological complications. Dissemination of AML cells to other marrow sites increases the frequency for AML cells to interact with normal marrow niches and extracellular matrix (ECM), such as stromal fibronectin, via surface integrins, which is one of the mechanisms responsible for minimal residual disease in AML (Matsunaga T *et al.*, 2003). Therefore, dissemination of acute leukemia cells must be considered a crucial step in leukemic progression (Figure 1). The current chemotherapies and molecular targeting drugs were designed to kill leukemia cells but none of them are able to antagonize their movement and trafficking. Understanding molecular mechanisms regulating aberrant leukemia cell trafficking will aid in developing innovative therapeutic modalities to block leukemic infiltration to secondary organs, and will lead to superior outcomes of leukemia treatment.
One of the major causative molecules associated with AML and poor prognosis is internal tandem duplication mutation of the Flt3 kinase gene (ITD-Flt3). Several Flt3 kinase inhibitors have been developed and evaluated in early clinical trials with varied degrees of success, achieving >50% blast reduction in 12.5 to 81.3% of patients, with the duration of response ranging from two weeks to five months (Fiedler W *et al.*, 2003, Smith BD *et al.*, 2004, Stirewalt DL & Radich JP, 2003), indicating that targeting cell autonomous mechanism alone by these therapies was not sufficient to produce a complete cure. In this regard, the discovery of the leukemia cell niche identifies a new concept and suggests potential therapeutic approaches to antagonize interaction between the leukemia cell and their niche in addition to those targeting cell autonomous mechanisms. The leukemia cells destroy the

normal hematopoietic niche and create their own niche by down-regulating SDF1 in the lesion where leukemia cells invade in the bone marrow (Colmone *et al.*, 2008). Extramedullary infiltration of AML to distant organs likely accompanies creation of new niches in secondary organs by the leukemia cells, which in turn protects them from various chemotherapeutic stimuli.

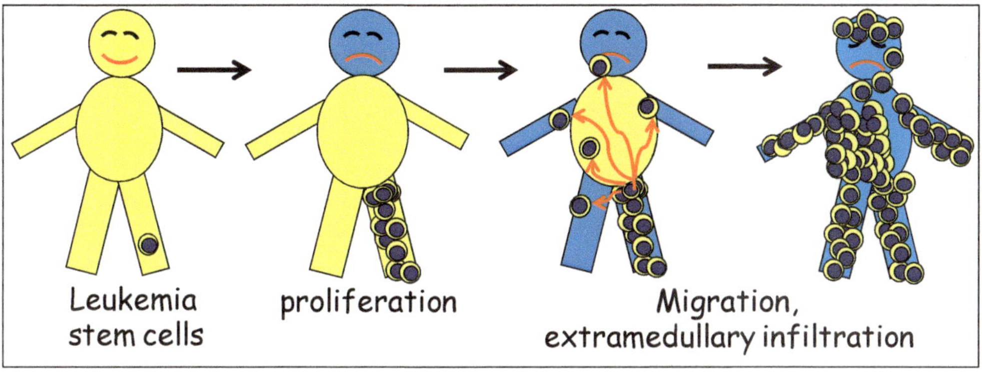

Fig. 1. Dissemination of leukemia cells is a crucial step for disease progression

Chemokines and their receptors play an important role in trafficking of hematopoietic stem cells (HSC) (Lapidot T & Petit I, 2000) and metastasis of tumor cells to distant organs (Muller A *et al.*, 2001). The major chemokine regulating homing and mobilization of HSC is stromal cell-derived factor-1 alpha (SDF1), a ligand for the cell surface CXCR4 receptor (Lapidot T & Petit I, 2000). SDF1 is expressed by osteoblasts, stromal cells and vascular endothelial cells in the bone marrow and attracts and retains HSC in the marrow niche (Lane SW, Scadden DT, & Gilliland DG, 2009). Within the niche, leukemia cells receive survival cues from osteoblasts and endothelial cells in the form of various cytokines and adhesion molecules provided by niche cells, which in turn increase their resistance to cytoreductive therapies (Lane SW, Scadden DT, & Gilliland DG, 2009). However, in skin, brain and visceral organs, extramedullary involvement is occasionally observed in patients with AML and ALL (Byrd JC, Edenfield WJ, Shields DJ, & Dawson NA, 1995, Pui CH & Howard SC, 2008). Leukemia cells need to leave their original bone marrow niche and find their home in the distant secondary niche for initiation of extramedullary dissemination. The mechanism for extramedullary infiltration of leukemia cells remains unexplored. Leukemia cells in the marrow express higher CXCR4 compared to their circulating counterparts, suggesting that interaction between SDF1 and CXCR4 facilitates retention of leukemia cells in the marrow niche (Spoo AC *et al.*, 2006). The majority of leukemia cells express CXCR4 and migrate in response to SDF1. Antagonizing CXCR4 inhibits engraftment and development of AML in a human xenograft human AML model, suggesting that CXCR4 is required for human AML to home to marrow niches (Tavor S *et al.*, 2004). Higher CXCR4 expression predicts extramedullary infiltration in pediatric patients with ALL (Crazzolara R *et al.*, 2001) and functional CXCR4 microparticles and SDF1 correlate with circulating AML (Kalinkovich *et al.*, 2006). These data suggest that chemokine signaling pathways are likely to play crucial roles in the dissemination of leukemia cells to secondary organs. Recent studies suggest that releasing leukemia cells from the marrow niche by blocking SDF1/CXCR4 interaction is effective in increasing their sensitivity to cytoreductive treatment (Nervi B *et al.*, 2009).

Instead of this strategy that principally targets aberrant leukemia cell proliferation, modulating functions of CXCR4 or other chemokine signaling in leukemia cells themselves may represent an alternative strategy to reduce their dissemination to secondary organs.

2.1 Physiological role of SDF1 and CXCR4

SDF1 is expressed in spleen, liver, lung, kidney, thymus, brain (Nervi B et al., 2009), stromal cells (Nagasawa T *et al.*, 1994) and osteoblasts (Jung Y *et al.*, 2006, Semerad CL *et al.*, 2005) in bone marrow and regulates development of hematopoietic cells, immune cells, blood vessels, heart and brain (Tachibana K *et al.*, 1998, Zou YR *et al.*, 1998). Targeted disruption of CXCR4 gene results in impaired bone marrow myelopoiesis and B-lymphopoiesis (Zou YR et al., 1998), which is a similar phenotype with SDF -/- mice (Nagasawa T *et al.*, 1996). One of the major physiological roles of the SDF1/CXCR4 axis is to regulate homing, retention, and survival of primitive hematopoietic stem and progenitor cells (HSPC) (Christopherson KW 2nd *et al.*, 2003, Kim CH & Broxmeyer HE, 1998, Levesque JP *et al.*, 2003, Liles WC *et al.*, 2003, Peled A *et al.*, 1999). Interaction between SDF1 and its receptor CXCR4 is believed to play an important role in these processes. SDF1 can attract HSPC that express CXCR4 to the marrow microenvironment (Kim CH & Broxmeyer HE, 1998, Peled A et al., 1999), while disruption of SDF1/CXCR4 interaction within marrow can under appropriate circumstances facilitate their mobilization to the peripheral circulation (Liles WC et al., 2003)(Figure 2).

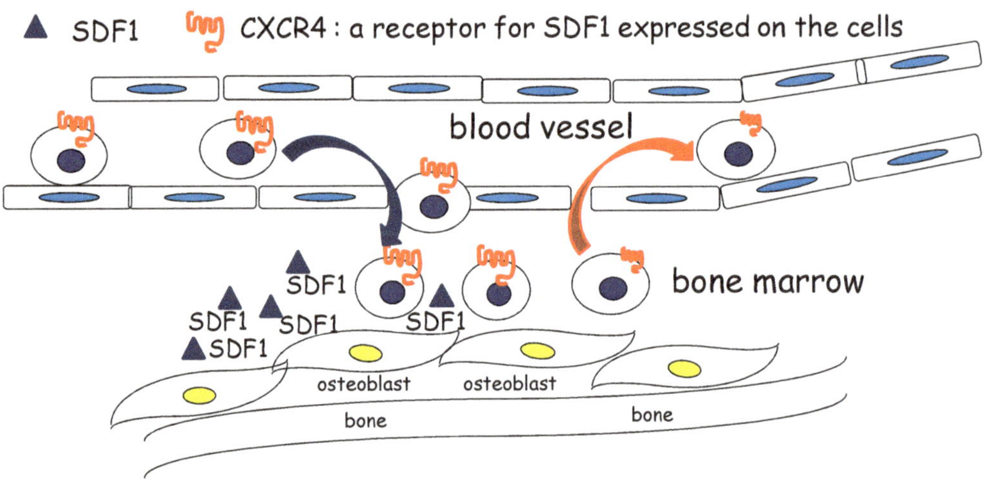

Fig. 2. SDF1 and CXCR4 regulate homing and mobilization of hematopoietic stem cells

HSCs can be found in contact with the cells expressing high amounts of SDF1 (Sugiyama T *et al.*, 2006). SDF1/CXCR4 signaling plays an essential role in maintaining the quiescent HSC pool (Sugiyama T et al., 2006). SDF1 can activate adhesion molecules, particularly very late antigen-4 (VLA-4) and lymphocyte function associated antigen-1 (LFA-1) on HSPC, which also regulate the homing process (Peled A *et al.*, 2000). SDF1 enhances survival or proliferation of normal hematopoietic progenitor cells (Broxmeyer HE *et al.*, 2003) and regulates development of B-cells (Ma Q *et al.*, 1999). Expression of CXCR4 is up-regulated by various cytokines, including stem cell factor (Peled A et al., 1999), VEGF, bFGF, EGF, IL2, IL4, IL6, IL7, IL10 and IL15 (Busillo JM & Benovic JL, 2007). In contrast, Flt3 ligand (Fukuda

S *et al.*, 2005), TNFα and INFγ down-regulate CXCR4 expression (Busillo JM & Benovic JL, 2007). Adrenergic inputs down-regulate SDF1 in the marrow environment during daytime (Mendez-Ferrer *et al.*, 2008), but up-regulate CXCR4 on HSC at night (Lucas D *et al.*, 2008). Although it was believed that CXCR4 was the only receptor for SDF1, a recent study identified CXCR7 as a secondary receptor for SDF1 (Balabanian K *et al.*, 2005). However, unlike CXCR4, CXCR7 mediates only cell survival, clustering and proliferation and lacks the ability to mediate chemotaxis (Burns JM *et al.*, 2006).

2.2 SDF1/CXCR4 in hematological malignancies

CXCR4 is expressed in most hematological malignancies including chronic lymphocytic leukemia (CLL), chronic myeloid leukemia (CML) (Burger JA *et al.*, 1999), acute lymphoblastic leukemia (ALL) (Bradstock KF *et al.*, 2000, Mohle R *et al.*, 2000), acute myeloid leukemia (AML) (Kalinkovich A *et al.*, 2006, Rombouts EJ *et al.*, 2004) (Voermans C *et al.*, 2002), B-cell lymphoma (Burger JA *et al.*, 1999, Trentin L *et al.*, 2004), T-cell non Hodgkin lymphoma (NHL) (Weng AP *et al.*, 2003) and multiple myeloma (Weng AP *et al.*, 2003). High expression of CXCR4 predicts extramedullary organ infiltration in childhood ALL (Crazzolara R *et al.*, 2001) and elevated CXCR4 expression is associated with poor prognosis of patients with AML (Rombouts EJ *et al.*, 2004, Spoo AC *et al.*, 2006). Extramedullary infiltration of M5 AML is associated with high CXCR4 expression (Mohle R *et al.*, 2000), suggesting that the SDF1/CXCR4 axis may be involved in the extramedullary disease of AML. In contrast, a recent report suggests that involvement of CXCR4 in skin infiltration of AML is unlikely (Faaij CMJM *et al.*, 2010). The extramedullary dissemination of AML may be associated with differentiation of AML that appears to affect CXCR4 expression, namely lower CXCR4 in undifferentiated M0, M1 and M2 compared to more differentiated M3, M4 and M5. Another study described that extramedullary dissemination of AML depends on single nucleotide polymorphism (SNP) of SDF1 (Dommange F *et al.*, 2006). Furthermore, SDF1 can recruit endothelial progenitor cells to the tumor microenvironment to facilitate neo-vascularization (Orimo A *et al.*, 2005), which may be required for continued growth of leukemia cells in the extramedullary niche. It has been suggested that targeting CXCR4 signaling pathways may be an important therapeutic strategy for ALL (Juarez J *et al.*, 2003), CLL (Burger M *et al.*, 2005a) and NHL (Bertolini F *et al.*, 2002). Recent data indicates that SDF1 plays an important role in protecting AML cells in the marrow niche, especially during intensive chemotherapy (Zeng ZH *et al.*, 2009). Blocking SDF1/CXCR4 signaling releases leukemia cells from marrow niches into blood circulation, dissociating them from the protective signal in the niche, and increases their sensitivity to chemotherapy (Nervi B *et al.*, 2009). Physiological circadian oscillation of SDF1 in the marrow niche and CXCR4 expression on HSC allows HSC to peripheralize into the blood circulation (Lucas D *et al.*, 2008, Mendez-Ferrer S *et al.*, 2008). It is likely that similar fluctuation in SDF1 and CXCR4 on leukemia stem cells that can affect their mobilization and homing may exist.

Similarly, recent evidence suggests that SDF1/CXCR4 signaling plays a central role in metastasis of solid tumors to the bone marrow or other tissues where SDF1 is expressed (Geminder H *et al.*, 2001, Muller A *et al.*, 2001) and serves as a survival factor for various solid tumor or leukemia cells (Burger JA *et al.*, 2000, Orimo A *et al.*, 2005, Zhou Y *et al.*, 2002). A growing body of evidence indicates that SDF1/CXCR4 signaling and oncogenic proteins, such as BCR/ABL in CML (Geay JF *et al.*, 2005, Mishra S *et al.*, 2006, Ptasznik A *et al.*, 2002, Salgia R *et al.*, 1999), HER2 in breast cancer (Cabioglu N *et al.*, 2006, Li YM *et al.*, 2004) and Internal Tandem Duplication (ITD)-Flt3 in AML (Fukuda S *et al.*, 2005, Fukuda S & Pelus

LM, 2006), functionally interact to modulate migration of malignant cells. Their concomitant expression with CXCR4 is often associated with poor patient prognosis (Li YM *et al.,* 2004, Mishra S *et al.,* 2006).

2.3 Hematopoietic growth factors that affect SDF1/CXCR4 signaling and migration of leukemia cells

While hematopoietic growth factors normally stimulate proliferation and survival of HSPC, some of them can stimulate migration. Stem cell factor (SCF) and Flt3 ligand (FL) are the respective ligands for the receptor tyrosine kinases c-kit and Flt3 that are expressed on HSPC. Although they have similar but distinct roles in HSPC proliferation and survival (Lyman SD & Jacobsen SEW, 1998), they both stimulate migration of human cord blood (UCB) $CD34^+$ cells (Fukuda S *et al.,* 2005, Kim CH & Broxmeyer HE, 1998). In contrast to the chemotactic activity of SDF1 that stimulates directional cell migration towards the chemokine (chemotaxis), SCF and FL stimulate random cell migration (chemokinesis). SCF increases SDF1-induced chemotaxis of the AML line MO7e cells when combined with SDF1 (Kim CH & Broxmeyer HE, 1998). Similarly, FL enhances migration of the RS4;11 bi-phenotypic acute leukemia cell lines to SDF1 (Fukuda S *et al.,* 2005). These data suggest that hematopoietic growth factors regulate migration of acute leukemia cells by modulating the SDF1/CXCR4 axis.

Although both SCF as well as FL enhance migration of human UCB $CD34^+$ cells induced by SDF1 in a similar manner, prolonged exposure the cells to SDF1 result in differential migratory responses. Prolonged incubation of UCB $CD34^+$ cells with SCF up-regulates CXCR4 expression and enhances subsequent migration to SDF1 (Peled A *et al.,* 1999). In contrast, incubation of UCB $CD34^+$ cells with FL over 24 hrs down-regulates CXCR4 expression coincident with a decrease in subsequent migration to SDF1 (Fukuda S *et al.,* 2005). Down-regulation of CXCR4 by incubation with FL is consistent with reduction of CXCR4 in $CD34^+$ cells transfected with ITD-Flt3 that activate Flt3 without ligand binding (Jacobi A *et al.,* 2010). Similar to human CD34+ cells, the differential migration to SDF1 modulated by FL was also observed in Ba/F3 cells expressing human wild-type Flt3 receptor. The synergistic cell migration in response to the combination of SDF1 and FL was associated with synergistic phosphorylation of ERK, Akt and CREB. These results suggest that ERK, Akt and CREB are involved in the synergistic increase in migration by the combination of SDF1 plus FL. On the other hand, pre-incubation of Ba/F3 cells expressing Flt3 with FL for 24 hours down-regulates CXCR4 and significantly diminishes their subsequent migration to SDF1 compared to control cells pre-incubated without FL. In contrast to synergistic response, phosphorylation of ERK, Akt and CREB in response to SDF1 was reduced in the cells pretreated with FL compared to untreated control cells, further validating the differential modulation of SDF1/CXCR4 signaling by FL/Flt3 (Fukuda S *et al.,* 2005). Down-regulation of CXCR4 by FL may explain one of the mechanisms of HPC mobilization by FL administration (Brasel K *et al.,* 1997). A similar effect by SCF is not known. These data indicate overlapping but distinct roles of c-kit and Flt3 signaling on $CD34^+$ cell migration induced by SDF1.

2.4 Bcr/abl alters signaling and chemotactic response mediated by SDF1/CXCR4

Chronic myeloid leukemia (CML) is caused by the Bcr/Abl oncogene with constitutive kinase activity, a result of a reciprocal translocation between chromosmes 9 and 22 (Kurzrock R *et al.,* 1988, Sawyers CL, 1999). Bcr/abl is occasionally observed in acute lymphoblastic leukemia cells (ALL) as well (Mishra S *et al.*, 2006). One of the characteristics of CML is an early release of myeloid cells from the marrow and their accumulation in the blood and spleen, suggesting that cell retention in the marrow or migration may be impaired. CML cells show reduced adhesion to stromal cells and extracellular matrix (Gordon MY *et al.*, 1987, Verfaillie CM *et al.*, 1992) that may concomitantly contribute to impaired retention. Ectopic Bcr/Abl increases spontaneous motility of hematopoietic cell lines; however, it significantly reduces chemotactic response to SDF1 (Salgia R *et al.*,1999). Homing of mouse hematopoietic Ba/F3 cells expressing Bcr/Abl to spleens in the mice that have been ectopically injected with SDF1 was significantly reduced compared to control cells, although their homing to the bone marrow, lung or blood was not affected. The migratory response of primary CML cells to SDF1 at blast crisis was profoundly reduced, which was associated with reduced CXCR4 expression, while $CD34^+$ cells at chronic phase migrate normally in response to SDF1 (Geay JF *et al.*, 2005). In addition, higher Bcr/abl expression induces a marked down regulation of CXCR4, while treatment with STI-571 (Imatinib), the Bcr/abl antagonist, that blocks Bcr/abl activity restores CXCR4 expression in $CD34^+$ cells from patients in blast crisis (Geay JF *et al.*,2005). The reduction in CXCR4 expression and loss of response to SDF1 mediated by Bcr/abl may allow CML cells to exit bone marrow, resulting in infiltration to secondary organs, including blood and spleen. These data suggest that Bcr/abl regulates trafficking of hematopoietic cells by modulating SDF1/CXCR4 function, which is associated with disease progression and extramedullary dissemination. Conversely, SDF1 can increase resistance of acute lymphoblastic leukemia cells expressing Bcr/abl to STI-571, suggesting that SDF1/CXCR4 signaling may augment Bcr/abl signaling that enhances resistance to the therapy (Mishra S *et al.*, 2006).

2.5 ITD-Flt3 alters chemotaxis induced by SDF1/CXCR4 signaling

Genetic mutations (Internal tandem duplication: ITD) of the Flt3 gene that pathologically auto-activate Flt3 tyrosine kinase activity have been found in ~25-30% of patients with AML and elevated CXCR4 receptor expression is associated with poor outcome in patients with acute myeloid leukemia (AML) (Levis M & Small D, 2003, Spoo AC et al., 2006), suggesting a role for ITD-Flt3 and CXCR4 in disease progression. Fifteen percent of patients with extramedullary AML were positive for ITD-Flt3 (Ansari-Lari *et al.*, 2004), suggesting that ITD-Flt3 may affect migration and trafficking of leukemia cells. ITD-Flt3 mutations cause extramedullary infiltration of hematopoietic cells with splenomegaly in a myeloproliferative disease model in mice (Kelly LM *et al.*, 2002). Consistent with this finding, ITD-Flt3 significantly increases accumulation of Ba/F3 cells in the spleen shortly after transplantation compared to wild-type Flt3 (Fukuda S & Pelus LM, 2006). Stable expression of ITD-Flt3 in mouse Ba/F3 and 32D cells significantly increases migration to SDF1 in addition to enhancing spontaneous motility (Figure 3) (Fukuda S *et al.*, 2005). This is in contrast to Bcr/abl that increases spontaneous motility while reducing migration in response to SDF1 (Geay JF *et al.*, 2005, Salgia R *et al.*, 1999). Importantly, CXCR4 expression on Ba/F3 cells harboring ITD-Flt3 mutations was significantly reduced, indicating that enhanced migration is not explained by CXCR4 expression (Fukuda S *et al.*, 2005) (Figure 3). This is consistent with down-regulation of CXCR4 in Ba/F3 cells expressing wild-type Flt3 or UCB CD34+ cells incubated with FL for over 24 hours. However, longer exposure to FL reduces migration to SDF1 (Fukuda S *et al.*, 2005). In contrast to synergistic phosphorylation of ERK, Akt or CREB coincident with enhanced migration to SDF1 and FL in Ba/F3 cells harboring wild-type Flt3, accentuated migration to SDF1 by ITD-Flt3 was not associated with an increase in phosphorylation of these molecules (Table 1). These findings suggest qualitative differences between ITD-Flt3 signaling and FL / wild type Flt3 signaling, even if both stimuli result in similar enhancement in migration to SDF1.

	FL	prolonged stimulation with FL	ITD-Flt3
CXCR4	no change →	decrease ↓	decrease ↓
Migration to SDF1	increase ↑	decrease ↓	increase ↑
Phospho ERK, Akt, CREB	increase ↑	decrease ↓	no change →

Table 1. Differential regulation on CXCR4 expression and migration to SDF1 by FL/wild-type Flt3 signaling or ITD-Flt3 in Ba/F3 cells

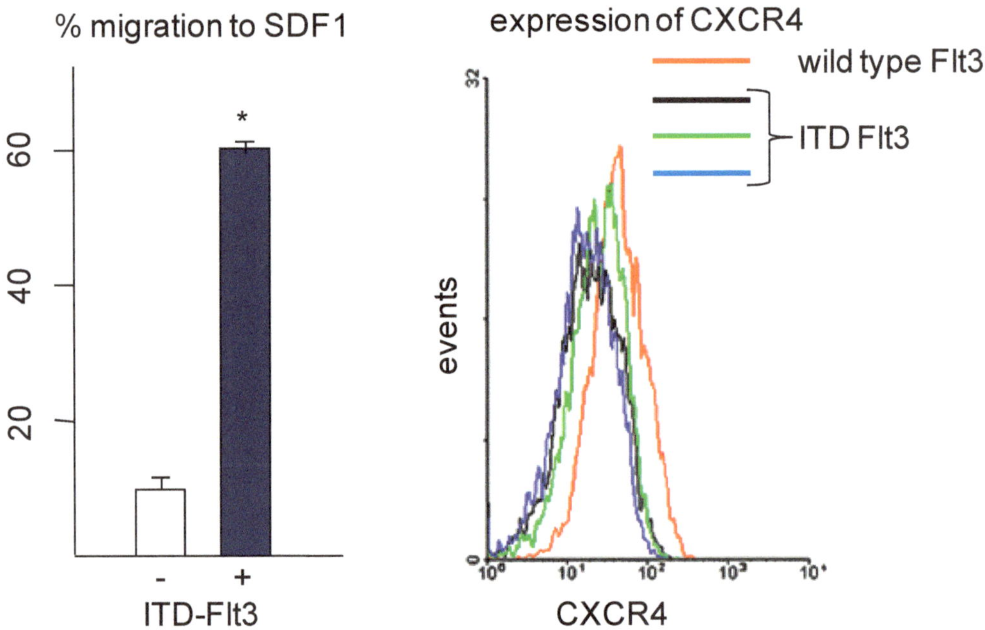

Fig. 3. Migration and CXCR4 expression of ITD-Flt3 + or ITD-Flt3 - Ba/F3 cells. Migration of ITD-Flt3+ cells towards SDF1 was significantly elevated compared to ITD-Flt3 - cells (* P<0.05: left panel). However, CXCR4 expression was significantly reduced in ITD-Flt3 + cells compared to ITD-Flt3 - cells (right panel), suggesting that the enhanced migration is not a quantitative increase of CXCR4 signaling but more likely to be a qualitative alteration of CXCR4 signaling by ITD-Flt3.

Enhanced chemotactic response to SDF1 is partially mediated through Ras signaling, since dominant negative H-Ras dramatically inhibits spontaneous and SDF-mediated migration of Ba/F3 cells, while constitutively active H-Ras expression in Ba/F3 cells harboring wild-type Flt3 increases chemotactic response to SDF1 to a similar extent as ITD-Flt3 (Fukuda S & Pelus LM, 2006). Accentuated migration of Ba/F3 cells to SDF1 induced by ITD-Flt3 was barely inhibited by the Flt3 inhibitor AG1296 or the CXCR4 antagonist AMD3100 alone, whereas it was partially inhibited by the combination of both compounds (Figure 4). Surprisingly, ITD-Flt3 mutations also increase cell migration away from an SDF1 gradient compared to control cells (Fukuda S *et al.*, 2005). This result implies that ITD-Flt3 may facilitate peripheralization of leukemia cells out of the bone marrow niche where SDF1 is present, in addition to the effects of enhancing cell homing towards SDF1 in the niche.

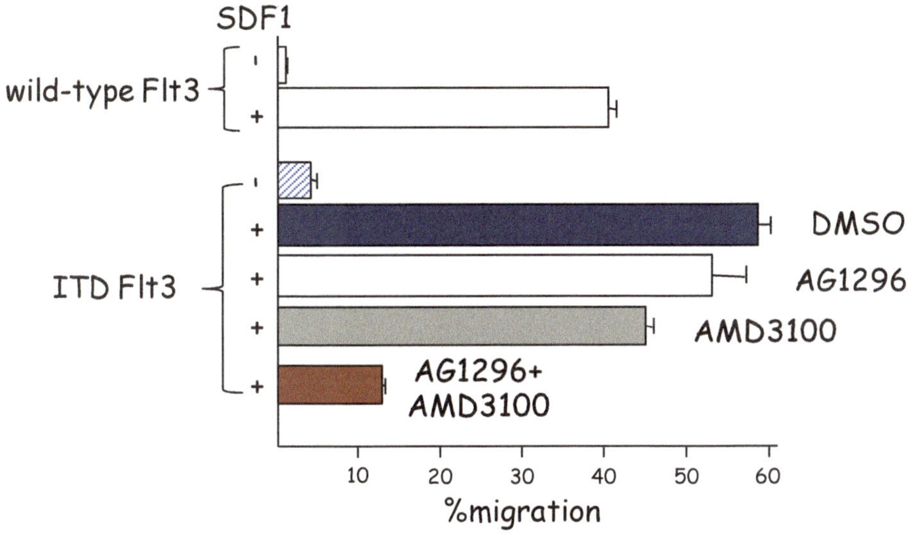

Fig. 4. Migration of Ba/F3 cells expressing ITD-Flt3 pretreated with AMD3100 and/or AG1296

In contrast to the mouse cell system where human ITD-Flt3 mutations were retrovirally transduced into Ba/F3 cells and 32D cells (Fukuda S *et al.*, 2005), a recent report has shown that transient expression of ITD-Flt3 in human $CD34^+$ cells inhibited migration to SDF1 concomitant with reduction in cell surface CXCR4 expression (Jacobi A *et al.*, 2010). While reduction in CXCR4 in $CD34^+$ cells by ITD-Flt3 is consistent with Ba/F3 cells transduced with ITD-Flt3, the differential effects on migration to SDF1 by these cells may reflect the timeframe of exposure to SDF1 following introduction of ITD-Flt3 into the cells. Shortly after introduction of ITD-Flt3, expression of CXCR4 is down-regulated, thereby inhibited migration to SDF1. In contrast, prolonged expression of ITD-Flt3 leads to functional activation of CXCR4 signaling pathways and increases cell migration, while maintaining lower CXCR4 expression, suggesting that ITD-Flt3 may differentially regulate chemotactic response to SDF1. These findings suggest that migration of leukemia cells to SDF1 may be diminished shortly after emergence of ITD-Flt3 in the patients due to reduction of CXCR4 level and concomitant quantitative decline in CXCR4 signaling. This does not accompany qualitative changes in CXCR4 signaling. In contrast, their migration to SDF1 is enhanced at a later stage of the disease long after ITD-Flt3 appearance, most likely due to subsequent functional alteration of CXCR4 signaling by ITD-Flt3 that is not coupled with CXCR4 expression level. Reduced migration to SDF1 by ITD-Flt3 can facilitate their peripheralization into blood at an early stage of the disease whereas enhanced migration to SDF1 may aid to increase homing of the leukemia cells to the organs where SDF1 is expressed at a later stage of the disease.

2.6 Identification of CXCR4 pathways that are selectively regulated by ITD-Flt3

CXCR4 is expressed in the majority of hematopoietic cells, including HSC, T-cells, B-cells and myeloid cells. While antagonizing CXCR4 has been shown to be a safe way to collect HSC from the healthy donors (Liles WC *et al.*, 2003), it is known that SDF1/CXCR4 signaling provides survival effects to the primitive hematopoietic cell compartment (Broxmeyer HE *et al.*, 2003), therefore the long term effect of CXCR4 antagonist on normal hematopoietic cell function should be monitored with caution. In this regard, concomitant use of a CXCR4 antagonist with chemotherapeutic drugs may enhance toxicity, not just to leukemia cells, but also to normal HSC. In order to minimize toxicity on HSC by CXCR4 antagonist, it would be necessary to identify selective signaling molecules downstream of CXCR4 that are specifically regulated in leukemia stem cells but not in normal HSC. Similarly, identification of selective CXCR4 related molecular pathways regulating homing of leukemia cells distinct from normal hematopoietic cells will aid to antagonize aberrant trafficking of leukemia cells without affecting normal hematopoiesis.

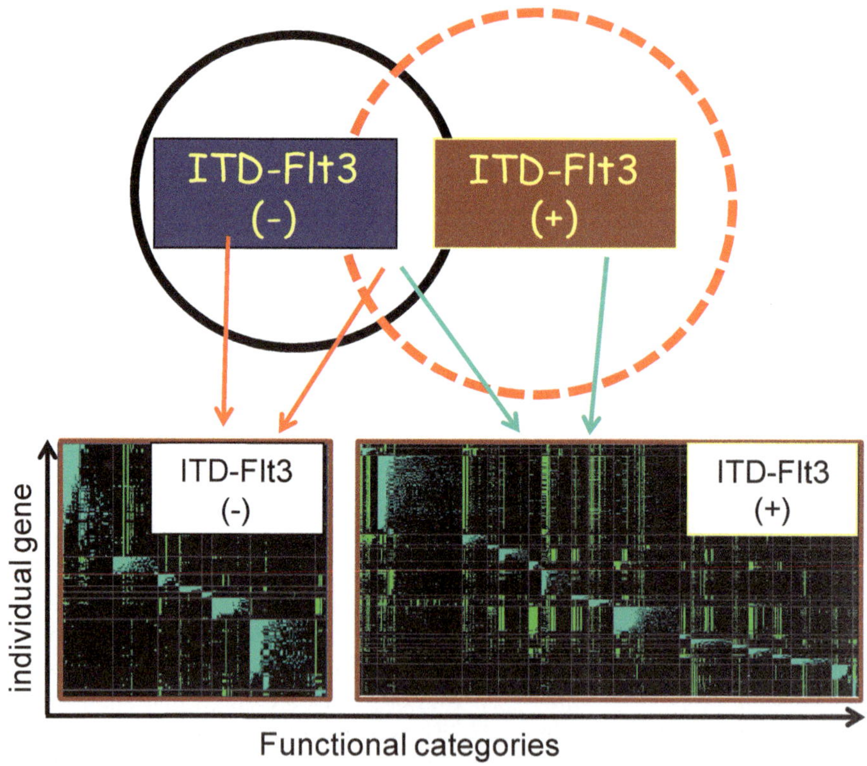

Fig. 5. Functional classification of genes downstream of SDF1/CXCR4 in ITD-Flt3 $^{+}$ versus ITD-Flt3 $^{-}$ mouse Ba/F3 cells.

As we previously described, ITD-Flt3 mutations enhance migration of hematopoietic cells to the chemokine SDF1 (Figure 3) (Fukuda S *et al.*, 2005), suggesting that ITD-Flt3 may facilitate dissemination of leukemia cells by modulating the SDF1/CXCR4 signaling pathway. The enhanced migration to SDF1 by ITD-Flt3 positive cells was associated with down regulation of CXCR4 compared to control cells lacking ITD-Flt3. This suggests that the enhanced migration to SDF1 by ITD-Flt3 is not a consequence of a quantitative increase in SDF1/CXCR4 signaling, which led us to investigate qualitative alteration of CXCR4 signaling by ITD-Flt3. Analysis of gene expression in ITD-Flt3$^-$ and ITD-Flt3$^+$ Ba/F3 cells migrating to SDF1 indicated that SDF1 modulates 4.0% of 40,000 genes analyzed in ITD-Flt3$^+$ cells, of which 2.5% were regulated by SDF1 exclusively in ITD- Flt3$^+$ cells. Figure 4 indicates comparison of changes in gene expression before and after migration to SDF1 (SDF1 responsive genes) between ITD-Flt3- and ITD-Flt3+ Ba/F3 cells. Genes modulated in ITD-Flt3- cells or ITD-Flt3+ cells following migration to SDF1 compared to these cells analyzed before migration were functionally classified based on Gene Ontology Term using DAVID software (Huang DW *et al.*, 2009)(Figure 5). X-axis represents functional categories of the individual genes analyzed in the Y-axis. Functional classification indicated that several functional signaling pathways were significantly enriched exclusively in ITD-Flt3 but not in control cells. These data indicate that enhanced cell migration to SDF1 induced by ITD-Flt3 is likely mediated through activation of selective CXCR4 signaling pathways that are functionally distinct from ITD-Flt3$^-$ cells and that are not coupled with CXCR4 expression. Importantly, several of these CXCR4 downstream molecules selectively regulated by ITD-Flt3 are products of genes known to be deregulated in AML stem cells (Majeti R *et al.*, 2009). Leukemia stem cells (LSC) are likely responsible for dissemination to secondary organs in addition to disease initiation and recurrence. Genes deregulated by LSC and regulated by SDF1 specifically in ITD-Flt3$^+$ cells may represent key targets to prevent unnecessary dissemination and invasion of ITD-Flt3$^+$ acute leukemia cells without affecting normal hematopoiesis. In addition to the genes selectively regulated by SDF1 in ITD-Flt3+ cells, approximately 30 mRNAs that are known to be functionally associated with cell motility or migration were deregulated in ITD-Flt3+ cells compared to ITD-Flt3- cells. This data suggests that ITD-Flt3 itself may affect cell migration. This is consistent with enhanced spontaneous migration by ITD-Flt3 in Ba/F3 cells (Fukuda S *et al.*, 2005).

Our working hypothesis on ITD-Flt3$^+$ AML cell trafficking regulated by interaction between ITD-Flt3 and SDF1/CXCR4 pathway is shown in Figure 6. The presence of ITD-Flt3 mutations decrease CXCR4 expression, thereby reducing interaction between SDF1 and AML cells and allowing their release from bone marrow. In addition, ITD-Flt3$^+$ cells can migrate away from SDF1 more efficiently compared to ITD-Flt3$^-$ cells, which can also contribute to their peripheralization/egress. Alternatively, migration to SDF1 may not be enhanced shortly after ITD-Flt3 emergence or at an early stage of the disease owing to the reduction of CXCR4 that without activation of CXCR4 signaling. Prolonged exposure to aberrant signaling generated by ITD-Flt3 functionally activates SDF1/CXCR4 signaling in the ITD-Flt3$^+$ cells that is different from ITD-Flt3$^-$ cells (Figure 5) while maintaining lower levels of CXCR4 expression (Figure 3). This suggests that enhanced migration to SDF1 is a consequence of functional alteration of CXCR4 signaling rather than CXCR4 up-regulation. This will help AML cells to home to the distant organs or secondary bone marrow where SDF1 is present. Circadian oscillation of SDF1 in the marrow niche and CXCR4 expression on HSC (Lucas D et al., et al 2008, Mendez-Ferrer S *et al.*, 2008) may also exist in the leukemia niche and leukemia stem cells expressing ITD-Flt3. This fluctuation of SDF1 and CXCR4 can also affect their mobilization and homing. De-sensitization of CXCR4 signaling following exposure to SDF1 may also be distinct in leukemia cells versus normal HSC, which can affect their response to SDF1.

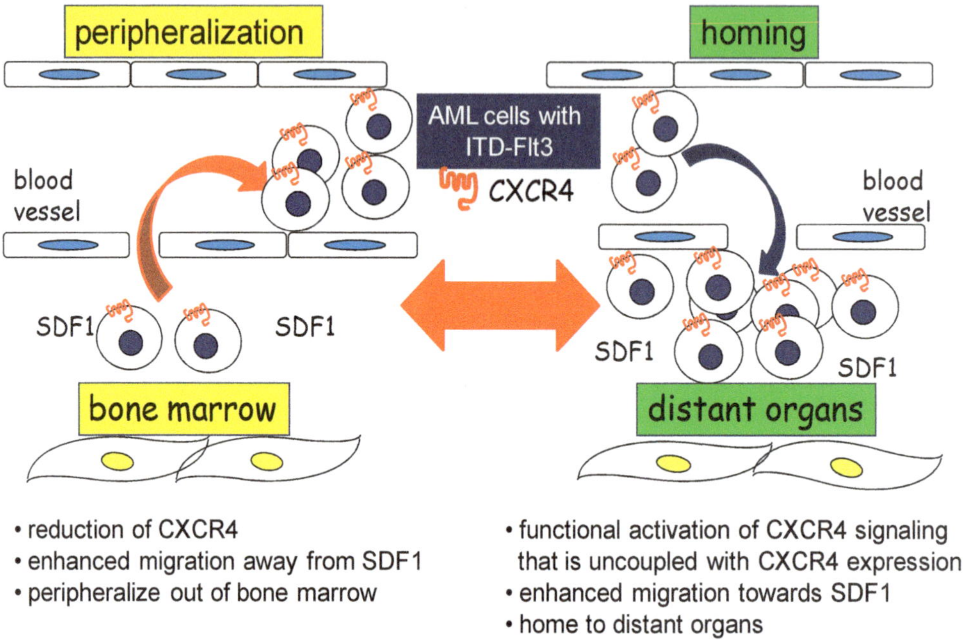

Fig. 6. Suggested model for ITD-Flt3+ AML cell trafficking regulated by interaction between ITD-Flt3 and SDF1/CXCR4 pathway

2.7 Role of other chemokines and their receptors for leukemia cell dissemination

Childhood T-ALL often relapses in the CNS (Pui CH & Howard SC, 2008). Oncogenic Notch1 signaling that is frequently activated in T-ALL regulates CCR7 expression. CCL19 expressed in central nervous system serves as a chemo-attractant for T-ALL cells with elevated expression of CCR7. Antagonizing CCR7 and its chemokine ligand CCL19 inhibit CNS infiltration of T-ALL in an animal model (Buonamici S *et al.*, 2009). On the other hand, overexpression of CCR7 was sufficient to recruit T-ALL cells into the CNS. The data indicates that CCL19/CCR7 signaling activated by oncogenic Notch1 regulates CNS infiltration of T-ALL and that targeting the CCR7 pathway may represent a novel therapeutic strategy for treatment of CNS prophylaxis of T-ALL (Buonamici S *et al.*, 2009) (Figure 7).

While antagonizing CCR7 signaling is a promising strategy to block invasion of T-ALL cells, it may impair immune surveillance by normal T-cells, since CCR7 is one of the chemokine receptors required for T-cell trafficking (Burger M *et al.*, 2005b). Unnecessary immune impairment that can cause serious life threatening infection by pathogens needs to be avoided during the intensified treatment for leukemia. In this regard, identification of selective signaling molecules in the CCR7 pathway in T-ALL that are functionally distinct from normal T-cells is important in order to develop selective strategy with minimal toxicity on T-cells.

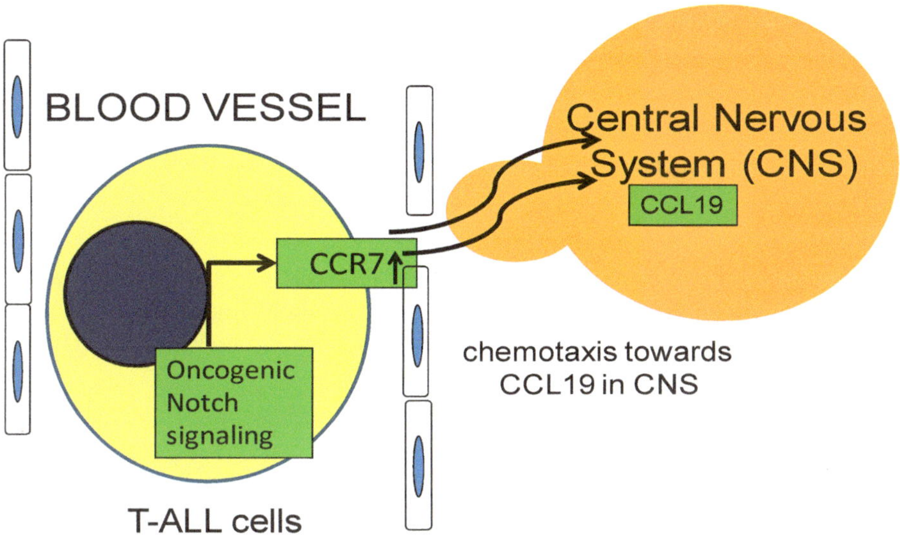

Fig. 7. Migration and invasion of T-ALL cells into central nervous system mediated through CCL19/CCR7 pathway

Mixed lineage leukemia (MLL) frequently found in infant ALL is caused by a chromosomal translocation that involves 11q23 (Pieters R, 2009). This is associated with poor outcome with relatively high frequency of central nervous involvement compared to older children, suggesting that MLL gene rearrangement modulates leukemia cell dissemination. A recent report indicates that MEF2C regulates homing and invasiveness of MLL/ENL leukemia cells without affecting establishment and maintenance of leukemia stem cells (Schwieger M *et al.*, 2009). MEF2 regulates expression of the chemokine receptors CXCR4, CCR2 and CCR5 and chemokines, such as CCL2, CCL3, CCL4 and CCL6 (Schwieger M *et al.*, 2009). This suggests that MLL gene rearrangement regulates homing and invasion of leukemia cells through MEF2C by affecting expression of chemokines and their receptors.
Chemokine receptor expression is differentially regulated in AML patients with skin involvement. Skin residing AML cells displayed a different set of chemokine receptors in situ, for instance: CCR5, CXCR4, CXCR7 and CX3CR1. However, a recent report indicates a high percentage of circulating CCR2 ^{pos} AML cells were only detected in patients with extramedullary disease (Faaij CMJM *et al.*, 2010). High expression of CCR2 was not observed in bone marrow blasts. This study showed that there was no difference in the expression of CXCR4, suggesting that CCR2 may be a dominant regulator for skin dissemination of AML.

3. Conclusion

Given that various oncogenic molecules responsible for hematological malignancies such as ITD-Flt3, Bcr-abl and Ras, modulate response to SDF1, these oncogenes likely modulate trafficking of leukemia cells. Although there is no definitive evidence that CXCR4 is indeed involved in the dissemination of acute leukemia, multiple data support that this is most likely the case. Blocking CXCR4 appears to be a promising strategy to sensitize leukemia cells to chemotherapy by releasing/mobilizing them into the peripheral blood circulation. Targeting CXCR4 signaling pathways may also be useful to minimize leukemia cell dissemination in addition to sensitizing them to chemotherapy by releasing them from marrow niches. This idea is consistent with targeting the CCR7 receptor in T-ALL that blocks their CNS dissemination (Buonamici S et al., 2009). Although promising, precautions need to be taken since antagonizing CXCR4 initiates mobilization of leukemia cells into circulation, which may facilitate secondary organ infiltration.

4. Acknowledgment

The authors have no conflict of interest associated with this work. This work was supported by Naito Memorial Foundation, the Mother and Child Health Foundation and the Grant-in-Aid for Scientific Research (B) (20390298) from Japan Society for the Promotion of Science (to SF).

5. References

Ansari-Lari, M. A., Yang, C. F., Tinawi-Aljundi, R., Cooper, L., Long, P., Allan, R. H., Borowitz, M. I., Berg, K. D., & Murphy, K. M. (2004). FLT3 mutations in myeloid sarcoma. *British Journal of Haematology 126*, 785-791

Balabanian, K., Lagane, B., Infantino, S., Chow, K. Y. C., Harriague, J., Moepps, B., Arenzana-Seisdedos, F., Thelen, M., & Bachelerie, F. (2005). The chemokine SDF-1/CXCL12 binds to and signals through the orphan receptor RDC1 in T lymphocytes. *Journal of Biological Chemistry 280*, 35760-35766

Bertolini F, Dell'Agnola C, Mancuso P, Rabascio C, Burlini A, Monestiroli S, Gobbi A, Pruneri G, & Martinelli G (2002). CXCR4 neutralization, a novel therapeutic approach for non-Hodgkin's lymphoma. *Cancer Res. 62*, 3106-12.

Bradstock KF, Makrynikola V, Bianchi A, Shen W, Hewson J, & Gottlieb DJ (2000). Effects of the chemokine stromal cell-derived factor-1 on the migration and localization of precursor-B acute lymphoblastic leukemia cells within bone marrow stromal layers. *Leukemia 14*, 882-8.

Brasel K, McKenna HJ, Charrier K, Morrissey PJ, Williams DE, & Lyman SD (1997). Flt3 ligand synergizes with granulocyte-macrophage colony-stimulating factor or granulocyte colony-stimulating factor to mobilize hematopoietic progenitor cells into the peripheral blood of mice. *Blood 90*, 3781-3788.

Broxmeyer HE, Kohli L, Kim CH, Lee Y, Mantel C, Cooper S, Hangoc G, Shaheen M, Li X, & Clapp DW (2003). Stromal cell-derived factor-1/CXCL12 directly enhances survival/antiapoptosis of myeloid progenitor cells through CXCR4 and G(alpha)i proteins and enhances engraftment of competitive, repopulating stem cells. *J Leukoc Biol. 73*, 630-8.

Buonamici, S., Trimarchi, T., Ruocco, M. G., Reavie, L., Cathelin, S., Mar, B. G., Klinakis, A., Lukyanov, Y., Tseng, J. C., Sen, F., Gehrie, E., Li, M. L., Newcomb, E., Zavadil, J., Meruelo, D., Lipp, M., Ibrahim, S., Efstratiadis, A., Zagzag, D., Bromberg, J. S., Dustin, M. L., & Aifantis, I. (2009). CCR7 signalling as an essential regulator of CNS infiltration in T-cell leukaemia. *Nature 459*, 1000-1005

Burger JA, Burger M, & Kipps TJ (1999). Chronic lymphocytic leukemia B cells express functional CXCR4 chemokine receptors that mediate spontaneous migration beneath bone marrow stromal cells. *Blood. 94*, 3658-67.

Burger JA, Tsukada N, Burger M, Zvaifler NJ, Dell'Aquila M, & Kipps TJ (2000). Blood-derived nurse-like cells protect chronic lymphocytic leukemia B cells from spontaneous apoptosis through stromal cell-derived factor-1. *Blood. 96*, 2655-63.

Burger M, Hartmann T, Krome M, Rawluk J, Tamamura H, Fujii N, Kipps TJ, & Burger JA (2005a). Small peptide inhibitors of the CXCR4 chemokine receptor (CD184) antagonize the activation, migration, and antiapoptotic responses of CXCL12 in chronic lymphocytic leukemia B cells. *Blood. 106*, 1824-30.

Burger M, Hartmann T, Krome M, Rawluk J, Tamamura H, Fujii N, Kipps TJ, & Burger JA (2005b). Small peptide inhibitors of the CXCR4 chemokine receptor (CD184) antagonize the activation, migration, and antiapoptotic responses of CXCL12 in chronic lymphocytic leukemia B cells. *Blood. 106*, 1824-30.

Burns, J. M., Summers, B. C., Wang, Y., Melikian, A., Berahovich, R., Miao, Z. H., Penfold, M. E. T., Sunshine, M. J., Littman, D. R., Kuo, C. J., Wei, K., McMaster, B. E., Wright, K., Howard, M. C., & Schall, T. J. (2006). A novel chemokine receptor for SDF-1 and I-TAC involved in cell survival, cell adhesion, and tumor development. *Journal of Experimental Medicine 203*, 2201-2213

Busillo, J. M. & Benovic, J. L. (2007). Regulation of CXCR4 signaling. *Biochimica et Biophysica Acta-Biomembranes 1768*, 952-963

Byrd JC, Edenfield WJ, Shields DJ, & Dawson NA (1995). Extramedullary myeloid cell tumors in acute nonlymphocytic leukemia: a clinical review. *J Clin Oncol. 13*, 1800-1816.

Cabioglu N, Summy J, Miller C, Parikh NU, Sahin AA, Tuzlali S, Pumiglia K, Gallick GE, & Price JE (2006). CXCL-12/stromal cell-derived factor-1alpha transactivates HER2-neu in breast cancer cells by a novel pathway involving Src kinase activation. *Cancer Res. 65*, 6493-7.

Christopherson KW 2nd, Cooper S, & Broxmeyer HE (2003). Cell surface peptidase CD26/DPPIV mediates G-CSF mobilization of mouse progenitor cells. *Blood. 101*, 4680-4686.

Colmone, A., Amorim, M., Pontier, A. L., Wang, S., Jablonski, E., & Sipkins, D. A. (2008). Leukemic Cells Create Bone Marrow Niches That Disrupt the Behavior of Normal Hematopoietic Progenitor Cells. *Science 322*, 1861-1865

Crazzolara R, Kreczy A, Mann G, Heitger A, Eibl G, Fink FM, Mohle R, & Meister B (2001). High expression of the chemokine receptor CXCR4 predicts extramedullary organ infiltration in childhood acute lymphoblastic leukaemia. *Br J Haematol. 115*, 545-53.

Dommange, F., Cartron, G., Espanel, C., Gallay, N., Domenech, J., Benboubker, L., Ohresser, M., Colombat, P., Binet, C., Watier, H., & Herault, O. (2006). CXCL12 polymorphism and malignant cell dissemination/tissue infiltration in acute myeloid leukemia. *Faseb Journal 20*, 1913-5

Faaij, C. M. J. M., Willemze, A. J., Revesz, T., Balzarolo, M., Tensen, C. P., Hoogeboom, M., Vermeer, M. H., van Wering, E., Zwaan, C. M., Kaspers, G. J. L., Story, C., van Halteren, A. G. S., Vossen, J. M., Egeler, R. M., van Tol, M. J. D., & Annels, N. E. (2010). Chemokine/Chemokine Receptor Interactions in Extramedullary

Leukaemia of the Skin in Childhood AML: Differential Roles for CCR2, CCR5, CXCR4 and CXCR7. *Pediatric Blood & Cancer 55*, 344-348,

Fiedler W, Mesters R, Tinnefeld H, Loges S, Staib P, Duhrsen U, Flasshove M, Ottmann OG, Jung W, Cavalli F, Kuse R, Thomalla J, Serve H, O'Farrell AM, Jacobs M, Brega NM, Scigalla P, Hossfeld DK, & Berdel WE (2003). A phase 2 clinical study of SU5416 in patients with refractory acute myeloid leukemia. *Blood 102*, 2763-2767.

Fukuda S, Broxmeyer, & Pelus (2005). Flt3 ligand and the Flt3 receptor regulate hematopoietic cell migration by modulating the SDF-1a(CXCL12)/CXCR4 axis. *Blood 105*, 3117-3126.

Fukuda S & Pelus LM (2006). Internal Tandem Duplication of Flt3 (ITD-Flt3) modulates chemotaxis and survival of hematopoietic cells by SDF1a but negatively regulates marrow homing in vivo. *Exp Hematol 34*, 1041-51.

Geay JF, Buet D, Zhang Y, Foudi A, Jarrier P, Berthebaud M, Turhan AG, Vainchenker W, & Louache F (2005). p210BCR-ABL inhibits SDF-1 chemotactic response via alteration of CXCR4 signaling and down-regulation of CXCR4 expression. *Cancer Res. 1*, 7-2676.

Geminder H, Sagi-Assif O, Goldberg L, Meshel T, Rechavi G, Witz IP, & Ben-Baruch A (2001). A possible role for CXCR4 and its ligand, the CXC chemokine stromal cell-derived factor-1, in the development of bone marrow metastases in neuroblastoma. *J Immunol. 167*, 4747-57.

Gordon MY, Dowding CR, Riley GP, Goldman JM, & Greaves MF (1987). Altered adhesive interactions with marrow stroma of haematopoietic progenitor cells in chronic myeloid leukaemia. *Nature. 328*, 342-4.

Huang, D. W., Sherman, B. T., & Lempicki, R. A. (2009). Systematic and integrative analysis of large gene lists using DAVID bioinformatics resources. *Nature Protocols 4*, 44-57

Jacobi, A., Thieme, S., Lehmann, R., Ugarte, F., Malech, H. L., Koch, S., Thiede, C., Muller, K., Bornhauser, M., Ryser, M., & Brenner, S. (2010). Impact of CXCR4 inhibition on FLT3-ITD-positive human AML blasts. *Experimental Hematology 38*, 180-190

Juarez J, Bradstock KF, Gottlieb DJ, & Bendall LJ (2003). Effects of inhibitors of the chemokine receptor CXCR4 on acute lymphoblastic leukemia cells in vitro. *Leukemia. 17*, 1294-1300.

Jung Y, Wang J, Schneider A, Sun YX, Koh-Paige AJ, Osman NI, McCauley LK, & Taichman RS (2006). Regulation of SDF-1 (CXCL12) production by osteoblasts; a possible mechanism for stem cell homing. *Bone. 38*, 497-508.

Kalinkovich, A., Tavor, S., Avigdor, A., Kahn, J., Brill, A., Petit, I., Goichberg, P., Tesio, M., Netzer, N., Naparstek, E., Hardan, I., Nagler, A., Resnick, I., Tsimanis, A., & Lapidot, T. (2006). Functional CXCR4-expressing microparticles and SDF-1 correlate with circulating acute myelogenous leukemia cells. *Cancer Research 66*, 11013-11020

Kaneider NC, Egger P, Wiedermann FJ, Ritter M, Woll E, & Wiedermann CJ (2002). Involvement of cyclic adenosine monophosphate-dependent protein kinase A and pertussis toxin-sensitive G proteins in the migratory response of human CD14+ mononuclear cells to katacalcin. *J Bone Miner Res. 17*, 1872-1882.

Kelly LM, Liu Q, Kutok JL, Williams IR, Boulton CL, & Gilliland DG (2002). FLT3 internal tandem duplication mutations associated with human acute myeloid leukemias induce myeloproliferative disease in a murine bone marrow transplant model. *Blood 99*, 310-318.

Kim CH & Broxmeyer HE (1998). In vitro behavior of hematopoietic progenitor cells under the influence of chemoattractants: stromal cell-derived factor-1, steel factor, and the bone marrow environment. *Blood. 91*, 100-110.

Kurzrock R, Gutterman JU, & Talpaz M (1988). The molecular genetics of Philadelphia chromosome-positive leukemias. *N Engl J Med. 319*, 990-8.

Lane, S. W., Scadden, D. T., & Gilliland, D. G. (2009). The leukemic stem cell niche: current concepts and therapeutic opportunities. *Blood 114*, 1150-1157

Lapidot T & Petit I (2000). Current understanding of stem cell mobilization: the roles of chemokines, proteolytic enzymes, adhesion molecules, cytokines, and stromal cells. *Exp Hematol 30*, 973-981.

Levesque JP, Hendy J, Takamatsu Y, Simmons PJ, & Bendall LJ (2003). Disruption of the CXCR4/CXCL12 chemotactic interaction during hematopoietic stem cell mobilization induced by G-CSF or cyclophosphamide. *J Clin Invest. 111*, 187-196.

Levis M & Small D (2003). FLT3: ITDoes matter in leukemia. *Leukemia. 17*, 1738-1752.

Li YM, Pan Y, Wei Y, Cheng X, Zhou BP, Tan M, Zhou X, Xia W, Hortobagyi GN, Yu D, & Hung MC (2004). Upregulation of CXCR4 is essential for HER2-mediated tumor metastasis. *Cancer Cell. 6*, 459-69.

Liles WC, Broxmeyer HE, Rodger E, Wood B, Hubel K, Cooper S, Hangoc G, Bridger GJ, Henson GW, Calandra G, & Dale DC (2003). Mobilization of hematopoietic progenitor cells in healthy volunteers by AMD3100, a CXCR4 antagonist. *Blood 102*, 2728-2730.

Lucas, D., Battista, M., Shi, P. A., Isola, L., & Frenette, P. S. (2008). Mobilized Hematopoietic Stem Cell Yield Depends on Species-Specific Circadian Timing. *Cell Stem Cell 3*, 364-366

Lyman, S. D. & Jacobsen, S. E. W. (1998). c-kit ligand and flt3 ligand: Stem/progenitor cell factors with overlapping yet distinct activities. *Blood 91*, 1101-1134.

Ma Q, Jones D, & Springer TA (1999). The chemokine receptor CXCR4 is required for the retention of B lineage and granulocytic precursors within the bone marrow microenvironment. *Immunity. 10*, 463-71.

Majeti, R., Becker, M. W., Tian, Q., Lee, T. L. M., Yan, X. W., Liu, R., Chiang, J. H., Hood, L., Clarke, M. F., & Weissman, I. L. (2009). Dysregulated gene expression networks in human acute myelogenous leukemia stem cells. *Proceedings of the National Academy of Sciences of the United States of America 106*, 3396-3401

Matsunaga T, Takemoto N, Sato T, Takimoto R, Tanaka I, Fujimi A, Akiyama T, Kuroda H, Kawano Y, Kobune M, Kato J, Hirayama Y, Sakamaki S, Kohda K, Miyake K, & Niitsu Y (2003). Interaction between leukemic-cell VLA-4 and stromal fibronectin is a decisive factor for minimal residual disease of acute myelogenous leukemia. *Nature Medicine 9*, 1158-1165.

Mendez-Ferrer, S., Lucas, D., Battista, M., & Frenette, P. S. (2008). Haematopoietic stem cell release is regulated by circadian oscillations. *Nature 452*, 442-444

Mishra S, Zhang B, Cunnick JM, Heisterkamp N, & Groffen J (2006). Resistance to imatinib of bcr/abl p190 lymphoblastic leukemia cells. *Cancer Res. 66*, 5387-93.

Mohle R, Schittenhelm M, Failenschmid C, Bautz F, Kratz-Albers K, Serve H, Brugger W, & Kanz L (2000). Functional response of leukaemic blasts to stromal cell-derived factor-1 correlates with preferential expression of the chemokine receptor CXCR4 in acute myelomonocytic and lymphoblastic leukaemia. *Br J Haematol. 110*, 563-572.

Muller A, Homey B, Soto H, Ge N, Catron D, Buchanan ME, McClanahan T, Murphy E, Yuan W, Wagner SN, Barrera JL, Mohar A, Verastegui E, & Zlotnik A (2001). Involvement of chemokine receptors in breast cancer metastasis. *Nature. 410*, 50-56.

Nagasawa T, Hirota S, Tachibana K, Takakura N, Nishikawa S, Kitamura Y, Yoshida N, Kikutani H, & Kishimoto T (1996). Defects of B-cell lymphopoiesis and bone-marrow myelopoiesis in mice lacking the CXC chemokine PBSF/SDF-1. *Nature. 382*, 635-8.

Nagasawa T, Kikutani H, & Kishimoto T (1994). Molecular cloning and structure of a pre-B-cell growth-stimulating factor. *Proc Natl Acad Sci U S A. 91*, 2305-9.

Nervi, B., Ramirez, P., Rettig, M. P., Uy, G. L., Holt, M. S., Ritchey, J. K., Prior, J. L., Piwnica-Worms, D., Bridger, G., Ley, T. J., & DiPersio, J. F. (2009). Chemosensitization of acute myeloid leukemia (AML) following mobilization by the CXCR4 antagonist AMD3100. *Blood 113*, 6206-6214

Orimo A, Gupta PB, Sgroi DC, Arenzana-Seisdedos F, Delaunay T, Naeem R, Carey VJ, Richardson AL, & Weinberg RA (2005). Stromal fibroblasts present in invasive human breast carcinomas promote tumor growth and angiogenesis through elevated SDF-1/CXCL12 secretion. *Cell. 121*, 335-48.

Peled A, Kollet O, Ponomaryov T, Petit I, Franitza S, Grabovsky V, Slav MM, Nagler A, Lider O, Alon R, Zipori D, & Lapidot T (2000). The chemokine SDF-1 activates the integrins LFA-1, VLA-4, and VLA-5 on immature human CD34(+) cells: role in transendothelial/stromal migration and engraftment of NOD/SCID mice. *Blood. 95*, 3289-3296.

Peled A, Petit I, Kollet O, Magid M, Ponomaryov T, Byk T, Nagler A, Ben-Hur H, Many A, Shultz L, Lider O, Alon R, Zipori D, & Lapidot T (1999). Dependence of human stem cell engraftment and repopulation of NOD/SCID mice on CXCR4. *Science 283*, 845-848.

Pieters R (2009). Infantile Acute Lymphoblastic Leukemia: Lessons Learned and Future Directions. *Current Hematology Malignancy Reports 4*, 167-174.

Ptasznik A, Urbanowska E, Chinta S, Costa MA, Katz BA, Stanislaus MA, Demir G, Linnekin D, Pan ZK, & Gewirtz AM (2002). Crosstalk between BCR/ABL oncoprotein and CXCR4 signaling through a Src family kinase in human leukemia cells. *J Exp Med. 196*, 667-78.

Pui CH & Howard SC (2008). Current management and challenges of malignant disease in the CNS in paediatric leukaemia. *Lancet Oncol 9*, 257-268.

Rombouts EJ, Pavic B, Lowenberg B, & Ploemacher RE (2004). Relation between CXCR-4 expression, Flt3 mutations, and unfavorable prognosis of adult acute myeloid leukemia. *Blood 104*, 550-557.

Salgia R, Quackenbush E, Lin J, Souchkova N, Sattler M, Ewaniuk DS, Klucher KM, Daley GQ, Kraeft SK, Sackstein R, Alyea EP, von Andrian UH, Chen LB, Gutierrez-Ramos JC, Pendergast AM, & Griffin JD (1999). The BCR/ABL oncogene alters the chemotactic response to stromal-derived factor-1alpha. *Blood 94*, 4233-4246.

Sawyers CL (1999). Chronic myeloid leukemia. *N Engl J Med. 340*, 1330-40.

Schwieger, M., Schuler, A., Forster, M., Engelmann, A., Arnold, M. A., Delwel, R., Valk, P. J., Lohler, J., Slany, R. K., Olson, E. N., & Stocking, C. (2009). Homing and invasiveness of MLL/ENL leukemic cells is regulated by MEF2C. *Blood 114*, 2476-2488

Semerad CL, Christopher MJ, Liu F, Short B, Simmons PJ, Winkler I, Levesque JP, Chappel J, Ross FP, & Link DC (2005). G-CSF potently inhibits osteoblast activity and CXCL12 mRNA expression in the bone marrow. *Blood. 106*, 3020-7.

Smith BD, Levis M, Beran M, Giles F, Kantarjian H, Berg K, Murphy KM, Dauses T, Allebach J, & Small D (2004). Single-agent CEP-701, a novel FLT3 inhibitor, shows biologic and clinical activity in patients with relapsed or refractory acute myeloid leukemia. *Blood 103*, 3669-3676.

Spoo AC, Lubbert M, Wierd WG, & Burger JA (2007). CXCR4 is a prognostic marker in Acute Myelogenous Leukemia. *Blood* 109, 786-91

Stirewalt DL & Radich JP (2003). The role of FLT3 in haematopoietic malignancies. *Nat Rev Cancer. 3*, 650-665.

Sugiyama, T., Kohara, H., Noda, M., & Nagasawa T (2006). Maintenance of the Hematopoietic Stem Cell Pool by CXCL12-CXCR4 Chemokine Signaling in Bone Marrow Stromal Cell Niches. *Immunity 25*, 977-988.

Tachibana K, Hirota S, Iizasa H, Yoshida H, Kawabata K, Kataoka Y, Kitamura Y, Matsushima K, Yoshida N, Nishikawa S, Kishimoto T, & Nagasawa T (1998). The chemokine receptor CXCR4 is essential for vascularization of the gastrointestinal tract. *Nature. 393*, 591-4.

Tavor S, Petit I, Porozov S, Avigdor A, Dar A, L.-T. L., Shemtov N, Deutsch V, Naparstek E, Nagler A, & Lapidot T (2004). CXCR4 regulates migration and development of human acute myelogenous leukemia stem cells in transplanted NOD/SCID mice. *Cancer Res. 64*, 2817-2824.

Trentin L, Cabrelle A, Facco M, Carollo D, Miorin M, Tosoni A, Pizzo P, Binotto G, Nicolardi L, Zambello R, Adami F, Agostini C, & Semenzato G (2004). Homeostatic chemokines drive migration of malignant B cells in patients with non-Hodgkin lymphomas. *Blood 104*, 502-8.

Verfaillie CM, McCarthy JB, & McGlave PB (1992). Mechanisms underlying abnormal trafficking of malignant progenitors in chronic myelogenous leukemia. Decreased adhesion to stroma and fibronectin but increased adhesion to the basement membrane components laminin and collagen type IV. *J Clin Invest. 90*, 1232-41.

Voermans C, van Heese WP, de Jong I, Gerritsen WR, & van Der Schoot CE (2002). Migratory behavior of leukemic cells from acute myeloid leukemia patients. *Leukemia. 16*, 650-657.

Weng AP, Shahsafaei A, & Dorfman DM (2003). CXCR4/CD184 immunoreactivity in T-cell non-Hodgkin lymphomas with an overall Th1- Th2+ immunophenotype. *Am J Clin Pathol. 119*, 424-30.

Zeng, Z. H., Shi, Y. X., Samudio, I. J., Wang, R. Y., Ling, X. Y., Frolova, O., Levis, M., Rubin, J. B., Negrin, R. R., Estey, E. H., Konoplev, S., Andreeff, M., & Konopleva, M. (2009). Targeting the leukemia microenvironment by CXCR4 inhibition overcomes resistance to kinase inhibitors and chemotherapy in AML. *Blood 113*, 6215-6224, doi:DOI 10.1182/blood-2008-05-158311.

Zhou Y, Larsen PH, Hao C, & Yong VW (2002). CXCR4 is a major chemokine receptor on glioma cells and mediates their survival. *J Biol Chem. 277*, 49481-7.

Zou YR, Kottmann AH, Kuroda M, Taniuchi I, & Littman DR (1998). Function of the chemokine receptor CXCR4 in haematopoiesis and in cerebellar development. *Nature*. *393*, 595-9.

Part 3

Pediatric Acute Leukemia

9

Diagnostics of Molecular Markers in Childhood Acute Leukaemia Using Biochips

Tatyana Nasedkina[1], Yuliya Yatsenko[1], Olga Gra[1], Natalia Guseva[1], Elena Samochatova[1,2] and Alexander Zasedatelev[1]
[1]*Engelhardt Institute of Molecular Biology, Russian Academy of Sciences,*
[2]*Federal Clinical Research Center of Pediatric Hematology, Oncology and Immunology, Russia*

1. Introduction

Acute leukemia is a very heterogeneous disease that can be divided in two major groups according to lymphoblastic or myeloblastic origin of leukemic blast cells: acute lymphoblastic leukemia (ALL) and acute myeloblastic leukemia (AML). ALL and AML, in their turn, are both subdivided into many subgroups with different clinical features.

ALL is more frequent in children and represents about 80% of all pediatric leukemia cases. Prognosis of newly diagnosed children with ALL has improved significantly mainly due to treatment with high-doses of chemotherapeutic drugs, but also a risk-stratification strategy and optimization of therapy. 5-year event-free survival (EFS) rates in different clinics range between 76% and 86%. Overall remission rates usually are 98% or higher (Pui et al., 2011). Age and white cell count at diagnosis have been used to predict a prognosis in ALL for many years, having been identified in early epidemiologic studies as predictors of an outcome (Smith et al., 1996). Children aged from 1 to 9 years have the best outcomes; children and adolescents aged from 10 to 20 years have slightly worse outcomes, which is associated in part with higher incidence of T-cell leukemia and lower incidence of favorable genetic abnormalities such as *TEL/AML1* and hyperdiploidy. Also, ALL blasts from older patients become more resistant to multiple antileukemic drugs than the blasts from younger children in the first decade of life (Pieters et al., 1998; Nachman et al., 2009). Infants diagnosed at age of less than 1 year have relatively poor outcomes, which is associated with high incidence of immature pro-B-ALL phenotype and presence of *MLL* gene rearrangements (Hilden et al., 2006). Another biologic factor of prognostic value besides immunophenotype is a rapidity of response to the induction therapy with glucocorticoides, for instance decrease in peripheral blood blast count after a week of treatment. It has been shown by flow cytometry and molecular techniques, that a level of minimal residual disease (MRD) in bone marrow during first months of therapy may have high prognostic value and is used for stratification in many protocols (Szczepanski et al., 2001). Further risk stratification has been achieved using cytogenetic and molecular genetic characteristics of leukemia. The *TEL-AML1* translocation and hyperdiploidy were found to predict a good prognosis; therefore they allow relative therapy reduction in carriers (Pui et al., 2000). Philadelphia-chromosome-positive ALL (Ph+-ALL) is associated with a poorer prognosis

and application of novel therapies may significantly improve clinical outcome (Arico et al., 2000). Introduction of tyrosine kinase inhibitors has completely changed therapy strategy for chronic myeloid leukemia (CML), potentially it may be a treatment of choice for Philadelphia positive ALL. Historically, the children with Ph+- ALL have been transplanted in their first complete remission (Davies & Mehta, 2010).
Acute myeloid leukemia (AML) is defined as a hematologic malignancy in which more than 20% of nucleated cells represent myeloid blasts by morphology and immunophenotype. Despite apparent phenotypic uniformity, it has become increasingly clear that AML is a heterogeneous group of neoplastic diseases (Watt & Bagg, 2010). To great extent, the heterogeneity is based upon its genetic complexity. The traditional parameters such as clinical features, blood counts, morphology, cytochemistry, immunophenotype are keeping their position in clinical evaluation, but genetic approaches are now firmly established as the central component in diagnostics and classification of AML. There are different, but recurrent, structural and numeric cytogenetic abnormalities, translocations, inversions and derivative chromosomes (Mitelman et al., 2011). Three broad prognostic groups in AML with either favorable, intermediate, or adverse prognosis are identified by specific cytogenetic abnormalities (Grimwade & Hills, 2009). Also there is a growing number of acquired gene mutations which are essential to pathogenesis of AML (Gaidzik & Dohner, 2008). In addition, aberrant gene expression and copy number variations have recently been recognized as a common phenomena that underlie malignant transformation (Eklund, 2010). The average EFS rate in AML is significantly lower comparing with ALL and usually ranges from 40% to 63% in most successful clinical trials, thus stimulating the search and implementation of new approaches to the treatment based on molecular genetic markers.
Molecular technologies continue to evolve and provide more profound comprehension of leukemia pathology. Many of them have rapidly moved into clinical laboratories, while others remain as important discovery tools. Eventually, molecular genetic approaches will play the leading role in future leukemia practice.

1.1 Clinically relevant genetic lesions in ALL

The World Health Organization (WHO) provides current diagnostic criteria for ALL as a precursor B-cell acute lymphoblastic leukemia (B-ALL) or as a precursor T-cell acute lymphoblastic leukemia (T-ALL) (Brunning et al., 2001). Of the annually diagnosed ALL cases in different countries, approximately 80–85% have the B-ALL phenotype, and remainder displays the T-ALL phenotype. This classification scheme does not subdivide ALL into molecular subtypes, but most often, ALL is subtyped and studied on the basis of particular underlying genetic abnormality. The genetic defects in ALL include chromosomal translocations that deregulate gene expression or create novel fusion genes, numerical chromosome copy number aberrations (especially hyperdiploidy), and gene-specific mutations (Teitell & Pandolfi, 2009).
Hyperdiploidy (more than 50 chromosomes per leukemia cell) is found in approximately 25% of children who have B-lineage ALL. This genome abnormality is associated with a favorable outcome, especially when extra copies of chromosome 4, 10 or 17 are presented (Heerema et al., 2000). The hyperdiploid ALL cells are highly sensitive to cytostatics and L-asparaginase, and accumulate high amounts of methotrexate derivates, so they are easily subjected to apoptosis (Kaspers et al., 1995).
The *TEL/AML1* (*ETV6/RUNX1*) fusion accounts for approximately 20-25% of cases and also is associated with a favorable outcome. It is formed by fusion of *TEL* gene on the

chromosome 12 encoding a member of the ETS family of transcription factors and *AML1* gene on the chromosome 21, a transcription factor gene encoding a part of core-binding factor (CBF). The *TEL/ AML1* fusion probably inhibits transcription activity of normal *AML1* gene involved in proliferation and differentiation of hematopoietic cells. The t(12;21) is cryptic and cannot be identified by conventional cytogenetics. It is associated with high sensitivity to chemotherapeutic drugs, especially to L-asparaginase, though the mechanism of the sensitivity is unclear (Ramakers-van Woerden et al., 2000). Also the sensitivity to other drugs especially anthracyclines and etoposide has been reported (Frost et al., 2004). Both hyperdiploidy and *TEL/AML1* translocation occur mainly in children younger than 10 years with common or pre-B-ALL.

Abnormalities of a mixed lineage leukemia (*MLL*) gene on the chromosome 11q23 occur in approximately 80% of infants with ALL, but only in 2% of children above age of 1 year. All types of *MLL* gene rearrangements, such as *MLL/AF4* derived from t(4;11), *MLL/MLLT1(ENL)* derived from t(11;19), and *MLL/MLLT3* derived from t(9;11), are associated with a poor outcome in infants (Pieters et al., 2007); but in older children the poor outcome likely remains only for *MLL/ AF4* fusion gene (Pui et al., 2002). The fusion products involving *MLL* are associated with an aberrant expression of *HOX* genes, which are involved in early embryogenesis and may influence normal development of hematopoietic stem cells (Armsrong et al., 2002). The blast cells with *MLL* rearrangements are highly resistant to glucocorticoids and L-asparaginase (Dordelmann et al., 1999; Ramakers-van Woerden et al., 2004). These cells however, show a noticeable sensitivity to nucleoside analogue cytarabine, that is probably related to high expression of a membrane nucleoside transporter ENT1 (Stam et al., 2003).

The translocation t(9;22) results in a fusion between *BCR* gene on the chromosome 22 and *ABL* gene on the chromosome 9 leading to over expression of the abnormal ABL tyrosine kinase, thus increasing proliferation and decreasing apoptosis (Kharas & Fruman, 2005). The *BCR/ABL* fusion is found mainly in common and pre-B ALL. Incidence of the *BCR/ABL* increases with age from approximately 3% of children with ALL up to approximately 25% in adult ALL cases. Presence of BCR/ ABL predicts a poor outcome; more often it is associated with a poor response to prednisone and high levels of residual blasts carrying the *BCR/ABL* fusion after induction therapy (Schrappe et al., 1998).

The prognostic value of genetic abnormalities in T-ALL is not so evident. The translocation t(1;14) resulted in *SIL/TAL1* fusion gene is found in approximately 25% of all T-ALL cases. The translocations t(10;14) and t(7;10) occur in approximately 10% of T-ALL cases leading to activation of *HOX11* gene (Graux et al., 2006). Two recently described abnormalities occur exclusively in T-ALL: an abnormal expression of HOX11L2 caused mainly by translocation t(5;14) in approximately 25% of T-ALL cases, and activating mutations in *NOTCH1* gene in 50% of T-ALL cases. The mutations in *NOTCH1* gene may be associated with a favorable outcome (Breit et al., 2006). Other recurrent genetic lesions occur in small subgroups of childhood ALL. The translocation t(1;19) leading to *E2A-PBX1* fusion occurs in less than 5% of precursor B-ALL, mainly pre-B-ALL cases and is associated with a more aggressive clinical course (Aspland et al., 2001). Hypodiploidy (<45 chromosomes) is detected in only 1% of children who have ALL and is associated with a poor outcome (Nachman,et al., 2007).

1.2 Clinically relevant genetic lesions an AML

The WHO classification of AML is based on genetically defined entities of this complex disease (Swerdlow, 2008). In 2008 seven groups based on recurrent translocations (AML with t(8;21) (q22;q22) *RUNX1/RUNX1T1*; AML with inv(16) (p13q22) or t(16;16) (p13;q22) *CBFB/MYH11*; AML with t(15;17) (q22;q12) *PML/RARA*; AML with t(9;11) (p22;q23) *MLLT3/MLL*; AML with t(6;9) (p23q34) *DEK/NUP214*; AML with inv(3) (q21q26.2) or t(3;3) (q21q26.2) *RPN1/EVI1* and AML with t(1;22) (p13;q130*RBM15/MKL1*) and two provisional groups characterized by gene mutations (AML with mutated *NPM1* and AML with mutated *CEBPA*) were included into the classification system. These nine diagnostic entities cover about two thirds of all AML cases, while additional subtypes of AML, in which genetic factors play the central role, include myelodysplastic syndrome and therapy-related myeloid neoplasms. The latter two subtypes typically represent cases with complex karyotype, which is defined as the coexistence of three and more clonal cytogenetic aberrations (Watt & Bagg, 2010).

1.2.1 Reccurent chromosomal aberrations

The t(8;21)(q22;q22) *RUNX1/RUNX1T1* is a specific genetic lesion. It occurs in approximately 8-10% of all cases of AML and usually is associated with the previously FAB-designated subtype AML-M2 (Peterson & Zhang, 2004; Swerdlow, 2008). *RUNX1* and *CBFB* encode two components of a heterodimeric transcription complex known as core binding factor (CBF). The CBF plays an important role in regulation of normal hematopoiesis, thus the disruption of these two genes becomes obviously pathogenic. One of two major recurrent translocations involving CBF is the t(8;21), another is the inv(16). A part of *RUNX1(AML1)* gene on 21q22 is fused with a part of the *RUNX1T1(ETO)* gene on 8q22. The subsequently derived fusion protein, RUNX1-RUNX1T1 (AML1/ETO), represents a protein with inhibitory function which represses transcription of a number of important hematopoietic genes. Clinically, the t(8;21) translocation is associated with a favorable prognosis (Heerema-McKenney & Arber, 2009).

The inv(16)(p13q22) or t(16;16)(p13;q22) *CBFB/MYH11* is a pericentric inversion or molecularly identical t(16;16) translocation. It represents approximately 5–10% of all cases of AML and is associated with the FAB entity of acute myelomonoblastic leukemia with eosinophilia (AML-M4Eo) (Heerema-McKenney & Arber, 2009). A part of *CBFB* gene is fused with a part of one of myosin heavy chain genes, *MYH11* and the fusion prevents the formation of a functional CBF transcription factor. The CBFB–MYH11 can act also as a transcriptional repressor in the nucleus (Shigesada et al., 2004). Although this genetic fusion is most often seen in M4Eo, it may also be found in other subtypes of AML, including those designated by FAB as M2 and M5. The inv(16) can sometimes be missed by cytogenetics as cryptic, so molecular methods have a particularly important role in the detection of this aberration. The breakpoints in *CBFB* gene occur in intron 5, while in *MYH11* gene breakpoints are involved seven different exons (7 through 13), yielding at least ten different fusion transcripts. The most common form, type A, accounts for approximately 90% of *CBFB/MYH11* cases, while two other transcripts (types D and E) account for an additional 5%. The aberration is associated with a favorable outcome.

The t(15;17)(q22;q12) *PML/RARA* is observed in approximately 5–8% of all cases of AML defining an unique entity acute promyelocytic leukemia (APL) (Swerdlow, 2008). Among all acute leukemias, APL represents one with the most stable genotype–phenotype correlation, in that the presence of specific translocation can frequently be expected based upon the characteristic morphology: the classic hypergranular form (FAB AML-M3) or the micrgranular variant (FAB AML-M3v). The part of *PML* gene on 15q22 is fused with *RARA* gene on 17q12 resulting in a *PML/RARA* gene. In the absence of retinoic acid the wild-type

RARA protein is a component of a heterodimeric transcriptional repressor complex, while binding with retinoic acid converts the RARA complex into a transcriptional activator. The chimeric protein PML/RARA becomes a potential transcriptional repressor with altered DNA-binding properties and the capacity to block myeloid differentiation. The treatment of PML/RARA carriers with pharmacologic doses of retinoic acid in the form of ATRA destroys the co-repressor complex and leads to differentiation of the malignant promyelocytes (Guidez et al., 1998). At least four rare variant translocations associated with APL phenotype have been described: t(11;17) (q23;q12) *ZBTB16/RARA*, t(11;17)(q13;q12) *NUMA1/RARA*, t(5;17)(q35;q12) *NPM1/RARA* and t(17;17)(q11.2;q12) *STAT5B/RARA*. Some of these variants, the t(11;17) *ZBTB16/RARA* and t(17;17) *STAT5B/RARA*, are not sensitive to ATRA, so the molecular characterization of APL is necessary.The breakpoints in *RARA* gene are restricted to intron 2, while in *PML* gene there are two major breakpoints leading to long (L-form, bcr 1) or short (S-form, bcr3) transcript variant.

MLL gene on the chromosome 11q23 is an exceptional target in AML; as it is involved in at least 73 different translocations with more than 50 different partner genes (Huret, 2011) including different leukemia subtypes, such as *de novo* AML, therapy-related AML, myelodysplastic syndromes and acute lymphoblastic leukemia. The protein MLL is a histone methyltransferase that modulates gene expression, especially the expression of *HOX* genes, via chromatin remodeling (Dou & Hess, 2008), while most fused partners are supposed to be transcription factors. An exact mechanism of leukemogenesis involved different *MLL* translocations has not been completely understood. The t(9;11) (p22;q23) *MLL/MLLT3* (*MLL/AF9*) is the most common, typically associated with subtype FAB-M5 having monocytic features. In contrast to most other *MLL* rearrangements that are associated with a poor prognosis, this translocation is associated with an intermediate prognosis. The breakpoints in *MLL* are clustered in a breakpoint cluster region, spanning exons 5-11. An extreme heterogeneity of translocations associated with *MLL* makes analysis using PCR diagnostic assay laborious. FISH is applicable for detection of *MLL* translocations in clinical practice (Keefe et al., 2010). Other significant *MLL* translocations in AML are t(6;11) *MLL/MLLT4 (MLL/AF6)*, t(11;19) *MLL/ELL*, t(10;11) *MLL/MLLT4 (MLL/AF10)*.

One of the rarer recurrent translocations the t(6;9)(p23;q34) occurs in approximately 1% of AML cases. The inv(3) and related t(3;3) translocation are found in approximately 1-2% of AML cases and associated with a poor clinical outcome (Swerdlow, 2008). AML with the t(1;22) translocation occurs primarily in infants representing less than 1% of all cases of AML. It is particularly associated with acute megakaryoblastic leukemia (FAB M7) and a good prognosis, if treated with intensive chemotherapy (Duchayne et al., 2003).

1.2.2 Gene mutations

Approximately 45% of AML cases have a normal karyotype but carry submicroscopic and cryptic genetic lesions that cannot be detected by conventional cytogenetics. Several acquired gene mutations have been described and characterized in AML. Two lesions (*NPM1* and *CEBPA* mutations) have obtained provisional status in the 2008 WHO classification (Swerdlow, 2008).

NPM1 encodes a 37 kDa protein with versatile biologic activity that shuttles between the nucleolus, nucleoplasm and the cytoplasm (Grisendi et al., 2006; Meani & Alcalay, 2009). Mutations in *NPM1* are common in AML, occurring with an overall frequency of 25-30% in adults and are associated with normal karyotype (Schnittger et al., 2005; Thiede et al., 2006). Most mutations in *NPM1* are small insertions (4-11bp) in the terminal coding region (exon

12). Although over 50 mutations have been described, three specific mutations (A, B and D) account for the majority of the changes observed in AML (Falini et al., 2009). As a general rule, the presence of an *NPM1* mutation is associated with a more favorable clinical outcome. However, the *NPM1* mutations are often found together with an internal tandem duplication *FLT3-ITD*, in this case the negative prognostic impact of a *FLT3-ITD* mutation may override the positive value of an *NPM1* mutation.

FLT3 is a class III receptor tyrosine kinase and a member of immunoglobulin receptor superfamily. It is expressed mostly in progenitor cells; the level of expression is lowered during differentiation. The ligand binding with FLT3 protein results in a phosphorylation of a juxtamembranous (JM) domain leading to the proliferation and inhibition of apoptosis. Two major types of lesions in *FLT3* gene have been described: an internal tandem duplication (ITD) of the JM domain and a missense mutation D835mut in the activation loop (PM). Functionally, these lesions result in the constitutive activation of the tyrosine kinase domains via autophosphorylation and, consequently, to permanent signaling through downstream effectors. FLT3-ITD is an independent predictor of poor clinical outcome (Meshinchi & Appelbaum, 2009). The prognostic value of the FLT3-PM is controversial (Yamamoto et al., 2001). Another important diagnostic target is *c-KIT* gene which encodes a type III tyrosine kinase involved in a signal transduction. The activating mutations, occurring in approximately 2-8% of all AML, lead to ligand independent signal transduction (Cairoli et al., 2006). In adults, the c-*KIT* mutations typically predict worse prognosis, but it may be different in children (Pollard et al., 2010).

Due to significant progress in our understanding of acute leukemia pathogenesis, risk stratification of patients more and more relies on molecular genetic markers. New molecular targets will be found to enrich a clinician's repertoire for making well-founded decisions regarding diagnosis, prognosis and therapy. This requires the establishment of appropriate and practical testing algorithms and development of standardized assays in order to obtain reliable and reproducible results.

1.3 Methods for detection of genetic lesions

Molecular diagnostics, first being a subsidiary tool in the clinical evaluation of acute leukemia, nowadays has been integrated rapidly into clinical laboratory practice. Genetic abnormalities associated with different leukemia subtypes can be detected by a variety of supplemental clinical methods, including conventional G-banded cytogenetics, FISH, PCR and DNA sequencing. The innovated technologies, such as gene-expression analysis, comparative genetic hybridization (CGH) and SNP arrays, still remaining at the experimental level, have a potential to hold a place in routine clinical evaluation and management of the disease. A brief overview of different methods allowing detection of different genetic lesions is presented in Table 1. Among them gel-based diagnostic biochips are considered, which are discussed further in more details.

A traditional karyotyping, based on Giemsa-stained metaphase chromosome spreads, continues to provide valuable information about translocations, as well as numerical changes in chromosome number and structure. Diagnostics of clonal process in a clinical sample is typically defined by the presence of at least two cells with the same structural abnormality, and at least three cells with the same abnormality in the case of a chromosomal loss. Despite limitations in analytic sensitivity and availability of dividing cells in a clinical sample, traditional karyotyping remains one of the most robust tools in molecular hematopathology.

Fluorescence *in situ* hybridization (FISH) involves fluorescently labeled probe binding to specific chromosome sequences that is visualized under fluorescent microscope. The structural microscopic or submicroscopic cryptic lesions, as well as different numeric chromosomal changes can be identified depending on a probe design (Wolff et al., 2007). FISH is more direct method to evaluate chromosomal lesions comparing with karyotyping, also it is more sensitive and can be applied to non-dividing interphase cells.

PCR is a popular and versatile tool in evaluation of acute leukemias. The technique is based on the exponential amplification of a target nucleic acid sequence; specific applications depend upon the type of initial nucleic acid and the detection method. The DNA-based allele-specific PCR is used for the detection of gene mutations. The RNA-based PCR assay, reverse-transcription PCR or RT-PCR, is extremely useful in the analysis of fusion genes which express chimeric transcripts. Also the measurement of gene expression is possible. The resulting amplicons are evaluated either quantitatively by a real-time PCR approach or qualitatively by gel electrophoresis after 30-35 cycles of amplification. Because of the exponential amplification of target, sensitivity of the method is very high allowing detection of 1 blast with specific lesion among 10^{-4}-10^{-5} normal cells (Rennert et al., 1999). Because of its increased analytical sensitivity regarding to karyotyping and FISH, RT-PCR is widely used for monitoring minimal residual disease in leukemia cases with recurrent translocations.

Feature	Target analyzed						Parameters		
Method	Sample type	Balanced translocations	Numeric chromosome changes	Gene mutation	Gene expression	CNV	MRD level, % of blasts	Time	Clinical usage
Karyotyping	Mitotic cells	Yes[1]	Yes	No	No	No	5-10	2-3 days	Yes
FISH	Any cells	Yes	Yes	No	No	No	1-5	1-2 days	Yes
PCR	DNA	Yes	No	Yes	No	No	0.0001	3-4 h	Yes
RT-PCR	RNA	Yes	No	Yes	Yes	No	0.0001	5-6 h	Yes
Sequencing	DNA	No	No	Yes	No	No	10-20	1 day	No
CGH array	DNA	No	Yes	No	No	Yes	10-30	2 days	No
Expression array	RNA	No	No	No	Yes	No	10-30	2 days	No
SNP arays	DNA	No	Yes	No	No	Yes	10-30	2 days	No
Gel-based biochips	RNA/DNA	Yes	No	Yes	No	No	0.001-5[2]	16-20 h	Yes

Table 1. Characteristics of different molecular genetic methods in the analysis of acute leukemias

The variability and complexity of mutations in some genes, like *NPM1* or *CEBPA*, make them ineligible for standard PCR assays, in such cases direct DNA sequencing can be used to search for the presence of a genetic lesion (Ahn et al., 2009). The traditional sequencing is a robust and flexible methodology that reliably detects the presence of mutations when approximately 20% of cells carry the genetic lesion. While not available clinically, next-generation DNA sequencing methods become more and more applicable regarding to time, money and data analysis. In 2010, it is feasible to sequence a human genome in

[1] (-except cryptic aberrations;

[2] - the MRD level is 0.001% for translocations and 5 % per gene mutations)

approximately 1 week for approximately US$15,000 (Aparicio & Huntsman, 2010). Different microarray-based methodologies are applied to profiling gene expression and measuring copy number variations (CNV) (Bacher al., 2010; Nasedkina et al., 2009). It has been shown that the gene expression measurement is independently capable of classifying many of the clinically relevant ALL and AML categories based on their distinct expression profiles (Bullinger et al., 2004; Radmacher et al., 2006). At the same time, expression arrays can not predict the mutation status of several prognostically relevant genes, such as *FLT3* (Kohlmann et al., 2010). Further standardization of these complex techniques is needed for successful introduction into clinical laboratories (Haferlach et al., 2010).

2. Diagnostics of molecular markers in childhood leukemia using biochips

The translation of research to practice has been stimulated the development of novel approaches to clinical diagnostics potentially capable to overcome the limitations of settled technologies, like karyotyping, FISH and RT-PCR. Complicated assays using high-density arrays hardly are used in daily routine diagnostics, especially in small clinical laboratories. To overlap this gap different low-density array-based techniques have been developed, which are less complex, less expensive and more reproducible systems with a few molecular markers comparing to high-density microarrays. Gel-based biochips are a good example of such a technology.

2.1 Gel-based biochip technology

Overviews of low-density gel-based biochip or hydrogel biochip technology and applications in different fields exemplifying diagnostics from infectious diseases to protein oncological markers have been published recently (Mikhailovich et al., 2008; Nasedkina et al., 2009; Rubina et al., 2008). Principal difference of gel-based biochip technology comparing with other matrix microarrays is an immobilization of identifying probes in semi-spherical three-dimensional (3-D) gel elements instead of the flat supporting surface. The solution containing oligonucleotide probes mixed with gel-forming monomer is placed on a activated plastic or glace surface by a standard robotic device. Oligonucleotide probes are modified and carry NH_2 -groups at their 3′ ends. Copolymerization of molecular probes and main gel components is processed under UV-light. As a result the immobilized molecules become covalently bound to monomers of a growing polymer chain and distribute evenly throughout each gel element, as shown by confocal microscopy (Rubina et al., 2004). The diameters of gel elements are ranged from 50 up to 300 μm with a distance between them from 100 up to 500 μm depending on experimental tasks. A number of gel elements vary from several tens up to several thousands depending on the complexity of target analyzed. The quality control of gel element disposition is performed using specialized optical device and computerized image analysis. Such quality control allows minimizing intra- and inter-array variation of a drop size on ready-to-use biochips and substantially increases the reproducibility of hybridization results with different series of biochips.

Fluorescent dyes are used as labels to register hybridization pattern. Different analogs of cyanine fluorescent dyes Cy3 and Cy5 have been synthesized to increase the sensitivity and efficacy of hybridization analysis (Kuznetsova et al., 2008). In the case of DNA sequence analysis the hybridization target represents a fragment of genome and the amplification of DNA is usually needed using PCR with simultaneous incorporation of fluorescent label. The size of amplified fragments is in range of 100-1000 b.p. For proteome analysis gel elements contain antigen or antibody and the fluorescent label is conjugated directly with target analyzed or with molecules of developing antibodies like in the sandwich immunoassay. A biochip photograph and view under light microscope are presented in Fig.1, A and B.

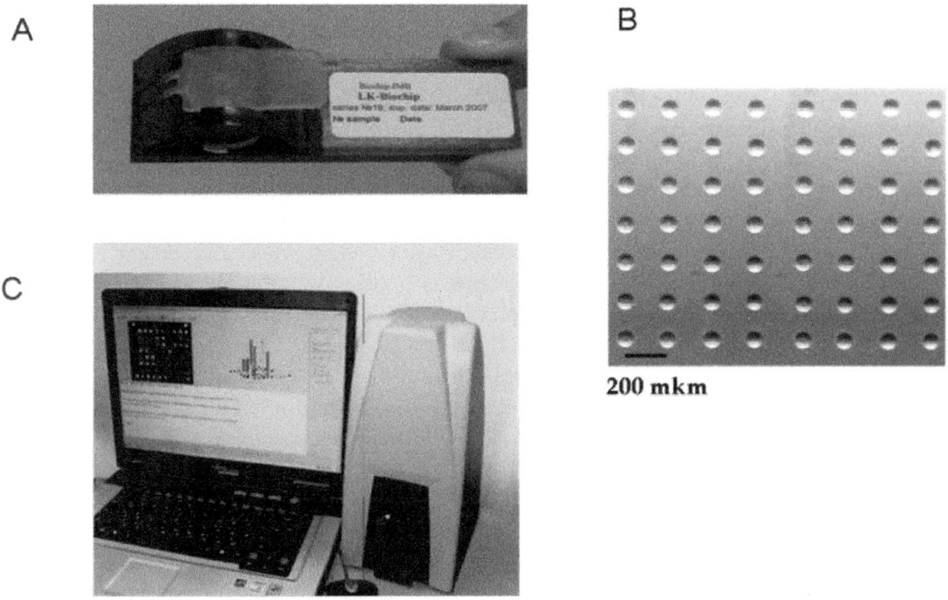

A - General view of biochip with hybridization chamber;
B - gel elements with a diameter of 100 μm under light microscope;
C - portable biochip analyzer (*on the right*). Scale bar = 200 μm.

Fig. 1. Gel-based biochips.

The higher probe concentration in gel drops compared with spots of 2-dimensional microarrays allows the use of a simple detection system consisting of a laser source equipped with lenses and charge-coupled device camera (Fig. 1, C). The portable biochip analyzer is certified for clinical use by a national regulatory agency, the Ministry of Public Health of the Russian Federation (Registration Certificate of Federal Service for Supervision in Public Health Sphere No. FS 022a2006/3777-06). Image analysis is performed using automated user-friendly software «Imageware»® , which measures the fluorescence intensities in gel elements after allele-specific hybridization and determines the gel elements where the formation of perfect duplexes is performed between complementary probe and target. Then the system presents a report about the presence of mutation, polymorphism or chromosome translocation in a sample under analysis.

The main features of the gel-based biochip analysis are its simplicity, and the low cost of equipment and biochips themselves (approximately 8 $US per chip in 2011), enabling their use by small diagnostic laboratories. One of the first clinical biochip applications was the analysis of chromosomal translocations occurring in leukemia.

2.2 Analysis of chromosomal translocations in leukemia

The recurrent chromosomal aberrations represent important diagnostic and prognostic markers of different types of disease requiring appropriate therapy and are taken into account in the risk-stratification of patients in different clinical trials (Look, 1997; Möricke et al., 2008; Rubnitz et al., 2008; Rabbits, 1994; Shrappe, 2004). When an aberration is found, it also serves as a reliable target for monitoring of minimal residual disease.

Traditionally, chromosomal translocations have been identified using cytogenetics and FISH. However, the analysis of chromosomal translocations with cytogenetic methods is not always accurate and representative, because of submicroscopic lesions and cryptic translocations. The FISH technique is comprehensive, reliable and available for clinics approach, but it requires expensive basic equipment, does not allow the detection of all targets of interest simultaneously and is not sensitive enough for effective monitoring of MRD. The reverse-transcription (RT)-PCR is another widely used method able to detect chimeric transcripts, which derive from fusion genes and represent an excellent molecular target expressed in leukemic blasts (Braziel et al., 2003; Haferlach et al., 2005). As far as the identification of each transcript requires an individual PCR reaction with specific primers, a scale of the study increases markedly when each patient is analyzed for several transcripts simultaneously. Thus, multiplex protocols have been developed to diminish time- and labor-intensity of the procedure (Pallisgaard et al., 1998; Scurto et al., 1998). The multiplex RT-PCR assay is usually multi-stage: the multiplex reaction is followed by series of identifying PCR reactions with primers specific for individual translocations. To facilitate the identification of recurrent translocations an oligonucleotide biochip has been developed and combined with multiplex RT-PCR assay. The hybridization step increases specificity of the assay while reduces associated costs and amount of patient material required. Taking into consideration the results of clinical trials, thirteen chromosomal aberrations considered the most important for diagnosis and prognosis, were chosen as targets (Mitiaeva et al., 2004; Nasedkina et al., 2003). The following translocations were included into the assay: t(9;22)p190 and p210, t(12;21), t(1;19), t(8;21), inv(16), t(15;17), t(4;11), t(6;11), t(9;11); t(10;11), t(11;19)*ELL*, t(11,19)*ENL*.

Oligonucleotide probes of 20–25 bp in length were spotted in duplicates in order to increase reproducibility of hybridization results. The biochip contains probes for the detection of wild type *ABL* gene, which is expressed in all cells. The detection of *ABL* transcript is used to control the quantity and quality of isolated RNA and to estimate the effectiveness of labeled target preparation. For each translocation, a set of probes was designed including a so-called common probe from one of the genes involved in the translocation, and also specific probes to identify the breakpoint variants. The procedure includes the isolation of RNA from bone marrow or peripheral blood cells, multiplex RT-PCR using primers specific for different translocations, labeling of single strand PCR product via incorporation of modified Cy5-dUTP in the course of asymmetric PCR, hybridization on the biochip, and registration of fluorescence intensities in gel elements of biochip using a biochip analyzer. Computer-based processing of fluorescent signals using a specially developed algorithm allows an automated image analysis. Examples of different hybridization patterns are presented in Fig. 2, A and B. The limit of sensitivity is one blast cell with a chromosomal translocation among 10^3–10^4 normal cells.

The MLL translocations represent a difficult subject for analysis by conventional cytogenetics or standard RT-PCR due to high diversity of gene partners involved in translocations with *MLL* gene. In MLL translocations the fusion results in a gene and transcript with the 5′ end belonging to *MLL* gene originally located in 11q23 region and the 3′ end belonging to one of more than 50 partner genes (Eguchi et al., 2005). In biochip-based assay a set of probes specific for different *MLL* exons and probes specific to different exons

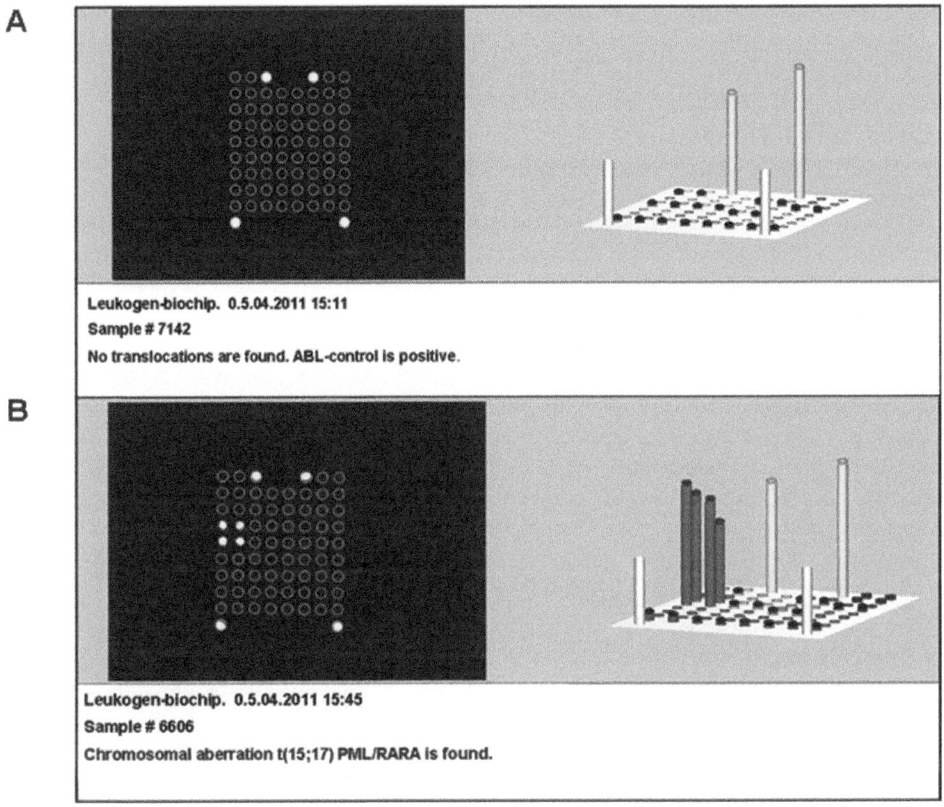

Fig. 2. Identification of chromosomal translocations by Leukogen-biochip. Two lower spots represent fluorescent marker, two upper spots correspond to ABL-gene specific signals. A – a sample of patient carrying no translocations; B- a sample of patient carrying translocation t(15;17), fusion gene *PML/RARA, bcr3* breakpoint variant.

of partner gene is used. The analysis was done as described previously (Mitiaeva et al., 2004). The biochip-based approach can indicate which *MLL* exon is involved in formation of a chimeric transcript, as well as identifies the partner gene. Most frequent translocations in ALL and AML are included into assay, namely t(4;11), t(6;11), t(9;11); t(10;11), t(11;19)*ELL*, t(11,19)*ENL*. They are included in the last version of Leukogen-biochip for the analysis of 13 translocations. Another diagnostic biochip has been described which allowed the analysis of about thirty different gene partners, but the sensitivity limit of the assay is significantly lower: 1 blast cell per 10 normal (Maroc et al., 2004).

During 2006-2009 the bone marrow samples of patients with leukemia of age 0 to 18 treated in hematological clinics were received and tested using the biochip-based approach for the presence of translocations. The hematologic malignancies ALL and AML were diagnosed according to standard criteria by cytomorphologic, cytochemical, and immunophenotypic studies of bone marrow cells. Totally, 1200 children with leukemia from different parts of Russia were included into assay: 912 patients were diagnosed with ALL and 282 with AML. In ALL patients the chromosomal aberrations analyzed were found in 24,4% of all cases. In

AML the portion of patients carrying specific translocations was 36,4% of all cases. The most frequent translocation in ALL was cryptic translocation t(12;21) (12,8%), fusion transcript *TEL/AML1* or *ETV6/RUNX1*. In AML most frequent translocations are t(8;21) (9,5%) with fusion gene AML/ETO or *RUNX1/RUNX1T1*; t(15;17) (8,0%) with fusion gene *PML/RARA* and t(9;11) (10,5 %) with *MLL/MLLT3*. The frequency of t(12;21) obtained in Russia is lower than the frequencies of 18-20% found in other countries (Hilden et al., 2006; Rubnitz et al., 2008; Vilmer et al., 2000).

Validation of the method was done using individual RT-PCR protocols for each translocation (Pallisgaard et al., 1998), in others words, for 325 patients the standard RT-PCR assay was performed parallel to biochip-based analysis. The concordance between the two methods was about 98%. The main source of false-positive signals on biochip may be contamination by amplified DNA fragments; the problem can be overcome by more accurate PCR handling. To avoid false-negative results, biochips were tested periodically with control samples carrying translocations. The results of the biochip analysis were also compared with clinical data and a morphologically determined leukemia variant. The patients carrying translocations were further monitored for minimal residual disease to follow efficacy of therapy and to predict a relapse. The Leukogen-biochip was certified by a national regulatory agency, the Ministry of Public Health of the Russian Federation, for clinical application (Registration Certificate of Federal Service for Supervision in Public Health Sphere No. FS 012b2006/4756-06).

2.3 Analysis of gene mutations using biochip

Gene mutation analysis using gel-based biochips included following steps: DNA isolation from biological sample, two-round multiplex PCR of gene fragments containing the mutations analyzed, labeling of PCR products with Cy-5-dUTP during an asymmetric PCR of the second round, hybridization on biochip, registration of fluorescent signals and image analysis of hybridization patterns. The hybridization with allele-specific probes allows distinguishing between wild-type and mutant alleles with high fidelity (Nasedkina et al., 2006). Mutations in *NPM1* gene are considered as genetic markers defining patient's subgroups with different clinical characteristics. The genetic lesions in *NPM1* gene are mostly presented by tetra nucleotide insertions in exon 12. A biochip has been developed for the analysis of about 20 different insertion types in *NPM1* gene. The biochip for the analysis of *NPM1* gene mutations and hybridization patterns is presented in Fig. 3.

A clinical screening was performed to identify the *NPM1* mutations in 188 de novo diagnosed pediatric AML cases previously investigated for the presence of aberrations with Leukogen-biochip. The *NPM1* mutations appeared only in patients without chromosomal aberrations and this association with normal karyotype was statistically significant ($p<0.05$). Frequency of mutations was 4.8% (9/186) of total AML patients group and 8.0% (9/112) of patients without aberrations. The mutations in *NPM1* gene were represented by 4 b.p. insertions: TCTG (type A), CATG (type B), CCTG (type D), TCGG (type Qm). The nomenclature of mutation types is given as described previously (Rau & Brown, 2009). All patients with mutations were heterozygote carrying one mutant and one wild-type alleles.

In adults, the mutations in *NPM1* gene are considered most frequent events in AML, especially in AML with normal karyotype. The mutation frequency is ranged between 12%-18% (Falini et al., 2005; Thiede et al., 2006; Rau & Brown, 2009). In childhood AML it seems to be relatively rare occurring in 2-7% of all cases (Brown et al., 2007; Cazzaniga et al., 2005;

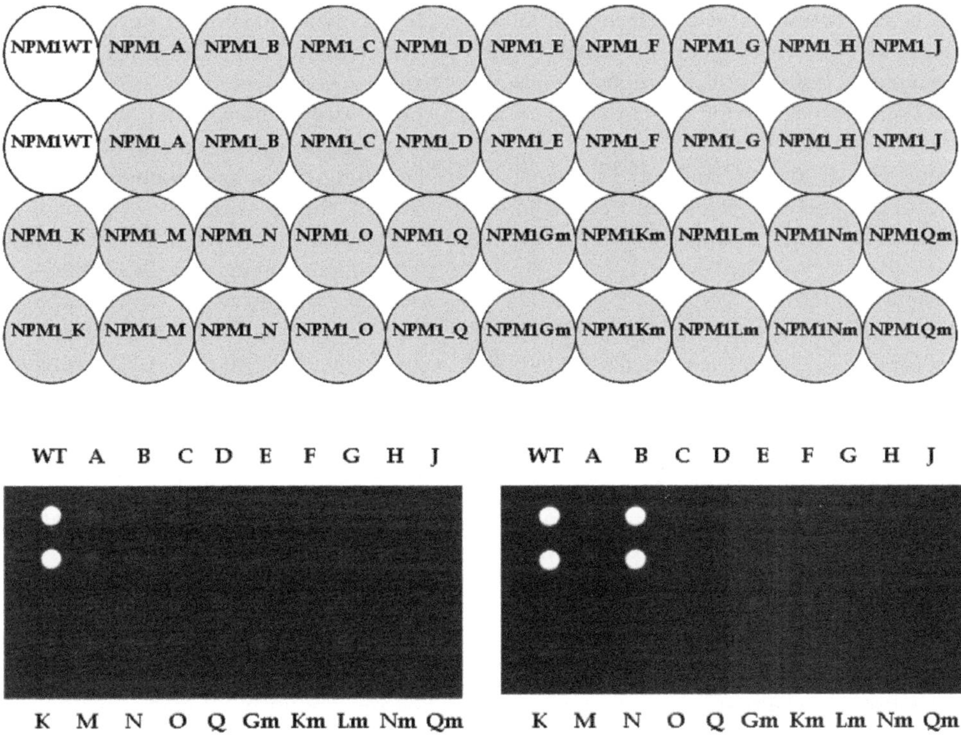

Fig. 3. Analysis of the mutations in *NPM1* gene. A - scheme of biochip, B – hybridization pattern for patient homozygous for wild-type NPM1 allele; C – hybridization pattern for patient carrying mutation type B, wild-type allele is also presented (WT - wildtype, A-Qm - mutation types).

Renneville et al., 2008). In our study the *NPM1* mutations were found in 4.8% of all patients and in 8.0% of patients without chromosomal aberrations, thus the data corresponded to those previously described. As far as *NPM1* mutations occur only in patients with normal karyotype it is possible to use them as potential diagnostic markers for MRD monitoring. The high diversity and complex nature of the *NPM1* mutations make difficult the analysis using PCR methods, more often direct sequencing is applied. In this case the biochip-based hybridization analysis may be a method of choice allowing detection of a wide spectrum of *NPM1* insertions. The usefulness of biochip-based approach becomes apparent in analysis of many mutations in different genes simultaneously. Further development of *NPM1*-biochip is suggested to include most important mutations in *FLT3* and *c-KIT* genes. The parallel usage of two kinds of diagnostic biochips, one for translocations and another for mutations may significantly improve molecular diagnostics of leukemia.

2.4 Pharmacogenetic testing and personalized treatment

Germline polymorphisms in genes, which hypothetically can mediate differential responses to drugs in leukemic patients, are perspective targets for investigation. Such genes are involved in drug absorption and excretion, metabolism, cellular transport and the drug targets and pathways of standard chemotherapeutics. Polymorphisms in these genes can potentially lead to higher or lower levels of chemotherapeutic drug response and consequently might affect toxicity or efficacy. Numerous studies have investigated an association of polymorphisms in different genes coding drug-metabolizing enzymes with patient responses to chemotherapy. The cytochrome P450 enzymes are involved in the Phase I metabolism of many antileukemic agents including cyclophosphamide, etoposide, doxorubicin and vincristine, and might influence on ALL therapy outcomes (Fleury et al., 2004; Rocha et al., 2005). A number of Phase II metabolism enzymes are involved in inactivation of antileukemic agents. Through glutathione conjugation, glutathione S-transferases (GSTs) generally inactivate glucocorticoids, vincristine, anthracyclines, cyclophosphamide and epipodophyllotoxins. Polymorphisms in various GST genes (*GSTT1, GSTM1, GSTP1*) have been extensively studied in prognosis of childhood ALL (Anderer et al., 2000; Davies et al., 2002; Kishi et al., 2004; Stanulla et al., 2000).

2.4.1 Biochip for the analysis of drug-metabolizing genes

To investigate association between polymorphisms in drug-metabolizing genes and response to therapy and clinical outcome a Pharmagen-biochip has been designed. The following targets were included into assay: genes *CYP1A1, CYP2D6, CYP2C9, CYP2C19,* coding cytochromes, enzymes of Phase I of biotransformation; genes *GSTT1* and *GSTM1,* coding glutathione S-transferases (GST), gene *NAT2,* coding N-arylamine acetyl transferase, gene *TPMT,* coding thiopurine-S-methyl transferase, which products are involved in different Phase II reactions; and also *MTHFR* gene, which product participates in folate metabolism. An example of sample analysis using Pharmagen-biochip is given on Fig. 4.

Finally, the Pharmagen-biochip allows analyzing 16 SNP's and 2 deletions in 10 genes *CYP1A1* (4887C>A, 4889A>G, 6235T>C), *CYP2D6* (1934G>A, 2637delA), *NAT2* (481C>T, 590G>A, 857G>A), *MTHFR* (677C>T), *CYP2C9* (430C>T, 1075C>T), *CYP2C19* (681G>A), , *TPMT* (238G>C, 460G>A, 719 A>G), *GSTT1* (deletion) and *GSTM1* (deletion). Accuracy of the analysis was found to be no less than 98% in experiments with control samples of known genotype. The Pharmagen-biochip was approved by the Ministry of Public Health of the Russian Federation for clinical testing of drug-metabolizing enzyme polymorphisms (Registration Certificate No. FS 012b2006/5317-06)

2.4.2 Polymorphism of thiopurine-S-methyltransferase 6-MP toxicity

One of the well known antileukemic drugs is 6-mercaptopurine (6-MP), which is used for supportive therapy in ALL. Within the cell thiopurines are metabolized into active thioguanine nucleotides (TGNs) which incorporate into DNA or RNA and result in cell cycle arrest and apoptosis. Like other thiopurine drugs, 6-MP is metabolized mainly by a highly polymorphic enzyme thiopurine-S-methyltransferase (TPMT) (Evans & McLeod, 2003). The relationship between *TPMT* polymorphisms and thiopurines efficacy and toxicity in children with ALL is a paradigm of the clinical application of pharmacogenetics (Evans & McLeod, 2003; Stanulla et al., 2005; Relling et al., 1999). The TPMT activity is inherited in an autosomal dominant manner and demonstrates genetic polymorphism: about 91% of people have polymorphic variants with high activity, an intermediate TPMT activity occurs in about 9% of the population and 0.3% have low or undetectable TPMT enzyme activity (Yates et al., 1997). The wild-type allele, *TPMT*1*, encodes an active TPMT enzyme. While

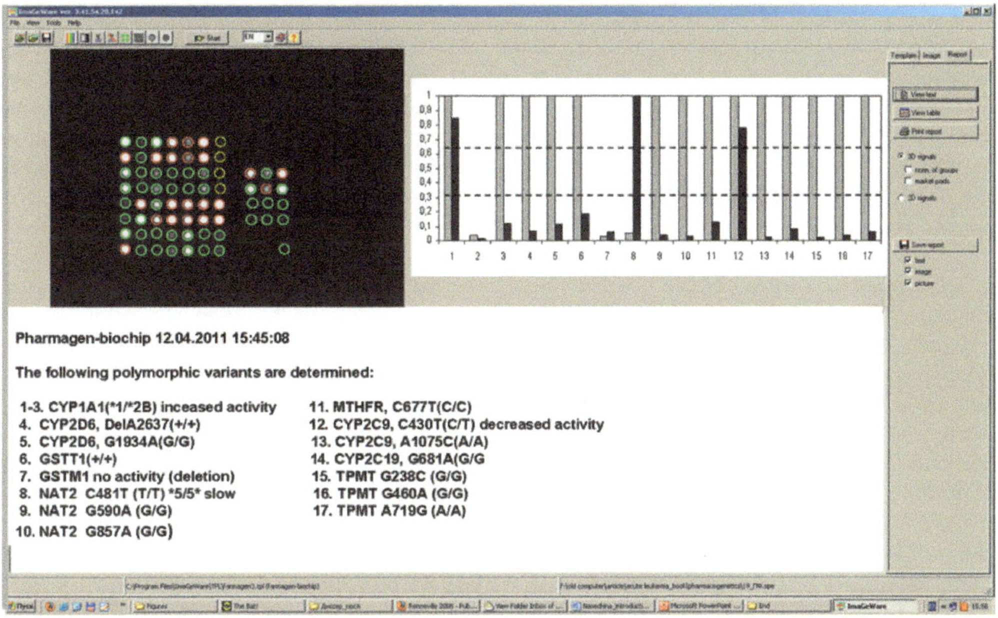

Fig. 4. Image analysis of hybridization pattern. For correct genotype assignment the average signals from two upper and two lower drops in each column are divided on the strongest signal and normalized signals are compared (*see diagram on the right*). Two threshold lines are used to distinguish between homozygotes and heterozygotes. For homozygotes one signal from wild-type or mutant allele is maximal and another should not exceed the lower threshold. The discrimination between positive and negative signals is more than 5 fold. For heterozygotes both signals from wild-type and mutant alleles should not descend below the upper threshold.

many variant alleles of TPMT have been identified, three account for more than 95% of inherited TPMT deficiency: *TPMT**2 (238G>C), *TPMT**3A (460G>A, 719A>G) and *TPMT**3C (719A>G) (Krynetski & Evans, 2003). It was demonstrated that specific TPMT variants have low activity due to aggregation of variant proteins, providing a structural explanation for the observed differences in TPMT activity (Wang et al., 2005). The patients with very low or undetectable TPMT activity are at high risk of severe, potentially fatal hematopoietic toxicity when they are treated with standard doses of thiopurines (Evans et al., 1991). At the same time they also have relatively lower levels of residual leukemic blasts and may be at lower risk of relapse (Lennard et al., 1990). The *TPMT* heterozygotes display a phenotype intermediate between the two homozygous states (Evans et al., 2001). Because of these data, the prospective testing of *TPMT* gene status in ALL patients is recommended to allow preventive dosage reductions in those with low enzyme activity to minimize the treatment toxicity. In some trials patients heterozygous for TPMT-deficient alleles received reduced 6MP dose, but the risk of relapse is not higher than for those with wild type TPMT, who were treated with full dose (Relling et al., 2006; Evans et al., 1998).

The most frequent *TPMT* gene mutations leading to enzyme deficiency in Russian population were analyzed using biochips (Nasedkina et al., 2006). The genotyping of patients included DNA isolation from peripheral blood leukocytes, multiplex PCR, hybridization with the biochip, and image analysis. A total of 446 children with hematologic malignancies were genotyped using the TPMT-biochip (Samochatova et al., 2009). Of 241 patients with ALL for whom molecular analysis has been performed, 18 patients (7.5%) were heterozygous carriers of polymorphic alleles with deficient enzyme activity. The most frequent deficient allele was *TPMT**3A (2.3%), while more rare alleles were *TPMT**3C (0.4%) and *TPMT**2 (0.1%); the wild-type allele *TPMT**1 accounted for 97.2%. Thus, spectrum of *TPMT* deficient alleles and their frequencies in Russian children with leukemia was close to those in European populations and in white population of USA. A retrospective analysis of the 6-MP therapy intolerance stratified by *TPMT* genotype was carried out using the TPMT-biochip. Dosages were adjusted to keep the WBC count between 2 and $3x10^9/Lm$, but not on the basis of *TPMT* genotype. Eighteen ALL patients heterozygous for *TPMT* deficient allele were characterized by decreased ability to tolerate the 6-MP therapy, and as a result they received significantly lower doses of this drug compared with patients with a homozygous wild-type genotype (average weekly dose of 6-MP was 264 vs 312 mg/m^2 respectively; p = 0,04). Also they received more erythrocyte and thrombocyte transfusions and had more infectious episodes. Despite all deviations from protocol, the results of treatment did not differ significantly between patients who did and did not have the *TPMT* gene variations. An EFS estimate was 90% for patients with variations and 83% for patients with wild-type genotype at a median follow-up of 31.3 months (p= 0,562). It may be explained by a fact that the treatment levels of intracellular TGN (the active metabolite of 6MP) were achieved in both cases, regardless *TPMT* genotype. Thus, *TPMT* genotyping can be highly recommended to those patients treated with 6MP, who is found to have repeated episodes of prolonged cytopenia, to adjust an individual drug dosage (Samochatova et al., 2009).

2.4.3 Polymorphism of drug-metabolizing enzyme genes and risk of relapse in ALL

Other different polymorphic enzyme variants that have decreased or increased activity can potentially modulate clinical response to anticancer therapy. This may lead to increased toxicity of the treatment, but also to the development of drug resistance or increased risk of relapse or secondary tumor development (Balta et al., 2003; Krajinovic et al., 2002; Rocha et al., 2005). The most important enzymes of phase I biotransformation enzymes, cytochromes of the P450 family (*CYP1A1, CYP2D6, CYP2C9,* and *CYP2C19*), which activate xenobiotics to yield genotoxic intermediates, and phase II enzymes, such as glutathione S-transferases (GSTs) and arylamine *N*-acetyltransferases (NATs), which convert genotoxic compounds to nontoxic compounds, were chosen for the analysis.

Using Pharmagen-biochip the frequencies of the polymorphic variants of *CYP1A1, CYP2D6, GSTT1, GSTM1, MTHFR, CYP2C9, CYP2C19,* and *NAT2* in 332 children with acute lymphoblastic leukemia (ALL) were determined. Among them, 258 patients with primary leukemia, having no relapse within 1 year of therapy, and 74 with relapse were included in the study. Our results demonstrated that some allelic variants of the drug-metabolizing genes were associated with a higher risk of relapse in childhood acute leukemia (Fig. 5). The association of polymorphic variant *CYP1A1*2A* with poor therapeutic prognosis has been shown in children with ALL (OR = 2.3, 95% CI = 1.09 – 4.8, p = 0.03) (Gra et al., 2009). Also it was found that the *GSTT1* null genotype occurred rarely in children with relapse as compared with those with one or two functional alleles (OR = 0.48, 95% CI = 0.26 – 0.90, p = 0.02), thus being protective. The presence of both risk genotypes has an additive effect: the frequency of relapse was higher among carriers of the combined *CYP1A1 *1/*2A* and *GSTT1* non-null genotype (OR = 2.36, CI = 1.02 - 5.46, p = 0.048).

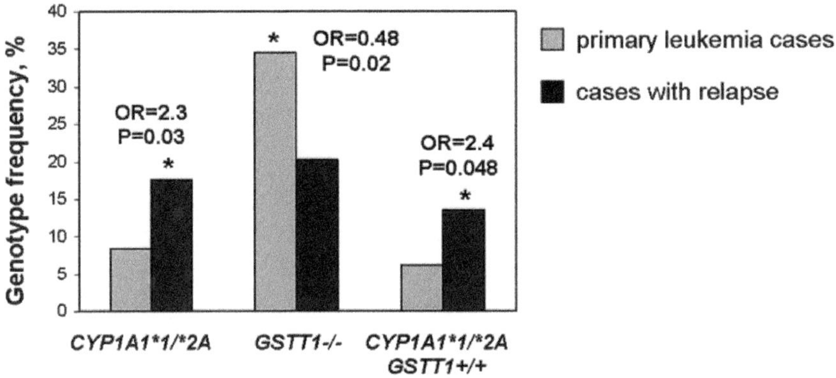

Fig. 5. The genotype frequencies in primary leukemia and relapsed patients with pediatric ALL (statistically significant difference is marked by asterisk).

The observed regularities corresponded to published data (Anderer et al., 2000; Stanulla et al., 2000; Voso et al., 2005). An increase in frequency of the *CYP1A1* genotype **1/*2A* in children with ALL relapse may be explained by the impact of synthetic glucocorticoids (such as dexametasone and prednisolone) being an important component of the ALL treatment protocol and induction therapy. They cause lymphopenia and involution of lymphoid tissue that lead to immunosuppression. The increased enzymatic activity of the *CYP1A1 *1/*2A* leads to the increased concentration of intermediate genotoxic metabolites and of total mutagenic activity (Voso et al., 2005). Since the formation of additional mutations may cause resistance of cancer cells towards therapy, it is likely that the *CYP1A1 *1/*2A* genotype may decrease the efficacy of therapy and promote the development of relapse. GSTs are involved in metabolism of many antitumor drugs, catalyzing conjugation of intermediate metabolites with reduced glutathione. The ALL children carrying *GSTT1* null genotype have been observed to respond well to induction therapy with prednisone, while carriers of at least one functional *GSTT1* allele displayed glucocorticoid resistance, a poor response to therapy, and a higher relapse rate (Anderer et al., 2000). It is likely, that in carriers of the *GSTT1* and/or *GSTM1* null genotype, lack of GSTT1 and/or GSTM1 enzymes leads to an accumulation of cytotoxic drugs that may enhance their efficacy and longer relapse-free survival.

3. Conclusion

The modern diagnostics of leukemia is multifaceted, including clinical characterization, histochemistry, cell morphology, immunophenotyping and also molecular genetic analysis. Molecular markers, recurrent chromosome aberrations and gene mutations, allow subdividing leukemia patients into biological groups with unique clinical features. The risk-stratification of patients based on genetics of leukemia blasts contributes not only to classification of leukemia subtypes, but can predict prognosis and clinical outcome. The molecular genetic analysis provides clinicians with an important knowledge for a decision making and a choice of appropriate therapy. Further progress in therapy of oncologic diseases is inseparable from individualization of the treatment based on the molecular characteristics of malignant cells and genetic features of a patient. An introduction of new technologies in routine clinical practice can significantly increase the power of modern diagnostics. Low-density gel-based biochips are a good example of such a technology. The diagnostic biochips may provide easily, rapid genotyping in clinics and be a useful tool in large screening programs. The properties of gel-based biochips are defined by immobilization in 3D-volume of hydrogel: high concentration of probe due to immobilization capacity of gel and high level of fluorescent signal enabling usage of a simple detecting device, like a portable biochip analyzer. Although hybridization on 2D-microarrays is slightly faster, gel-based biochips provide better discrimination between perfect and imperfect duplexes (5- to 20-fold difference). Thus, unambiguous interpretation of results is attained that can be crucial for clinical diagnostics. Different genetic abnormalities may be identified successfully with diagnostic biochips: from balanced translocations forming fusion genes to gene mutations or polymorphic variants.

4. Acknowledgment

The authors are thankful to their colleagues from the Laboratory for biological microchips of Engelhardt Institute of Molecular Biology, Russian Academy of Sciences, and to clinicians of Russian Children Clinical Hospital and other clinics for their invaluable contribution to the studies. The work was supported by the Russian Foundation for Basic Research (projects 08-04-01480 and 11-04-01950).

5. References

Ahn, JY., Seo, K., Weinberg, O., Boyd, SD., & Arber, DA. (2009). A comparison of two methods for screening *CEBPA* mutations in patients with acute myeloid leukemia. *J. Mol. Diagn.* Vol.11, No.4, pp. 319–323, ISSN 1525-1578

Anderer, G., Schrappe, M., Brechlin, AM., Brechlin, AM., Lauten, M., Muti, P., Welte, K., & Stanulla, M. (2000). Polymorphisms within glutathione S-transferase genes and initial response to glucocorticoids in childhood acute lymphoblastic leukaemia. *Pharmacogenetics*. Vol.10, No.8, pp.715-26, ISSN 0960-314X

Aparicio, SA., & Huntsman, DG. (2010). Does massively parallel DNA resequencing signify the end of histopathology as we know it? *J. Pathol.* Vol.220, No.2, pp. 307–315, ISSN 0022-3417

Arico, M., Valsecchi, MG., Camitta, B., Schrappe, M., Chessells, J., Baruchel, A., Gaynon, P., Silverman, L., Janka-Schaub, G., Kamps, W., Pui, CH., & Masera, G. (2000). Outcome of treatment in children with Philadelphia chromosome-positive acute lymphoblastic leukemia. *N Engl J Med* Vol.342, No.14, pp. 998–1006, ISSN 1533-4406

Armstrong, SA., Staunton, JE., Silverman, LB., Pieters, R., den Boer, ML., Minden, MD., Sallan, SE., Lander, ES., Golub, TR., & Korsmeyer, SJ. (2002). MLL translocations specify a distinct gene expression profile that distinguishes a unique leukemia. *Nat Genet.* Vol.30, No.1, pp.41–7, ISSN 1061-4036

Aspland, S., Bendall, H., & Murre, C. (2001). The role of E2A-PBX1 in leukemogenesis. *Oncogene*; Vol.20, No.40, pp.5708-5717. ISSN 0950-9232

Bacher, U., Kohlmann, A., & Haferlach, T. (2009). Perspectives of gene expression profiling for diagnosis and therapy in haematological malignancies. *Brief Funct. Genomic Proteomic.* Vol.8, No.3, pp. 184–193, ISSN 2041-2649

Balta, G., Yuksek N., Ozyurek, E., Ertem, U., Hicsonmez G., Altay, C., & Gurgey, A. (2003). Characterization of MTHFR, GSTM1, GSTT1, GSTP1, and CYP1A1 genotypes in childhood acute leukemia. *Am J Hematol*. Vol.73, No.3, pp.154-60, ISSN 0361-8609

Braziel, RM., Shipp, MA., Feldman., AL, Espina, V., Winters, M., Jaffe, ES., Petricoin, EF., & Liotta LA. (2003). Molecular diagnostics. Hematology Am Soc Hematol Educ Program. pp.279-93, ISSN 1520-4391

Breit, S., Stanulla, M., Flohr, T., Schrappe, M., Ludwig, WD., Tolle, G., Happich, M., Muckenthaler, MU., & Kulozik, AE. (2006). Activating NOTCH1 mutations predict favorable early treatment response and long-term outcome in childhood precursor T-cell lymphoblastic leukemia. *Blood* Vol. 108, No. 4, pp. 1151–7. ISSN 0006-4971

Brown, P., McIntyre, E., Rau, R., Meshinchi, S., Lacayo, N., Dahl, G., Alonzo, TA., Chang, M., Arceci, RJ., & Small, D. (2007). The incidence and clinical significance of nucleophosmin mutations in childhood AML. Blood. Vol.110, No.3, pp.979-85, ISSN 0006-4971

Brunning, RD., Flandrin, G., Borowitz, M., Swerdlow, SH., & Matutes, E. (2001). WHO histological classification of precursor B cell and T cell neoplasms. In *Pathology and Genetics of Tumours of Haematopoietic and Lymphoid Tissues*, ed. Jaffe, E.S., Harris. N.L., Stein, H., Vardiman, J.W., pp. 110–17. Lyon: IARC, 2001.

Bullinger, L., Dohner, K., Bair, E., Frųhling, S., Schlenk, RF., Tibshirani, R., Dųhner, H., & Pollack, JR. (2004). Use of gene-expression profiling to identify prognostic subclasses in adult acute myeloid leukemia. *N. Engl. J. Med.* Vol.350, No.16, pp.1605–1616, ISSN 0028-4793

Cairoli, R., Beghini, A., Grillo, G., Nadali, G., Elice, F., Ripamonti, CB., Colapietro, P., Nichelatti, M., Pezzetti, L., Lunghi, M., Cuneo, A., Viola, A., Ferrara, F., Lazzarino, M., Rodeghiero, F., Pizzolo, G., Larizza, L., & Morra, E. (2006). Prognostic impact of *c-KIT* mutations in core binding factor leukemias: an Italian retrospective study. *Blood.* Vol.107, No.9, pp. 3463–3468, ISSN 0006-4971

Cazzaniga, G., Dell'Oro, MG., Mecucci, C., Giarin, E., Masetti, R., Rossi, V., Locatelli, F., Martelli, MF., Basso, G., Pession, A., Biondi, A., & Falini, B. (2005). Nucleophosmin mutations in childhood acute myelogenous leukemia with normal karyotype. Blood. Aug 15; Vol.106, No.4, pp.1419-22, ISSN 0006-4971

Davies, SM., Bhatia, S., Ross, JA., Kiffmeyer, WR., Gaynon, PS., Radloff, GA., Robison, LL., & Perentesis, JP. (2002). Glutathione S-transferase genotypes, genetic susceptibility, and outcome of therapy in childhood acute lymphoblastic leukemia. *Blood.* Vol.100, No.1, pp.67-71, ISSN 0006-4971

Davies, SM., & Mehta, PA. (2010). Pediatric acute lymphoblastic leukemia: is their still a role for transplant. *Hematol. Am. Soc. Hematol. Educ. Program.* pp. 363-367, ISSN 1466-4860

Dohner, K., Schlenk, RF., Habdank, M., Scholl, C., Rьcker, FG., Corbacioglu, A., Bullinger, L., Frцhling, S., & Dцhner, H. (2005). Mutant nucleophosmin (*NPM1*) predicts favorable prognosis in younger adults with acute myeloid leukemia and normal cytogenetics: interaction with other gene mutations. *Blood.* Vol.106, No. 12, pp.3740–3746, ISSN 0006-4971

Dordelmann, M., Reiter, A., Borkhardt, A., Ludwig, WD., Gцtz, N., Viehmann, S., Gadner, H., Riehm, H., & Schrappe, M. (1999). Prednisone response is the strongest predictor of treatment outcome in infant acute lymphoblastic leukemia. *Blood.* Vol.94, No.4, pp.1209–17. ISSN 0006-4971

Dou, Y., & Hess, JL. (2008). Mechanisms of transcriptional regulation by MLL and its disruption in acute leukemia. *Int. J. Hematol.* Vol.87, No.1, pp.10–18, ISSN: 0925-5710

Duchayne, E., Fenneteau, O., Pages MP., Sainty D., Arnoulet C., Dastugue N., Garand R., Flandrin G., Groupe Franзais d'Hйmatologie Cellulaire, & Groupe Franзais de Cytogйnйtique Hйmatologique. (2003). Acute megakaryoblastic leukaemia: a national clinical and biological study of 53 adult and childhood cases by the Groupe Francais d'Hematologie Cellulaire (GFHC). *Leuk. Lymphoma.* Vol.44, No.1, pp. 49–58, ISSN 1042-8194

Eguchi, M., Eguchi-Ishimae, M., & Greaves, M. (2005). Molecular pathogenesis of MLL-associated leukemias. *Int J Hematol.* Vol.82, No.1, pp.9-20, ISSN 0925-5710

Eklund, EA. (2010). Genomic analysis of acute myeloid leukemia: potential for new prognostic indicators. *Curr. Opin. Hematol.* Vol.17, No.2, pp.75–78, ISSN 1065-6251

Evans, WE., Horner, M., Chu, YQ., Kalwinsky, D., & Roberts, WM. (1991). Altered mercaptopurine metabolism, toxic effects, and dosage requirement in a thiopurine methyltransferase-deficient child with acute lymphocytic leukemia. *J Pediatr.* Vol.119, No.6, pp.985-9, ISSN 0192-8562

Evans, WE., Relling, MV., Rodman, JH., Crom, WR., Boyett, JM., & Pui, CH. (1998). Conventional compared with individualized chemotherapy for childhood acute lymphoblastic leukemia. *N Engl J Med.* Vol.338, No.8, pp.499-505, ISSN 0028-4793

Evans, WE., Hon, YY., Bomgaars, L., Coutre, S., Holdsworth, M., Janco, R., Kalwinsky, D., Keller, F., Khatib, Z., Margolin, J., Murray, J., Quinn, J., Ravindranath, Y., Ritchey, K., Roberts, W., Rogers, ZR., Schiff, D., Steuber, C., Tucci, F., Kornegay, N., Krynetski, EY., & Relling, MV. (2001). Preponderance of thiopurine S-methyltransferase deficiency and heterozygosity among patients intolerant to mercaptopurine or azathioprine. *J Clin Oncol.* Vol.19, No.8, pp.2293-301, ISSN 0732–183X

Evans, WE., & McLeod, HL. (2003). Pharmacogenomics -- drug disposition, drug targets, and side effects. *N Engl J Med.* Vol.348, No.6, pp.538-49, ISSN 0028-4793

Falini, B., Mecucci, C., Tiacci, E., Alcalay, M., Rosati, R., Pasqualucci, L., La Starza, R., Diverio, D., Colombo, E., Santucci, A., Bigerna, B., Pacini, R., Pucciarini, A., Liso A., Vignetti, M., Fazi, P., Meani, N., Pettirossi, V, Saglio, G., Mandelli, F., Lo-Coco, F., Pelicci, PG., Martelli MF., & GIMEMA Acute Leukemia Working Party. (2005). Cytoplasmic nucleophosmin in acute myelogenous leukemia with a normal karyotype. *N Engl J Med.* Vol.352, No.3, pp.254–266, ISSN 0028-4793

Falini, B., Sportoletti, P., & Martelli, MP. (2009). Acute myeloid leukemia with mutated *NPM1*: diagnosis, prognosis and therapeutic perspectives. *Curr. Opin. Oncol.* Vol.21, No.6, pp. 573–581, ISSN 1040-8746

Fleury, I., Primeau, M., Doreau, A., Costea, I., Moghrabi, A., Sinnett, D., & Krajinovic, M. (2004). Polymorphisms in genes involved in the corticosteroid response and the outcome of childhood acute lymphoblastic leukemia. *Am J Pharmacogenomics.* Vol.4, No.5, pp.331-41 ISSN 1462-2416

Frost, BM., Froestier, E., Gustafsson, G., Nygren, P., Hellebostad, M., Jonsson, OG., Kanerva, J., Schmiegelow, K., Larsson, R., & Lцnnerholm, G.. (2004). Translocation t(12;21) is related to in vitro cellular drug sensitivity to doxorubicin and etoposide in childhood acute lymphoblastic leukemia. *Blood.* Vol.104, No.8, pp.2452–7, ISSN 0006-4971

Gaidzik, V., & Dohner, K. (2008). Prognostic implications of gene mutations in acute myeloid leukemia with normal cytogenetics. *Semin. Oncol.* Vol.35, No.4, pp.346–355, ISSN 0093-7754

Gra, O.A., Kozhekbaeva, Zh.M., Makarova, O.V., Samochatova, H.V., & Nasedkina, T.V. (2009). Polymorphism of biotransformation genes and risk of relapse in childhood acute leukemia. *Balkan Journal of Medical Genetics.* Vol. 12, No. 1, pp. 21-35, ISSN 1311-0160

Graux, C., Cools, J., Michaux, L., Vandenberghe, P., & Hagemeijer A. (2006). Cytogenetics and molecular genetics of T-cell acute lymphoblastic leukemia: from thymocyte to lymphoblast. *Leukemia.* Vol.20, No.9, pp.1496–510, ISSN 0887-6924

Grimwade, D., & Hills, RK. (2009). Independent prognostic factors for AML outcome. *Hematol. Am. Soc. Hematol. Educ. Program.* pp. 385–395. ISSN 1466-4860

Grisendi, S., Mecucci, C., Falini, B., & Pandolfi, PP. (2006). Nucleophosmin and cancer. *Nat. Rev. Cancer* Vol. 6, No.7, pp. 493–505, ISSN 1474-175X

Guidez, F., Ivins, S., Zhu, J., Soderstrom, M., Waxman, S., & Zelent, A. (1998). Reduced retinoic acid-sensitivities of nuclear receptor corepressor binding to PML- and PLZF-RARa underlie molecular pathogenesis and treatment of acute promyelocytic leukemia. *Blood* Vol.91, No.8, pp.2634–2642, ISSN 0006-4971

Haferlach, T., Kern, W., Schnittger, S., & Schoch C. (2005). Modern diagnostics in acute leukemias. *Crit Rev Oncol Hematol.* Vol.56, No.2, pp.223-34, ISSN 1040-8428

Haferlach, T., Kohlmann, A., Wieczorek, L., Basso, G., Kronnie, GT., Bйпй, MC., De Vos, J., Hernбndez, JM., Hofmann, WK., Mills, KI., Gilkes, A., Chiaretti, S., Shurtleff, SA., Kipps, TJ., Rassenti, LZ., Yeoh, AE., Papenhausen, PR., Liu, WM., Williams, PM., & Foa, R. (2010). Clinical utility of microarray-based gene expression profiling in the diagnosis and subclassification of leukemia: report from the International Microarray Innovations in Leukemia Study Group. *J. Clin. Oncol.* Vol.28, No.15, pp.2529–2537, ISSN 0732-183X

Heerema, NA., Sather, HN., Sensel, MG., Zhang, T., Hutchinson, RJ., Nachman, JB., Lange, BJ., Steinherz, PG., Bostrom, BC., Reaman, GH., Gaynon, PS., & Uckun, FM. (2000). Prognostic impact of trisomies of chromosomes 10, 17, and 5 among children with acute lymphoblastic leukemia and high hyperdiploidy (>50 chromosomes). *J Clin Oncol.* Vol.18, No.9, pp.1876–87, ISSN 0732-183X

Heerema-McKenney, A., & Arber, DA. (2009). Acute myeloid leukemia. *Hematol. Oncol. Clin. North Am.* Vol.23, No.4, pp. 633–654, ISSN 0889-8588

Hilden, JM., Dinndorf, PA., Meerbaum, SO., Sather, H., Villaluna, D., Heerema, NA., McGlennen, R., Smith, FO., Woods, WG., Salzer, WL., Johnstone, HS., Dreyer, Z., Reaman, GH., & Children's Oncology Group. (2006). Analysis of prognostic factors of acute lymphoblastic leukemia in infants: report on CCG 1953 from the Children's Oncology Group. *Blood.* Vol.108, No.2, pp. 441- 451., ISSN 0006-4971

Huret, JL. (2011). MLL (myeloid/lymphoid or mixed lineage leukemia). *Atlas of Genetics and Cytogenetics in Oncology and Haematology.* http://atlasgeneticsoncology.org/Genes/MLL.html

Kaspers, GJ., Smets, LA., Pieters, R., Van Zantwijk, CH., Van Wering, ER., & Veerman, AJ. (1995). Favorable prognosis of hyperdiploid common acute lymphoblastic leukemia may be explained by sensitivity to antimetabolites and other drugs: results of an in vitro study. *Blood.* Vol.85, No.3, pp.751–6, ISSN 0006-4971

Keefe, JG., Sukov, WR., Knudson RA., Nguyen, LP., Williamson, C., Sinnwell, JP., & Ketterling RP. (2010). Development of five dual-color, doublefusion fluorescence *in situ* hybridization assays for the detection of common MLL translocation partners. *J. Mol. Diagn.* Vol.12, No.4, pp., 441–452, ISSN 1525-1578

Kharas, MG., & Fruman, DA. (2005). ABL oncogenes and phosphoinositide 3-kinase: mechanism of activation and downstream effectors. *Cancer Res.* Vol. 65, No.6, pp.2047-53, ISSN 0008-5472

Kishi, S., Yang, W., Boureau, B., Morand, S., Das, S., Chen, P., Cook, EH., Rosner, GL., Schuetz, E., Pui, CH., & Relling, MV. (2004). Effects of prednisone and genetic polymorphisms on etoposide disposition in children with acute lymphoblastic leukemia. *Blood.* Vol.103, No.1, pp.67-72, ISSN 0006-4971

Kohlmann, A., Bullinger, L., Thiede, C., Schaich, M., Schnittger, S., Dцhner, K., Dugas, M., Klein, HU., Dцhner, H., Ehninger, G., & Haferlach, T. (2010). Gene expression profiling in AML with normal karyotype can predict mutations for molecular markers and allows novel insights into perturbed biological pathways. *Leukemia* Vol.24, No.6, pp.1216–1220, ISSN 0887-6924

Krajinovic, M., Labuda, D., Mathonnet, G., Labuda, M., Moghrabi, A., Champagne, J., & Sinnett, D. (2002). Polymorphisms in genes encoding drugs and xenobiotic metabolizing enzymes, DNA repair enzymes, and response to treatment of childhood acute lymphoblastic leukemia. *Clin Cancer Res.* Vol.8, No.3, pp.802-10, ISSN 1078-0432

Krynetski, E., & Evans, WE. (2003). Drug methylation in cancer therapy: lessons from the TPMT polymorphism. *Oncogene.* Vol.22, No.47, pp.7403-13, ISSN 0950-9232

Kuznetsova, V., Vasiliskov, V., Antonova, O., Mikhaнlovich, V., Zasedatelev, A., & Chudinov, A. (2008). New indodicarbocyanine dyes for the biological microchip technology. *Bioorg Khim.* Vol.34, No.1, pp.141-4 [In Russian], ISSN 0132-3423

Lennard, L., Lilleyman, JS., Van Loon, J., & Weinshilboum, RM. (1990). Genetic variation in response to 6-mercaptopurine for childhood acute lymphoblastic leukaemia. *Lancet.* Vol.336, No.8709, pp.225-9, ISSN 0140-6736

Look, AT. (1997). Oncogenic transcription factors in the human acute leukemias. *Science.* Vol.278, No.5340, pp.1059-64, ISSN 0036-8075

Maroc, N., Morel, A., Beillard, E., De La Chapelle, AL., Fund, X., Mozziconacci, MJ., Dupont, M., Cayuela, JM., Gabert, J., Koki, A., Fert, V., & Hermitte, F. (2004). A diagnostic biochip for the comprehensive analysis of MLL translocations in acute leukemia. *Leukemia*. Vol.18, No.9, pp.1522-30, ISSN 0887-6924

Mead, AJ., Linch, DC., Hills, RK., Wheatley, K., Burnett, AK., & Gale, RE. (2007). *FLT3* tyrosine kinase domain mutations are biologically distinct from and have a significantly more favorable prognosis than *FLT3* internal tandem duplications in patients with acute myeloid leukemia. *Blood*. Vol.110, No.4, pp.1262–1270, ISSN 0006-4971

Meani, N., & Alcalay, M. (2009). Role of nucleophosmin in acute myeloid leukemia. *Expert Rev. Anticancer Ther*. Vol. 9, No. 9, pp. 1283–1294, ISSN 1473-7140

Meshinchi, S, & Appelbaum, FR. (2009). Structural and functional alterations of FLT3 in acute myeloid leukemia. *Clin. Cancer Res*. Vol.15, No.13, pp.4263–4269, ISSN 1078-0432

Mikhailovich, V., Gryadunov, D., Kolchinsky, A., Makarov, A., & Zasedatelev, A. (2008). DNA microarrays in the clinic: infectious diseases. *Bioessays*. Vol.30, No.7, pp.673-82, ISSN 0265-9247

Mitelman, F., Johansson, B., & Merrens, F. (Eds). Reccurent chromosome aberrations in cancer. http://cgap.nci.nih.gov/Chromosomes/Mitelman

Mitiaeva, ON., Nasedkina, TV., Zharinov, VS., Isaeva, EA., Turygin, AIu., Chupeeva, VV., Kreĭndlin, E., & Mirzabekov, A. (2004). Analysis of chromosome translocations involving MLL by hybridization with an oligonucleotide microarray. *Mol Biol* [in Russian] Vol.38, No.3, pp.449-56, ISSN 0026-8984

Möricke, A., Reiter, A., Zimmermann, M., Gadner, H., Stanulla, M., Dцrdelmann, M., Lцning, L., Beier, R., Ludwig, WD., Ratei, R., Harbott, J., Boos, J., Mann, G., Niggli, F., Feldges, A., Henze, G., Welte, K., Beck, JD., Klingebiel, T., Niemeyer, C., Zintl, F., Bode, U., Urban, C., Wehinger, H., Niethammer, D., Riehm, H., Schrappe, M., & German-Austrian-Swiss ALL-BFM Study Group. (2008). Risk-adjusted therapy of acute lymphoblastic leukemia can decrease treatment burden and improve survival: treatment results of 2169 unselected pediatric and adolescent patients enrolled in the trial ALL-BFM 95. *Blood*. Vol.111, No.9, pp.4477-89, ISSN 0006-4971

Nachman, JB., Heerema, NA., Sather H, Camitta., B, Forestier, E., Harrison, CJ., Dastugue, N., Schrappe, M., Pui CH., Basso, G., Silverman, LB., & Janka-Schaub, GE. (2007). Outcome of treatment in children with hypodiploid acute lymphoblastic leukemia. *Blood*. Vol.110, No.4, pp. 1112–5. ISSN 0006-4971

Nachman, JB., La, MK., Hunger, SP., Heerema, NA., Gaynon, PS., Hastings, C., Mattano, LA Jr., Sather, H., Devidas, M., Freyer, DR., Steinherz, PG., & Seibel, NL. (2009). Young adults with acute lymphoblastic leukemia have an excellent outcome with chemotherapy alone and benefit from intensive postinduction treatment: a report from the children's oncology group. *J Clin Oncol*. Vol.27, No.31, pp. 5189–5194, ISSN 0732-183X

Nasedkina, TV., Zharinov, VS., Isaeva, EA., Mityaeva, ON., Yurasov, RN., Surzhikov, SA., Turigin, AY., Rubina, AY., Karachunskii, AI., Gartenhaus, RB., & Mirzabekov, AD. (2003). Clinical screening of gene rearrangements in childhood leukemia by using a multiplex polymerase chain reaction-microarray approach. *Clin Cancer Res.* Vol.9, No.15, pp.5620-9, ISSN ISSN 1078-0432

Nasedkina, T.V., Fedorova, O.E., Glotov, A.S., Chupova, N.V., Samochatova E.V., Maiorova O.A., Zemlyakova, V.V., Roudneva, A.E., Chudinov, A.V., Yurasov, A.E., Kozhekbaeva, J.M., Barsky, V.E., Krusnetskiy, E.Y., Krusnetskaia, N.F., Cheng, Ch., Ribeiro, R.C., Evans, W.E., Roumyantsev, A.G., & Zasedatelev, A.S. (2006). Rapid genotyping of common deficient thiopurine S-methyltransferase (TPMT) alleles using the DNA-microchip technique. *Eur. J. Human Genetics.* Vol.14, No.9, pp. 991-998, ISSN 1018-4813

Nasedkina, T., Guseva, N., Gra, O., Mityaeva, O., Chudinov, A., & Zasedatelev, A. (2009). Diagnostic Microarrays in hematologic oncology. *Molecular Diagnosis and Therapy.* Vol.13, No.2, pp.1-12, ISSN 1177-1062

Pallisgaard, N., Hokland, P., Riishoj, DC., Pedersen, B., & Jııırgensen, P. (1998). Multiplex reverse transcription-polymerase chain reaction for simultaneous screening of 29 translocations and chromosomal aberrations in acute leukemia. *Blood.* Vol.92, No.2, pp.574-88, ISSN 0006-4971

Peterson, LF., & Zhang, DE. (2004). The (8;21) translocation in leukemogenesis. *Oncogene* Vol.23, No.24, pp. 4255–4262, ISSN 0950-9232

Pieters, R., den Boer, ML., Durian, M., Janka, G., Schmiegelow, K., Kaspers, GJ., van Wering, ER., & Veerman, AJ. (1998). Relation between age, immunophenotype and in vitro drug resistance in 395 children with acute lymphoblastic leukemia—implications for treatment of infants. *Leukemia.* Vol.12, No.9, pp. 1344–8, ISSN 0887-6924

Pieters, R., Schrappe, M., De Lorenzo, P., Hann, I., De Rossi, G., Felice, M., Hovi, L., LeBlanc, T., Szczepanski, T., Ferster, A., Janka, G., Rubnitz, J., Silverman, L., Stary, J., Campbell, M., Li, CK., Mann, G., Suppiah, R., Biondi, A., Vora, A., & Valsecchi, MG. (2007). A treatment protocol for infants younger than 1 year with acute lymphoblastic leukaemia (Interfant-99): and observational study and a multicentre randomised trial. *Lancet.* Vol.370, No.9583, pp. 240–50, ISSN 0140-6736

Pollard, JA., Alonzo, TA., Gerbing, RB., Gerbing, RB., Miller, KL., Pollard, JA., Stirewalt, DL., Heerema, NA., Raimondi, SC., Hirsch, B., Franklin, JL., Lange, B., & Meshinchi, S. (2010). Prevalence and prognostic significance of *KIT* mutations in pediatric patients with core binding factor AML enrolled on serial pediatric cooperative trials for *de novo* AML. *Blood.* Vol.115, No.12, pp. 2372–2379, ISSN 0006-4971

Pui, CH, Boyett, JM, Rivera, GK, Hancock, ML, Sandlund, JT, Ribeiro, RC, Rubnitz, JE, Behm, FG, Raimondi, SC, Gajjar, A, Razzouk, B, Campana, D, Kun, LE, Relling, MV, & Evans, WE. (2000). Long-term results of total therapy studies 11, 12 and 13A for childhood acute lymphoblastic leukemia at St Jude Children's Research Hospital. *Leukemia.* Vol.14, No.12, pp.2286–94, ISSN 0887-6924

Pui, CH., Gaynon, PS., Boyett, JM., Chessells, JM., Baruchel, A., Kamps, W., Silverman, LB., Biondi, A., Harms, DO., Vilmer, E., Schrappe, M., & Camitta B. (2002). Outcome of treatment in childhood acute lymphoblastic leukaemia with rearrangements of the 11q23 chromosomal region. *Lancet.* Vol.359, No.9321, pp.1909–15, ISSN 0140-6736

Pui, CH., Carroll, WL., Meshinchi, S.,& Arceci, RJ. (2011). Biology, risk stratification, and therapy of pediatric acute leukemias: an update. *J Clin Oncol.* Vol.29, No.5 pp. 551-565, ISSN 0732-183X

Rabbits, TH. (1994). Chromosomal translocations in human cancer. *Nature*. Vol.372, No.6502, pp.143-9, ISSN 0028-0836

Radmacher, MD., Marcucci, G., Ruppert, AS., Mryzek K., Whitman, SP., Vardiman, JW., Paschka, P., Vukosavljevic, T., Baldus, CD., Kolitz, JE., Caligiuri, MA., Larson, RA, Bloomfield, CD., & Cancer and Leukemia Group B. (2006). Independent confirmation of a prognostic gene-expression signature in adult acute myeloid leukemia with a normal karyotype: a Cancer and Leukemia Group B study. *Blood.* Vol.108, No.5, pp.1677–1683, ISSN 0006-4971

Ramakers-van Woerden, NL., Pieters, R., Loonen, AH., Hubeek, I., van Drunen, E., Beverloo, HB., Slater, RM., Harbott, J., Seyfarth, J., van Wering, ER., Hдhlen, K., Schmiegelow, K., Janka-Schaub, GE., & Veerman, AJ. (2000). TEL/AML1 gene fusion is related to in vitro drug sensitivity for L-asparaginase in childhood acute lymphoblastic leukemia. *Blood*. Vol.96, No.3, pp.1094–9. ISSN 0006-4971

Ramakers-van Woerden, NL., Beverloo, HB., Veerman, AJ., Camitta, BM., Loonen, AH., van Wering, ER., Slater, RM., Harbott, J., den Boer, ML., Ludwig, WD., Haas, OA., Janka-Schaub, GE., & Pieters, R. (2004). In vitro drug-resistance profile in infant acute lymphoblastic leukemia in relation to age, MLL rearrangements and immunophenotype. *Leukemia*. Vol.18, No.3, pp.521–9, ISSN 0887-6924

Rau, R., & Brown, P. (2009). Nucleophosmin (*NPM1*) mutations in adult and childhood acute myeloid leukaemia: towards definition of a new leukaemia entity. *Hematol Oncol*. Vol.27, No.4, pp.171-81, ISSN 1543-0790

Relling, MV., Hancock, ML., Boyett, JM., Pui, CH., & Evans, WE. (1999). Prognostic importance of 6-mercaptopurine dose intensity in acute lymphoblastic leukemia. *Blood*. Vol.93, No.9, pp.2817-23, ISSN 0006-4971

Relling, MV., Pui, CH., Cheng, C., & Evans, WE. (2006). Thiopurine methyltransferase in acute lymphoblastic leukemia. *Blood*. Vol.107, No.2, pp.843-4, ISSN 0006-4971

Rennert, H., Golde, T., Wilson, RB., Spitalnik, SL., Van Deerlin, VM., & Leonard, DG. (1999). A novel, non-nested reverse-transcriptase polymerase chain reaction (RT-PCR) test for the detection of the t(15;17) translocation: a comparative study of RT-PCR cytogenetics, and fluorescence *in situ* hybridization. *J. Mol. Diagn.* Vol.4, No.3, pp. 195–209, ISSN 1525-1578

Renneville, A., Roumier, C., Biggio, V., Nibourel, O., Boissel, N., Fenaux, P., & Preudhomme, C. (2008). Cooperating gene mutations in acute myeloid leukemia: a review of the literature. *Leukemia*. Vol.22, No.5, pp.915-31, ISSN 0887-6924

Rocha, JC., Cheng, C., Liu, W., Kishi, S., Das, S., Cook, EH., Sandlund, JT., Rubnitz, J., Ribeiro; R., Campana, D., Pui, CH., Evans, WE., & Relling, MV. (2005). Pharmacogenetics of outcome in children with acute lymphoblastic leukemia. *Blood*. Vol.105, No.12, pp.4752-8, ISSN 0006-4971

Rubina, A., Pan'kov, S., Dementieva, E., Pen'kov D., Butygin A., Vasiliskov V., Chudinov A., Mikheikin A., Mikhailovich V., & Mirzabekov A. (2004). Hydrogel drop microchips with immobilized DNA: properties and methods for large-scale production. *Anal Biochem*. Vol.325, No.1, pp.92-106, ISSN 0003-2697

Rubina, A., Kolchinsky, A., Makarov, A., & Zasedatelev A. (2008). Why 3-D? Gel-based microarrays in proteomics. *Proteomics*. Vol.8, No.4, pp.817-31, ISSN 1615-9861

Rubnitz, JE., Wichlan, D., Devidas, M., Shuster J., Linda SB., Kurtzberg J., Bell B., Hunger SP., Chauvenet A., Pui CH., Camitta B., Pullen J., & Children's Oncology Group. (2008). Prospective analysis of TEL gene rearrangements in childhood acute lymphoblastic leukemia: a Children's Oncology Group study. *J Clin Oncol*. Vol.26, No.13, pp.2186-91, ISSN 0732-183X

Samochatova, E.V., Chupova, N.V., Rudneva, A.E., Makarova, O.A., Nasedkina, T.V., Fedorova, O.E., Glotov, A.S., Kozhekbaeva, Zh.M., Maiorova, O.A., Roumyantsev, A.G., Krynetski, E.Y., Krynetskaia, N.F., Evans, W.E., & Ribeiro, R.C. (2009). TPMT genetic variations in populations of the Russian Federation. *Pediatr Blood Cancer*, Vol.52, No.2, pp.203-208, ISSN 545-5009

Schnittger, S., Schoch, C., Kern, W., Mecucci, C., Tschulik, C., Martelli, MF., Haferlach, T., Hiddemann, W., & Falini B. (2005). Nucleophosmin gene mutations are predictors of favorable prognosis in acutemyelogenous leukemia with a normal karyotype. *Blood* Vol.106, No.12, pp. 3733–3739, ISSN 0006-4971

Schrappe, M., Arico, M., Harbott, J., Biondi A., Zimmermann, M., Conter, V., Reiter, A., Valsecchi, MG., Gadner, H., Basso, G., Bartram, CR., Lampert, F., Riehm, H., & Masera, G. (1998). Philadelphia chromosome-positive (Ph1) childhood acute lymphoblastic leukemia: good initial steroid response allows early prediction of a favorable treatment outcome. *Blood*. Vol.92, No.8, pp.2730–41. ISSN 0006-4971

Scurto, P., Rocha, MH., Kane, JR., Williams, WK., Haney, DM., Conn, WP., Shurtleff, SA., & Downing, JR. (1998). A multiplex RT-PCR assay for the detection of chimeric transcripts encoded by the risk-stratifying translocations of pediatric acute lymphoblastic leukemia. *Leukemia*. Vol.12, No.12, pp.1994-2005, ISSN 0887-6924

Shigesada, K., van de Sluis, B., & Liu, PP. (2004). Mechanism of leukemogenesis by the inv(16) chimeric gene *CBFB/PEBP2B-MHY11. Oncogene* Vol.23, No.24, pp. 4297–4307, ISSN 0950-9232

Shrappe, M. (2004). Evolution of BFM trials for childhood ALL. *Ann Hematol*. Vol.83, No.1, pp.121-3, ISSN 0939-5555

Smith, M., Arthur, D., Camitta, B., Carroll, AJ., Crist, W., Gaynon, P., Gelber, R., Heerema, N., Korn, EL., Link, M., Murphy, S., Pui, CH., Pullen, J., Reamon, G., Sallan, SE., Sather, H., Shuster, J., Simon, R., Trigg, M., Tubergen, D., Uckun, F., & Ungerleider, R. (1996). Uniform approach to risk classification and treatment assignment for children with acute lymphoblastic leukemia. *J Clin Oncol*. Vol.14, No.1, pp. 18–24, ISSN 0732-183X

Stam, RW., den Boer, ML., Meijerink, JP., Ebus, ME., Peters, GJ., Noordhuis, P., Janka-Schaub, GE., Armstrong, SA., Korsmeyer, SJ., & Pieters, R. (2003). Differential mRNA expression of Ara-C-metabolizing enzymes explains Ara-C sensitivity in MLL gene-rearranged infant acute lymphoblastic leukemia. *Blood*. Vol.101, No.4, pp.1270–6. ISSN 0006-4971

Stanulla, M., Schrappe, M., Brechlin, AM., Zimmermann, M., & Welte, K. (2000). Polymorphisms within glutathione S-transferase genes (GSTM1, GSTT1, GSTP1) and risk of relapse in childhood B-cell precursor acute lymphoblastic leukemia: a case-control study. *Blood*. Vol.95, No.4, pp.1222-8, ISSN 0006-4971

Stanulla, M., Schaeffeler, E., Flohr, T., Cario, G., Schrauder, A., Zimmerman, M., Welte, K., Ludwig, WD., Bartram, CR., Zanger, UM., Eichelbaum, M., Schrappe, M., & Schwab, M. (2005). Thiopurine methyltransferase (TPMT) genotype and early treatment response to mercaptopurine in childhood acute lymphoblastic leukemia. *JAMA*. Vol.293, No.12, pp.1485-9, ISSN 0098-7484

Swerdlow, SH. (2008). International Agency for Research on Cancer. *WHO Classification of Tumours of Haematopoietic and Lymphoid Tissues*. International Agency for Research on Cancer, Lyon, France.

Szczepanski, T., Orfao, A., van der Velden, VH., San Miguel, JF., & van Dongen, JJ. (2001). Minimal residual disease in leukaemia patients. *Lancet Oncol* Vol.2, No.7, pp. 409–17, ISSN 1470-2045

Teitell, MA., & Pandolfi, PP. (2009). Molecular genetics of acute lymphoblastic leukemia. *Annu Rev Pathol Mech Dis*. Vol.4, pp. 175-198, ISSN 1553-4014

Thiede, C., Koch, S., & Creutzig, E. (2006). Prevalence and prognostic impact of *NPM1* mutations in 1485 adult patients with acute myeloid leukemia (AML). *Blood*. Vol.107, No.10, pp. 4011–4020, ISSN 0006-4971

Vilmer, E., Suciu, S., Ferster, A., Bertrand, Y., Cavũ, H., Thyss, A., Benoit, Y., Dastugue, N., Fournier, M., Souillet, G., Manel, AM., Robert, A., Nelken, B., Millot, F., Lutz, P., Rialland, X., Mechinaud, F., Boutard, P., Behar, C., Chantraine, JM., Plouvier, E., Laureys, G., Brock, P., Uyttebroeck, A., Margueritte, G., Plantaz, D., Norton, L., Francotte, N., Gyselinck, J., Waterkeyn, C., Solbu, G., Philippe, N., & Otten, J. (2000). Long-term results of three randomized trials (58831, 58832, 58881) in childhood acute lymphoblastic leukemia: a CLCGEORTC report. Children Leukemia Cooperative Group. *Leukemia*. Vol.14, No.12, pp.2257–66, ISSN 0887-6924

Voso, MT., D'Alo, F., Gumiero, D., Guidi, F., Hohaus, S., & Leone, G. (2005). The CYP1A1*2a allele is an independent prognostic factor for acute myeloid leukemia. *Haematologica*. Vol. 90, No.7, pp. 982-984, ISSN 0390-6078

Wang, L., Nguyen, TV., McLaughlin, RW., Sikkink, LA., Ramirez-Alvarado, M., & Weinshilboum, RM. (2005). Human thiopurine S-methyltransferase pharmacogenetics: variant allozyme misfolding and aggresome formation. *Proc Natl Acad Sci USA*. Vol.102 No.26, pp.9394-9, ISSN 0027-8424

Watt, CD., & Bagg, A. Molecular diagnosis of acute myeloid leukemia. (2010). *Expert Rev Mol Diagn*. Vol.10, No. 8, pp. 993-1012, ISSN 1473-7159

Wolff, DJ., Bagg, A., Cooley, LD., Dewald, GW., Hirsch, BA., Jacky, PB., Rao, KW., Rao, PN., Association for Molecular Pathology Clinical Practice Committee, & American College of Medical Genetics Laboratory Quality Assurance Committee. (2007). Guidance for fluorescence *in situ* hybridization testing in hematologic disorders. *J. Mol. Diagn*. Vol.9, No.2, pp. 134–143, ISSN 1525-1578

Yamamoto, Y., Kiyoi, H., Nakano, Y., Suzuki, R., Kodera, Y., Miyawaki, S., Asou, N., Kuriyama, K., Yagasaki, F., Shimazaki, C., Akiyama, H., Saito, K., Nishimura, M., Motoji, T., Shinagawa, K., Takeshita, A., Saito, H., Ueda, R., Ohno, R., & Naoe, T. (2001). Activating mutation of *D835* within the activation loop of *FLT3* in human hematologic malignancies. *Blood*. Vol.97, No.8, pp. 2434–2439, ISSN 0006-4971

Yates, CR., Krynetski, EY., Loennechen, T., Fessing, MY., Tai, HL., Pui, CH., Relling, MV., & Evans, WE. (1997). Molecular diagnosis of thiopurine S-methyltransferase deficiency: genetic basis for azathioprine and mercaptopurine intolera nce. *Ann Intern Med*. Vol.126, No.8, pp.608-14, ISSN 0003-4819

10

Pediatric Natural Killer Cell Malignancy

Yoshiko Hashii
Department of Developmental Medicine, Osaka University Graduate School of Medicine
Japan

1. Introduction

Natural killer (NK) cell malignancy is a heterogeneous disorder and rare, representing <1% of non-Hodgkin lymphomas for most of the world, except in Asia and Latin America. In Asia, especially, the incidence of NK-cell lymphomas is approximately 7%–10% of lymphomas [Au et al., 2005].
The pathogenesis of NK-cell malignancies has not yet been fully elucidated. In the 2008 World Health Organization (WHO) classification of tumors of hematopoietic and lymphoid tissues, there are two entities associated with NK cells: mature T-cell and NK-cell neoplasms (including chronic lymphoproliferative disorder of NK cells, aggressive NK-cell leukemia, and extranodal NK/T-cell lymphoma, nasal type) and NK-cell lymphoblastic leukemia/lymphoma, which is included provisionally in the category of acute leukemias of ambiguous lineage (Table 1) [Swedlow et al., 2008]. What was previously described as blastic NK-cell leukemia is defined as blastic plasmacytoid dendritic cell neoplasm in the WHO 2008 classification [Swedlow et al., 2008]. In pediatric patients, the four NK cell neoplasms are rare, with blastic NK-cell lymphoma being the most prevalent.

- Acute leukemias of ambiguous lineage
  - NK-cell lymphoblastic leukemia/lymphoma
- Mature T-cell and NK-cell neoplasms
  - Chronic lymphoproliferative disorder of NK cells
  - Aggressive NK-cell leukemia
  - Extranodal NK/T-cell lymphoma, nasal type

Table 1. WHO classification of hematopoietic and lymphoid neoplasms associated with NK cells [Swerdlow et al., 2008]

A rigorous review of the literature to date is required to adequately understand and manage the various pediatric NK-cell malignant entities. The clinical characteristics of pediatric cases with these NK-cell malignant entities defined according to the 2008 WHO classification are discussed in this paper and compared to adult cases.

2. Pathology of NK-cell neoplasms in pediatric patients

The 2008 WHO classification of tumors of hematopoietic and lymphoid tissue recognizes four categories of NK-cell neoplasms: NK-cell lymphoblastic leukemia/lymphoma, chronic lymphoproliferative disorder of NK cells, aggressive NK-cell leukemia (ANKL), and extranodal NK/T-cell lymphoma, nasal type (ENKL) (Table 1). NK-cell lymphoblastic leukemia involves immature NK cells, while chronic lymphoblastic leukemia/lymphoma, chronic lymphoproliferative disorder of NK cells, and aggressive NK-cell leukemia are mainly neoplasms of mature NK cells. ENKL is the main neoplasm of mature NK cells. Among the four entities, ANKL and ENKL are associated with Epstein-Barr virus (EBV).

2.1 NK-cell lymphoblastic leukemia/lymphoma

NK-cell lymphoblastic leukemia/lymphoma is a very rare disease in both adults and children. Because of limitations in NK-cell-specific markers, it is included as acute leukemia of ambiguous lineage according to the WHO 2008 classification [Swerdlow et al., 2008]. This neoplasm has been difficult to define. CD56 is the most important and sensitive NK-cell marker, but CD56 is not specific for NK cells. Previously, many cases were reported as NK-cell leukemia because of the expression of CD57 but are plasmacytoid dendritic cell leukemia in the WHO 2008 classification. This issue is discussed below.

2.2 Chronic lymphoproliferative disorder of NK cells

Chronic lymphoproliferative disorder of NK cells is rare, especially in pediatric patients. It occurs in adults at a median age of 60 years. This provisional entity in the WHO 2008 classification is characterized by a persistent (>6 months) increase in peripheral blood NK cells (usually $2 \times 10^9/L$) without a clearly identified cause. It is very difficult to distinguish between neoplastic and reactive NK cells. Cells have an NK-cell phenotype: CD16$^+$, CD56$^+$, CD2$^-$, CD7$^-$, surface CD3 (sCD3)$^-$, and cytoplasmic CD3 (CD3ε)$^+$. Cytotoxic markers including T-cell-restricted intracellular antigen-1 (TIA-1), granzyme B, and granzyme M are positive. EBV is negative. One pediatric case has been reported from China [Kwong et al., 1995]. CD2 was positive and CD3 was weakly positive. EBV status was not described. The case was a 3-year-old female who presented hepatosplenomegaly. She died 11 days after diagnosis because of uncontrolled disease and did not receive chemotherapy. The clinical course of the majority of cases with chronic lymphoproliferative disorder of NK cells shows a good prognosis and transformation to aggressive disease has been rarely reported [Ohno et al., 1998].

2.3 Aggressive NK-cell leukemia

ANKL is a systemic proliferation of NK cells with primary involvement of peripheral blood and bone marrow, and shows a fulminant clinical course. The age distribution of ANKL patients has been reported to show two peaks, one at 20 years and the other at 40 years of age [Suzuki et al., 2004b]. The disease typically affects patients at a younger age compared to other NK-cell malignancies. The clinical features, and cytological and immunohistochemical findings of this rare pediatric NK-cell malignancy are summarized in Tables 2 and 3. EBV is closely associated with the pathogenesis of this disease. Latent EBV shows monoclonality and causes EBV-infected NK-cell lymphoproliferative disease.

2.3.1 Diagnosis

Patients are diagnosed with ANKL when a proliferation of large granular lymphoblasts of an NK-cell phenotype is found in peripheral blood and/or bone marrow exceeding 30% of the total nucleated cells [Suzuki et al., 2004b]. The immunophenotype of ANKL is typically defined by $CD2^+$, $sCD3^-$, $CD3\varepsilon^+$, and $CD56^+$. Loss of CD7 is occasionally observed. This immunophenotype is almost identical to that for extranodal NK/T-cell lymphoma, except for $CD16^+$. T-cell receptor (TCR) genes are in germline configuration. Some cases are $CD11b^+$ and $CD57^-$. These neoplastic cells express FAS ligand and high levels of FAS ligand can found in the serum of affected patients [Kato et al., 1998].

2.3.2 Clinical features and immunohistochemical findings in pediatric and adolescent patients

To date, 19 pediatric and adolescent cases (<19 years of age) have been reported in the literature from 1986 to 2010. Most patients have been reported from Japan and Korea. Table 2 summarizes the clinical findings of these 19 pediatric cases. Median age at diagnosis was 14 years (range, 2–19 years). Gender distribution was equal (9 females and 10 males), which is the same in adult patients. Acute lymphoblastic leukemia typically affects children at 2–6 years of age, while the median age of ANKL patients is generally higher.

Pediatric ANKL patients presented acute and rapidly progressive symptomatology. The most common presenting symptom is fever (12/13, 92%). Hepatomegaly (10/13, 77%), splenomegaly (12/16, 75%), and lymphoadenopathy (6/16, 37%) are also frequently observed. The incidence of these symptoms is almost same as that of adult patients [Yoo et al., 2009]. Two patients (cases 3 and 5) presented a chronic course and spontaneous regression was seen and transformation to ANKL. In adult patients, transformation from chronic lymphoproliferative disorder of NK cells to ANKL has been rarely reported. Pediatric patients manifest features of chronic active EBV infection, leading to overlap with EBV-positive T-cell lymphoproliferative disorders [Suzuki et al., 2004a]. The clinical presentation of ANKL has a resemblance to EBV-associated hemophagocytic lymphohistiocytosis. Chronic active EBV infection occurs predominantly in children and young adults and the incidence of hemophagocytosis as a clinical feature is frequently observed in cases of pediatric ANKL. Hypersensitivity to mosquito bites is sometimes seen as a preceding feature of ANKL in pediatric and adolescent patients.

This disease is typically resistant to chemotherapy and successful treatment has been infrequently reported. The complete response rate is below 20% and 2-year overall survival rate is 5% in adult patients [Suzuki, 2010; Suzuki et al., 2010]. There is insufficient data to interpret complete remission and overall survival rates in pediatric ANKL patients. Results have been unsatisfactory using combination chemotherapy regimens that are typically used for acute lymphoblastic leukemia or non-Hodgkin lymphoma. In adults, chemotherapy with L-asparaginase-containing regimens has been reported to be effective in some cases [Ichikawa et al., 2010]. Among pediatric ANKL cases, only two patients were reported as being alive and one patient died with complete remission, while 13 cases died and one (case 15) died of graft-versus-host disease (GVHD) and infection without relapse. The median survival time for patients who died is 4 months. Two cases received allogeneic stem cell transplantation: one died due to GVHD without disease and one was alive. Chemotherapy with L-asparaginase-containing regimens and subsequent allogeneic stem cell transplantation led to prolonged survival in a few young adult patients, even when the stem cell transplantation was performed in patients who did not have a complete response [Ito et al., 2008]. Better outcome is suggested among patients who received allogeneic stem cell transplantation.

Case	Age/ gender	Fever	Hepato- megaly	Spleno- megaly	Lymph- adenopathy	Other sites	Treatment	Prognosis	Reference
1	6 y/M	+	+	+	+		NHL-BFM 90/Allo-SCT	Alive	Ohnuma et al., 1997
2	14 y/F	+	+	+	+	Skin	VCR/Dox/Cy /CA	Aggressive, died 4 mo	Koizumi et al., 1986
3	13 y/M	ND	ND	+	ND		ND	ND	Kawa-Ha et al., 1989
4	15 y/M	ND	ND	+	ND		ND	ND	Kawa-Ha et al., 1989
5	16 y/F	ND	ND	+	ND		ND	ND	Kawa-Ha et al., 1989
6	16 y/F	+	+	+	–		ND	Aggressive, died 32 mo	Imamura et al., 1990
7	13 y/F	+	+	+	+		ND	Aggressive, died 26 mo	Imamura et al., 1990
8	18 y/M	+	+	+	+	Lung	VDS/THP-ADR/Cy/PSL	Aggressive, died 4 mo	Furuno et al., 1994
9	13 y/M	+	+	+	–		PSL	Aggressive, died 47 d	Kaizu et al., 2004
10	19 y/F	+	+	–	–	HPS	DHAP	Aggressive, died 14 d	Kohrt & Advani, 2004
11	17 y/F	+	+	+	–		COP/BLM	Aggressive, died 1 mo	Suzuki et al., 2004b
12	12 y/M	+	-	-	+	Lung	DNR/Cy/VCR /L-Asp/PSL	Aggressive, died 5 mo	Suzuki et al., 2004b
13	16 y/F	+	+	+	–	Kidney	PSL	Aggressive, died 1 d	Suzuki et al., 2004b
14	18 y/F	+	–	–	+	Tonsil	CHOP/Allo-SCT	Died due to GVHD 39 mo	Suzuki et al., 2004b
15	13 y/M	–	–	+	–		AIEOP-95	Alive, CCR 1447 d	Patel et al., 2010
16	14 y/F	ND	ND	ND	ND		ND	Aggressive, died 1 mo	Yoo et al., 2009
17	2 y/M	ND	ND	ND	ND		ND	Aggressive, died 5 d	Yoo et al., 2009
18	16 y/M	ND	ND	ND	ND		ND	Aggressive, died 11 mo	Yoo et al., 2009
19	5 y/M	+	+	–	–	HPS	HLH2004	Aggressive, died 4 mo	Petterson et al., 2008

Abbreviations: ADR, adriamycin; AIEOP-95, Associazione Italiana Ematologia Oncologia Pediatrica 95 protocol; Allo-SCT, allogeneic stem cell transplantation; BLM, bleomycin; CA, cytarabine; CCR, clinical complete response; CHOP, cyclophosphamide, doxorubicin, vincristine, prednisolone; COP, cyclophosphamide, vincristine, prednisolone; Cy, cyclophosphamide; d, days; DHAP, dexamethasone, high-dose cytarabine, cisplatin; Dox, doxorubicin; F, female; GVHD, graft-versus-host disease; HLH2004, hemophagocytic lymphohistiocytosis 2004 protocol; HPS, hemophagocytosis; L-Asp, L-asparaginase; M, male; mo, months; ND, not determined; NHL-BFM 90, non-Hodgkin lymphoma-Berlin-Frankfurt-Munster 90 protocol; mo, month; PSL, prednisolone; THP-ADR, pirarubicin; VCR, vincristine; VDS, vindesine; y, year.

Table 2. Clinical characteristics of pediatric patients with aggressive NK leukemia

Yoo et al. have reported that CD7 antigen loss is frequently observed among adult ANKL patients and the absence of CD7 may serve as a reliable marker for the diagnosis of ANKL in adults [Yoo et al., 2009]. However, $CD7^{+}$ is shown in 13 of 16 pediatric ANKL patients (Table 3). Immunophenotypic analysis of CD7 expression is therefore not useful in the diagnosis of ANKL in pediatric patients. EBV DNA is detected in almost all pediatric patients.

Case	CD2	CD3ε	sCD3	CD4	CD7	CD8	CD16	CD56	CD57	EBV DNA	Reference
1	+	ND	-	-	+	-	-	+	-	+	Ohnuma et al., 1997
2	+	ND	-	-	ND	-	+	-	-	+	Koizumi et al., 1986
3	+	ND	-	-	ND	-	+	ND	ND	+	Kawa-Ha et al., 1989
4	+	+	-	-	+	-	-	+	ND	+	Kawa-Ha et al., 1989
5	+	ND	-	-	+	-	+	+	ND	+	Kawa-Ha et al., 1989
6	+	ND	-	-	+	-	+	ND	-	ND	Imamura et al., 1990
7	+	ND	-	-	+	-	ND	+	ND	ND	Imamura et al., 1990
8	+	ND	-	-	+	-	+	ND	ND	+	Furuno et al., 1994
9	+	ND	-	ND	+	ND	-	+	-	+	Kaizu et al., 2004
10	ND	+	-	ND	ND	ND	ND	+	ND	ND	Kohrt & Advani, 2004
11	+	ND	-	-	+	+	ND	+	ND	+	Suzuki et al., 2004b
12	+	ND	-	-	-	-	+	+	ND	+	Suzuki et al., 2004b
13	+	ND	-	-	+	-	+	+	ND	+	Suzuki et al., 2004b
14	+	-	-	-	+	-	ND	+	-	ND	Suzuki et al., 2004b
15	-	+	-	-	-	-	-	+	ND	ND	Patel et al., 2010
16	+	+	-	-	+	-	+	+	ND	ND	Yoo et al., 2009
17	+	+	-	ND	+	ND	+	+	ND	ND	Yoo et al., 2009
18	+	+	-	-	+	-	+	+	ND	-	Yoo et al., 2009
19	+	+	-	-	-	+	ND	+	ND	+	Petterson et al., 2008

Abbreviations: EBV, Epstein-Barr virus; ND, not determined.

Table 3. Phenotypic characteristics of pediatric patients with aggressive NK leukemia. Case numbers correspond with those in Table 2

2.4 Nasal and extranodal NK-cell lymphoma

ENKL is characterized by vascular damage and destruction, prominent necrosis, a cytotoxic phenotype, and an association with EBV. ENKL typically presents in the nasal cavity or nasopharynx, with most cases having tumors localized in the upper aerodigestive tract (UAT) including nasal cavity, nasopharynx, oral cavity, oropharynx, and hypopharynx. Primary tumors that present outside the UAT, but share identical histologic features with the UAT disease, have also been categorized as non-nasal-type NK/T-cell lymphoma (NUAT-ENKL). There is clinical heterogeneity between nasal and extranasal UAT-ENKL or between UAT-ENKL and NUAT-ENKL [Kohrt et al., 2009; Kim et al., 2008]. Kim et al. reported that NUAT-ENKL had significantly higher proportions of disseminated disease, aggressive biologic features, and worse prognosis than UAT-ENKL [Kim et al., 2008]. In the UAT-ENKL group, there are differences in clinical prognostic factors between nasal UAT and extranasal UAT. Patients with extranasal UAT showed a higher proportion of advanced disease (stages III and IV on the Ann Arbor system) and regional lympohadenopathy. However, there did not seem to be any difference between extranasal UAT-ENKL and nasal UAT-ENKL with respect to survival rate. Compared to patients with UAT-ENKL (including both nasal and extranasal UAT ENKL), patients with NUAT-ENKL showed significantly higher proportions of advanced-stage disease, two or more extranodal sites, positive regional lymphadenopathy, presence of B symptoms, and poor Eastern Cooperative Oncology Group performance status. As a result of the aggressive features of NUAT-ENKL, survival rates were lower than those of UAT-ENKL (5-year overall survival rate: 22% versus 41%, $P < 0.001$) [Kim et al., 2008].

ENKL is rare in Western countries, but is more frequent in East Asia, and Central and South America [Oshimi, 1996]. It represents 3.3% of all non-Hodgkin lymphoma in Japan, 6% in Hong Kong, 8% in Korea, and 5% in Taiwan [Lymphoma Study Group of Japanese Pathologists, 2000]. ENKL is the most common lymphoma type among primary nasal-type lymphomas in Asian patients. The male:female ratio in approximately 3:1 and the median age of presentation is middle age [Ishida & Kwong, 2010]. ENKL shows onset at an older age than ANKL.

2.4.1 Diagnosis

The immunophenotype of ENKL is typically $CD2^+$, $CD56^+$, $CD3\varepsilon^+$, $sCD3^-$, $CD4^-$, $CD20^-$, and $CD30^-$. CD56, a highly useful marker for NK cells, is not specific for ENKL and can be expressed in peripheral T-cell lymphomas. Occasional cases are $CD7^+$ or $CD30^+$. ENKL shares many feature with ANKL, such as the presence of azurophilic granules in the cytoplasm of the neoplastic cells and identical immunophenotype except for CD16 expression. CD16 is negative in ENKL cases, but is positive in most ANKL cases [Nava & Jaffe, 2005]. As with ANKL, ENKL tumor cells are usually EBV positive. Cytotoxic molecules are positive (granzyme B, TIA-1, and perforin). Lymphomas that demonstrate a $CD3\varepsilon^+$ and $CD56^-$ immunophenotype are also classified ENKL if both cytotoxic molecules and EBV are positive. TCR rearrangement is in the germline configuration. CD56 is a highly useful marker of NK cells but is not specific for ENKL. CD56 is expressed in peripheral T-cell lymphomas, particularly those that show the gamma delta TCR configuration.

2.4.2 Clinical features and Immunohistochemical findings in pediatric and adolescent patients

In this literature review, all journals were searched from 1996 to date for ENKL cases (Tables 4 and 5). Twenty-one pediatric cases with ENKL were reported: seven from Asia, 11 from

Case	Age/ gender	Stage (Ann Arbor)	Fever	Subtype (primary site)	Sites involved	Other signs	Treatment	Prognosis	Reference
1	17 y/M	IV	+	NUAT	L/S/LN	HPS	mBACOD, 2-CdA	Aggressive, died 2 mo	Kwong et al., 1997
2	17 y/F	I	-	UAT (nasal)			CHOP	Alive 27 mo	Kwong et al., 1997
3	18 y/F	I	-	UAT (nasal)			CHOP	Alive 107 mo	Kwong et al., 1997
4	16 y/F	II	+	NUAT	Cecum		CHOP	Aggressive, died 7 mo	Lei et al., 1997
5	15 y/F	IV	+	NUAT	L/S/Meso/BM		-	Aggressive, died 59 d	Catlin et al., 1999
6	1 mo/M	IV	+	NUAT	L/S/BM		IFN-α	Aggressive, died 6 d	Catlin et al., 1999
7	9 y/M	II	-	NUAT	Sk/LN		POG9219/ CCG1883/ HDC	Alive, 41 mo	Shaw et al., 2001
8	12 y/M	II	-	NUAT	M/LN		POG9219/ICE/HDC	Alive, 15 mo	Shaw et al., 2001
9	17 y/M	IV	ND	NUAT	Sk	HPS	ND	Died 33 mo	Ko et al., 2004
10	17 y/M	IV	-	NUAT	L/Sk/LN		GEM/IRI	Aggressive, died 67 d	Pol-Rodriguez et al., 2006
11	17 y/F	IV	+	NUAT	LN/Sk/S/K/P/O	HPS/HMB	CHOP	Aggressive, died 3 mo	Aydin et al., 2007
12	0.7 y/F	I	ND	UAT (mastoid)			POG9219	Alive	Hutchinson et al., 2008
13	16.3 y/M	I	ND	UAT (nasal)			POG9219	Died	Hutchinson et al., 2008
14	16.3 y/F	II	ND	UAT (nasal)	Sk		POG9219	Alive	Hutchinson et al., 2008
15	16.6 y/M	II	ND	UAT (nasal)			POG9219	Died	Hutchinson et al., 2008
16	16 y/M	I	-	UAT (nasal)			CHOP	Alive, CCR >24 mo	Chang et al., 2008
17	12 y/F	I	-	UAT (nasal)			CHOP/IR	Alive, CCR 8 mo	Lee et al., 2008
18	11 y/M	IV	+	UAT (nasal)	BM	HPS	-	Aggressive, died 5 mo	Brodkin et al., 2008
19	9 y/F	I	+	UAT (nasopharynx)		HMB	CHOP	ND	Zhang et al., 2009
20	15 y/F	IV	+	UAT (tonsil)		HPS/Li/S	CHOP	Died 1 mo	Pellier et al., 2009
21	4 y/M	I	+	UAT (nasal)			CHOP	Aggressive, died 18 d	Miles et al., 2010

Abbreviations: BM, bone marrow; CCG1883, Childhood Cancer Group 1883 protocol; CCR, clinical complete response; CHOP, cyclophosphamide, doxorubicin, vincristine, prednisolone; d, days; F, female; GEM, gemcitabine; HDC, high-dose chemotherapy; HMB, hypersensitivity to mosquito bites; HPS, hemophagocytosis; ICE, ifosfamide, carboplatin, etoposide; IFN-α, interferon alpha; IR, irinotecan; K, kidney; L, lung; Li, liver; LN, lymph node; M, mastoid; mo, months; P, pancreas; POG9219, Pediatric Onocology Group 9219 protocol; M, male; mBACOD; bleomycin, adriamycin, cyclophosphamide, vincristine, dexamethasone, methotrexate; meso, mesosalpinx; ND, not determined; NUAT; non-upper aerodigestive tract; O, oral; S, spleen; Sk, skin; UAT; upper aerodigestive tract; y, years; 2-CdA, 2-chlorodeoxyadenosine.

Table 4. Clinical characteristics of pediatric patients with extranodal NK leukemia

Case	CD2	CD3ε	sCD3	CD4	CD7	CD8	CD16	CD56	Cytotoxic markers	TCR re-arrangement	EBV DNA	Reference
1	+	ND	–	–	–	–	–	+	ND	ND	ND	Kwong et al., 1997
2	+	ND	–	–	–	–	–	+	ND	ND	ND	Kwong et al., 1997
3	+	ND	–	–	–	–	–	+	ND	ND	ND	Kwong et al., 1997
4	+	–	–	–	+	–		+	ND	–	ND	Lei et al., 1997
5	–	–	–	–	NT	–	–	+	ND	NT	+	Catlin et al., 1999
6	–	–	–	+	+	+	+	+	ND	NT	+	Catlin et al., 1999
7	+	–	–	–	–	–	–	+	ND	–	–	Shaw et al., 2001
8	–	–	–	–	–	–	–	+	ND	ND	+	Shaw et al., 2001
9	ND	ND	ND	ND	ND	ND	ND	ND	ND	–	+	Ko et al., 2004
10	+	+	+	+	+	+	+	+	TIA-1+	NT	+	Pol-Rodriguez et al., 2006
11	+	+	ND	–	ND	–	ND	–	Granzyme B+	–	–	Aydin et al., 2007
12	ND	ND	ND	ND	ND	ND	ND	ND	ND	ND	ND	Hutchinson et al., 2008
13	ND	ND	ND	ND	ND	ND	ND	ND	ND	ND	ND	Hutchinson et al., 2008
14	ND	ND	ND	ND	ND	ND	ND	ND	ND	ND	ND	Hutchinson et al., 2008
15	ND	ND	ND	ND	ND	ND	ND	ND	ND	ND	ND	Hutchinson et al., 2008
16	+	+	NT	+	+	–	NT	–	TIA-1, granzyme B+	+	+	Chang et al., 2008
17	NT	+	+	NT	NT	NT	+	+	NT	NT	–	Lee et al., 2008
18	+	+	+	NT	NT	-	NT	+	NT	NT	+	Brodkin et al., 2008
19	+	NT	+	NT	+	+	NT	-	TIA-1 +	–	+	Zhang et al., 2009
20	+	+	+	+	+	+	–	+	ND	+	+	Pellier et al., 2009
21	+	+	NT	–	+	+	NT	–	TIA-1+	+	+	Miles et al., 2010

Abbreviations: EBV, Epstein Barr virus; ND, not determined; NT, not tested; TCR, T-cell antigen receptor; TIA-1, T-cell-restricted intracellular antigen-1.

Table 5. Phenotypic characteristics of pediatric patients with extranodal NK leukemia. Case numbers correspond with those in Table 4

US (including one with acquired disease), and one each from Turkey, South America, and France. In adult patients, the International Peripheral T-cell Lymphoma Project reported a four-fold higher relative frequency of ENKL among lymphoma in Asian countries compared to Western countries [Au et al., 2009]. For peripheral T-cell lymphoma, ENKL was the most common histology in Asian countries (range 34%-56%) except for Japan (11%) [Au et al., 2009]. In children and adolescents, the frequency of Asian cases is the same as in adults. Median age is 16 years (range, 0.7–18 years excluding the infant with acquired disease) and the mean age is 13 years. ENKL presents at a higher age than other forms of pediatric leukemia/lymphoma in a similar manner to other NK-lineage leukemias/lymphomas. There were 11 males and 9 females (male to female ratio, 1.22:1) and male predominance has been reported in adults.

Of the 21 pediatric patients, 14 patients had local disease (stage I and II) and seven had disseminated disease (stage III and IV) on the Ann Arbor staging system. The ratio of patients with UAT-ENKL as compared to those with NUAT-ENKL is 7:2 in adults and 2:1 in pediatric patients (Table 4). In pediatric patients, the frequency of NUAT-ENKL patients is higher than in adults [Oshimi et al., 2005]. In pediatric ENKL patients, about half of them presented UAT-ENKL: nine patients had a nasal site and three patients had an extranasal site, including mastoid, tonsil, and skin. UAT patients have been regarded as having no dissemination to other sites [Kim & Heo, 2009]. Cases 18 and 21 are therefore exceptional cases. They had significant hepatomegaly and lymphadenopathy. Their condition deteriorated progressively and lymph node biopsy and bone marrow aspiration presented the invasion of ENKL cells. Case 18 died after 4 days and case 20 died after 30 days from onset [Brodkin et al., 2008]. In adult patients, only 16% of UAT-ENKL patients are reported to have involvement of an extranodal site [Kim et al., 2008].

The proportion of pediatric NUAT-ENKL with a primary tumor outside the UAT is higher than that in adults. In adults, Kim et al. reported three patients with local disease (stage II) and six with disseminated disease (stage IV) [Kim et al., 2008]. Patients with NUAT-ENKL showed higher proportions of advanced-stage disease than adult patients with NUAT-ENKL. In pediatric patients tumor tended to disseminate. The sites involved were lymph node (5 cases), spleen (5 cases), lung (4 cases), bone marrow (2 cases), and skin (2 cases). The predominant site of adult NUAT-ENKL group is skin (37%), liver or spleen (31%), and the GI tract (24%).

Hemophagocytosis (HPS) can be a complication in ENKL (2%-8% of patients) [Kim et al., 2008]. In pediatric patients, four (1 UAT and 3 NUAT) of 20 cases were reported with HPS (Table 4). The frequency of HPS in pediatric patients may be higher than that of adults.

2.4.3 Hypersensitivity to Mosquito Bite syndrome and ENKL

Hypersensitivity to mosquito bite (HMB) syndrome is characterized by an intense skin reaction and systemic symptomatology such as high fever, lymphadenopathy, and hepatosplenomegaly. This condition has been mostly reported in Japanese children. HMB syndrome occurs in association with NK-cell lymphocytosis-related chronic EBV infection. $CD4^+$ T cells from patients respond markedly to mosquito salivary gland extracts, and $CD4^+$ T cells stimulated by mosquito bites may play a key role in the development of HMB syndrome and NK-cell oncogenesis. It is unclear how stimulated $CD4^+$ T cells are involved in viral reactivation of viral oncogene expression in NK cells (Fig. 1) [Asada, 2007]. In the 20 pediatric ENKL cases in this review, two cases may have exhibited HMB syndrome before ENKL; one from China and the other from Turkey.

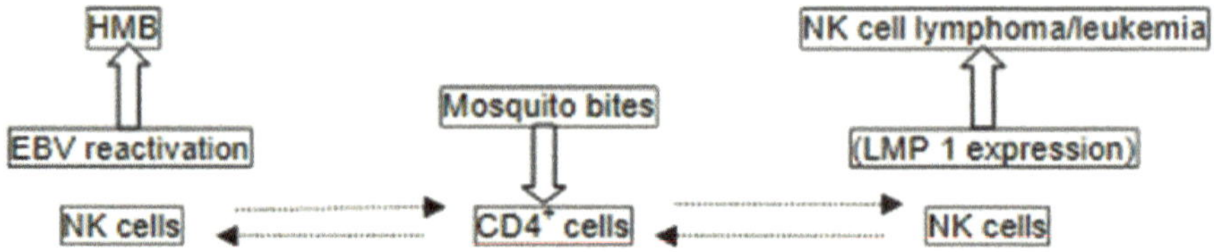

Fig. 1. CD4+ T cells stimulated by mosquito bites may play a key role in the development of hypersensitivity to mosquito bites (HMB) and NK-cell oncogenesis via the induction of Epstein-Barr virus (EBV) reactivation and EBV-oncogene latent membrane protein 1 (LMP1) expression, respectively [Asada 2007]

2.4.4 Treatment and outcome

There remains a lack of consensus on the treatment of ENKL and there is no standard therapy in adults or pediatric patients. ENKL shows an aggressive clinical course with various clinicopathologic characteristics. Due to this clinical heterogeneity of ENKL, optimal treatment and prognostic factors have been difficult to determine with the conventional Ann Arbor staging system. NUAT-ENKL has a pathologic similarity to UAT-ENKL but is a clinically distinct subtype.

2.4.4.1 Radiotherapy

For early-stage ENKL, both UAT and NUAT, experience with radiation therapy, chemotherapy, and combined therapy has been reported. The largest study with radiotherapy or radiotherapy plus chemotherapy was reported by Kim et al. [2001]. In this report of 143 patients, 104 received upfront radiotherapy alone with a median dose of 50.4 Gy (range, 20–70 Gy). Of those who received radiotherapy alone, 69% of patients achieved a complete response (CR), while only 8% of those who received chemotherapy prior to radiotherapy achieved CR [Kim et al., 2001; Korht & Advani 2009]. Huang et al. reported CR and 5-year overall survival (OS) rates of 100% in patients who received radiotherapy alone, while those who received chemotherapy (CHOP) alone had rates of 25% and 90%, respectively [Huang et al., 2008]. Li et al. reported overall response in 85 of 87 (97.7%) patients with stage I UAT-ENKL who received radiotherapy with 50–56 Gy (standard is 50 Gy). The 5-year OS, 5-year progression-free survival (PFS), and local control rates for all patients were 80%, 69%, and 93%, respectively [Li et al., 2011b].

The dose and field of radiation in stage I or II ENKL is an important factor with respect to outcome. A radiation dose of at least 54 Gy is seen as being associated with better outcome. Comparing those who received ≥54 Gy versus <54 Gy, 5-year OS and disease-free survival (DFS) rates were higher with the former: 75% vs 46% and 60% vs 46%, respectively [Huang et al., 2008]. Systemic failure is shown in 25% to 30% of patients with stage II and II disease treated with radiotherapy alone. This shows the role of chemotherapy in control of clinically occult disease.

2.4.4.2 Chemotherapy

There are few studies that included patients treated with chemotherapy alone. Studies of chemotherapy regimens including cyclophosphamide, doxorubicin, vincristine, and prednisone (CHOP) are disappointing because of high rates of refractory disease or early relapse: the CR rate with chemotherapy alone was <33% and 2-year DFS and OS were 23%

and 44%, respectively [Kim et al., 2003]. This poor prognosis with chemotherapy alone appears related to high P-glycoprotein (P-gp) expression in this NK-cell neoplasm. P-gp is associated drug efflux and treatment resistance.

2.4.4.3 Combined modality therapy

For the control of clinically occult early-stage disease, a combined modality therapy is anticipated to reduce distant failure and overall risk of relapse. In a series of 108 patients with early-stage ENKL receiving radiotherapy followed by chemotherapy consisting with cyclophosphamide, epirubicin, vincristine, prednisolone, and bleomycin [Avilés et al., 2003], combined therapy demonstrated high efficacy with a 92% overall response rate and 8-year OS of 86%. In early-stage ENKL, Guo et al. reported that patients who received CHOP followed by radiotherapy (45 Gy) had a CR rate of only 49% as compared to 100% for those who received radiotherapy prior to CHOP [Guo et al., 2008]. Li et al. reported that patients with early-stage UAT-ENKL (stages I and II) treated with radiotherapy or radiotherapy plus chemotherapy had 5-year OS and PFS rates of 72% and 65%, respectively, overall. The cumulative rates of 5-year systemic failure and OS, respectively, were 24% and 74% for combined modality therapy as compared to 28% and 70% for radiotherapy alone. There was no significant difference between radiotherapy alone and combined modality therapy. A very low incidence of cervical lymph node or CNS relapse was observed. As a result, the addition of chemotherapy did not significantly decrease the systemic failure rate or improve survival [Li et al., 2011a]. In the Japanese JCOG 0211 study [Yamaguchi et al. 2008], 27 patients received radiotherapy (50 Gy) and reduced-dose chemotherapy (carboplatin etoposide, ifosfamide, and dexamethasone). The CR rate was 77% and overall response rate was 81%. Of the ten patients with disease recurrence, nine failed at a distant site. These studies demonstrate that local control using radiotherapy should precede systemic chemotherapy. Prospective studies are needed to clarify the role of chemotherapy.

2.4.4.4 Advanced-stage disease

Combined chemotherapy and radiotherapy is the most commonly used approach for advanced-stage disease. Due to the limited number and size of series, the efficacy of intensive therapy has not been demonstrated. For CHOP or m-BACOD (bleomycin, vincristine, dexamethasone, and methotrexate) followed by radiotherapy, the CR rate in patients with advanced-stage disease was 25% and median OS was 2 months as compared to 75% and 12 months, respectively, in those with early-stage disease [Kwong et al., 1997].

L-asparaginase has been reported as a novel approach for the treatment of advanced-stage ENKL. NK-cell tumors appear highly sensitive to L-asparaginase *in vitro*, as NK cells express low levels of asparaginase synthase. In a series of 15 patients with relapsed or refractory ENKL treated with L-asparaginase monotherapy, seven achieved a CR with an overall response rate of 87% [Jaccard et al., 2009]. Yamaguchi et al. have reported the efficacy of the SMILE regimen consisting with steroids, methotrexate, ifosfamide, L-asparaginase, and etoposide. These agents are independent of the multidrug resistant mechanism (mediated by P-gp) in tumor cells. This phase I study included six patients with advanced-stage disease. The overall response rate after 2 cycles of SMILE therapy was 67%, with 50% achieving CR [Yamaguchi et al., 2008].

2.4.4.5 Stem cell transplantation

Autologous and allogeneic stem cell transplantation (SCT) have been evaluated for consolidation and for relapsed or refractory disease. Suzuki et al. reported 25 CR patients who received SCT and 4-year OS was 68% [Suzuki et al., 2006]. This demonstrated a significant benefit compared to 188 historical controls who had 4-year OS of 21%. As there have been few reports of SCT, the ability to define its role as therapy for relapsed or refractory disease remains limited. For refractory and relapsed ENKL patients, Yokoyama et al. reported a retrospective analysis of five cases treated with allogeneic SCT [Yokoyama et al., 2010]. All five patients received a myeloablative conditioning regimen (total body irradiation/cyclophosphamide with or without cytarabine) and survived without disease (median follow-up period of 1,911 days). This small case series suggests that allogeneic SCT might improve the outcome of advanced-stage ENKL.

2.4.4.6 Pediatric study

In the pediatric ENKL patients (excluding case 19 whose prognosis was not reported), eight of 12 patients with early-stage (stage I and II) disease including UAT and NUAT were alive (Table 4). Two cases were not described in detail and another two cases died within 1 year. The CR rate is 61%. Case 21 had nasal and right cervical lymphadenopathy and his tumor was not controlled; he died despite CHOP and more intensive chemotherapy. The outcome of pediatric early-stage patients was worse than in adults. The reason is that most cases did not receive radiotherapy and received chemotherapy alone, generally CHOP.

In advanced-stage disease (stage IV), all cases died and average survival was 181 days (6 days to 33 months). Both UAT and NUAT cases show very progressive disease and poor prognosis. Two cases with NUAT received high-dose chemotherapy, had complete remission, and were alive. Case 9 received cord blood SCT after a conditioning regimen consisting of total body irradiation (12 Gy), thiotepa, and cyclophosphamide, while case 10 received autologous SCT after thiotepa and cyclophosphamide.

There have been no large studies in pediatric patients. The largest is a report from China. Wang et al. reported the outcome of 37 pediatric and adolescent UAT-ENKL patients. Among the patients with stage I and II disease, 19 patients received primary radiotherapy with or without chemotherapy, and 14 patients received chemotherapy followed by radiotherapy. The CR rate after initial radiotherapy was 74%, which was significantly higher than the response rate after initial chemotherapy (17%). The median radiation dose for the primary tumor was 50 Gy (range, 15–60 Gy), with dose fractions of 1.8–2 Gy. They reported no late side effects, e.g. secondary malignancy [Wang et al., 2009].

2.5 Blastic plasmacytoid dendritic cell neoplasm and blastic NK-cell lymphoma

Blastic plasmacytoid dendritic cell neoplasm (pDCL) defines leukemia/lymphoma with expression of CD4 and CD56 without any other lineage-specific markers. pDCL is rare and presents a <1% of acute leukemias and 0.7% of cutaneous lymphomas [Garnache-Ottou et al., 2007]. It primarily affects the elderly (median age 69 years) [Feuillard et al., 2002]. The clinical course is very aggressive and rapidly fatal [Reimer et al., 2003]. Histologically, this malignancy is classified as blastic NK-cell lymphoma/leukemia. The 2000 WHO classification considers this malignancy as blastic NK-cell lymphoma [Harris et al., 2000].

The ontogenic origin of this malignancy has not been clearly identified. Chaperot et al. have demonstrated the origin of these tumor cells as dendritic cells [Chaperot et al., 2001]. These malignant cells express interleukin-3 (IL-3) receptor maturation with IL-3 and produce interferon alpha (IFN-α) in response to influenza virus. These cells become a powerful inducer of naïve $CD4^+$ T-cell proliferation and promote T-helper 2 polarization. Finally, these authors concluded the origin of this neoplasm is a plasmacytoid dendritic cell subset. Feuilliard et al. reported 23 cases with $CD4^+$, $CD56^+$ leukemia. The majority of patients were elderly adults, but three children were included in their report. At diagnosis, most patients had cutaneous involvement, with disseminated purple lesions on the dermis. Lymphadenopathy and/or splenomegaly were frequent [Chaperot et al., 2001]. Morphologic and cytochemical analysis revealed a high frequency of vacuolization with pseudopodia-like cytoplasmic expansions. Myeloperoxidase and monocytic esterase activity were never detected.

However, all cases of pDCL do not produce IFN-α and secretion levels of IFN-α have been lower than their normal counterparts. pDCL cells proved incapable of differentiating into NK cells, B cells, myeloid cells, or monocytes, and differentiation into mature pDC was only possible. Furthermore, a subset of pDCL demonstrated the expression of blood dendritic cell antigen 2 (BDCA-2), a specific dendritic cell marker. This fact supports that the origin of pDCL as dendritic cells [Jaye et al., 2006]. However, some other reports remain undetermined concerning the possible origin of pDCL. More investigation is required to establish the definitive nature of these CD4$^+$/CD56$^+$ tumor cells.

2.5.1 Differential diagnosis

Table 6 shows the differential diagnosis. ENKL is associated with EBV infection, while this has not been reported for pDCL. Although expression of CD56$^+$, CD2$^+$, CD7$^+$, and intraplasmic granzyme B can be in common between ENKL and pDCL, ENKL never expresses CD4$^+$ [Harris et al., 1997]. In about 10% to 20% of acute myelogenous leukemia patients, tumor cells express CD33$^+$, CD4$^+$, and CD56$^+$. Very undifferentiated acute myelogenous leukemia weakly shows myelocytic or monoblastic markers. In these cases, identification of pDC-specific markers (e.g. BDCA-2) is useful [Garnache-Outtu et al., 2007]

Mixed myeloblastic/NK-cell leukemia are defined as types of myeloid leukemia in the WHO 2008 classification [Swerdlow et al., 2008]. These leukemias express CD7$^+$, CD33$^+$, and CD56$^+$. They correspond to proliferation of animmature precursor with myeloid and NK potential [Suzuki et al., 1997]. The leukemia phenotype is different from pDCL as they do not express CD4 and CD36 in reported cases [Suzuki et al., 1997]. Furthermore, in pDCL, there is no expression of CD34 , while its expression has always shown in mixed myeloblastic/NK-cell leukemia cells.

Marker	pDCL	ENKL	AML	Mixed myeloblastic/NK-cell leukemia
CD2	-	+	-	
CD7	-	+	±	+
CD56	+	+	+	+
CD4	+	-	+	-
Granzyme B	-	+		
CD33	-	-	+	+
CD117	-	-	+	
CD34	-	-	±	+
CD36	+	-	-	-
BDCA-2	+	-	-	-

Abbreviations: AML, acute myelogenous leukemia; BDCA-2, blood dendritic cell antigen 2; ENKL, extranodal NK-cell leukemia; pDCL, blastic plasmacytoid dendritic cell neoplasm.

Table 6. Differential diagnosis of blastic plasmacytoid dendritic cell neoplasms

2.5.2 Pediatric cases

Pediatric pDCL is very rare and limited to a few case reports and small case series. Jegalian et al. reported 25 pediatric cases (20 in the literature, 9 at their institution) with pDCL [Jegalian et al., 2010]. They demonstrated the clinical features and prognosis of pediatric patients. In pediatric patients, 24% of patients lacked cutaneous involvement, which is slightly higher rate than adults. In adult patients, pDCL clinical presentation at the time of diagnosis usually consists of a cutaneous involvement and the patients without cutaneous involvement are very rare. In adult patients, especially the elderly, prognosis is very poor. Median OS was only 13 months for all patients. Allogeneic SCT is a useful treatment in younger adult patients. They reported a regimen suited to acute lymphoblastic leukemia followed by SCT is more effective than using an acute myelogenous leukemia or non-Hodgkin lymphoma regimen. While the OS of pediatric patients receiving SCT was 67% (4 of 6 patients), that for patients without SCT was 74%. In pediatric patients, treatment with a high-risk regimen appears effective without SCT. SCT was useful for only relapsed or secondary remission disease. Outcome of pediatric patients was more favorable than that of adults [Jegalian et al., 2010].

3. Conclusion

NK-cell malignancy is difficult to define and there is confusion in diagnosis. One of the reasons for the confusion is that CD56 is not only expressed in NK-cell malignancy but in various other hematopoietic malignancies, e.g. acute myelogenous leukemia non-Hodgkin lymphoma, pDCL. It is hoped that more specific markers for NK-cell malignancy will assist in defining these malignancies. NK-cell precursor tumors with lymphomatous presentation that expressed NK-specific CD94A1 transcripts have been described [Lin et al., 2005]. I used this method and clarified the origin of one case [Hashii et al., 2010]. Antibodies against killer immunoglobulin-like receptors (KIRs) will hopefully provide a useful tool for clarification of the diagnosis of the NK-cell malignancies. Currently, these antibodies are not commonly used. Although, BDCA-2 is useful for clarifying the difference between NK-cell malignancy and pDCL, it is not commonly used. The diagnosis of precursor NK-cell lymphoblastic leukemia/lymphoma may be considered in cases that express $CD56^+$ along with immature T-cell markers ($CD2^+$, $CD7^+$, and $CD3\varepsilon^+$) without B-cell or myeloid markers.

4. References

Asada, H. (2007). Hypersensitivity to mosquito bites: a unique pathogenic mechanism linking Epstein-Barr virus infection, allergy and oncogenesis, *Journal of Dermatological Science* 45(3): 153–160.

Au, W.Y., Ma, S.Y., Chim, C.S., et al. (2005). Clinicopathologic features and treatment outcome of mature T-cell and natural killer-cell lymphomas diagnosed according to the World Health Organization classification scheme: a single center experience of 10 years, *Annals of Oncology* 16(2): 206–214.

Au, W.Y. & Weisenburger, D.D., Intragumtornchai, T., et al. (2009). Clinical differences between nasal and extranasal natural killer/T-cell lymphoma: a study of 136 cases from the International Peripheral T-Cell Lymphoma Project, *Blood* 113(17): 3931–3937.

Avilés, A., Neri, N., Fernández, R., et al. (2003). Nasal NK/T-cell lymphoma with disseminated disease treated with aggressive combined therapy, *Medical Oncology* 20(1): 13–17.

Aydin, G.B., Akyuz, C., Talim, B., et al. (2007). Extranodal type T/NK-cell lymphoma with an atypical clinical presentation, *Pediatric Hematology-Oncology* 24(4): 291–299.

Brodkin, D.E., Hobohm, D.W., Nigam, R. (2008). Nasal-type NK/T-cell lymphoma presenting as hemophagocytic syndrome in an 11-year-old Mexican boy, *Journal of Pediatric Hematology and Oncology* 30(12): 938–940.

Catlin, E.A., Roberts, J.D. Jr., Erana, R., et al. (1999). Transplacental transmission of natural-killer-cell lymphoma, *New England Journal of Medicine* 341(2): 85–91.

Chang, B.H., Stork, L. & Fan, G. (2008). A unique case of adolescent CD56-negative extranodal NK/T-cell lymphoma, nasal type, *Pediatric and Developmental Pathology* 11(1): 50–54.

Chaperot, L., Bendriss, N., Manches, O., et al. (2001). Identification of a leukemic counterpart of the plasmacytoid dendritic cells, *Blood* 97(10): 3210–3217.

Feuillard, J., Jacob, M.C., Valensi, F., et al. (2002). Clinical and biologic features of CD4(+)CD56(+) malignancies, *Blood* 99(5): 1556–1563.

Furuno, T., Hara, N., Hagimoto, N., et al. (1994). Multiple pulmonary nodules manifested in a patient with NK cell granular lymphocyte proliferative disorder, *Chest* 105(6): 1893–1895.

Garnache-Ottou, F., Feuillard, J. & Saas, P. (2007). Plasmacytoid dendritic cell leukaemia/lymphoma: towards a well defined entity? *British Journal of Haematology* 136(4): 539–548.

Guo, Y., Lu, J.J., Ma, X., et al. (2008). Combined chemoradiation for the management of nasal natural killer (NK)/T-cell lymphoma: elucidating the significance of systemic chemotherapy, *Oral Oncology* 44(1):23–30.

Harris, N.L., Jaffe, E.S., Diebold, J., et al. (2000). The World Health Organization classification of neoplasms of the hematopoietic and lymphoid tissues: report of the Clinical Advisory Committee meeting-Airlie House, Virginia, November, 1997, The *Hematology Journal* 1(1): 53–66.

Hashii, Y., Okuda, T., Ohta, H., et al. (2010). Pediatric myeloid/NK cell precursor lymphoma/leukemia expressing T/NK immunophenotype markers, *International Journal of Hematology* 91(3): 525–529.

Huang, M.J., Jiang, Y., Liu, W.P., et al. (2008). Early or up-front radiotherapy improved survival of localized extranodal NK/T-cell lymphoma, nasal-type in the upper aerodigestive tract, *International Journal of Radiation Oncology Biology Physics* 70(1): 166–174.

Hutchison, R.E., Laver, J.H., Chang, M., et al. (2008). Non-anaplastic peripheral t-cell lymphoma in childhood and adolescence: a Children's Oncology Group study, *Pediatric Blood Cancer* 51(1): 29–33.

Ichikawa, S., Fukuhara, N., Yamamoto, J., et al. (2010). Successful allogeneic hematopoietic stem cell transplantation for aggressive NK cell leukemia, *Internal Medicine* 49(17): 1907–1910.

Imamura, N., Kusunoki, Y., Kawa-Ha, K., et al. (1990). Aggressive natural killer cell leukaemia/lymphoma: report of four cases and review of the literature. Possible existence of a new clinical entity originating from the third lineage of lymphoid cells, *British Journal of Haematology* 75(1): 49–59.

Ishida, F. & Kwong, Y.L. (2010). Diagnosis and management of natural killer-cell malignancies, *Expert Review of Hematology* 3(5): 593–602.

Ito, T., Makishima H., Nakazawa, H., et al. (2008). Promising approach for aggressive NK cell leukaemia with allogeneic haematopoietic cell transplantation, *European Journal of Haematology* 81(2): 107–111.

Jaccard, A., Petit, B., Girault, S., et al. (2009). L-asparaginase-based treatment of 15 western patients with extranodal NK/T-cell lymphoma and leukemia and a review of the literature, *Annals of Oncology* 20(1): 110–116.

Jaye, D.L., Geigerman, C.M., Herling, M., et al. (2006). Expression of the plasmacytoid dendritic cell marker BDCA-2 supports a spectrum of maturation among CD4+ CD56+ hematodermic neoplasms, *Modern Pathology* 19(12): 1555–1562.

Jegalian, A.G., Buxbaum, N.P., Facchetti, F., et al. (2010). Blastic plasmacytoid dendritic cell neoplasm in children: diagnostic features and clinical implications, *Haematologica* 95(11): 1873–1879.

Kaizu, K., Maeda, M., Ohkawa, T., et al. (2004). Marked elevation of soluble fas ligand and cytokine secretion after splenectomy in aggressive natural killer cell leukemia/lymphoma, *Leukemia and Lymphoma* 45(11): 2291–2294.

Kato K., Ohshima K., Ishihara S., et al. (1998). Elevated serum soluble Fas ligand in natural killer cell proliferative disorders, *British Journal of Haematology* 103(4):1164–1166.

Kawa-Ha, K., Ishihara, S., Ninomiya, T., et al. (1989). CD3-negative lymphoproliferative disease of granular lymphocytes containing Epstein-Barr viral DNA, *Journal of Clinical Investigation* 84(1): 51–55.

Kim, B.S., Kim, T.Y., Kim, C.W., et al. (2003). Therapeutic outcome of extranodal NK/T-cell lymphoma initially treated with chemotherapy–result of chemotherapy in NK/T-cell lymphoma, *Acta Oncologica* 42(7): 779–783.

Kim, G.E., Lee, S.W., Chang, S.K., et al. (2001). Combined chemotherapy and radiation versus radiation alone in the management of localized angiocentric lymphoma of the head and neck, *Radiotherapy and Oncology* 61(3): 261–269.

Kim, T.M. & Heo, D.S. (2009). Extranodal NK/T-cell lymphoma, nasal type: new staging system and treatment strategies, *Cancer Science* 100(12): 2242–2248.

Kim, T.M., Lee, S.Y., Jeon, Y.K., et al. (2008). Clinical heterogeneity of extranodal NK/T-cell lymphoma, nasal type: a national survey of the Korean Cancer Study Group, *Annals of Oncology* 19(8): 1477–1484.

Ko, Y.H., Cho, E.Y., Kim, J.E., et al. (2004). NK and NK-like T-cell lymphoma in extranasal sites: a comparative clinicopathological study according to site and EBV status, *Histopathology* 44(5): 480–489.

Kohrt, H. & Advani, R. (2009). Extranodal natural killer/T-cell lymphoma: current concepts in biology and treatment, *Leukemia and Lymphoma* 50(11): 1773–1784.

Koizumi, S., Seki, H., Tachinami, T., et al. (1986). Malignant clonal expansion of large granular lymphocytes with a Leu-11+, Leu-7- surface phenotype: in vitro responsiveness of malignant cells to recombinant human interleukin 2, *Blood* 68(5): 1065–1073.

Kwong, Y.L., Chan, A.C., Liang, R., et al. (1997). CD56+ NK lymphomas: clinicopathological features and prognosis, *British Journal of Haematology* 97(4): 821–829.

Kwong, Y.L., Wong, K.F., Chan, L.C., et al. (1995). Large granular lymphocyte leukemia. A study of nine cases in a Chinese population, *American Journal of Clinical Pathology* 103(1): 76–81.

Lee, J.Y., Jang, Y.D. & Kim, H.K. (2008). The primary role of the otolaryngologist in managing pediatric sinonasal malignancies: an extranodal NK/T-cell lymphoma originating from the inferior turbinate mucosa of the nasal cavity, *Journal of Pediatric Hematology and Oncology* 30(5): 401–404.

Lei, K.I., Chow, J.H. & Johnson P.J. (1997). Aggressive primary natural killer cell lymphoma of the caecum: a case report and literature review, *Clinical Oncology (Royal College of Radiology)* 9(3): 191–194.

Li, Y.X., Liu, Q.F., Wang, W.H., et al. (2011a). Failure patterns and clinical implications in early stage nasal natural killer/T-cell lymphoma treated with primary radiotherapy, *Cancer* doi: 10.1002/cncr.26167 [Epub ahead of print].

Li, Y.X., Wang, H., Jin, J., et al. (2011b). Radiotherapy Alone With Curative Intent in Patients With Stage I Extranodal Nasal-type NK/T-cell Lymphoma, *International Journal of Radiation Oncology Biology Physics* [Epub ahead of print].

Lin, C.W., Liu, T.Y., Chen, S.U., et al. (2005). CD94 1A transcripts characterize lymphoblastic lymphoma/leukemia of immature natural killer cell origin with distinct clinical features, *Blood* 106: 3567–3574.

Miles, R.R., Afify Z., Yaish, H., et al. (2010). CD56-negative extranodal nasal type NK/T-cell lymphoma, *Pediatric Blood Cancer* 55: 186-189.

Nava, V.E. & Jaffe, E.S. (2005). The pathology of NK-cell lymphomas and leukemias, *Advances in Anatomic Pathology* 12: 27–34.

Ohno, Y., Amakawa, R., Fukuhara, S., et al. (1989). Acute transformation of chronic large granular lymphocyte leukemia associated with additional chromosome abnormality, *Cancer* 64: 63–67.

Ohnuma, K., Toyoda, Y., Nishihira, H., et al. (1997). Aggressive natural killer (NK) cell lymphoma: report of a pediatric case and review of the literature, *Leukemia and Lymphoma* 25: 387–392.

Oshimi, K., Kawa, K., Nakamura, S., et al. (2005). NK-cell neoplasms in Japan, *Hematology* 10(3): 237–245.

Oshimi, K. (1996). Lymphoproliferative disorders of natural killer cells, *International Journal of Hematology* 63(4): 279–290.

Patel, A.P., Ghatak, S.B. & Patel, J.A. (2010). Long term survival in aggressive NK cell leukemia. *Indian Pediatrics* 47(9): 807–808.

Lymphoma Study Group of Japanese Pathologists. (2000). The World Health Organization classification of malignant lymphomas in Japan: incidence of recently recognized entities, *Pathology International* 50(9): 696–702.

Pellier, I., N'Golet, L., Rachieru, P., et al. (2009). Disseminated nasal-type natural killer/T-cell lymphoma in a child: a case report, *Journal of Pediatric Hematology and Oncology* 31(5): 362–366.

Petterson, T.E., Bosco, A.A. & Cohn, R.J. (2008). Aggressive natural killer cell leukemia presenting with hemophagocytic lymphohistiocytosis, *Pediatric Blood Cancer* 50(3): 654–657.

Pol-Rodriguez, M.M., Fox, L.P., Sulis, M.L., et al. (2006). Extranodal nasal-type natural killer T-cell lymphoma in an adolescent from Bangladesh, *Journal of the American Academy of Dermatology* 54(5 Suppl): S192–S197.

Reimer, P., Rüdiger, T., Kraemer, D., et al. (2003). What is CD4+CD56+ malignancy and how should it be treated? *Bone Marrow Transplantation* 32(7): 637–646.

Shaw, P.H., Cohn, S.L., Morgan, E.R., et al. (2001). Natural killer cell lymphoma: report of two pediatric cases, therapeutic options, and review of the literature, *Cancer* 91(4): 642–646.

Suzuki, K., Ohshima, K., Karube, K., et al. (2004a). Clinicopathological states of Epstein-Barr virus-associated T/NK-cell lymphoproliferative disorders (severe chronic active EBV infection) of children and young adults, *International Journal of Oncology* 24(5): 1165–1174.

Suzuki, R., Suzumiya, J., Nakamura, S., et al. (2004b). Aggressive natural killer-cell leukemia revisited: large granular lymphocyte leukemia of cytotoxic NK cells, *Leukemia* 18(4): 763–770.

Suzuki, R., Suzumiya, J., Nakamura, S., et al. (2006). Hematopoietic stem cell transplantation for natural killer-cell lineage neoplasms, *Bone Marrow Transplant* 37(4): 425-431.

Suzuki, R., Suzumiya, J., Yamaguchi, M., et al. (2010). Prognostic factors for mature natural killer (NK) cell neoplasms: aggressive NK cell leukemia and extranodal NK cell lymphoma, nasal type, *Annals of Oncology* 21(5): 1032–1040.

Suzuki, R., Yamamoto, K., Seto, M., et al. (1997). CD7+ and CD56+ myeloid/natural killer cell precursor acute leukemia: a distinct hematolymphoid disease entity, *Blood* 90(6): 2417–2428.

Suzuki, R. (2010). Treatment of advanced extranodal NK/T cell lymphoma, nasal-type and aggressive NK-cell leukemia, *International Journal of Hematology* 92(5): 697–701.

Swerdlow, S.H., Campo, E. & Harris, N.L. (2008). WHO Classification of Tumours of Haematopoietic and Lymphoid Tissues. IARC, Lyon.

Wang, Z.Y., Li, Y.X., Wang, W.H., et al. (2009). Primary radiotherapy showed favorable outcome in treating extranodal nasal-type NK/T-cell lymphoma in children and adolescents, *Blood* 114(23): 4771–4776.

Yamaguchi, M., Suzuki, R., Kwong, Y.L., et al. (2008). Phase I study of dexamethasone, methotrexate, ifosfamide, L-asparaginase, and etoposide (SMILE) chemotherapy for advanced-stage, relapsed or refractory extranodal natural killer (NK)/T-cell lymphoma and leukemia, *Cancer Science* 99(5): 1016–1020.

Yokoyama, H., Yamamoto, J., Tohmiya, Y., et al. (2010). Allogeneic hematopoietic stem cell transplant following chemotherapy containing l-asparaginase as a promising treatment for patients with relapsed or refractory extranodal natural killer/T cell lymphoma, nasal type, *Leukemia and Lymphoma* 51(8): 1509–1512.

Yoo, E.H., Kim, H.J., Lee, S.T., et al. (2009). Frequent CD7 antigen loss in aggressive natural killer-cell leukemia: a useful diagnostic marker, *The Korean Journal of Laboratory Medicine* 29(6): 491–496.

Zhang, Z., Shi, Q., An, X., et al. (2009). NK/T-cell lymphoma in a child with hypersensitivity to mosquito bites, *Journal of Pediatric Hematology/Oncology* 31(11): 855–857.

11

Pediatric Acute Myeloid Leukemia

C. Michel Zwaan and Marry M. van den Heuvel-Eibrink
Erasmus MC-Sophia Children's Hospital, Rotterdam, The Netherlands

1. Introduction

Acute leukemias are clonal diseases characterized by a maturation arrest and by enhanced proliferation of hematopoietic precursor cells, which normally would differentiate into mature blood cells. The leukemic cells are released from the bone marrow into the peripheral blood and may accumulate in vital organs such as the spleen, liver, skin, central nervous system and lymph nodes. Chronic leukemias arise form hyperproliferation without a clear maturation arrest. In children, chronic leukemias are rare, and most cases are classified as acute leukemias. (Pui, *et al* 2011) Acute leukemias can be further subdivided in acute lymphoblastic leukemias (ALL, either from precursor T- or B-cells), and in acute myeloid leukemias (AML, either from red blood cell precursors, platelet precursors, or granulocytic or monocytic precursors). In children, approximately 80% of cases are ALL, and 15-20% AML. There is a peak in the incidence of AML in infants under one year of age, after which the incidence is low throughout childhood. (Creutzig, *et al* 2010a, Kaspers and Zwaan 2007) AML may even be present in newborn babies. (Bresters, *et al* 2002) In adolescents the incidence of AML starts to rise and rises further throughout adult life (1-3 per 10^5 each year in childhood, rising to 15 per 10^5 in early adulthood to 35 per 10^5 at the age of 90 years). (Ries, *et al* 1999)
AML may either arise de novo or occur following underlying diseases such as myelodysplastic syndrome, which is much more frequent in elderly patients with AML than in children. Other underlying diseases may be chromosomal-breakage syndromes such as Fanconi anemia. (Tonnies, *et al* 2003) Moreover, AML may be secondary to previous exposure to irradiation or to chemotherapy, including both alkylating chemotherapy and epipodopyllotoxins. (Sandler, *et al* 1997, Weiss, *et al* 2003) A specific type of AML arises in children with Down syndrome. (Zwaan, *et al* 2008) Exposure to environmental factors has also been described as a potential cause of AML. (Smith, *et al* 2011) Infrequently, families with an unexplained high risk of AML have been described which suggests that germ-line mutations such as *RUNX1* and *CEBPA* may play a role in leukemogenesis. (Owen, *et al* 2008)

1.1 Clinical presentation

AML has a variable clinical presentation. The history of a child with AML is often relatively short and at most a few weeks. Children with AML usually present with signs of inadequate production of normal blood cells, such as pallor and tiredness or feeding problems due to anemia, spontaneous bleeding due to al low platelet count, and fever/infections due to low white blood cells. High white counts can give rise to hyperviscosity and sludging and hence to pulmonary complaints (dyspnea) or central nervous system related symptoms (lowered consciousness, coma, convulsions). Bone pain due to high intra-osseous pressure often occurs. Extramedullary disease due to infiltration of leukemic cells has been reported in 4-10 percent of all cases, and may either present as skin infiltrates (referred to as 'blue-berry muffin' skin lesions) or solid leukemic masses, also referred to as chloromas. Organs prone for accumulation of leukemic cells and subsequent organomegaly are the spleen, liver, gingiva and lymph nodes. Leukemia in the central nervous system may occur either as liquor pleiocytosis or as solid tumors in the central nervous system. A specific type of AML, acute promyelocytic leukemia (APL), often presents with serious life threatening bleeding disorders, which is due to abnormal coagulation factors, and not just to thrombocytopenia. (Creutzig, *et al* 2010c)

2. Diagnostics

2.1 Morphology and immunophenotyping

The first step to diagnose leukemia is to study the morphology of the peripheral blood and the bone marrow aspirate using light microscopy. A classical morphological feature distinguishing AML from ALL are the so-called Auer rods (see Figure 1), which are mainly seen in leukemias derived from granulocytic precursors. However, differentiation between AML and ALL is nowadays usually done with flow cytometry. Typically, AML blasts are positive for CD13 or CD33, and negative for lymphocyte markers such as CD3/CD7 (T-cells) or CD19/CD20/CD2 (B-cell precursors). Myeloperoxidase (MPO) staining can be used to differentiate AML from ALL, although MPO-positivity is mainly confined to granuclocytic leukemias. Esterase staining is helpful to identify monocytic types of leukemia.

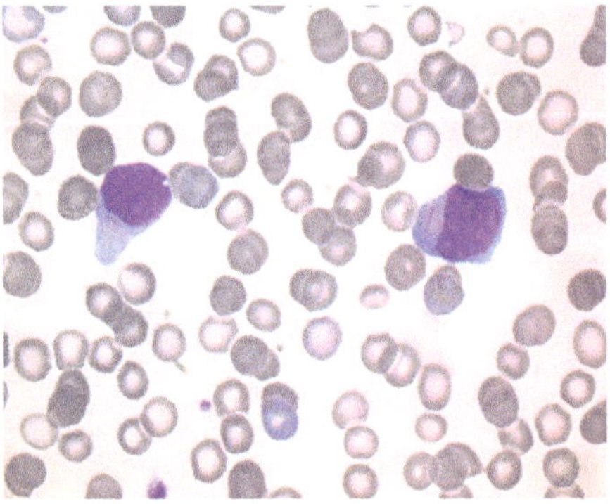

Fig. 1. Auer rods present in the 2 AML blasts visible in a peripheral blood smear.

The morphological classification of AML is referred to as the French-American-British or FAB-classification (see table 1), and is based on the cell-line of origin. (Bennett, *et al* 1985a, Bennett, *et al* 1985b, Bennett, *et al* 1991) Certain morphological subtypes need confirmation with flowcytometry, such as minimally differentiated AML (FAB M0) and acute megakaryoblastic leukemia (FAB M7). (Bennett, *et al* 1985a, Bennett, *et al* 1991) Morphological assessment should also focus on the occurrence of myelodysplasia, and differentiation between AML and advanced myelodysplastic syndromes (MDS) may be difficult. In adults, a blast threshold of 20% is used to differentiate between these 2 diseases, but in children we still use the 30% cut-off. (Hasle, *et al* 2003) Other characteristics may also be helpful: AML-specific translocations, organomegaly, rapid progression and CNS-localization are indicative or AML rather than MDS.

FAB type	Name	Relationship with specific cytogenetic abnormalities
M0	minimally differentiated acute myeloblastic leukemia	
M1	acute myeloblastic leukemia, without maturation	
M2	acute myeloblastic leukemia, with granulocytic maturation	t(8;21)(q22;q22), t(6;9)(p23;q34)
M3	promyelocytic, or acute promyelocytic leukemia (APL)	t(15;17)(q22;q12)
M4	acute myelomonocytic leukemia	
M4Eo	myelomonocytic together with bone marrow eosinophilia	inv(16)(p13.1q22) or t(16;16)(p13.1;q22)
M5	acute monoblastic leukemia	*MLL*-gene rearrangements
M6	acute erythroid leukemias	
M7	acute megakaryoblastic leukemia	t(1;22)(p13;q13)

Table 1. FAB-classification of AML, and relationship between FAB-types and specific cytogenetic abnormalities. (Bennett, *et al* 1985a, Bennett, *et al* 1985b, Bennett, *et al* 1991). *MLL*=mixed-lineage leukemia

2.2 Cytogenetics and molecular genetic screening

AML is a genetically very heterogeneous disease. Genetic aberrations in AML can be subdivided in type 1 and type 2 aberrations, based on the Gilliland hypothesis that at least two different collaborative types of abnormalities are needed in the pathogenesis of AML. Kelly, L.M. & Gilliland, D.G. (2002a) Genetics of myeloid leukemias. *Annu.Rev.Genomics Hum.Genet.*, 3, 179-198. Type 1 abnormalities mainly induce proliferation, and consist for instance of mutations in tyrosine kinase receptors such as the *FLT3*-gene(Zwaan, *et al* 2003a) or *KIT*-mutations(Goemans, *et al* 2005, Pollard, *et al* 2010), and type 2 abnormalities induce maturation arrest and mainly result from genetic aberrations in hematopoietic transcription factors, either resulting from translocations, or from mutations in genes such as *NPM1*, *GATA1* and *CEBPA*. (Ahmed, *et al* 2004, Hollink, *et al* 2011, Hollink, *et al* 2009c) Evidence for this model is supported by several factors: 1) AML-specific translocations can already be demonstrated in cord-blood (Wiemels, *et al* 2002), and may only cause AML several years later, 2) fusion transcripts may be demonstrated using sensitive techniques in patients in long-term clinical remission of AML (Leroy, *et al* 2005), 3) *FLT3* mutations induce a myeloproliferative disorder in mice but lack the maturation arrest typical of full-blown AML (Kelly, *et al* 2002b), and 4) certain type I and II genetic aberrations cluster together in a non-random fashion.

Conventional karyotyping may identify AML-specific abnormalities, which are not only of use in diagnosis and the correct classification of the leukemia, but may also provide prognostic information used for risk-group stratification of pediatric AML. (Harrison, *et al* 2010, von Neuhoff, *et al* 2010) One of the recurrent aberrations in pediatric AML is the group of 'core binding factor (CBF)' leukemias, including t(8;21)(q22;q22) and

Major categories	Subdivided in the following categories:
Acute myeloid leukemia with recurrent genetic abnormalities	t(8;21)(q22;q22); *RUNX1-RUNX1T1* inv(16)(p13.1q22) or t(16;16)(p13.1;q22); *CBFB-MYH11* t(15;17)(q22;q12); *PML-RARA* t(9;11)(p22;q23); *MLLT3-MLL* t(6;9)(p23;q34); *DEK-NUP214* inv(3)(q21q26.2) or t(3;3)(q21;q26.2); *RPN1-EVI1* t(1;22)(p13;q13); *RBM15-MKL1* *Provisional entity: AML with mutated NPM1* *Provisional entity: AML with mutated CEBPA*
Acute myeloid leukemia with myelodysplasia-related changes	
Therapy-related myeloid neoplasms	
Acute myeloid leukemia, not otherwise specified	AML with minimal differentiation AML without maturation AML with maturation Acute myelomonocytic leukemia Acute monoblastic/monocytic leukemia Acute erythroid leukemia Pure erythroid leukemia Erythroleukemia, erythroid/myeloid Acute megakaryoblastic leukemia Acute basophilic leukemia Acute panmyelosis with myelofibrosis
Myeloid sarcoma	
Myeloid proliferations related to Down syndrome	

Table 2. The new WHO-classification of AML (Vardiman, *et al* 2009)

inv16/t(16;16)(p13/p13;q22), which are considered as good-risk abnormalities by most collaborative groups. (Creutzig, *et al* 1993a, Grimwade, *et al* 1998) CBF-AML is present in approximately 20-25% of pediatric AML cases, which is a higher frequency than found in adults. Rearrangements of the *Mixed Lineage Leukemia (MLL)*-gene, localized at chromosome 11q23, are associated with >50 different fusion partners, and are considered as intermediate or poor risk. *MLL*-gene rearrangements are usually screened for with fluorescent in-situ hybridization (FISH), which does not identify the translocation partner. However, prognosis may depend on the translocation partner, and therefore certain translocation partners need to be specifically searched for with reverse-transcriptase polymerase chain reaction (RT-PCR), such as the t(1;11)(q21;q23), t(6;11)(q27;q23) and t(10;11)(p12;p23). (Balgobind, *et al*

2009) Other abnormalities involve deletion of chromosome 7q or monosomy 7, which are generally considered as poor risk abnormalities. (Hasle, *et al* 2007) Some abnormalities are only found in pediatric AML, such as t(7;12)(q36;p13) and t(1;22)(p13;q13), which both occur in infants with AML. (Bernard, *et al* 2009, von Bergh, *et al* 2006) On the other hand, certain abnormalities such as inv(3)(q21q26.2), which is associated with poor clinical outcome, are rare in children and more frequently found in adults. (Balgobind, *et al* 2010a)

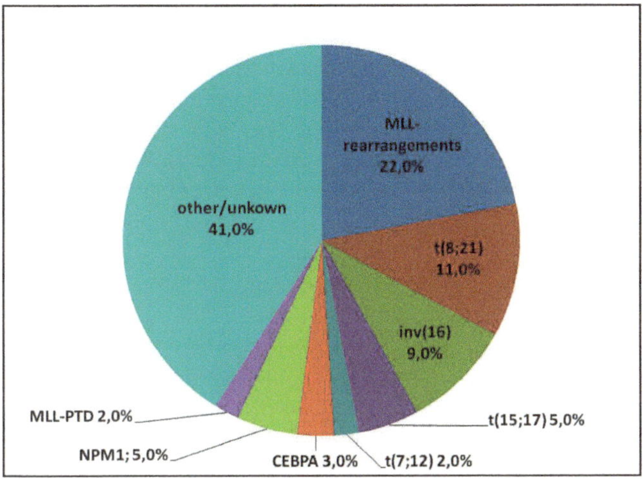

Type 2 abnormalities in pediatric AML

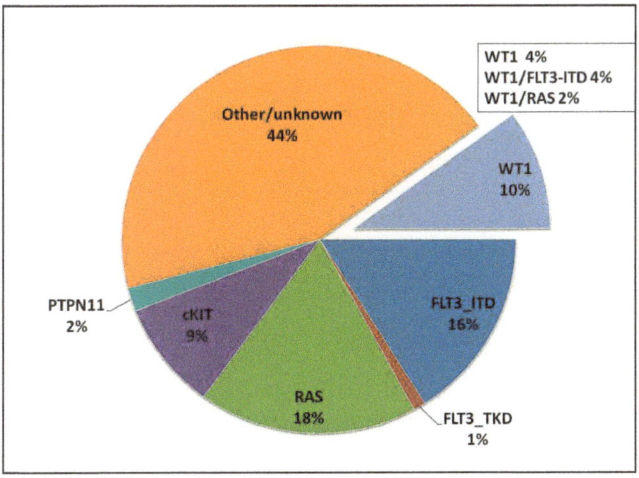

Type 1 abnormalities in pediatric AML.

Fig. 2. Genetic abnormalities in pediatric AML, subdivided as type 1 and type 2 abnormalities. WT1 mutations were included in this graph as type I aberrations, please see text for comments.

In the revised WHO-2008 classification of myeloid neoplasms (Table 2), the category of AML with recurrent genetic abnormalities was further expanded and *NPM1* and *CEBPA* mutated AML were added as provisional categories. (Vardiman, *et al* 2009)
Apart from cytogenetic aberrations, AML is characterized by various gene mutations. Some of these mutations cluster in cytogenetically-normal AML, which is found in 20-25% of pediatric AML cases, which is a lower frequency than in adults, where approximately 50% of cases do not have cytogenetic abnormalities. (Balgobind, et al 2011a, Marcucci, et al 2011) *NPM1* and *CEBPA* gene mutations confer good clinical outcome, whereas mutations in the *FLT3* and *WT1*-genes confer poor clinical outcome. (Ho, et al 2009, Ho, et al 2010b, Hollink, et al 2011, Hollink, et al 2009a, Hollink, et al 2009c, Meshinchi, et al 2006, Zwaan, et al 2003a) Figure 2 shows the distribution of type 1 and 2 abnormalities, as identified in >400 cases of pediatric AML. We have arbitrarily included the WT1 mutations as type I aberrations, however, their role in AML still has to be elucidated. (Hollink, et al 2009a, Yang, et al 2007) Moreover, they are not mutually exclusive with some other typical type I aberrations, as shown in the graph.

2.3 Gene expression profiling as a diagnostic tool

Recently, in pediatric AML, several gene expression profiling studies have been performed with the aim to study their diagnostic potential, and whether they could replace the current diagnostics mentioned above. In a seminal study of 130 *de novo* pediatric AML patients, Ross and colleagues discriminated successfully between acute lymphoblastic leukemia (ALL) and AML by gene expression signatures. (Ross, *et al* 2004) Likewise, the major prognostic AML subclasses, i.e. t(15;17), t(8;21), inv(16), and t(11q23)/*MLL*, as well as cases classified as acute megakaryoblastic leukemia were correctly predicted with an overall classification accuracy greater than 93% using supervised learning algorithms. (Ross, *et al* 2004) This was confirmed by Balgobind et al. in an independent study of 237 children with pediatric AML (specificity and sensitivity for discovery of the indicated cytogenetic subclasses was 92% and 99%, respectively). (Balgobind, *et al* 2011b) However, in the latter study no general predictive gene expression signatures were found for the molecular genetic aberrations *NPM1, CEBPA, FLT3*-ITD, *or KIT.* This may have been caused either by a low frequency of certain mutations, but also by underlying cytogenetics or cell line of origin. For instance, distinct gene expression signatures were discovered for *FLT3*-ITD in patients with normal cytogenetics and in those with t(15;17)(q21;q22)-positive AML. (Balgobind, *et al* 2011b) Therefore, the value of gene expression profiling for use in routine diagnostics is limited to the 40% of cases with clearly discriminative profiles.

3. Current treatment of pediatric AML

3.1 Chemotherapy

Chemotherapy treatment for pediatric AML can be subdivided in several treatment phases: a) induction chemotherapy - which typically consists of 2 courses of intensive chemotherapy; b) consolidation chemotherapy, which may again consist of 2 or 3 courses of chemotherapy; and c) maintenance therapy, which is currently only applied by some groups; and d) hematopoietic stem cell transplantation, which is subject to debate, and is discussed in more detail in paragraph 5.2. Almost all modern protocols include risk-group stratification based on a combination of cytogenetics (defining a good-risk group consisting of CBF-AML and acute promyelocytic leukemia or FAB M3) and early response to therapy (either day 15 bone marrow results, or CR after course 1, or minimal-residual disease status after course 1, which is discussed further in paragraph 6 below).

The former protocols of the Children's Cancer Group (CCG-2891) were based on 'timed sequential induction chemotherapy', which involved a 4-day cycle of five different chemotherapeutic agents, with the second cycle administered either 10 days after the first cycle, despite low or dropping blood counts (intensive timing), or 14 days or later from the beginning of the first cycle, depending on bone marrow status (standard timing). (Woods, *et al* 1996) This concept, however, was inferior to results obtained with other regimens in that era from the MRC and BFM-AML groups(Gibson, *et al* 2005, Stevens, *et al* 1998), and hence this was abandoned. One explanation for the differences in outcome between the CCG 2891 study and the MRC and BFM protocols may have been differences in ethnicity between the populations enrolled on these studies, as Hispanic and black children have poorer outcome compared to white children on CCG 2891, and are over represented in the CCG compared to the Northern-European protocols. (Aplenc, *et al* 2006)

Most protocols nowadays use a typical '3+10 day induction course' (3 days of anthracyclines + 10 days of cytarabine ± a third drug) followed by a second '3+7 or 3+8 course' (3 days of anthracyclines plus 7 or 8 days of cytarabine ± a third drug). The NOPHO group uses a different format which resembles the aforementioned CCG-approach, but is response based. (Abrahamsson, *et al* 2011) The first induction course in their protocols lasts 6 days and contains only 4 days of cytarabine. The timing of the 2nd course then depends on the bone marrow response at day 15. All patients with <5% blast are allowed hematological recovery, all others start with the 2nd course at day 15. The total CR rate was 92% after 2 courses, which is very similar to the CR rates with MRC or BFM approaches. (Creutzig, *et al* 2010b, Gibson, *et al* 2005) Most protocols nowadays consist of a total of 4-5 courses of intensive chemotherapy, although the optimal number of cycles has not been established. (Creutzig, *et al* 2005b, Gibson, *et al* 2005, Kaspers and Creutzig 2005, Kaspers and Zwaan 2007) In protocol MRC AML 12 this question was addressed (see Table 4). Maintenance therapy in AML is subject to debate, but there are several studies showing that if any effect it leads to worse retrieval at relapse, and is therefore probably not indicated. (Perel, *et al* 2002, Wells, *et al* 1994)

Chemotherapy for AML is intensive and consists of a cytarabine/anthracycline backbone to which other drugs may be added, for instance epipodophyllotoxins (i.e. etoposide) or anti-metabolites (i.e. 6-thioguanine). In some protocols asparaginase is applied, which seems mainly effective against monoblastic leukemias (Zwaan, *et al* 2002a), and is usually given in combination with cytarabine (also referred to as the Capizzi regimen). (Capizzi, *et al* 1988, Zwaan, *et al* 2002b) Some protocols use 2-chlorodeoxyadenosine as nucleoside analog instead of cytarabine. Other protocols aim at potentiating cytarabine by combining it with fludarabine (often combined with GCSF and then referred to as a FLAG course) or 2-chlorodeoxyadenosine, which leads to increased Ara-CTP levels (the active metabolite). (Burnett, *et al* 2011, Creutzig, *et al* 2010b, Rubnitz, *et al* 2009) In more recent studies gemtuzumab ozogamicin has been evaluated together with standard chemotherapy in induction and consolidation, but results for children have not been reported as yet. (Burnett, *et al* 2011) In older protocols, steroids were sometimes included, but steroids may (at least in-vitro) induce proliferation of AML cells, and hence are no longer applied. (Zwaan, *et al* 2002b)

Prevention of CNS-relapse is mainly based on intrathecal chemotherapy, which is given on top of intensive IV cytarabine courses. There is no evidence that low numbers of blasts in the

Study	Randomized comparison	Era	CR rate	EFS	OS	Ref
AML-BFM 2004	Liposomal DNR 3x80 mg/m² vs. idarubicin 3x12 mg/m²	2004-2010	NA	L-DNR 60% vs. Ida 54% (p=0.17)	L-DNR 78% vs. Ida 70% (p=0.15)	(Creutzig, *et al* 2010b)
St Jude AML02	High-dose vs. low dose cytarabine (18 vs. 2 gr/m²)	2002-2008	MRD-positivity high 34% vs. low 42%, p=0.17	High: 60.2% vs. low 65.7%, p=-p.41	High 68.8% vs. low 73.4%, p=0.41	(Rubnitz, *et al* 2010)
MRC-AML 12	DNR 3x50 mg/m² vs. Mitoxantrone 3x12 mg/m²	1995-2002	DNR 92% vs. Mitox 90%, p=0.3	NA	DNR 65% vs. Mitox 70%, p=0.1	(Gibson, *et al* 2005)
POG-9421	Standard dose (100 mg/m²x7 days) versus high dose (1 gram/m²/x7 days) cytarabine	1995-1999	Standard 87.9% vs. high 91%, p=0.23	Standard 35% vs. high dose 40%, p=0.28	NA	(Becton, *et al* 2006)
AML-BFM 1993	DNR3x60mg/m² vs. idarubicin 3x12 mg/m²	1993-1998	>5% blasts in day 15 BMA: Ida 17% vs DNR 31%, p=0.01	Ida 51 *vs* DNR 50%, p=0.72	Ida 60% *vs* DNR 57, p=0.55	(Creutzig, *et al* 2001)
CCG 2891	Standard versus intensive timing	1989-1995	Standard 70% vs. intensive 75%, p=0.18	Standard 27% vs. intensive 42%, p=0.0005	Standard 39% vs. intensive 51%, p=0.07	(Woods, *et al* 1996)
MRC-AML 10	6-thioguanine 75 mg/m², 12-h, d1-10 vs. etoposide 100 mg/m² IV day 1-5	1988-1995	6-TG 90% vs Etoposide 93%, p=0.3	6-TG 48% vs Etoposide 45%, p=0.3	6-TG 57% vs Etoposide 51%, p=0.5	(Gibson, *et al* 2005)

CR=complete remission, EFS=event free survival, OS=overall survival, Ref=reference, DNR=daunorubicn, Ida=idarubicin, Mitox=mitoxantrone, 6-TG=6-thioguanine, NA=not available, BMA=bone-marrow aspirate, MRD=minimal residual disease.

Table 3. Randomized induction questions in pediatric AML studies.

cerebrospinal fluid (CNS-2 status) are clinically relevant in AML, and hence additional intrathecal therapy is not needed in case of CNS-2. (Abbott, *et al* 2003) Most groups do not apply prophylactic CNS-irradiation in pediatric AML patients, apart from the BFM-group. In their AML-BFM 87 study, which was initially set-up as a randomized study but failed due to non-compliance with this randomization, it was found that irradiated patients had fewer bone marrow relapses, and hence prophylactic irradiation was continued. (Creutzig, *et al* 1993b) Patients with clear CNS-involvement (CNS-3) are given irradiation in most treatment protocols, although this may be replaced by frequent intrathecal injections in younger children, with the aim to avoid late effects or cranial irradiation on neurocognitive development.

Several randomized studies have been performed addressing either induction or consolidation chemotherapy questions over the past few years. Table 3 summarizes the induction randomizations that were performed. As can be seen most randomizations were negative, although it remains difficult to interpret the results for the anthracyclines, as it is not known whether the randomized dosages are in fact dose-equivalent. Considering consolidation, the randomized questions are summarized in Table 4, and again most of these do not provide statistically significant results.

Study	Era	Randomized comparison	EFS	OS	Ref.
AML-BFM 2004	2004-2010	Cytarabine/idarubicin ± 2-chlorodeoxyadenosine (2-CDA)	2-CDA 51% vs. no 2-CDA 51%, p=0.98	2-CDA: 75% vs. no 2-CDA 65%, p=0.18	(Creutzig, *et al* 2010b)
AML-BFM 98	1998-2004	6-week consolidation vs. 2 short cycles	6-week 51% vs 2 cycles 50%, p=0.66		(Creutzig, *et al* 2006)
AML-BFM 93	1993-1998	Early HAM course in consolidation versus late	Early: 49% vs. Late 41% (p=non-significant)	Early: 57% vs. Late 54% (p=non-significant)	(Creutzig, *et al* 2005b)
POG-9421	1995-1999	Ciclosporin A (CsA) added to consolidation chemotherapy	DFS: CsA 40.6% vs. no CsA 33.9%, p=0.24	NA	(Becton, *et al* 2006)
MRC-AML12	1995-2002	4 versus 5 courses (MIDAC vs. MIDAC plus CLASP)	NA	4 courses 81% vs. 5 courses 78%, p=0.5	(Gibson, *et al* 2005)

EFS=event free survival, OS=overall survival, Ref=reference, NA=not available, DFS=disease free survival

Table 4. Chemotherapy-based consolidation randomizations in pediatric AML (excluding stem-cell transplant related questions).

3.2 Stem-cell transplantation

The principle of stem-cell transplantation is to eradicate minimal residual disease using high-dose chemotherapy and/or total body irradiation. (Bleakley, *et al* 2002, Niewerth, *et al* 2010) Allogeneic SCT also has an immunological effect, as the graft may induce a 'graft-versus-leukemia effect (GVL)', and hence may be able to prevent leukemia relapse. Autologous SCT has also been used in pediatric AML, but there is basically no evidence that this is superior to intensive chemotherapy consolidation. (Aplenc, *et al* 2006, Pession, *et al* 2005) Two reviews have addressed the issue of allo-SCT versus chemotherapy in pediatric AML, and both conclude that although allo-SCT reduces relapse risk this is counterbalanced by increased procedure-related mortality and by poorer retrieval at relapse. (Bleakley, *et al* 2002, Niewerth, *et al* 2010) Hence, in most studies overall survival does not improve. It should also be emphasized that 'older' studies may show more benefit from SCT than more recent studies, given that the beneficial effect of SCT is likely to be greater with less intensive induction chemotherapy. (Creutzig and Reinhardt 2002, Woods, *et al* 2001) In most current protocols SCT in 1st complete remission is therefore only recommended for selected high-risk cases, although there is little evidence that this in fact improves outcome in these cases. (Creutzig and Reinhardt 2002, Reinhardt, *et al* 2006) In first relapse, most patients are transplanted after achieving a 2nd CR. (Kaspers, *et al* 2009) There is limited evidence that pre-emptive therapy post-SCT may be effective in reducing the frequency of overt relapse. (Bader, *et al* 2004)

3.3 Supportive care

The current intensity of pediatric AML treatment is only possible with rigorous supportive care, including (but not limited to) blood transfusions, antibiotic and antifungal prophylaxis, viral surveillance, early diagnostics of fungal infections with high-resolution CT-scans, prevention of nephropathy using rasburicase in hyperleucocytosis, GCSF use in life-threatening infections, tube feeding and total parenteral nutrition. (Goldman, *et al* 2001, Inaba, *et al* 2011, Lehrnbecher, *et al* 2009, Lehrnbecher, *et al* 2004, van de Wetering, *et al* 2005) In fact, a substantial part of the progress in pediatric AML over the last decades is due to improvements in supportive care. Despite this progress, a a significant number of patients still do not survive as a result of early death or due to treatment related mortality, as summarized in Table 5. Therefore, further intensification of AML studies is currently not considered feasible. This was also demonstrated in a French study from the LAME group, who tried to further intensify induction therapy by a timed-sequential approach, but this pilot was stopped given the time needed for hematological recovery until consolidation, which was median 98 days in the timed-sequential approach versus 76 days using their regular 2 induction courses. (Perel, *et al* 2005)

	Early death	Treatment related mortality	Cumulative incidence of death	References
DCOG 83, 87 and 92/94 studies	13.1%	4.4%	NA	(Slats, *et al* 2005)
BFM 93- and 98 studies	3.5%	8%	NA	(Creutzig, *et al* 2004)
St Jude	NA	NA	7.6%	(Rubnitz, *et al* 2004)
NOPHO 84, 88 and 93 studies	3%	10%	NA	(Molgaard-Hansen, *et al* 2010b)

NA=not available

Table 5. Summary of early death and treatment related deaths in pediatric AML studies.

4. Outcome of pediatric AML

4.1 Newly diagnosed pediatric AML

The outcome of newly diagnosed pediatric AML has increased significantly over the past decades. Contemporary studies show survival rates in the range of at least 65-75%, as detailed in Table 6.

4.2 Relapsed AML

The cumulative incidence of relapse is around 30% with modern intensive chemotherapy protocols used in newly diagnosed disease. (Creutzig, *et al* 2005b, Gibson, *et al* 2005, Sander, *et al* 2010) Relapsed AML is usually treated with similar chemotherapy as given upfront, hence intensive cytarabine/anthracyline based chemotherapy. Following a second remission induction patients are usually transplanted. A summary of studies in relapsed pediatric AML is provided in table 7. As can be seen, outcome is poor, and the largest and most recent study of the International BFM-Study Group reported 35% overall survival. (Kaspers, *et al*

2009) Outcome for patients with late relapse and/or good risk cytogenetics is better, as well as for patients who have not been transplanted in CR1 and for those achieving CR2 with re-induction chemotherapy. (Sander, *et al* 2010, Webb 1999) Patients with refractory first relapse or with second relapse are considered candidates for experimental therapy. (Zwaan, *et al* 2010b)

Study Group	**Years**	**No of patients**	**EFS (5yrs)**	**OS (5yrs)**	**References**
LAME 91	1991-1998	262	47%	61%	(Perel, *et al* 2005)
AIEOP LAM 92	1992-2001	160	54%	60%	(Pession, *et al* 2005)
GATLA AML 90	1993-2000	179	31%	41%	(Armendariz, *et al* 2005)
EORTC 58921	1993-2000	177	49%	62%	(Entz-Werle, *et al* 2005)
MRC AML 12	1994-2002	455	56%	66%	(Gibson, *et al* 2005)
POG 9421	1995-1999	565	36% (3-year EFS)	54% (3-year OS)	(Becton, *et al* 2006)
AML PPLLSG 98	1998-2002	147	47%	50%	(Dluzniewska, *et al* 2005)
BMF 98	1998-2003	473	49%	62%	(Creutzig, *et al* 2006)
AML 99 Japan	2000-2002	240	62%	76%	(Tsukimoto, *et al* 2009)
SJCRH AML	2002-2008	230	63%	71%	(Rubnitz, *et al* 2010)
NOPHO AML 2004	2004-2009	151	57% (3-year EFS)	69% (3-year OS)	(Abrahamsson, *et al* 2011)
AML-BFM 2004	2004-2010	566	54%	72%	(Creutzig, *et al* 2010b)

Table 6. Overall outcome data for pediatric AML studies started from 1990 onwards.

Study Group	**Years**	**No of patients**	**DFS (5yrs)**	**EFS (5yrs)**	**OS(5yrs)**	**Ref**
TACL institutions	1995-2004	99	43%	24%	29%	(Gorman, *et al* 2010)
LAME group	Relapse following LAME 89/91	106	45%	NA	33%	(Aladjidi, *et al* 2003)
MRC group	Relapse following MRC AML-10	125	44%	NA	24% (3 yrs)	(Webb, *et al* 1999)
BFM-group	Relapse following AML-BFM 87, 93 and 98	379	NA	NA	23%	(Sander, *et al* 2010)
I-BFM	2002-2009	360	NA	NA	35% (3-year OS)	(Kaspers, *et al* 2009)

Table 7. Studies in relapsed pediatric AML.

4.3 Late effects of treatment

The major long-term toxicity in AML patients treated without stem cell transplantation is long-term cardiac toxicity. (Creutzig, *et al* 2007, Temming, *et al* 2011) This is associated with higher cumulative dosages of anthracyclines. (Nysom, *et al* 1998) The use of liposomal formulations may be an option to reduce cardiac toxicity, as discussed below in paragraph 7.2. Stem cell transplantation is associated with many late effects, mainly depending on the type of conditioning regimen (type of chemotherapy and/or total body irradiation), and the occurrence of graft-versus-host disease. Toxicities include growth arrest, infertility, other endocrine abnormalities, secondary cancers and cataracts. (Leung, *et al* 2000, Leung, *et al* 2001) Neurocognitive sequelae may be anticipated in patients receiving cranial irradiation, depending on dose and age of radiotherapy administration. (Reinhardt, *et al* 2002b, Temming and Jenney 2010) A quality-of-life study form the NOPHO group showed that self-reported health was considered excellent or very good in 77% of ex-patients, and comparable to that of siblings, with a median follow-up of 11 years. (Molgaard-Hansen, *et al* 2010a)

5. Specific subgroups in pediatric AML

5.1 Children with Down syndrome

Children with Down syndrome have an increased risk (approximately 150-fold) of developing myeloid leukemia, which is often preceded by a so-called 'transient leukemia (TL)' in neonatal life. (Hasle, *et al* 2000, Zwaan, *et al* 2008) This Down syndrome associated myeloid-leukemia (ML-DS) is a unique disease entity characterized by occurrence at young age (before the age of 4 years), a smoldering disease course, megakaryocytic features, and mutations in the *GATA1* transcription factor gene localized on the X-chromosome. (Ahmed, *et al* 2004, Creutzig, *et al* 2005a, Hitzler, *et al* 2003, Lange, *et al* 1998, Zwaan, *et al* 2008) Interestingly, ML-DS is a highly curable disease, when reduced-intensity treatment protocols are used, avoiding excessive treatment-related mortality. (Creutzig, *et al* 2005a, Gamis, *et al* 2006) This is probably due to enhanced sensitivity to chemotherapy, as was determined with in-vitro cell-kill assays. (Ge, *et al* 2004, Zwaan, *et al* 2002b) This also implicates that these patients should not be transplanted in CR1, and that longer intervals between courses are necessary and acceptable if the patient needs to recover from a prior course of chemotherapy. TL occurs in approximately 10% of children with DS, and is probably derived from trisomy 21 induced expansion of fetal liver megakarocyte precursors, which become 'leukemic' once a *GATA1* mutation occurs. (Chou, *et al* 2008, Klusmann, *et al* 2008, Tunstall-Pedoe, *et al* 2008) In most cases (~80%) TL resolves spontaneously without development of ML-DS later in life, however, in 20% of children TL is followed by ML-DS between 1-4 years of age (Figure 3). (Hasle, *et al* 2008) It is currently unknown whether ML-DS may also occur without preceding TL, although it is perhaps unlikely. Moreover, it is unknown which factors exactly drive clonal evolution to ML-DS in these 20% of children, although research is ongoing to unravel this. (Chen, *et al* 2010, Klusmann, *et al* 2010a, Klusmann, *et al* 2010b) Of interest, a recent paper shows that lower protein expression of GATA1s predicts a higher chance of ML-DS development after TL. (Kanezaki, *et al* 2010) Current efforts in TL are focused on 2 aspects: 1) Treatment of children with symptomatic TL to avoid TL-related deaths, which may occur from either fluid overload, organomegaly and high WBC, or from liver failure which is believed to result from cytokines produced by the leukemic blasts infiltrating the liver. (Klusmann, *et al* 2008) Treatment can consist of (repetitive) courses of low dose cytarabine (Al Ahmari, *et al* 2006), and 2) the potential to avoid clonal evolution to ML-DS by treating children with low clearance of TL as assessed by MRD measurements at pre-defined time-points. Results from the latter studies are not yet available, and hence this cannot be considered standard of care as yet.

5.2 Infants with AML

There is a peak in the incidence of AML in children below the age of 1 year. These leukemias have a different genetic profile compared to older children with AML, as approximately 50% of these cases are characterized by *MLL*-rearrangements. (Creutzig, *et al* 2010a, Vormoor, *et al* 1992) Moreover, certain specific chromosomal aberrations are only found in children below one year of age, such as the *OTT-MAL* fusion gene found in young children with megakaryoblastic leukemia and t(1;22)(p13;q13)(Reinhardt, *et al* 2005), and the t(7;12)(q36,p13), which is characterized by very poor clinical outcome. (von Bergh, *et al* 2006) Clinically, children below the age of one year more often present with high WBC, organomegaly and CNS-involvement. (Pui, *et al* 2000, Vormoor, *et al* 1992) In ALL, outcome of infants is worse compared to older children, which led to the introduction of specific treatment protocols, but there is no evidence that this is the case in AML. (Creutzig, *et al* 2010a, Pieters, *et al* 2007) Most protocols advise dose-reduction in infants with AML, and chemotherapy is usually calculated on a mg/kg basis rather than using body surface area.

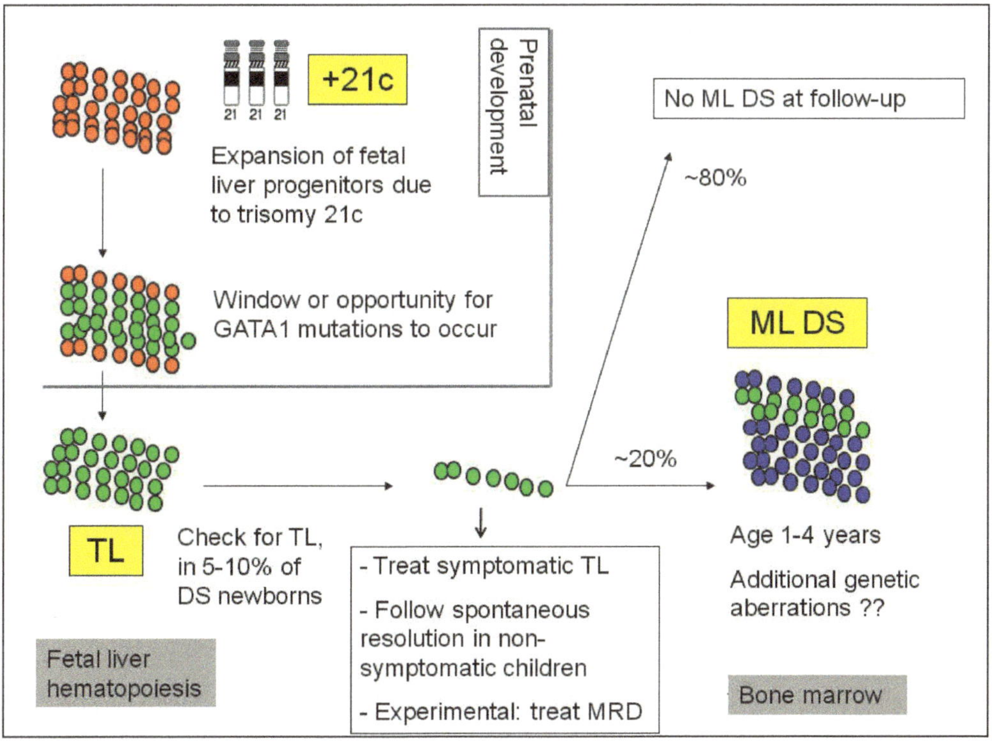

Fig. 3. Development of ML-DS from transient leukemia.

5.3 Adolescents and young adults with AML

In ALL, it appeared that adolescents and younger adults fared much better on pediatric treatment protocols than on adult treatment regimens. (Boissel, *et al* 2003, de Bont, *et al* 2004) Subsequently, this was also investigated for AML. Creuztig et al. could not find differences in outcome between patients treated on a pediatric and an adult treatment protocol. (Creutzig, *et al* 2008) In an Australian study, for cases diagnosed between 2000 and 2004, there was no difference in outcome for children, adolescents and young adults (20-29 years). (Pinkerton, *et al* 2010) This is probably due to a greater similarity between pediatric and adult AML protocols, whereas there are major differences between pediatric and adult ALL protocols. Prognosis however declines with age, as a consequences of a reduction of good-risk cytogenetic abnormalities, and reduced host-tolerance to chemotherapy.

5.4 Cytogenetically normal AML

In children, approximately 15-20% of AML cases present without karyotypic abnormalities, which is a much lower frequency than in adults. (Balgobind, *et al* 2011a, Harrison, *et al* 2010, von Neuhoff, *et al* 2010) Over the past few years many gene mutations or overexpression of specific genes have been identified in CN-AML, with clear prognostic impact. (Hollink, *et al* 2009b) This includes typical type II aberrations such as *NPM1* mutations in ~20%, *CEPBA* double mutations in ~15-20% of cases. (Balgobind, *et al* 2011a) The *NPM1* and *CEBPA* double mutations confer good clinical outcome, allowing risk-stratification with the "good risk" cytogenetic subgroups. (Brown, *et al* 2007, Ho, *et al* 2009, Hollink, *et al* 2011, Hollink, *et al* 2009c) In addition, the following type-1 mutations were identified: *FLT3*-internal tandem duplications (*FLT3*-ITD), found in ~30-40% of cases, *FLT3*-tyrosine kinase domain mutations (*FLT3*-TKD) in ~2% and *N*- or *K-RAS* mutations in ~15-20% of CN-AML cases. (Balgobind, *et al* 2011a, Goemans, *et al* 2005, Meshinchi, *et al* 2006) *WT1* mutations were found in 20-25% of pediatric CN-AML cases, in approximately half of the cases together with a *FLT3*-ITD, and in a quarter together with a *RAS*-mutation. (Balgobind, *et al* 2011a, Ho, *et al* 2010b, Hollink, *et al* 2009a) In 20-25% of cases no type-I aberration can be detected so far. The Children's Oncology Group published similar data, although they could not confirm the poor outcome of patients with *WT1* mutations. In adults, specific prognostic paradigms are being developed for CN-AML, which is not yet the case in children, in part because numbers are small. (Damm, *et al* 2011, Mrozek, *et al* 2007)

5.5 MLL-rearranged AML

MLL-rearrangements are typically found in younger children with AML. The true incidence of *MLL*-rearrangements in pediatric AML is considered to be in the range of 15-25% according to the latest trials, since cryptic *MLL*-rearrangements were not always identified in the past with conventional karyotyping only. (Harrison, *et al* 2010, von Neuhoff, *et al* 2010) In the past, *MLL*-rearranged AML has been related to poor outcome despite intensive chemotherapy. However recent studies showed that outcome in *MLL*-rearranged AML is dependent on different factors, e.g. translocation partner, age, WBC and additional cytogenetic aberrations. (Balgobind, *et al* 2009) Cases with a t(1;11)(q21;q23) have an excellent outcome and may benefit from less intensive treatment, whereas cases with a t(6;11)(q27;q23) or t(10;11)(p21;q23) have a poor outcome and do need adjusted and alternative treatment strategies to improve outcome. This means that these abnormalities need to be specifically screened for, as suggested in Figure 4. Although cooperating events are a hallmark of developing AML, additional genetic aberrations in *MLL*-rearranged AML are hardly identified. Roughly 50% of the *MLL*-rearranged AML cases harbor a known type-I mutation, and most of these mutations were identified in genes involved in the RAS-pathway, including mutations in *NRAS, KRAS, PTPN11* and *NF1*. (Balgobind, *et al* 2008) Recently, novel aberrantly expressed genes have been identified that are involved in MLL-gene rearranged AML leukemogenesis, such as *IGSF4, BRE* and *EVI1*. (Balgobind, *et al* 2010a, Balgobind, *et al* 2010b, Kuipers, *et al* 2011) Upregulation of *HOX* genes is one of the most important hallmarks of *MLL*-rearranged leukemias, and may be a target for epigenetic therapy. (Krivtsov, *et al* 2008)

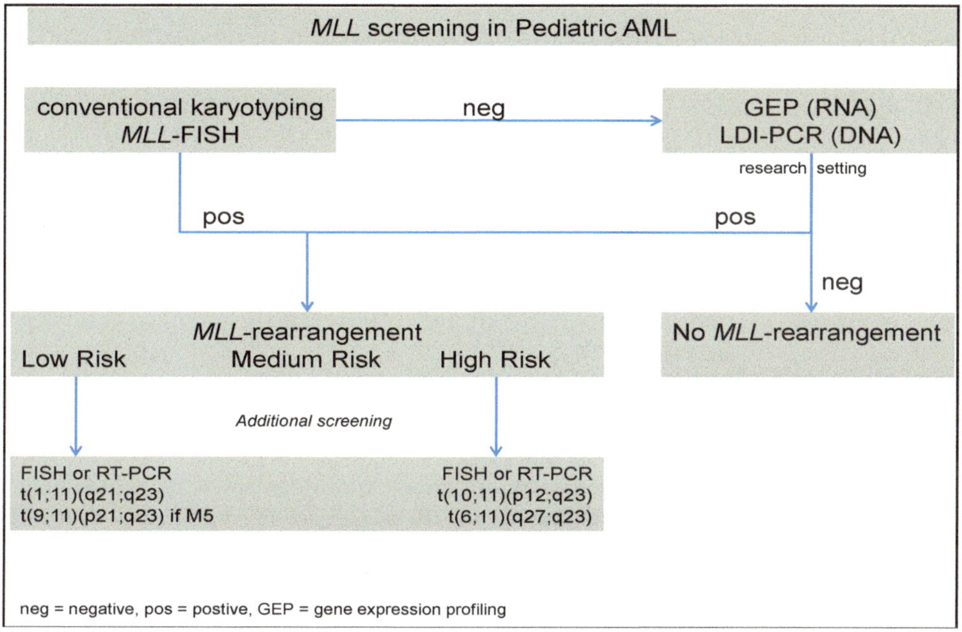

Fig. 4. Screening for *MLL*-rearrangements in pediatric AML.

5.6 Acute promyelocytic leukemia

Acute promyelocytic leukemia (APL) is a distinct pathological entity that occurs in only 4-8% of all AML cases in children. The disease is characterized by a specific morphological subtype (FAB M3), although in a small percentage morphology is different, referred to as 'microgranular variant morphology (M3V)'. (Tallman, *et al* 2010) Furthermore, APL is characterized by the presence of the chromosomal translocation t(15;17)(1q22;q21), which results in the *PML-RARa* fusion transcript, and its reciprocal product *RARa-PML*. (Sanz, *et al* 2009) In a minority of cases (<5%), *RARa* is fused to an alternative partner, most commonly *NPM1* resulting from a t(5;17)(q35;q21) or *NuMA* in t(11;17)(q13;q21). (Grimwade, *et al* 2000) The diagnostic white blood cell count is the most important prognostic factor in APL. The hallmarks of the disease is the sensitivity for all-trans-retinoic acid (ATRA), which is now considered standard of care for APL in induction and in maintenance in combination with chemotherapy, or arsenic trioxide (ATO), which is mostly used in salvage treatment.

(Soignet 2001) Both drugs induce differentiation and apoptosis of leukemic cells, and have reduced the incidence of early fatal bleeding complications that APL is associated with. (Sanz, *et al* 2009, Stein, *et al* 2009) Currently, overall survival rates in children with APL are in the range of 80-90% (see table 8). (Creutzig, *et al* 2010c, Testi, *et al* 2005) Based on these results, the International-BFM Group has launched a 'standard of care' protocol for children with APL (the ICC APL study 01). The main aim of this study is to lower the cumulative dose of anthracyclines used in the treatment of APL, which is very high in some adult protocols that pediatric regimens were based upon. (Testi, *et al* 2005) Given the risk of severe long-term cardiac toxicity, the ICC APL 01 study combines a lower dose of anthracyclines with cytarabine and ATRA, as has been used previously by the BFM group. (Creutzig, *et al* 2010c)

Study Group	Years	No of patients	EFS (5yrs)	OS(5yrs)	References
AML-BFM SG	1993-2010	81	73%	89%	(Creutzig, *et al* 2010c)
GIMEMEA-AEIOPAIDA	1993-2000	107	76%	89%	(Testi, *et al* 2005)
North-American Intergroup Trial*	1992-1995	53	NA	69%	(Gregory, *et al* 2009)
AML-99 M3 (Japan)	1997-2004	58	91%	93%	(Imaizumi, *et al* 2011)

* ATRA was not given to all patients

Table 8. Outcome results in APL in children.

Several adult studies have now also introduced arsenic trioxide in newly diagnosed patients, either in combination with chemotherapy, or as single-agent, or in combination with ATRA. (Hu, *et al* 2009, Mathews, *et al* 2010, Powell, *et al* 2011) Using arsenic alone, Mathews et al. reported durable responses with almost 70% event-free survival. (Mathews, *et al* 2010) This has also been piloted in 11 children, with similar encouraging findings. (George, *et al* 2004) When this is confirmed in larger studies treatment of APL without chemotherapy may be feasible, especially when no long-term toxicities from arsenic treatment emerge.

6. Minimal Residual Disease

In acute lymphoblastic leukemia risk group stratification is based on assessment of minimal residual disease (MRD) in modern treatment protocols, as this is superior to any of the classical prognostic factors (age, WBC, cytogenetics, immunophenotype). (Flohr, *et al* 2008, Van Dongen, *et al* 1998) In ALL, this can either be done using flow cytometry, or by using quantative polymerase chain reaction of immunoglobulin or T-cell receptor rearrangements. (van der Velden and van Dongen 2009) In AML, MRD assessment is more complicated. (Goulden, *et al* 2006) Flow cytometry is used by several investigators, and leukemia-specific aberrant immunophenotypes can be detected in the majority of patients. (van der Velden, *et al* 2010) However, flow cytometry may not always have sufficient sensitivity. For instance, investigators from the AML-BFM SG analysed MRD in their AML-98 study. (Langebrake, *et al* 2006) Using 4-color immunophenotyping, they could not show that MRD was superior to the traditional BFM-risk group classification (based on cytogenetics at diagnosis and morphological assessment of bone marrow blasts at day 15 and 28) to predict clinical outcome. However, other groups have reported independent prognostic significance of MRD assessment. Van der Velden et al. have monitored MRD in the context of the MRC12 protocol, and showed that 3-year relapse-free survival was 85% for MRD-negative patients (MRD<0.1%) and 64% for MRD-low-positive patients (0.1%<or=MRD<0.5%) and only 14% for MRD-high-positive patients (MRD>or=0.5%; P<0.001). (van der Velden, *et al* 2010) In the AML02 study from St Jude Children's Research Hospital MRD was used for patient stratification. (Rubnitz, *et al* 2010) High MRD at the end of induction was the only independent risk-factor for survival, with a cut—off level for MRD-positivity of 0.1%. In conclusion, there is an increasing amount of evidence that flow cytometry based MRD stratification is superior to using more conventional parameters to risk-stratify patients. Molecular MRD assessment in pediatric AML has been based on the quantative assessment of fusion-genes using RQ-PCR. Only rising MRD values are clinically relevant, as it is known that for instance *AML1-ETO* and *CBF*beta-*MYH11* can still be detected with sensitive methods in patients in long-lasting continuous complete remission. (Leroy, *et al* 2005, Miyamoto, *et al* 1996, Perea, *et al* 2006, Viehmann, *et al* 2003) Using fusion genes as MRD targets has the limitation that only a subset of patients (approximately 40-50%) can be studied. However, the newly discovered molecular mutations, such as *NPM1* or *GATA1* mutations, may also be suitable MRD-targets. (Pine, *et al* 2005, Schnittger, *et al* 2009) Some of these targets, such as *FLT3* mutations, may not be stable between diagnosis and relapse, and this may result in false-negative results(Bachas, *et al* 2010), which may also occur in flow-cytometry based MRD assessment due to immunophenotypic shifts. (Langebrake, *et al* 2005) Another important issue is the frequency of required sampling post-treatment, as leukemias may differ in the lag-time between molecular and overt relapse, which appears to be translocation/molecular marker dependent. (Ommen, *et al* 2010) Given this heterogeneity a more ubiquitously expressed MRD target would be more practical, and several investigators have chosen *WT1*-expression as a suitable MRD-target, given that *WT1* is overexpressed in the majority of pediatric AML patients. (Cilloni, *et al* 2009, Lapillonne, *et al* 2006, Willasch, *et al* 2009) Despite all these technical advantages, MRD in pediatric AML is still mainly an area of research rather than a standardized approach implemented as standard of care in clinical treatment protocols, in contrast to pediatric ALL. The one exception in AML is acute promyelocytic leukemia, where MRD-follow-up is nowadays considered standard, and where it has been shown that pre-emptive therapy of molecular relapse may prevent the occurrence of overt relapse. (Grimwade, *et al* 2009, Testi, *et al* 2005)

7. New treatment options

7.1 Gemtuzumab ozogamicin

Gemtuzumab ozogamicin (GO) is a conjugated antibody in which an anti-CD33 antibody is linked to the anti-tumor antibiotic calichemicin. (Sievers, *et al* 1999, Zwaan, *et al* 2003b) After binding to CD33 the complex is internalized and calicheamicin is spliced off and exterts its cytotoxic activity. In studies in adults, the main side-effects of GO were hematological and liver toxicity, referred to as sinusoidal obstruction syndrome (SOS). (Rajvanshi, *et al* 2002, Sievers, *et al* 2001) Although the initial development in adults concerned single-agent high-dose GO (2 dosages of GO 9 mg/m^2 IV given with a 14 day-interval), combination studies showed that dosages in the range of 3-5 mg/m^2 could be incorporated in existing AML chemotherapy regimens. (Kell, *et al* 2003) In AML in adults, several large randomized studies were performed. This includes the addition of GO in induction therapy in the MRC-AML 15 study, which showed an improvement in survival mainly for patients with good-risk cytogenetics. (Burnett, *et al* 2011) Löwenberg et al. gave 3 cycles of GO (6 mg/m2 at 4 week intervals) as post-remission treatment in elderly AML patients, which failed to show a benefit in this population. (Lowenberg, *et al* 2010a)

In children, phase I studies showed that 6-7.5 mg/m^2 was the maximum tolerated dose. (Arceci, *et al* 2005) Several phase II studies have been performed, either as single-agent or in combination with cytarabine, showing response rates in the range of 30-40%. (Brethon, *et al* 2008, Zwaan, *et al* 2010b) GO seems better tolerable in children, in that lower frequencies of SOD were seen. Aplenc et al. published safety data of GO in combination with either cytarabine and mitoxantrone or cytarabine and asparaginase in relapsed pediatric AML patients, and showed that the MTD for the 1st combination was 3 mg/m^2 of GO, versus 2 mg/m^2 for the latter combination. (Aplenc, *et al* 2008) The results of a study in newly diagnosed AML patients as conducted by the Children's Oncology Group are awaited. Rubnitz et al. gave GO in combination with induction chemotherapy to slow early responders (non-randomized). (Rubnitz, *et al* 2010) Given the results of the phase II studies mentioned above, the International-BFM AML group will perform a randomized study in relapsed/refractory AML patients in which standard chemotherapy is given with or without one infusion of GO. Considering its use in pediatric AML the current phase II results suggest better activity and less side-effects than in adults, but no randomized studies have been performed as yet. The current registration status of GO is a major obstacle in its use, as it is only licensed for use in Japan, and hence is not commercially available in Europe or the US. Its prior accelerated approval in the US was withdrawn in 2010 after a follow-up study in adults with relapsed AML (study SWOG S0106) was interrupted as it did not show sufficient benefit and caused safety concerns. (FDA 2010)

7.2 Liposomal drugs

A major concern in children is the development of long-term cardiac toxicity following exposure to high dosages of anthracyclines. (Creutzig, *et al* 2007, Lipshultz and Adams 2010, van Dalen, *et al* 2006) It is hypothesized that liposomal daunorubicin (DNX) has less cardiac toxicity, as the liposomal formulation prohibits its accumulation in cardiac tissue. A cardio-protective effect has been shown for liposomal doxorubicin in solid tumors,(van Dalen, *et al* 2010) however no long-term follow-up studies are available for liposomal daunorubicin to show that it is indeed cardioprotective as well. In adults, a randomized trial between 80 mg/m^2 DNX compared to 45 mg/m^2 of daunorubicin showed a survival advantage for the DNX-arm because of a reduction in late relapses, despite increased treatment related deaths in the DNX-arm. (Latagliata, *et al* 2008) In children, DNX was piloted by the BFM-group in the relapsed AML-98 trial, and was used in all subsequent relapse studies. (Reinhardt, *et al* 2002a) Population pharmacokinetic data showed a lower volume of distribution and lower clearance compared to free daunorubicin. (Hempel, *et al* 2003) DNX is currently considered standard of care in relapsed pediatric AML, given the results of the I-BFM Relapsed AML 2001/01 randomized study showing a significant benefit in terms of early treatment response in patients randomized to the FLAG plus DNX arm (60 mg/m^2 on day 1, 3 and 5), versus those randomized to FLAG alone. (Kaspers, *et al* 2009) Moreover, in the AML-BFM SG upfront studies, DNX was introduced in the 2004 protocol at a dose of 80 mg/m^2 and randomized against idarubicin. (Creutzig, *et al* 2010b) Patients randomized to DNX had

better outcome, although the results were not statistically significant. DNX appeared somewhat less toxic than idarubicin, which included less cases of acute cardiac toxity. (Creutzig, *et al* 2010b) Perhaps further dose-escalation of DNX is possible given the improved therapeutic index for acute cardiac and other toxicity(Creutzig, *et al* 2010b, Kaspers, *et al* 2009), as it is expected that a higher anthracycline dose will translate in better survival, as recently demonstrated in a randomized study in elderly patients with AML (45 versus 90 mg/m^2 for 3 days in induction). (Lowenberg, *et al* 2009)
A new liposomal formulation (CPX-351) combines bot cytarabine and daunorubicin in a 5:1 ratio. (Feldman, *et al* 2011) Recently, a phase I study in adults with relapsed/refractory AML was completed, showing responses in approximately 25% of patients. The recommended phase II dose was 101 U/m^2, following toxicities including hypertensive crisis, congestive heart failure, and prolonged cytopenias at higher dosages.

7.3 Nucleoside analogs

2-Chlorodeoxyadenosine (2-CDA) is a synthetic nucleoside analog that inhibits ribonucloetide reductase and increases the activity of deoxycitidine kinase. In vitro, the drug was more potent than cytarabine, and especially monoblastic leukemias appeared sensitive to this compound. (Hubeek, *et al* 2006) This nucleoside analog has mainly been incorporated in studies from St Jude Children's Research Hospital, showing clear anti-leukemic efficacy against relapsed and newly diagnosed AML. (Krance, *et al* 2001, Santana, *et al* 1991, Santana, *et al* 1992) In later studies it was combined with cytarabine to potentiate the efficacy of cytarabine, and enhanced cytarabine-triphosphate levels (the active metabolite of cytarabine) were demonstrated in patients treated with the combination. (Crews, *et al* 2002, Rubnitz, *et al* 2009) The AML-BFM SG has randomized 2-CDA in consolidation in high risk patients in their AML-BFM 2004 study and compared activity to cytarabine, and no significant difference was found. (Creutzig, *et al* 2010b)
Clofarabine is a new nucleoside analog, which was synthesized to improve the properties of its ancestors fludarabine and cladribine. The phase I study in children showed that the maximum tolerated dose was 52 mg/m2, once daily for 5 consecutive days. (Jeha, *et al* 2004) Liver toxicity and skin rash were the main dose-limiting toxicities. Based on its activity in relapsed pediatric ALL, this drug was approved for this indication in 2004. A phase II study in pediatric AML showed mainly partial responses, perhaps reflecting the resistant phenotype of the leukemias that were included. (Jeha, *et al* 2009) However, in adults with AML clofarabine appears to be an active agent. (Burnett, *et al* 2010) Several phase II studies in pediatric AML are currently ongoing which combine clofarabine with standard AML drugs such as cytarabine, anthracyclines and/or etopside aiming at the development of a new treatment block that could be randomized against other AML blocks. (Jeha, *et al* 2006) A head-to-head comparison to cytarabine or to a FLAG-course should demonstrate whether clofarabine has indeed superior activity, and is not available at the moment.
Elacytarabine is a lipophilic fatty acid derivative of cytarabine, which is in phase II development in adults, and may retain activity in cells with deficient nucleoside membrane transport, and hence be able to overcome cytarabine resistance. Currently, no pediatric studies have been performed. (O'Brien, *et al* 2009)

7.4 Signal transduction inhibitors

7.4.1 FLT3-inhibitors

Several activated tyrosine kinase pathways are described in pediatric AML, which have led to the development of targeted therapy options. Most of the attention has been focused on

FLT3 mutations and small molecule inhibitors, and pediatric development in general follows adult development programs. There are several *FLT3*-inhibitors available on the market, with different selectivity against *FLT3*. This includes for instance the relatively selective inhibitors AC220 and sorafenib, the intermediate selective inhibitor sunitinib, and the less selective inhibitors such as midostaurin and lestaurtinib. In vitro, comparing the properties of these compounds, Pratz et al. reported that in newly diagnosed samples the less selective inhibitors appeared more effective in terms of cytotoxicity, but it is unknown whether this assay is a reliable predictor of clinical responses. (Pratz, *et al* 2010) Moreover, they showed that the presence of dephosphorylation not always predicted cytotoxicity, which may be explained by the lack of oncogenic addiction in some AML cases despite an activation of this pathway, or the activation of parallel pathways at the same time.
Several of these compounds are currently being evaluated in children with leukemia. There is an ongoing phase I study with midostaurin in patients with relapsed pediatric AML and an activating *FLT3*-mutation (NCT00866281). This study builds on the results of studies in adults, which showed moderate activity as a single-agent. (Fischer, *et al* 2010) However, a randomized trial of midostaurin in combination with chemotherapy is ongoing. Sorafenib is evaluated in children with de novo or relapsed *FLT3*-mutant AML, and preliminary results in 15 children are reported. (Inaba, *et al* 2010) In this study most children are treated with combination therapy together with sorafenib, and hence it is difficult to draw conclusions regarding its activity. At 200 mg/m2 twice daily for 20 days 3/6 children had DLTs, but no DLTs were observed on the next lower dose-level of 150 mg/m2 twice daily. Several reports are available on the use of sorafenib in adults with AML. Metzelder et al. observed responses using single-agent sorafenib on compassionate use basis. (Metzelder, *et al* 2009) Ravandi et al performed a phase I/II study of sorafenib in conjunction with chemotherapy. (Ravandi, *et al* 2010) In the phase I portion they escalated sorafenib to 400 mg twice daily together with idarubicin 12 mg/m2 for 3 days and cytarabine 1.5 gram/m2 for 4 days. They found a 93% CR rate in the phase II part of the study for the 15 *FLT3*-mutated patients, versus 66% in *FLT3*-wild type patients. Serve et al. reported initial results of a placebo-controlled trial in elderly AML patients in combination with standard chemotherapy. (Serve, *et al* 2010) No beneficial effect of sorafenib was found, also not in the small subset of patients with a *FLT3*-mutation (n=28 of the 197 patients in the total study). Lestaurtinib is evaluated in children and younger adults with relapsed/refractory AML (NCT00469859), but no results have been presented as yet. In an adult trial in *FLT3*-mutant AML in 1st relapse patients were treated with chemotherapy alone plus or minus lestaurtinib during aplasia between courses and/or following chemotherapy. (Levis, *et al* 2011) Patients treated with lestaurtinib did not achieve better responses, and survival was not prolonged. Of interest, only 58% of patients had sufficient target inhibition in the lestaurtinib arm. This was considered due to the unfavorable pharmacokinetic properties of lestaurtinib, but also to increasing*FLT3*-ligand levels after intensive chemotherapy. (Sato, *et al* 2011) Especially the latter might be a problem that may cause resistance to all *FLT3*-small molecule inhibitors. Other resistance-mechanisms may consist of secondary mutations in the *FLT3*-gene, that impair with binding of the inhibitors.

7.4.2 KIT-inhibitors

Dasatinib may be of use for inhibition of KIT, especially as it also has activity against the D816V mutant, and hence is an option in core-binding factor leukemias which are frequently associated with these mutations. (Goemans, *et al* 2005, Pollard, *et al* 2010) There is an ongoing study in adults with CBF-AML and dasatinib, and no results have been reported to date. In the pediatric phase I study with dasatinib no responses were observed in AML-patients, but none of the included patients was *KIT*-mutated. (Zwaan, *et al* 2006)

7.5 Others

Tosedostat is a compound with a new mechanisms of action, i.e. it is an orally available aminopeptidase inhibitor. In a phase II study in adult relapsed/refractory AML, using the 130 mg/m2 dose level for 28-days blocks, an overall response rate of 27% was noted. (Lowenberg, *et al* 2010b) There are, to the best of our knowledge, no pediatric studies ongoing at this moment.

8. Genome-wide approaches in AML

Genome-wide approaches proved to be a powerful tool to further dissect AML, providing insight in the heterogeneity of AML, and directing the development of *novel* treatment strategies. The use of high resolution array-based comparative genome hybridization (A-CGH) and single nucleotide polymorphism arrays (SNP-A) led to the identification of recurrent copy number aberrations (CNAs) and regions with loss of heterozygosity. However, the frequency of CNAs in AML appeared to be relatively low, which suggests that AML is a genomically stable disease. (Bullinger, *et al* 2010, Radtke, *et al* 2009) However, using such techniques, aberrations in the tumor suppressor gene *TET2* were discovered in 26% of adult MDS patients, as well as in AML. (Delhommeau, *et al* 2009, Langemeijer, *et al* 2009) Pediatric data show that this mutation is rare *in children with AML.* (Langemeijer, *et al* 2011) Also, the *WT1* mutations and *NF1*-mutations described in pediatric AML were detected with genomic profiling. (Balgobind, *et al* 2008, Hollink, *et al* 2009a)
The development of high-throughput sequencing methods aims at identifying new mutations involved in AML. The sequencing of the first AML genome led to the identification of repetitive *IDH1*-mutations, although again they appeared to be rare in pediatric AML. (Ho, *et al* 2010a, Mardis, *et al* 2009) Moreover, *DNMT3A* mutations (encoding DNA methyltransferase 3A) were identified in this way, which appeared highly recurrent and associated with poor clinical outcome. (Ley, *et al* 2010, Yan, *et al* 2011) Recently, Greif et al. sequenced all transcriptionally active genes in another AML genome. (Greif, *et al* 2011) Five mutations specific to the tumor sample were found.
Novel information on the molecular pathogenesis underlying paediatric AML, can also be found by gene-expression profiling. For example, *NPM1*-mutated AML was associated with deregulation of homeobox genes, different from *HOX* gene deregulation in *MLL*-rearranged paediatric AML, thereby suggesting for the first time different routes of perturbed *HOX* gene expression in paediatric AML subclasses. (Mullighan, *et al* 2007) In addition *novel* genes involved in the pathogenesis of MLL-gene rearranged pediatric AML were identified, such as the *IGSF4* and *BRE* genes. (Balgobind, *et al* 2010b, Kuipers, *et al* 2011) Insights into the function of leukemia-associated antigens were recently gained from investigating the expression levels of the *PRAME* (Preferentially Expressed Antigen of MElanoma) gene in paediatric AML, showing cases with *PRAME*-overexpression to also harbour an increased expression of genes encoding ABC transporters such as multidrug resistance (MDR) proteins, and a decreased expression of genes encoding apoptotic proteins. (Goellner, *et al* 2006)

9. Conclusion and perspectives

In conclusion, pediatric AML is a heterogeneous disease, which currently can be cured in approximately 70% of children. Despite the heterogeneity most cases of AML are treated on uniform treatment protocols, as a result of the historical division between lymphoblastic and non-lymphoblastic leukemia. Improvement in prognosis may have reached a plateau as further intensification of therapy is not considered feasible, due to the relatively high rate of treatment-related deaths. Therefore, further improvements should come from understanding the underlying biology of pediatric AML and the development of more targeted therapy options. For many of the new therapeutic developments we are dependent on data obtained in adults, given the small number of available patients for studies. Nonetheless, pediatric safety studies should always be performed, as children are not small adults when it comes to drug development, especially given the risk of long term toxicity on growth and development. (Zwaan, *et al* 2010a) In the end this will require large international collaboration, especially for smaller subgroups characterized by specific genetic abnormalities, such as *FLT3*-mutated or *KIT*-mutated AML. That this is feasible is shown by current available treatment protocols specifically for Down syndrome AML and APL.

10. References

Abbott, B.L., Rubnitz, J.E., Tong, X., Srivastava, D.K., Pui, C.H., Ribeiro, R.C. & Razzouk, B.I. (2003) Clinical significance of central nervous system involvement at diagnosis of pediatric acute myeloid leukemia: a single institution's experience. *Leukemia,* 17, 2090-2096.

Abrahamsson, J., Forestier, E., Heldrup, J., Jahnukainen, K., Jonsson, O.G., Lausen, B., Palle, J., Zeller, B. & Hasle, H. (2011) Response-guided induction therapy in pediatric acute myeloid leukemia with excellent remission rate. *J Clin Oncol,* 29, 310-315.

Ahmed, M., Sternberg, A., Hall, G., Thomas, A., Smith, O., O'Marcaigh, A., Wynn, R., Stevens, R., Addison, M., King, D., Stewart, B., Gibson, B., Roberts, I. & Vyas, P. (2004) Natural history of GATA1 mutations in Down syndrome. *Blood,* 103, 2480-2489.

Al Ahmari, A., Shah, N., Sung, L., Zipursky, A. & Hitzler, J. (2006) Long-term results of an ultra low-dose cytarabine-based regimen for the treatment of acute megakaryoblastic leukaemia in children with Down syndrome. *Br.J.Haematol.,* 133, 646-648.

Aladjidi, N., Auvrignon, A., Leblanc, T., Perel, Y., Benard, A., Bordigoni, P., Gandemer, V., Thuret, I., Dalle, J.H., Piguet, C., Pautard, B., Baruchel, A. & Leverger, G. (2003) Outcome in children with relapsed acute myeloid leukemia after initial treatment with the French Leucemie Aique Myeloide Enfant (LAME) 89/91 protocol of the French Society of Pediatric Hematology and Immunology. *J.Clin.Oncol.,* 21, 4377-4385.

Aplenc, R., Alonzo, T.A., Gerbing, R.B., Lange, B.J., Hurwitz, C.A., Wells, R.J., Bernstein, I., Buckley, P., Krimmel, K., Smith, F.O., Sievers, E.L. & Arceci, R.J. (2008) Safety and efficacy of gemtuzumab ozogamicin in combination with chemotherapy for pediatric acute myeloid leukemia: a report from the Children's Oncology Group. *J Clin Oncol,* 26, 2390-3295.

Aplenc, R., Alonzo, T.A., Gerbing, R.B., Smith, F.O., Meshinchi, S., Ross, J.A., Perentesis, J., Woods, W.G., Lange, B.J. & Davies, S.M. (2006) Ethnicity and survival in childhood acute myeloid leukemia: a report from the Children's Oncology Group. *Blood,* 108, 74-80.

Arceci, R.J., Sande, J., Lange, B., Shannon, K., Franklin, J., Hutchinson, R., Vik, T.A., Flowers, D., Aplenc, R., Berger, M.S., Sherman, M.L., Smith, F.O., Bernstein, I. & Sievers, E.L. (2005) Safety and efficacy of gemtuzumab ozogamicin (Mylotarg(R)) in pediatric patients with advanced CD33-positive acute myeloid leukemia. *Blood,* 106, 1181-1188.

Armendariz, H., Barbieri, M.A., Freigeiro, D., Lastiri, F., Felice, M.S. & Dibar, E. (2005) Treatment strategy and long-term results in pediatric patients treated in two consecutive AML-GATLA trials. *Leukemia,* 19, 2139-2142.

Bachas, C., Schuurhuis, G.J., Hollink, I.H., Kwidama, Z.J., Goemans, B.F., Zwaan, C.M., van den Heuvel-Eibrink, M.M., de Bont, E.S., Reinhardt, D., Creutzig, U., de Haas, V., Assaraf, Y.G., Kaspers, G.J. & Cloos, J. (2010) High-frequency type I/II mutational shifts between diagnosis and relapse are associated with outcome in pediatric AML: implications for personalized medicine. *Blood,* 116, 2752-2758.

Bader, P., Kreyenberg, H., Hoelle, W., Dueckers, G., Kremens, B., Dilloo, D., Sykora, K.W., Niemeyer, C., Reinhardt, D., Vormoor, J., Gruhn, B., Lang, P., Greil, J., Handgretinger, R., Niethammer, D., Klingebiel, T. & Beck, J.F. (2004) Increasing mixed chimerism defines a high-risk group of childhood acute myelogenous leukemia patients after allogeneic stem cell transplantation where pre-emptive immunotherapy may be effective. *Bone Marrow Transplant.,* 33, 815-821.

Balgobind, B.V., Hollink, I.H., Arentsen-Peters, S.T., Zimmerman, M., Harbott, J., Beverloo, B., Von Bergh, A.R., Cloos, J., Kaspers, G.J.L., De Haas, V., Zemanova, Z., Stary, J., Cayuela, J.M., Baruchel, A., Creutzig, U., Reinhardt, D., Pieters, R., Zwaan, C.M. & Van den Heuvel-Eibrink, M. (2011a) "Integrative analysis of type-I and type-II aberrations underscores the genetic heterogeneity of pediatric acute myeloid leukemia." Haematologica, Jul 26, E-pub ahead of print.

Balgobind, B.V., Lugthart, S., Hollink, I.H., Arentsen-Peters, S.T., van Wering, E.R., de Graaf, S.S., Reinhardt, D., Creutzig, U., Kaspers, G.J., de Bont, E.S., Stary, J., Trka, J., Zimmermann, M., Beverloo, H.B., Pieters, R., Delwel, R., Zwaan, C.M. & van den Heuvel-Eibrink, M.M. (2010a) EVI1 overexpression in distinct subtypes of pediatric acute myeloid leukemia. *Leukemia,* 24, 942-949.

Balgobind, B.V., Raimondi, S.C., Harbott, J., Zimmermann, M., Alonzo, T.A., Auvrignon, A., Beverloo, H.B., Chang, M., Creutzig, U., Dworzak, M.N., Forestier, E., Gibson, B., Hasle, H., Harrison, C.J., Heerema, N.A., Kaspers, G.J., Leszl, A., Litvinko, N., Nigro, L.L., Morimoto, A., Perot, C., Pieters, R., Reinhardt, D., Rubnitz, J.E., Smith, F.O., Stary, J., Stasevich, I., Strehl, S., Taga, T., Tomizawa, D., Webb, D., Zemanova, Z., Zwaan, C.M. & van den Heuvel-Eibrink, M.M. (2009) Novel prognostic subgroups in childhood 11q23/MLL-rearranged acute myeloid leukemia: results of an international retrospective study. *Blood,* 114, 2489-2496.

Balgobind, B.V., Van den Heuvel-Eibrink, M.M., De Menezes, R.X., Reinhardt, D., Hollink, I.H., Arentsen-Peters, S.T., van Wering, E.R., Kaspers, G.J., Cloos, J., de Bont, E.S., Cayuela, J.M., Baruchel, A., Meyer, C., Marschalek, R., Trka, J., Stary, J., Beverloo, H.B., Pieters, R., Zwaan, C.M. & den Boer, M.L. (2011b) Evaluation of gene expression signatures predictive of cytogenetic and molecular subtypes of pediatric acute myeloid leukemia. *Haematologica,* 96, 221-230.

Balgobind, B.V., Van Vlierberghe, P., van den Ouweland, A.M., Beverloo, H.B., Terlouw-Kromosoeto, J.N., van Wering, E.R., Reinhardt, D., Horstmann, M., Kaspers, G.J., Pieters, R., Zwaan, C.M., Van den Heuvel-Eibrink, M.M. & Meijerink, J.P. (2008) Leukemia-associated NF1 inactivation in patients with pediatric T-ALL and AML lacking evidence for neurofibromatosis. *Blood,* 111, 4322-4328.

Balgobind, B.V., Zwaan, C.M., Reinhardt, D., Arentsen-Peters, T.J., Hollink, I.H., de Haas, V., Kaspers, G.J., de Bont, E.S., Baruchel, A., Stary, J., Meyer, C., Marschalek, R., Creutzig, U., den Boer, M.L., Pieters, R. & van den Heuvel-Eibrink, M.M. (2010b) High BRE expression in pediatric MLL-rearranged AML is associated with favorable outcome. *Leukemia,* 24, 2048-2055.

Becton, D., Dahl, G.V., Ravindranath, Y., Chang, M.N., Behm, F.G., Raimondi, S.C., Head, D.R., Stine, K.C., Lacayo, N.J., Sikic, B.I., Arceci, R.J. & Weinstein, H. (2006) Randomized use of Cyclosporin A (CSA) to modulate P-glycoprotein in children with AML in remission: pediatric oncology group study 9421. *Blood,* 107, 1315-1324.

Bennett, J.M., Catovsky, D., Daniel, M.T., Flandrin, G., Galton, D.A., Gralnick, H.R. & Sultan, C. (1985a) Criteria for the diagnosis of acute leukemia of megakaryocyte lineage (M7). A report of the French-American-British Cooperative Group. *Ann.Intern.Med.,* 103, 460-462.

Bennett, J.M., Catovsky, D., Daniel, M.T., Flandrin, G., Galton, D.A., Gralnick, H.R. & Sultan, C. (1985b) Proposed revised criteria for the classification of acute myeloid leukemia. A report of the French-American-British Cooperative Group. *Ann.Intern.Med.,* 103, 620-625.

Bennett, J.M., Catovsky, D., Daniel, M.T., Flandrin, G., Galton, D.A., Gralnick, H.R. & Sultan, C. (1991) Proposal for the recognition of minimally differentiated acute myeloid leukaemia (AML-MO). *Br.J.Haematol.,* 78, 325-329.

Bernard, O.A., Gilliland, D.G. & Mercher, T. (2009) [The OTT-MAL fusion oncogene: another Notch in megakaryoblastic leukemia]. *Med Sci (Paris),* 25, 676-678.

Bleakley, M., Lau, L., Shaw, P.J. & Kaufman, A. (2002) Bone marrow transplantation for paediatric AML in first remission: a systematic review and meta-analysis. *Bone Marrow Transplant.,* 29, 843-852.

Boissel, N., Auclerc, M.F., Lheritier, V., Perel, Y., Thomas, X., Leblanc, T., Rousselot, P., Cayuela, J.M., Gabert, J., Fegueux, N., Piguet, C., Huguet-Rigal, F., Berthou, C., Boiron, J.M., Pautas, C., Michel, G., Fiere, D., Leverger, G., Dombret, H. & Baruchel, A. (2003) Should adolescents with acute lymphoblastic leukemia be treated as old children or young adults? Comparison of the French FRALLE-93 and LALA-94 trials. *J Clin Oncol,* 21, 774-780.

Bresters, D., Reus, A.C., Veerman, A.J., Van Wering, E.R., Van Der Does-Van Den, B. & Kaspers, G.J. (2002) Congenital leukaemia: the Dutch experience and review of the literature. *Br.J.Haematol.,* 117, 513-524.

Brethon, B., Yakouben, K., Oudot, C., Boutard, P., Bruno, B., Jerome, C., Nelken, B., de Lumley, L., Bertrand, Y., Dalle, J.H., Chevret, S., Leblanc, T. & Baruchel, A. (2008) Efficacy of fractionated gemtuzumab ozogamicin combined with cytarabine in advanced childhood myeloid leukaemia. *Br J Haematol,* 143, 541-547.

Brown, P., McIntyre, E., Rau, R., Meshinchi, S., Lacayo, N., Dahl, G., Alonzo, T.A., Chang, M., Arceci, R.J. & Small, D. (2007) The incidence and clinical significance of nucleophosmin mutations in childhood AML. *Blood*, 110, 979-985.

Bullinger, L., Kronke, J., Schon, C., Radtke, I., Urlbauer, K., Botzenhardt, U., Gaidzik, V., Cario, A., Senger, C., Schlenk, R.F., Downing, J.R., Holzmann, K., Dohner, K. & Dohner, H. (2010) Identification of acquired copy number alterations and uniparental disomies in cytogenetically normal acute myeloid leukemia using high-resolution single-nucleotide polymorphism analysis. *Leukemia*, 24, 438-449.

Burnett, A.K., Hills, R.K., Milligan, D., Kjeldsen, L., Kell, J., Russell, N.H., Yin, J.A., Hunter, A., Goldstone, A.H. & Wheatley, K. (2011) Identification of patients with acute myeloblastic leukemia who benefit from the addition of gemtuzumab ozogamicin: results of the MRC AML15 trial. *J Clin Oncol*, 29, 369-377.

Burnett, A.K., Russell, N.H., Kell, J., Dennis, M., Milligan, D., Paolini, S., Yin, J., Culligan, D., Johnston, P., Murphy, J., McMullin, M.F., Hunter, A., Das-Gupta, E., Clark, R., Carr, R. & Hills, R.K. (2010) European development of clofarabine as treatment for older patients with acute myeloid leukemia considered unsuitable for intensive chemotherapy. *J Clin Oncol*, 28, 2389-2395.

Capizzi, R.L., Davis, R., Powell, B., Cuttner, J., Ellison, R.R., Cooper, M.R., Dillman, R., Major, W.B., Dupre, E. & McIntyre, O.R. (1988) Synergy between high-dose cytarabine and asparaginase in the treatment of adults with refractory and relapsed acute myelogenous leukemia--a Cancer and Leukemia Group B Study. *J.Clin.Oncol.*, 6, 499-508.

Chen, J., Li, Y., Doedens, M., Wang, P., Shago, M., Dick, J.E. & Hitzler, J.K. (2010) Functional differences between myeloid leukemia-initiating and transient leukemia cells in Down's syndrome. *Leukemia*, 24, 1012-1017.

Chou, S.T., Opalinska, J.B., Yao, Y., Fernandes, M.A., Kalota, A., Brooks, J.S., Choi, J.K., Gewirtz, A.M., Danet-Desnoyers, G.A., Nemiroff, R.L. & Weiss, M.J. (2008) Trisomy 21 enhances human fetal erythro-megakaryocytic development. *Blood*, 112, 4503-4506.

Cilloni, D., Renneville, A., Hermitte, F., Hills, R.K., Daly, S., Jovanovic, J.V., Gottardi, E., Fava, M., Schnittger, S., Weiss, T., Izzo, B., Nomdedeu, J., van der Heijden, A., van der Reijden, B.A., Jansen, J.H., van der Velden, V.H., Ommen, H., Preudhomme, C., Saglio, G. & Grimwade, D. (2009) Real-time quantitative polymerase chain reaction detection of minimal residual disease by standardized WT1 assay to enhance risk stratification in acute myeloid leukemia: a European LeukemiaNet study. *J Clin Oncol*, 27, 5195-5201.

Creutzig, U., Buchner, T., Sauerland, M.C., Zimmermann, M., Reinhardt, D., Dohner, H. & Schlenk, R.F. (2008) Significance of age in acute myeloid leukemia patients younger than 30 years: a common analysis of the pediatric trials AML-BFM 93/98 and the adult trials AMLCG 92/99 and AMLSG HD93/98A. *Cancer*, 112, 562-571.

Creutzig, U., Diekamp, S., Zimmermann, M. & Reinhardt, D. (2007) Longitudinal evaluation of early and late anthracycline cardiotoxicity in children with AML. *Pediatr.Blood Cancer*, 48, 651-662.

Creutzig, U. & Reinhardt, D. (2002) Current controversies: which patients with acute myeloid leukaemia should receive a bone marrow transplantation?--a European view. *Br.J.Haematol.*, 118, 365-377.

Creutzig, U., Reinhardt, D., Diekamp, S., Dworzak, M., Stary, J. & Zimmermann, M. (2005a) AML patients with Down syndrome have a high cure rate with AML-BFM therapy with reduced dose intensity. *Leukemia,* 19, 1355-1360.

Creutzig, U., Ritter, J., Ludwig, W.D., Harbott, J., Löffler, H. & Schellong, G. (1993a) Classification of AML by morphologic, immunologic and cytogenetic criteria. Review with reference to subtypes in the AML-BFM-87 study. *Klin.Padiatr.,* 205, 272-280.

Creutzig, U., Ritter, J., Zimmermann, M., Hermann, J., Gadner, H., Sawatzki, D.B., Niemeyer, C.M., Schwabe, D., Selle, B., Boos, J., Kuhl, J. & Feldges, A. (2001) Idarubicin improves blast cell clearance during induction therapy in children with AML: results of study AML-BFM 93. AML-BFM Study Group. *Leukemia,* 15, 348-354.

Creutzig, U., Ritter, J., Zimmermann, M. & Schellong, G. (1993b) Does cranial irradiation reduce the risk for bone marrow relapse in acute myelogenous leukemia? Unexpected results of the Childhood Acute Myelogenous Leukemia Study BFM-87. *J.Clin.Oncol.,* 11, 279-286.

Creutzig, U., Zimmermann, M., Dworzak, M., Bourquin, J.P., Neuhoff, C., Sander, A., Stary, J. & Reinhardt, D. (2010a) *Excellent Outcome In Infants below One Year of Age with AML – Results of Studies AML-BFM -98 and -2004. Blood,* 116, abstract 17.

Creutzig, U., Zimmermann, M., Dworzak, M., Bourquin, J.P., Neuhoff, C., Sander, A., Stary, J. & Reinhardt, D. (2010b) *Study AML-BFM 2004: Improved Survival In Childhood Acute Myeloid Leukemia without Increased Toxicity. Blood,* 116, abstract 181.

Creutzig, U., Zimmermann, M., Dworzak, M., Urban, C., Henze, G., Kremens, B., Lakomek, M., Bourquin, J.P., Stary, J. & Reinhardt, D. (2010c) Favourable outcome of patients with childhood acute promyelocytic leukaemia after treatment with reduced cumulative anthracycline doses. *Br J Haematol,* 149, 399-409.

Creutzig, U., Zimmermann, M., Lehrnbecher, T., Graf, N., Hermann, J., Niemeyer, C.M., Reiter, A., Ritter, J., Dworzak, M., Stary, J. & Reinhardt, D. (2006) Less toxicity by optimizing chemotherapy, but not by addition of granulocyte colony-stimulating factor in children and adolescents with acute myeloid leukemia: results of AML-BFM 98. *J.Clin.Oncol.,* 24, 4499-4506.

Creutzig, U., Zimmermann, M., Reinhardt, D., Dworzak, M., Stary, J. & Lehrnbecher, T. (2004) Early deaths and treatment-related mortality in children undergoing therapy for acute myeloid leukemia: analysis of the multicenter clinical trials AML-BFM 93 and AML-BFM 98. *J.Clin.Oncol.,* 22, 4384-4393.

Creutzig, U., Zimmermann, M., Ritter, J., Reinhardt, D., Hermann, J., Henze, G., J rgens, H., Kabisch, H., Reiter, A., Riehm, H., Gadner, H., Schellong, G. & for the, A.M.L.B.F.M.S.G. (2005b) Treatment strategy and long-term results in pediatric patients treated in four consecutive AMl-BFM trials. *Leukemia,* 19, 2030-2042.

Crews, K.R., Gandhi, V., Srivastava, D.K., Razzouk, B.I., Tong, X., Behm, F.G., Plunkett, W., Raimondi, S.C., Pui, C.H., Rubnitz, J.E., Stewart, C.F. & Ribeiro, R.C. (2002) Interim comparison of a continuous infusion versus a short daily infusion of cytarabine given in combination with cladribine for pediatric acute myeloid leukemia. *J.Clin.Oncol.,* 20, 4217-4224.

Damm, F., Heuser, M., Morgan, M., Wagner, K., Gorlich, K., Grosshennig, A., Hamwi, I., Thol, F., Surdziel, E., Fiedler, W., Lubbert, M., Kanz, L., Reuter, C., Heil, G., Delwel,

R., Lowenberg, B., Valk, P.J., Krauter, J. & Ganser, A. (2011) Integrative prognostic risk score in acute myeloid leukemia with normal karyotype. *Blood,* 117, 4561-4568.

de Bont, J.M., Holt, B., Dekker, A.W., Van Der Does-Van Den, B., Sonneveld, P. & Pieters, R. (2004) Significant difference in outcome for adolescents with acute lymphoblastic leukemia treated on pediatric vs adult protocols in the Netherlands. *Leukemia,* 18, 2032-2035.

Delhommeau, F., Dupont, S., Della Valle, V., James, C., Trannoy, S., Masse, A., Kosmider, O., Le Couedic, J.P., Robert, F., Alberdi, A., Lecluse, Y., Plo, I., Dreyfus, F.J., Marzac, C., Casadevall, N., Lacombe, C., Romana, S.P., Dessen, P., Soulier, J., Viguie, F., Fontenay, M., Vainchenker, W. & Bernard, O.A. (2009) Mutation in TET2 in myeloid cancers. *N Engl J Med,* 360, 2289-2301.

Dluzniewska, A., Balwierz, W., Armata, J., Balcerska, A., Chybicka, A., Kowalczyk, J., Matysiak, M., Ochocka, M., Radwanska, U., Rokicka-Milewska, R., Sonta-Jakimczyk, D., Wachowiak, J. & Wysocki, M. (2005) Twenty years of Polish experience with three consecutive protocols for treatment of childhood acute myelogenous leukemia. *Leukemia,* 19, 2117-2124.

Entz-Werle, N., Suciu, S., van der Werff ten, B., Vilmer, E., Bertrand, Y., Benoit, Y., Margueritte, G., Plouvier, E., Boutard, P., Vandecruys, E., Ferster, A., Lutz, P., Uyttebroeck, A., Hoyoux, C., Thyss, A., Rialland, X., Norton, L., Pages, M.P., Philippe, N., Otten, J. & Behar, C. (2005) Results of 58872 and 58921 trials in acute myeloblastic leukemia and relative value of chemotherapy vs allogeneic bone marrow transplantation in first complete remission: the EORTC Children Leukemia Group report. *Leukemia,* 19, 2072-2081.

FDA (2010) Mylotarg (gemtuzumab ozogamicin): Market Withdrawal. *http://www.fda.gov/Safety/MedWatch/SafetyInformation/SafetyAlertsforHumanMedicalProducts/ucm216458.htm.*

Feldman, E.J., Lancet, J.E., Kolitz, J.E., Ritchie, E.K., Roboz, G.J., List, A.F., Allen, S.L., Asatiani, E., Mayer, L.D., Swenson, C. & Louie, A.C. (2011) First-In-Man Study of CPX-351: A Liposomal Carrier Containing Cytarabine and Daunorubicin in a Fixed 5:1 Molar Ratio for the Treatment of Relapsed and Refractory Acute Myeloid Leukemia. *J Clin Oncol,* 29, 979-985.

Fischer, T., Stone, R.M., Deangelo, D.J., Galinsky, I., Estey, E., Lanza, C., Fox, E., Ehninger, G., Feldman, E.J., Schiller, G.J., Klimek, V.M., Nimer, S.D., Gilliland, D.G., Dutreix, C., Huntsman-Labed, A., Virkus, J. & Giles, F.J. (2010) Phase IIB trial of oral Midostaurin (PKC412), the FMS-like tyrosine kinase 3 receptor (FLT3) and multi-targeted kinase inhibitor, in patients with acute myeloid leukemia and high-risk myelodysplastic syndrome with either wild-type or mutated FLT3. *J Clin Oncol,* 28, 4339-4345.

Flohr, T., Schrauder, A., Cazzaniga, G., Panzer-Grumayer, R., van der Velden, V., Fischer, S., Stanulla, M., Basso, G., Niggli, F.K., Schafer, B.W., Sutton, R., Koehler, R., Zimmermann, M., Valsecchi, M.G., Gadner, H., Masera, G., Schrappe, M., van Dongen, J.J., Biondi, A. & Bartram, C.R. (2008) Minimal residual disease-directed risk stratification using real-time quantitative PCR analysis of immunoglobulin and T-cell receptor gene rearrangements in the international multicenter trial AIEOP-BFM ALL 2000 for childhood acute lymphoblastic leukemia. *Leukemia,* 22, 771-782.

Gamis, A.S., Alonzo, T., Hiden, J.M., Gerbing, R.B., Loew, T.W., Hathaway, L., McGavran, L., Barnard, D., Taub, J.W., Ravindranath, Y., Smith, F. & Arceci, R. (2006) Outcome of Down syndrome children with acute myeloid leukemia (AML) or myelodysplasia (MDS) treated with a uniform prospective trial - initial report of the COG trial A2971. *Blood*, 108, abstract 15.

Ge, Y., Jensen, T.L., Stout, M.L., Flatley, R.M., Grohar, P.J., Ravindranath, Y., Matherly, L.H. & Taub, J.W. (2004) The role of cytidine deaminase and GATA1 mutations in the increased cytosine arabinoside sensitivity of Down syndrome myeloblasts and leukemia cell lines. *Cancer Res.*, 64, 728-735.

George, B., Mathews, V., Poonkuzhali, B., Shaji, R.V., Srivastava, A. & Chandy, M. (2004) Treatment of children with newly diagnosed acute promyelocytic leukemia with arsenic trioxide: a single center experience. *Leukemia*, 18, 1587-1590.

Gibson, B.E., Wheatley, K., Hann, I.M., Stevens, R.F., Webb, D., Hills, R.K., de Graaf, S.S. & Harrison, C.J. (2005) Treatment strategy and long-term results in paediatric patients treated in consecutive UK AML trials. *Leukemia*, 19, 2130-2138.

Goellner, S., Steinbach, D., Schenk, T., Gruhn, B., Zintl, F., Ramsay, E. & Saluz, H.P. (2006) Childhood acute myelogenous leukaemia: association between PRAME, apoptosis- and MDR-related gene expression. *Eur J Cancer*, 42, 2807-2814.

Goemans, B.F., Zwaan, C., Miller, M., Zimmermann, M., Harlow, A., Meshinchi, S., Loonen, A.H., Hahlen, K., Reinhardt, D., Creutzig, U., Kaspers, G.J. & Heinrich, M.C. (2005) Mutations in KIT and RAS are frequent events in pediatric core-binding factor acute myeloid leukemia. *Leukemia*, 19, 1536-1542.

Goldman, S.C., Holcenberg, J.S., Finklestein, J.Z., Hutchinson, R., Kreissman, S., Johnson, F.L., Tou, C., Harvey, E., Morris, E. & Cairo, M.S. (2001) A randomized comparison between rasburicase and allopurinol in children with lymphoma or leukemia at high risk for tumor lysis. *Blood*, 97, 2998-3003.

Gorman, M.F., Ji, L., Ko, R.H., Barnette, P., Bostrom, B., Hutchinson, R., Raetz, E., Seibel, N.L., Twist, C.J., Eckroth, E., Sposto, R., Gaynon, P.S. & Loh, M.L. (2010) Outcome for children treated for relapsed or refractory acute myelogenous leukemia (rAML): a Therapeutic Advances in Childhood Leukemia (TACL) Consortium study. *Pediatr Blood Cancer*, 55, 421-429.

Goulden, N., Virgo, P. & Grimwade, D. (2006) Minimal residual disease directed therapy for childhood acute myeloid leukaemia: the time is now. *Br.J.Haematol.*, 134, 273-282.

Gregory, J., Kim, H., Alonzo, T., Gerbing, R., Woods, W., Weinstein, H., Shepherd, L., Schiffer, C., Appelbaum, F., Willman, C., Wiernik, P., Rowe, J., Tallman, M. & Feusner, J. (2009) Treatment of children with acute promyelocytic leukemia: results of the first North American Intergroup trial INT0129. *Pediatr Blood Cancer*, 53, 1005-1010.

Greif, P.A., Eck, S.H., Konstandin, N.P., Benet-Pages, A., Ksienzyk, B., Dufour, A., Vetter, A.T., Popp, H.D., Lorenz-Depiereux, B., Meitinger, T., Bohlander, S.K. & Strom, T.M. (2011) Identification of recurring tumor-specific somatic mutations in acute myeloid leukemia by transcriptome sequencing. Leukemia, 25, 821-827.

Grimwade, D., Biondi, A., Mozziconacci, M.J., Hagemeijer, A., Berger, R., Neat, M., Howe, K., Dastugue, N., Jansen, J., Radford-Weiss, I., Lo Coco, F., Lessard, M., Hernandez, J.M., Delabesse, E., Head, D., Liso, V., Sainty, D., Flandrin, G., Solomon, E., Birg, F. & Lafage-Pochitaloff, M. (2000) Characterization of acute promyelocytic leukemia cases lacking the classic t(15;17): results of the European Working Party. Groupe Francais de Cytogenetique Hematologique, Groupe de Francais d'Hematologie Cellulaire, UK Cancer Cytogenetics Group and BIOMED 1 European Community-Concerted Action "Molecular Cytogenetic Diagnosis in Haematological Malignancies". *Blood,* 96, 1297-1308.

Grimwade, D., Jovanovic, J.V., Hills, R.K., Nugent, E.A., Patel, Y., Flora, R., Diverio, D., Jones, K., Aslett, H., Batson, E., Rennie, K., Angell, R., Clark, R.E., Solomon, E., Lo-Coco, F., Wheatley, K. & Burnett, A.K. (2009) Prospective minimal residual disease monitoring to predict relapse of acute promyelocytic leukemia and to direct pre-emptive arsenic trioxide therapy. *J Clin Oncol,* 27, 3650-3658.

Grimwade, D., Walker, H., Oliver, F., Wheatley, K., Harrison, C., Harrison, G., Rees, J., Hann, I., Stevens, R., Burnett, A. & Goldstone, A. (1998) The importance of diagnostic cytogenetics on outcome in AML: analysis of 1,612 patients entered into the MRC AML 10 trial. The Medical Research Council Adult and Children's Leukaemia Working Parties. *Blood,* 92, 2322-2333.

Harrison, C.J., Hills, R.K., Moorman, A.V., Grimwade, D.J., Hann, I., Webb, D.K., Wheatley, K., de Graaf, S.S., van den Berg, E., Burnett, A.K. & Gibson, B.E. (2010) Cytogenetics of childhood acute myeloid leukemia: United Kingdom Medical Research Council Treatment trials AML 10 and 12. *J Clin Oncol,* 28, 2674-2681.

Hasle, H., Alonzo, T.A., Auvrignon, A., Behar, C., Chang, M., Creutzig, U., Fischer, A., Forestier, E., Fynn, A., Haas, O.A., Harbott, J., Harrison, C.J., Heerema, N.A., van den Heuvel-Eibrink, M.M., Kaspers, G.J., Locatelli, F., Noellke, P., Polychronopoulou, S., Ravindranath, Y., Razzouk, B., Reinhardt, D., Savva, N.N., Stark, B., Suciu, S., Tsukimoto, I., Webb, D.K., Wojcik, D., Woods, W.G., Zimmermann, M., Niemeyer, C.M. & Raimondi, S.C. (2007) Monosomy 7 and deletion 7q in children and adolescents with acute myeloid leukemia: an international retrospective study. *Blood,* 109, 4641-4647.

Hasle, H., Clemmensen, I.H. & Mikkelsen, M. (2000) Risks of leukaemia and solid tumours in individuals with Down's syndrome. *Lancet,* 355, 165-169.

Hasle, H., Abrahamsson, J., Arola, M., Karow, A., O'Marcaigh, A., Reinhardt, D., Webb, D.K., van Wering, E., Zeller, B., Zwaan, C.M. & Vyas, P. (2008) Myeloid leukemia in children 4 years or older with Down syndrome often lacks GATA1 mutation and cytogenetics and risk of relapse are more akin to sporadic AML. Leukemia, 22, 1428-1430.

Hasle, H., Niemeyer, C.M., Chessells, J.M., Baumann, I., Bennett, J.M., Kerndrup, G. & Head, D.R. (2003) A pediatric approach to the WHO classification of myelodysplastic and myeloproliferative diseases. *Leukemia,* 17, 277-282.

Hempel, G., Reinhardt, D., Creutzig, U. & Boos, J. (2003) Population pharmacokinetics of liposomal daunorubicin in children. *Br.J.Clin.Pharmacol.,* 56, 370-377.

Hitzler, J.K., Cheung, J., Li, Y., Scherer, S.W. & Zipursky, A. (2003) GATA1 mutations in transient leukemia and acute megakaryoblastic leukemia of Down syndrome. *Blood,* 101, 4301-4304.

Ho, P.A., Alonzo, T.A., Gerbing, R.B., Pollard, J., Stirewalt, D.L., Hurwitz, C., Heerema, N.A., Hirsch, B., Raimondi, S.C., Lange, B., Franklin, J.L., Radich, J.P. & Meshinchi, S. (2009) Prevalence and prognostic implications of CEBPA mutations in pediatric AML: a report from the Children's Oncology Group. *Blood, 113, 6558-6566.*

Ho, P.A., Alonzo, T.A., Kopecky, K.J., Miller, K.L., Kuhn, J., Zeng, R., Gerbing, R.B., Raimondi, S.C., Hirsch, B.A., Oehler, V., Hurwitz, C.A., Franklin, J.L., Gamis, A.S., Petersdorf, S.H., Anderson, J.E., Reaman, G.H., Baker, L.H., Willman, C.L., Bernstein, I.D., Radich, J.P., Appelbaum, F.R., Stirewalt, D.L. & Meshinchi, S. (2010a) Molecular alterations of the IDH1 gene in AML: a Children's Oncology Group and Southwest Oncology Group study. *Leukemia*, 24, 909-913.

Ho, P.A., Zeng, R., Alonzo, T.A., Gerbing, R.B., Miller, K.L., Pollard, J.A., Stirewalt, D.L., Heerema, N.A., Raimondi, S.C., Hirsch, B., Franklin, J.L., Lange, B. & Meshinchi, S. (2010b) Prevalence and prognostic implications of WT1 mutations in pediatric acute myeloid leukemia (AML): a report from the Children's Oncology Group. *Blood*, 116, 702-710.

Hollink, I.H., van den Heuvel-Eibrink, M.M., Arentsen-Peters, S.T., Zimmermann, M., Peeters, J.K., Valk, P.J., Balgobind, B.V., Sonneveld, E., Kaspers, G.J., de Bont, E.S., Trka, J., Baruchel, A., Creutzig, U., Pieters, R., Reinhardt, D. & Zwaan, C.M. (2011) Characterization of CEBPA mutations and promoter hypermethylation in pediatric acute myeloid leukemia. *Haematologica*, 96, 384-392.

Hollink, I.H., van den Heuvel-Eibrink, M.M., Zimmermann, M., Balgobind, B.V., Arentsen-Peters, S.T., Alders, M., Willasch, A., Kaspers, G.J., Trka, J., Baruchel, A., de Graaf, S.S., Creutzig, U., Pieters, R., Reinhardt, D. & Zwaan, C.M. (2009a) Clinical relevance of Wilms' tumor 1 gene mutations in childhood acute myeloid leukemia. *Blood, 113, 5951-5960.*

Hollink, I.H., van den Heuvel-Eibrink, M.M. & Zwaan, C.M. (2009b) CEBPA resembles Roman god Janus. *Blood*, 113, 6501-6502.

Hollink, I.H., Zwaan, C.M., Zimmermann, M., Arentsen-Peters, T.C., Pieters, R., Cloos, J., Kaspers, G.J., de Graaf, S.S., Harbott, J., Creutzig, U., Reinhardt, D., van den Heuvel-Eibrink, M.M. & Thiede, C. (2009c) Favorable prognostic impact of NPM1 gene mutations in childhood acute myeloid leukemia, with emphasis on cytogenetically normal AML. *Leukemia*, 23, 262-270.

Hu, J., Liu, Y.F., Wu, C.F., Xu, F., Shen, Z.X., Zhu, Y.M., Li, J.M., Tang, W., Zhao, W.L., Wu, W., Sun, H.P., Chen, Q.S., Chen, B., Zhou, G.B., Zelent, A., Waxman, S., Wang, Z.Y., Chen, S.J. & Chen, Z. (2009) Long-term efficacy and safety of all-trans retinoic acid/arsenic trioxide-based therapy in newly diagnosed acute promyelocytic leukemia. *Proc Natl Acad Sci U S A*, 106, 3342-3347.

Hubeek, I., Peters, G.J., Broekhuizen, R., Zwaan, C.M., Kaaijk, P., van Wering, E.S., Gibson, B.E., Creutzig, U., Janka-Schaub, G.E., Den Boer, M.L., Pieters, R. & Kaspers, G.J. (2006) In vitro sensitivity and cross-resistance to deoxynucleoside analogs in childhood acute leukemia. *Haematologica*, 91, 17-23.

Imaizumi, M., Tawa, A., Hanada, R., Tsuchida, M., Tabuchi, K., Kigasawa, H., Kobayashi, R., Morimoto, A., Nakayama, H., Hamamoto, K., Kudo, K., Yabe, H., Horibe, K., Tsuchiya, S. & Tsukimoto, I. (2011) Prospective study of a therapeutic regimen with all-trans retinoic acid and anthracyclines in combination of cytarabine in children with acute promyelocytic leukaemia: the Japanese childhood acute myeloid leukaemia cooperative study. *Br J Haematol*, 152, 89-98.

Inaba, H., Cao, X., Pounds, S., Pui, C.H., Rubnitz, J.E., Ribeiro, R.C. & Razzouk, B.I. (2011) Randomized trial of 2 dosages of prophylactic granulocyte-colony-stimulating factor after induction chemotherapy in pediatric acute myeloid leukemia. *Cancer,* 117, 1313-1320.

Inaba, H., Rubnitz, J.E., Coustan-Smith, E., Li, L., Furmanski, B.D., Maskara, G.P., Shurtleff, S.A., Pounds, S., Pui, C.H., Ribeiro, R.C., Campana, D. & Baker, S.D. (2010) Clinical Activity, Pharmacokinetics, and Pharmacodynamics of Sorafenib In Pediatric Acute Myeloid Leukemia. *Blood,* 116, abstract 1073.

Jeha, S., Gandhi, V., Chan, K.W., McDonald, L., Ramirez, I., Madden, R., Rytting, M., Brandt, M., Keating, M., Plunkett, W. & Kantarjian, H. (2004) Clofarabine, a novel nucleoside analog, is active in pediatric patients with advanced leukemia. *Blood,* 103, 784-789.

Jeha, S., Gaynon, P.S., Razzouk, B.I., Franklin, J., Kadota, R., Shen, V., Luchtman-Jones, L., Rytting, M., Bomgaars, L.R., Rheingold, S., Ritchey, K., Albano, E., Arceci, R.J., Goldman, S., Griffin, T., Altman, A., Gordon, B., Steinherz, L., Weitman, S. & Steinherz, P. (2006) Phase II study of clofarabine in pediatric patients with refractory or relapsed acute lymphoblastic leukemia. *J.Clin.Oncol.,* 24, 1917-1923.

Jeha, S., Razzouk, B., Rytting, M., Rheingold, S., Albano, E., Kadota, R., Luchtman-Jones, L., Bomgaars, L., Gaynon, P., Goldman, S., Ritchey, K., Arceci, R., Altman, A., Stine, K., Steinherz, L. & Steinherz, P. (2009) Phase II study of clofarabine in pediatric patients with refractory or relapsed acute myeloid leukemia. *J Clin Oncol,* 27, 4392-4397.

Kanezaki, R., Toki, T., Terui, K., Xu, G., Wang, R., Shimada, A., Hama, A., Kanegane, H., Kawakami, K., Endo, M., Hasegawa, D., Kogawa, K., Adachi, S., Ikeda, Y., Iwamoto, S., Taga, T., Kosaka, Y., Kojima, S., Hayashi, Y. & Ito, E. (2010) Down syndrome and GATA1 mutations in transient abnormal myeloproliferative disorder: mutation classes correlate with progression to myeloid leukemia. *Blood,* 116, 4631-4638.

Kaspers, G.J. & Creutzig, U. (2005) Pediatric acute myeloid leukemia: international progress and future directions. *Leukemia,* 19, 2025-2029.

Kaspers, G.J., Zimmermann, M., Reinhardt, D., Gibson, B., Tamminga, R., Aleinkova, O., Armendariz, H., Dworzak, M., Ha, S., Hovi, L., Maschan, A., Baruchel, A., Bertrand, Y., Razzouk, B., Rizzari, C., Smisek, P., Smith, O., Stark, B. & Creutzig, U. (2009) Addition of Liposomal Daunorubicin (DaunoXome(R)) to FLAG Significantly Improves Treatment Response in Pediatric Relapsed AML: Final Results From the International Randomised Phase III Study Relapsed AML 2001/01. Blood, 114, abstract 18.

Kaspers, G.J. & Zwaan, C.M. (2007) Pediatric acute myeloid leukemia: towards high-quality cure of all patients. *Haematologica,* 92, 1519-1532.

Kell, W.J., Burnett, A.K., Chopra, R., Yin, J.A., Clark, R.E., Rohatiner, A., Culligan, D., Hunter, A., Prentice, A.G. & Milligan, D.W. (2003) A feasibility study of simultaneous administration of gemtuzumab ozogamicin with intensive chemotherapy in induction and consolidation in younger patients with acute myeloid leukemia. *Blood,* 102, 4277-4283.

Kelly, L.M., Liu, Q., Kutok, J.L., Williams, I.R., Boulton, C.L. & Gilliland, D.G. (2002b) FLT3 internal tandem duplication mutations associated with human acute myeloid leukemias induce myeloproliferative disease in a murine bone marrow transplant model. *Blood,* 99, 310-318.

Kelly, L.M. & Gilliland, D.G. (2002a) Genetics of myeloid leukemias. *Annu.Rev.Genomics Hum.Genet.*, 3, 179-198.

Klusmann, J.H., Creutzig, U., Zimmermann, M., Dworzak, M., Jorch, N., Langebrake, C., Pekrun, A., Macakova-Reinhardt, K. & Reinhardt, D. (2008) Treatment and prognostic impact of transient leukemia in neonates with Down syndrome. *Blood*, 111, 2991-2998.

Klusmann, J.H., Godinho, F.J., Heitmann, K., Maroz, A., Koch, M.L., Reinhardt, D., Orkin, S.H. & Li, Z. (2010a) Developmental stage-specific interplay of GATA1 and IGF signaling in fetal megakaryopoiesis and leukemogenesis. *Genes Dev*, 24, 1659-1672.

Klusmann, J.H., Li, Z., Bohmer, K., Maroz, A., Koch, M.L., Emmrich, S., Godinho, F.J., Orkin, S.H. & Reinhardt, D. (2010b) miR-125b-2 is a potential oncomiR on human chromosome 21 in megakaryoblastic leukemia. *Genes Dev*, 24, 478-490.

Krance, R.A., Hurwitz, C.A., Head, D.R., Raimondi, S.C., Behm, F.G., Crews, K.R., Srivastava, D.K., Mahmoud, H., Roberts, W.M., Tong, X., Blakley, R.L. & Ribeiro, R.C. (2001) Experience with 2-chlorodeoxyadenosine in previously untreated children with newly diagnosed acute myeloid leukemia and myelodysplastic diseases. *J.Clin.Oncol.*, 19, 2804-2811.

Krivtsov, A.V., Feng, Z., Lemieux, M.E., Faber, J., Vempati, S., Sinha, A.U., Xia, X., Jesneck, J., Bracken, A.P., Silverman, L.B., Kutok, J.L., Kung, A.L. & Armstrong, S.A. (2008) H3K79 methylation profiles define murine and human MLL-AF4 leukemias. *Cancer Cell*, 14, 355-368.

Kuipers, J.E., Coenen, E.A., Balgobind, B.V., Stary, J., Baruchel, A., de Haas, V., de Bont, E.S., Reinhardt, D., Kaspers, G.J., Cloos, J., Danen-van Oorschot, A.A., den Boer, M.L., Marschalek, R., Meyer, C., Pieters, R., Zwaan, C.M. & van den Heuvel-Eibrink, M.M. (2011) High IGSF4 expression in pediatric M5 acute myeloid leukemia with t(9;11)(p22;q23). *Blood*, 117, 928-935.

Lange, B.J., Kobrinsky, N., Barnard, D.R., Arthur, D.C., Buckley, J.D., Howells, W.B., Gold, S., Sanders, J., Neudorf, S., Smith, F.O. & Woods, W.G. (1998) Distinctive demography, biology, and outcome of acute myeloid leukemia and myelodysplastic syndrome in children with Down syndrome: Children's Cancer Group Studies 2861 and 2891. *Blood*, 91, 608-615.

Langebrake, C., Brinkmann, I., Teigler-Schlegel, A., Creutzig, U., Griesinger, F., Puhlmann, U. & Reinhardt, D. (2005) Immunophenotypic differences between diagnosis and relapse in childhood AML: Implications for MRD monitoring. *Cytometry B Clin Cytom*, 63, 1-9.

Langebrake, C., Creutzig, U., Dworzak, M., Hrusak, O., Mejstrikova, E., Griesinger, F., Zimmermann, M. & Reinhardt, D. (2006) Residual disease monitoring in childhood acute myeloid leukemia by multiparameter flow cytometry: the MRD-AML-BFM Study Group. *J.Clin.Oncol.*, 24, 3686-3692.

Langemeijer, S.M., Jansen, J.H., Hooijer, J., van Hoogen, P., Stevens-Linders, E., Massop, M., Waanders, E., van Reijmersdal, S.V., Stevens-Kroef, M.J., Zwaan, C.M., van den Heuvel-Eibrink, M.M., Sonneveld, E., Hoogerbrugge, P.M., Geurts van Kessel, A. & Kuiper, R.P. (2011) TET2 mutations in childhood leukemia. *Leukemia, 25, 189-192*

Langemeijer, S.M., Kuiper, R.P., Berends, M., Knops, R., Aslanyan, M.G., Massop, M., Stevens-Linders, E., van Hoogen, P., van Kessel, A.G., Raymakers, R.A., Kamping, E.J., Verhoef, G.E., Verburgh, E., Hagemeijer, A., Vandenberghe, P., de Witte, T., van der Reijden, B.A. & Jansen, J.H. (2009) Acquired mutations in TET2 are common in myelodysplastic syndromes. *Nat Genet,* 41, 838-842.

Lapillonne, H., Renneville, A., Auvrignon, A., Flamant, C., Blaise, A., Perot, C., Lai, J.L., Ballerini, P., Mazingue, F., Fasola, S., Dehee, A., Bellman, F., Adam, M., Labopin, M., Douay, L., Leverger, G., Preudhomme, C. & Landman-Parker, J. (2006) High WT1 expression after induction therapy predicts high risk of relapse and death in pediatric acute myeloid leukemia. *J.Clin.Oncol.,* 24, 1507-1515.

Latagliata, R., Breccia, M., Fazi, P., Iacobelli, S., Martinelli, G., Di Raimondo, F., Sborgia, M., Fabbiano, F., Pirrotta, M.T., Zaccaria, A., Amadori, S., Caramatti, C., Falzetti, F., Candoni, A., Mattei, D., Morselli, M., Alimena, G., Vignetti, M., Baccarani, M. & Mandelli, F. (2008) Liposomal daunorubicin versus standard daunorubicin: long term follow-up of the GIMEMA GSI 103 AMLE randomized trial in patients older than 60 years with acute myelogenous leukaemia. *Br J Haematol,* 143, 681-689.

Lehrnbecher, T., Ethier, M.C., Zaoutis, T., Creutzig, U., Gamis, A., Reinhardt, D., Aplenc, R. & Sung, L. (2009) International variations in infection supportive care practices for paediatric patients with acute myeloid leukaemia. *Br J Haematol,* 147, 125-128.

Lehrnbecher, T., Varwig, D., Kaiser, J., Reinhardt, D., Klingebiel, T. & Creutzig, U. (2004) Infectious complications in pediatric acute myeloid leukemia: analysis of the prospective multi-institutional clinical trial AML-BFM 93. *Leukemia,* 18, 72-77.

Leroy, H., De Botton, S., Grardel-Duflos, N., Darre, S., Leleu, X., Roumier, C., Morschhauser, F., Lai, J.L., Bauters, F., Fenaux, P. & Preudhomme, C. (2005) Prognostic value of real-time quantitative PCR (RQ-PCR) in AML with t(8;21). *Leukemia,* 19, 367-372.

Leung, W., Hudson, M.M., Strickland, D.K., Phipps, S., Srivastava, D.K., Ribeiro, R.C., Rubnitz, J.E., Sandlund, J.T., Kun, L.E., Bowman, L.C., Razzouk, B.I., Mathew, P., Shearer, P., Evans, W.E. & Pui, C.H. (2000) Late effects of treatment in survivors of childhood acute myeloid leukemia. *J.Clin.Oncol.,* 18, 3273-3279.

Leung, W., Ribeiro, R.C., Hudson, M., Tong, X., Srivastava, D.K., Rubnitz, J.E., Sandlund, J.T., Razzouk, B.I., Evans, W.E. & Pui, C.H. (2001) Second malignancy after treatment of childhood acute myeloid leukemia. *Leukemia,* 15, 41-45.

Levis, M., Ravandi, F., Wang, E.S., Baer, M.R., Perl, A., Coutre, S., Erba, H., Stuart, R.K., Baccarani, M., Cripe, L.D., Tallman, M.S., Meloni, G., Godley, L.A., Langston, A.A., Amadori, S., Lewis, I.D., Nagler, A., Stone, R., Yee, K., Advani, A., Douer, D., Wiktor-Jedrzejczak, W., Juliusson, G., Litzow, M.R., Petersdorf, S., Sanz, M., Kantarjian, H.M., Sato, T., Tremmel, L., Bensen-Kennedy, D.M., Small, D. & Smith, B.D. (2011) Results from a randomized trial of salvage chemotherapy followed by lestaurtinib for patients with FLT3 mutant AML in first relapse. *Blood,* 117, 3294-3301.

Ley, T.J., Ding, L., Walter, M.J., McLellan, M.D., Lamprecht, T., Larson, D.E., Kandoth, C., Payton, J.E., Baty, J., Welch, J., Harris, C.C., Lichti, C.F., Townsend, R.R., Fulton, R.S., Dooling, D.J., Koboldt, D.C., Schmidt, H., Zhang, Q., Osborne, J.R., Lin, L., O'Laughlin, M., McMichael, J.F., Delehaunty, K.D., McGrath, S.D., Fulton, L.A., Magrini, V.J., Vickery, T.L., Hundal, J., Cook, L.L., Conyers, J.J., Swift, G.W., Reed, J.P., Alldredge, P.A., Wylie, T., Walker, J., Kalicki, J., Watson, M.A., Heath, S., Shannon, W.D., Varghese, N., Nagarajan, R., Westervelt, P., Tomasson, M.H., Link, D.C., Graubert, T.A., DiPersio, J.F., Mardis, E.R. & Wilson, R.K. (2010) DNMT3A mutations in acute myeloid leukemia. *N Engl J Med,* 363, 2424-2433.

Lipshultz, S.E. & Adams, M.J. (2010) Cardiotoxicity after childhood cancer: beginning with the end in mind. *J Clin Oncol,* 28, 1276-1281.

Löwenberg, B., Beck, J., Graux, C., van Putten, W., Schouten, H.C., Verdonck, L.F., Ferrant, A., Sonneveld, P., Jongen-Lavrencic, M., von Lilienfeld-Toal, M., Biemond, B.J., Vellenga, E., Breems, D., de Muijnck, H., Schaafsma, R., Verhoef, G., Dohner, H., Gratwohl, A., Pabst, T., Ossenkoppele, G.J. & Maertens, J. (2010a) Gemtuzumab ozogamicin as postremission treatment in AML at 60 years of age or more: results of a multicenter phase 3 study. *Blood,* 115, 2586-2591.

Löwenberg, B., Morgan, G., Ossenkoppele, G.J., Burnett, A.K., Zachee, P., Duhrsen, U., Dierickx, D., Muller-Tidow, C., Sonneveld, P., Krug, U., Bone, E., Flores, N., Richardson, A.F., Hooftman, L., Jenkins, C., Zweegman, S. & Davies, F. (2010b) Phase I/II clinical study of Tosedostat, an inhibitor of aminopeptidases, in patients with acute myeloid leukemia and myelodysplasia. *J Clin Oncol,* 28, 4333-4338.

Löwenberg, B., Ossenkoppele, G.J., van Putten, W., Schouten, H.C., Graux, C., Ferrant, A., Sonneveld, P., Maertens, J., Jongen-Lavrencic, M., von Lilienfeld-Toal, M., Biemond, B.J., Vellenga, E., van Marwijk Kooy, M., Verdonck, L.F., Beck, J., Dohner, H., Gratwohl, A., Pabst, T. & Verhoef, G. (2009) High-dose daunorubicin in older patients with acute myeloid leukemia. *N Engl J Med,* 361, 1235-1248.

Marcucci, G., Haferlach, T. & Dohner, H. (2011) Molecular genetics of adult acute myeloid leukemia: prognostic and therapeutic implications. *J Clin Oncol,* 29, 475-486.

Mardis, E.R., Ding, L., Dooling, D.J., Larson, D.E., McLellan, M.D., Chen, K., Koboldt, D.C., Fulton, R.S., Delehaunty, K.D., McGrath, S.D., Fulton, L.A., Locke, D.P., Magrini, V.J., Abbott, R.M., Vickery, T.L., Reed, J.S., Robinson, J.S., Wylie, T., Smith, S.M., Carmichael, L., Eldred, J.M., Harris, C.C., Walker, J., Peck, J.B., Du, F., Dukes, A.F., Sanderson, G.E., Brummett, A.M., Clark, E., McMichael, J.F., Meyer, R.J., Schindler, J.K., Pohl, C.S., Wallis, J.W., Shi, X., Lin, L., Schmidt, H., Tang, Y., Haipek, C., Wiechert, M.E., Ivy, J.V., Kalicki, J., Elliott, G., Ries, R.E., Payton, J.E., Westervelt, P., Tomasson, M.H., Watson, M.A., Baty, J., Heath, S., Shannon, W.D., Nagarajan, R., Link, D.C., Walter, M.J., Graubert, T.A., DiPersio, J.F., Wilson, R.K. & Ley, T.J. (2009) Recurring mutations found by sequencing an acute myeloid leukemia genome. *N Engl J Med,* 361, 1058-1066.

Mathews, V., George, B., Chendamarai, E., Lakshmi, K.M., Desire, S., Balasubramanian, P., Viswabandya, A., Thirugnanam, R., Abraham, A., Shaji, R.V., Srivastava, A. & Chandy, M. (2010) Single-agent arsenic trioxide in the treatment of newly diagnosed acute promyelocytic leukemia: long-term follow-up data. *J Clin Oncol,* 28, 3866-3871.

Meshinchi, S., Alonzo, T., Stirewalt, D.L., Zwaan, C.M., Zimmermann, M., Reinhardt, D., Kaspers, G.J.L., Heerema, N.A., Gerbing, R.B., Lange, B.J. & Radich, J.P. (2006) Clinical implications of FLT3 mutations in pediatric AML. *Blood,* 108, 3654-3661.

Metzelder, S., Wang, Y., Wollmer, E., Wanzel, M., Teichler, S., Chaturvedi, A., Eilers, M., Enghofer, E., Neubauer, A. & Burchert, A. (2009) Compassionate use of sorafenib in FLT3-ITD-positive acute myeloid leukemia: sustained regression before and after allogeneic stem cell transplantation. *Blood,* 113, 6567-6571.

Miyamoto, T., Nagafuji, K., Akashi, K., Harada, M., Kyo, T., Akashi, T., Takenaka, K., Mizuno, S., Gondo, H., Okamura, T., Dohy, H. & Niho, Y. (1996) Persistence of multipotent progenitors expressing AML1/ETO transcripts in long-term remission patients with t(8;21) acute myelogenous leukemia. *Blood,* 87, 4789-4796.

Molgaard-Hansen, L., Glosli, H., Jahnukainen, K., Jarfelt, M., Jonmundsson, G.K., Malmros-Svennilson, J., Nysom, K. & Hasle, H. (2010a) Quality of health in survivors of childhood acute myeloid leukemia treated with chemotherapy only: A NOPHO-AML study. *Pediatr Blood Cancer,* E-pub ahead of print, Dec 22nd.

Molgaard-Hansen, L., Mottonen, M., Glosli, H., Jonmundsson, G.K., Abrahamsson, J. & Hasle, H. (2010b) Early and treatment-related deaths in childhood acute myeloid leukaemia in the Nordic countries: 1984-2003. *Br J Haematol,* 151, 447-459.

Mrozek, K., Marcucci, G., Paschka, P., Whitman, S.P. & Bloomfield, C.D. (2007) Clinical relevance of mutations and gene-expression changes in adult acute myeloid leukemia with normal cytogenetics: are we ready for a prognostically prioritized molecular classification? *Blood,* 109, 431-438.

Mullighan, C.G., Kennedy, A., Zhou, X., Radtke, I., Phillips, L.A., Shurtleff, S.A. & Downing, J.R. (2007) Pediatric acute myeloid leukemia with NPM1 mutations is characterized by a gene expression profile with dysregulated HOX gene expression distinct from MLL-rearranged leukemias. *Leukemia,* 21, 2000-2009.

Niewerth, D., Creutzig, U., Bierings, M.B. & Kaspers, G.J. (2010) A review on allogeneic stem cell transplantation for newly diagnosed pediatric acute myeloid leukemia. *Blood,* 116, 2205-2214.

Nysom, K., Holm, K., Lipsitz, S.R., Mone, S.M., Colan, S.D., Orav, E.J., Sallan, S.E., Olsen, J.H., Hertz, H., Jacobsen, J.R. & Lipshultz, S.E. (1998) Relationship between cumulative anthracycline dose and late cardiotoxicity in childhood acute lymphoblastic leukemia. *J.Clin.Oncol.,* 16, 545-550.

O'Brien, S., Rizzieri, D.A., Vey, N., Ravandi, F., Krug, U., Sekeres, M.A., Dennis, M., Venditti, A., Jacobsen, T.F., Staudacher, K. & Nilsson, B.I. (2009) A Phase II Multicentre Study with Elacytarabine as Second Salvage Therapy in Patients with AML. *Blood,* 114, abstract 1042.

Ommen, H.B., Schnittger, S., Jovanovic, J.V., Ommen, I.B., Hasle, H., Ostergaard, M., Grimwade, D. & Hokland, P. (2010) Strikingly different molecular relapse kinetics in NPM1c, PML-RARA, RUNX1-RUNX1T1, and CBFB-MYH11 acute myeloid leukemias. *Blood,* 115, 198-205.

Owen, C., Barnett, M. & Fitzgibbon, J. (2008) Familial myelodysplasia and acute myeloid leukaemia--a review. *Br J Haematol,* 140, 123-132.

Perea, G., Lasa, A., Aventin, A., Domingo, A., Villamor, N., Queipo de Llano, M.P., Llorente, A., Junca, J., Palacios, C., Fernandez, C., Gallart, M., Font, L., Tormo, M., Florensa, L., Bargay, J., Marti, J.M., Vivancos, P., Torres, P., Berlanga, J.J., Badell, I., Brunet, S., Sierra, J. & Nomdedeu, J.F. (2006) Prognostic value of minimal residual disease (MRD) in acute myeloid leukemia (AML) with favorable cytogenetics [t(8;21) and inv(16)]. *Leukemia,* 20, 87-94.

Perel, Y., Auvrignon, A., Leblanc, T., Michel, G., Reguerre, Y., Vannier, J.P., Dalle, J.H., Gandemer, V., Schmitt, C., Mechinaud, F., Lejars, O., Piguet, C., Couillaud, G., Pautard, B., Landman-Parker, J., Thuret, I., Aladjidi, N., Baruchel, A. & Leverger, G. (2005) Treatment of childhood acute myeloblastic leukemia: dose intensification improves outcome and maintenance therapy is of no benefit--multicenter studies of the French LAME (Leucemie Aigue Myeloblastique Enfant) Cooperative Group. *Leukemia,* 19, 2082-2089.

Perel, Y., Auvrignon, A., Leblanc, T., Vannier, J.P., Michel, G., Nelken, B., Gandemer, V., Schmitt, C., Lamagnere, J.P., De Lumley, L., Bader-Meunier, B., Couillaud, G., Schaison, G., Landman-Parker, J., Thuret, I., Dalle, J.H., Baruchel, A. & Leverger, G. (2002) Impact of addition of maintenance therapy to intensive induction and consolidation chemotherapy for childhood acute myeloblastic leukemia: results of a prospective randomized trial, LAME 89/91. Leucamie Aique Myeloide Enfant. *J.Clin.Oncol.,* 20, 2774-2782.

Pession, A., Rondelli, R., Basso, G., Rizzari, C., Testi, A.M., Fagioli, F., De Stefano, P. & Locatelli, F. (2005) Treatment and long-term results in children with acute myeloid leukaemia treated according to the AIEOP AML protocols. *Leukemia,* 19, 2043-2053.

Pieters, R., Schrappe, M., De Lorenzo, P., Hann, I., De Rossi, G., Felice, M., Hovi, L., Leblanc, T., Szczepanski, T., Ferster, A., Janka, G., Rubnitz, J., Silverman, L., Stary, J., Campbell, M., Li, C.K., Mann, G., Suppiah, R., Biondi, A., Vora, A. & Valsecchi, M.G. (2007) A treatment protocol for infants younger than 1 year with acute lymphoblastic leukaemia (Interfant-99): an observational study and a multicentre randomised trial. *Lancet,* 370, 240-250.

Pine, S.R., Guo, Q., Yin, C., Jayabose, S., Levendoglu-Tugal, O., Ozkaynak, M.F. & Sandoval, C. (2005) GATA1 as a new target to detect minimal residual disease in both transient leukemia and megakaryoblastic leukemia of Down syndrome. *Leuk.Res.,* 29, 1353-1356.

Pinkerton, R., Wills, R.A., Coory, M.D. & Fraser, C.J. (2010) Survival from haematological malignancy in childhood, adolescence and young adulthood in Australia: is the age-related gap narrowing? *Med J Aust,* 193, 217-221.

Pollard, J.A., Alonzo, T.A., Gerbing, R.B., Ho, P.A., Zeng, R., Ravindranath, Y., Dahl, G., Lacayo, N.J., Becton, D., Chang, M., Weinstein, H.J., Hirsch, B., Raimondi, S.C., Heerema, N.A., Woods, W.G., Lange, B.J., Hurwitz, C., Arceci, R.J., Radich, J.P., Bernstein, I.D., Heinrich, M.C. & Meshinchi, S. (2010) Prevalence and prognostic significance of KIT mutations in pediatric patients with core binding factor AML enrolled on serial pediatric cooperative trials for de novo AML. *Blood,* 115, 2372-2379.

Powell, B.L., Moser, B., Stock, W., Gallagher, R.E., Willman, C.L., Stone, R.M., Rowe, J.M., Coutre, S., Feusner, J.H., Gregory, J., Couban, S., Appelbaum, F.R., Tallman, M.S. & Larson, R.A. (2011) Arsenic trioxide improves event-free and overall survival for adults with acute promyelocytic leukemia: North American Leukemia Intergroup Study C9710. *Blood,* 116, 3751-3757.

Pratz, K.W., Sato, T., Murphy, K.M., Stine, A., Rajkhowa, T. & Levis, M. (2010) FLT3-mutant allelic burden and clinical status are predictive of response to FLT3 inhibitors in AML. *Blood,* 115, 1425-1432.

Pui, C.H., Carroll, W.L., Meshinchi, S. & Arceci, R.J. (2011) Biology, risk stratification, and therapy of pediatric acute leukemias: an update. *J Clin Oncol,* 29, 551-565.

Pui, C.H., Raimondi, S.C., Srivastava, D.K., Tong, X., Behm, F.G., Razzouk, B.I., Rubnitz, J.E., Sandlund, J.T., Evans, W.E. & Ribeiro, R. (2000) Prognostic factors in infants with acute myeloid leukemia. *Leukemia,* 14, 684-687.

Radtke, I., Mullighan, C.G., Ishii, M., Su, X., Cheng, J., Ma, J., Ganti, R., Cai, Z., Goorha, S., Pounds, S.B., Cao, X., Obert, C., Armstrong, J., Zhang, J., Song, G., Ribeiro, R.C., Rubnitz, J.E., Raimondi, S.C., Shurtleff, S.A. & Downing, J.R. (2009) Genomic analysis reveals few genetic alterations in pediatric acute myeloid leukemia. *Proc Natl Acad Sci U S A*, 106, 12944-12949.

Rajvanshi, P., Shulman, H.M., Sievers, E.L. & McDonald, G.B. (2002) Hepatic sinusoidal obstruction after gemtuzumab ozogamicin (Mylotarg) therapy. *Blood*, 99, 2310-2314.

Ravandi, F., Cortes, J.E., Jones, D., Faderl, S., Garcia-Manero, G., Konopleva, M.Y., O'Brien, S., Estrov, Z., Borthakur, G., Thomas, D., Pierce, S.R., Brandt, M., Byrd, A., Bekele, B.N., Pratz, K., Luthra, R., Levis, M., Andreeff, M. & Kantarjian, H.M. (2010) Phase I/II study of combination therapy with sorafenib, idarubicin, and cytarabine in younger patients with acute myeloid leukemia. *J Clin Oncol*, 28, 1856-1862.

Reinhardt, D., Diekamp, S., Langebrake, C., Ritter, J., Stary, J., Dworzak, M., Schrauder, A., Zimmermann, M., Fleischhack, G., Ludwig, W.D., Harbott, J. & Creutzig, U. (2005) Acute megakaryoblastic leukemia in children and adolescents, excluding Down's syndrome: improved outcome with intensified induction treatment. *Leukemia*, 19, 1495-1496.

Reinhardt, D., Hempel, G., Fleischhack, G., Schulz, A., Boos, J. & Creutzig, U. (2002a) Liposomal daunorubicine combined with cytarabine in the treatment of relapsed/refractory acute myeloid leukemia in children. *Klin. Pädiatr.*, 214, 188-194.

Reinhardt, D., Kremens, B., Zimmermann, M., Vormoor, J., Dworzak, M., Peters, C., Creutzig, U. & Klingebiel, T. (2006) No improvement of overall survival in children with high-risk acute myeloid leukemia by stem-cell transplantation in 1st complete remission. Blood, 108, abstract 320

Reinhardt, D., Thiele, C. & Creutzig, U. (2002b) Neuropsychological sequelae in children with AML treated with or without prophylactic CNS-irradiation. *Klin. Pädiatr.*, 214, 22-29.

Ries, L.A.G., Smith, M.A., Gurney, J.G., Linet, M., Tamra, T., Young, J.L. & Bunin, G.R.e. (1999) *Cancer Incidence and Survival among Children and Adolescents: United States SEER Program 1975-1995.* National Cancer Institute, SEER program, Bethesda.

Ross, M.E., Mahfouz, R., Onciu, M., Liu, H.C., Zhou, X., Song, G., Shurtleff, S.A., Pounds, S., Cheng, C., Ma, J., Ribeiro, R.C., Rubnitz, J.E., Girtman, K., Williams, W.K., Raimondi, S.C., Liang, D.C., Shih, L.Y., Pui, C.H. & Downing, J.R. (2004) Gene Expression Profiling of Pediatric Acute Myelogenous Leukemia. *Blood*, 104, 3679-3687.

Rubnitz, J.E., Crews, K.R., Pounds, S., Yang, S., Campana, D., Gandhi, V.V., Raimondi, S.C., Downing, J.R., Razzouk, B.I., Pui, C.H. & Ribeiro, R.C. (2009) Combination of cladribine and cytarabine is effective for childhood acute myeloid leukemia: results of the St Jude AML97 trial. *Leukemia*, 23, 1410-1416.

Rubnitz, J.E., Inaba, H., Dahl, G., Ribeiro, R.C., Bowman, W.P., Taub, J., Pounds, S., Razzouk, B.I., Lacayo, N.J., Cao, X., Meshinchi, S., Degar, B., Airewele, G., Raimondi, S.C., Onciu, M., Coustan-Smith, E., Downing, J.R., Leung, W., Pui, C.H. & Campana, D. (2010) Minimal residual disease-directed therapy for childhood acute myeloid leukaemia: results of the AML02 multicentre trial. *Lancet Oncol*, 11, 543-552.

Rubnitz, J.E., Lensing, S., Zhou, Y., Sandlund, J.T., Razzouk, B.I., Ribeiro, R.C. & Pui, C.H. (2004) Death during induction therapy and first remission of acute leukemia in childhood: the St. Jude experience. *Cancer,* 101, 1677-1684.

Sander, A., Zimmermann, M., Dworzak, M., Fleischhack, G., von Neuhoff, C., Reinhardt, D., Kaspers, G.J. & Creutzig, U. (2010) Consequent and intensified relapse therapy improved survival in pediatric AML: results of relapse treatment in 379 patients of three consecutive AML-BFM trials. *Leukemia,* 24, 1422-1428.

Sandler, E.S., Friedman, D.J., Mustafa, M.M., Winick, N.J., Bowman, W.P. & Buchanan, G.R. (1997) Treatment of children with epipodophyllotoxin-induced secondary acute myeloid leukemia. *Cancer,* 79, 1049-1054.

Santana, V.M., Mirro, J., Jr., Harwood, F.C., Cherrie, J., Schell, M., Kalwinsky, D. & Blakley, R.L. (1991) A phase I clinical trial of 2-chlorodeoxyadenosine in pediatric patients with acute leukemia. *J.Clin.Oncol.,* 9, 416-422.

Santana, V.M., Mirro, J., Jr., Kearns, C., Schell, M.J., Crom, W. & Blakley, R.L. (1992) 2-Chlorodeoxyadenosine produces a high rate of complete hematologic remission in relapsed acute myeloid leukemia. *J.Clin.Oncol.,* 10, 364-370.

Sanz, M.A., Grimwade, D., Tallman, M.S., Lowenberg, B., Fenaux, P., Estey, E.H., Naoe, T., Lengfelder, E., Buchner, T., Dohner, H., Burnett, A.K. & Lo-Coco, F. (2009) Management of acute promyelocytic leukemia: recommendations from an expert panel on behalf of the European LeukemiaNet. *Blood,* 113, 1875-1891.

Sato, T., Yang, X., Knapper, S., White, P., Smith, B.D., Galkin, S., Small, D., Burnett, A. & Levis, M. (2011) FLT3 ligand impedes the efficacy of FLT3 inhibitors in vitro and in vivo. *Blood,* 117, 3286-3293.

Schnittger, S., Kern, W., Tschulik, C., Weiss, T., Dicker, F., Falini, B., Haferlach, C. & Haferlach, T. (2009) Minimal residual disease levels assessed by NPM1 mutation-specific RQ-PCR provide important prognostic information in AML. *Blood,* 114, 2220-2231.

Serve, H., Wagner, R., Sauerland, C., Brunnberg, U., Krug, U., Schaich, M., Ottmann, O., Duyster, J., Wandt, H., Herr, W., Giaganoudis, A.A.N., Neubauer, A., Reichle, A., Aulitzky, W.E., Noppeney, R., Blau, I.W., Kunzmann, V., Schmitz, N., Kreuzer, K.A., Kramer, A., Brandts, C., Steffen, B., Heinecke, A., Thiede, C., Muller-Tidow, C., Ehninger, G. & Berdel, W.E. (2010) Sorafenib In Combination with Standard Induction and Consolidation Therapy In Elderly AML Patients: Results From a Randomized, Placebo-Controlled Phase II Trial. *Blood,* 116, abstract 333.

Sievers, E.L., Appelbaum, F.R., Spielberger, R.T., Forman, S.J., Flowers, D., Smith, F.O., Shannon-Dorcy, K., Berger, M.S. & Bernstein, I.D. (1999) Selective ablation of acute myeloid leukemia using antibody-targeted chemotherapy: a phase I study of an anti-CD33 calicheamicin immunoconjugate. *Blood,* 93, 3678-3684.

Sievers, E.L., Larson, R.A., Stadtmauer, E.A., Estey, E., Lowenberg, B., Dombret, H., Karanes, C., Theobald, M., Bennett, J.M., Sherman, M.L., Berger, M.S., Eten, C.B., Loken, M.R., van Dongen, J.J., Bernstein, I.D. & Appelbaum, F.R. (2001) Efficacy and safety of gemtuzumab ozogamicin in patients with CD33-positive acute myeloid leukemia in first relapse. *J.Clin.Oncol.,* 19, 3244-3254.

Slats, A.M., Egeler, R.M., Van Der Does-Van Den Berg, A., Korbijn, C., H„hlen, K., Kamps, W.A., Veerman, A.J.P. & Zwaan, C.M. (2005) Causes of death - other than progressive leukemia - in childhood acute lymphoblastic (ALL) and myeloid leukemia (AML): the Dutch Childhood Oncology Group experience *Leukemia,* 19, 537-544.

Smith, M.T., Zhang, L., McHale, C.M., Skibola, C.F. & Rappaport, S.M. (2011) Benzene, the exposome and future investigations of leukemia etiology. *Chem Biol Interact, 192, 155-159.*

Soignet, S.L. (2001) Clinical experience of arsenic trioxide in relapsed acute promyelocytic leukemia. *Oncologist,* 6 Suppl 2, 11-16.

Stein, E., McMahon, B., Kwaan, H., Altman, J.K., Frankfurt, O. & Tallman, M.S. (2009) The coagulopathy of acute promyelocytic leukaemia revisited. *Best Pract Res Clin Haematol,* 22, 153-163.

Stevens, R.F., Hann, I.M., Wheatley, K., Gray, R.G. & on behalf of the, M.R.C.C.L.W.P. (1998) Marked improvements in outcome with chemotherapy alone in paediatric acute myeloid leukemia: results of the United Kingdom Medical Research Council's 10th AML trial. *Br.J.Haematol.,* 101, 130-140.

Tallman, M.S., Kim, H.T., Montesinos, P., Appelbaum, F.R., de la Serna, J., Bennett, J.M., Deben, G., Bloomfield, C.D., Gonzalez, J., Feusner, J.H., Gonzalez, M., Gallagher, R., Miguel, J.D., Larson, R.A., Milone, G., Paietta, E., Rayon, C., Rowe, J.M., Rivas, C., Schiffer, C.A., Vellenga, E., Shepherd, L., Slack, J.L., Wiernik, P.H., Willman, C.L. & Sanz, M.A. (2010) Does microgranular variant morphology of acute promyelocytic leukemia independently predict a less favorable outcome compared with classical M3 APL? A joint study of the North American Intergroup and the PETHEMA Group. *Blood,* 116, 5650-5659.

Temming, P. & Jenney, M.E. (2010) The neurodevelopmental sequelae of childhood leukaemia and its treatment. *Arch Dis Child,* 95, 936-940.

Temming, P., Qureshi, A., Hardt, J., Leiper, A.D., Levitt, G., Ancliff, P.J. & Webb, D.K. (2011) Prevalence and predictors of anthracycline cardiotoxicity in children treated for acute myeloid leukaemia: retrospective cohort study in a single centre in the United Kingdom. *Pediatr Blood Cancer,* 56, 625-630.

Testi, A.M., Biondi, A., Lo, C.F., Moleti, M.L., Giona, F., Vignetti, M., Menna, G., Locatelli, F., Pession, A., Barisone, E., De Rossi, G., Diverio, D., Micalizzi, C., Arico, M., Basso, G., Foa, R. & Mandelli, F. (2005) GIMEMA-AIEOPAIDA protocol for the treatment of newly diagnosed acute promyelocytic leukemia (APL) in children. *Blood,* 106, 447-453.

Tonnies, H., Huber, S., Kuhl, J.S., Gerlach, A., Ebell, W. & Neitzel, H. (2003) Clonal chromosome aberrations in bone marrow cells of Fanconi anemia patients: gains of the chromosomal segment 3q26q29 as an adverse risk factor. *Blood,* 101, 3872-3874.

Tsukimoto, I., Tawa, A., Horibe, K., Tabuchi, K., Kigasawa, H., Tsuchida, M., Yabe, H., Nakayama, H., Kudo, K., Kobayashi, R., Hamamoto, K., Imaizumi, M., Morimoto, A., Tsuchiya, S. & Hanada, R. (2009) Risk-stratified therapy and the intensive use of cytarabine improves the outcome in childhood acute myeloid leukemia: the AML99 trial from the Japanese Childhood AML Cooperative Study Group. *J Clin Oncol,* 27, 4007-4013.

Tunstall-Pedoe, O., Roy, A., Karadimitris, A., de la Fuente, J., Fisk, N.M., Bennett, P., Norton, A., Vyas, P. & Roberts, I. (2008) Abnormalities in the myeloid progenitor compartment in Down syndrome fetal liver precede acquisition of GATA1 mutations. *Blood,* 112, 4507-4511.

van Dalen, E.C., Michiels, E.M., Caron, H.N. & Kremer, L.C. (2010) Different anthracycline derivates for reducing cardiotoxicity in cancer patients. *Cochrane Database Syst Rev,* CD005006.

van Dalen, E.C., van der Pal, H.J., Kok, W.E., Caron, H.N. & Kremer, L.C. (2006) Clinical heart failure in a cohort of children treated with anthracyclines: a long-term follow-up study. *Eur.J.Cancer,* 42, 3191-3198.

van de Wetering, M.D., de Witte, M.A., Kremer, L.C., Offringa, M., Scholten, R.J. & Caron, H.N. (2005) Efficacy of oral prophylactic antibiotics in neutropenic afebrile oncology patients: a systematic review of randomised controlled trials. *Eur J Cancer,* 41, 1372-1382.

van der Velden, V.H., van der Sluijs-Geling, A., Gibson, B.E., te Marvelde, J.G., Hoogeveen, P.G., Hop, W.C., Wheatley, K., Bierings, M.B., Schuurhuis, G.J., de Graaf, S.S., van Wering, E.R. & van Dongen, J.J. (2010) Clinical significance of flowcytometric minimal residual disease detection in pediatric acute myeloid leukemia patients treated according to the DCOG ANLL97/MRC AML12 protocol. *Leukemia,* 24, 1599-1606.

van der Velden, V.H. & van Dongen, J.J. (2009) MRD detection in acute lymphoblastic leukemia patients using Ig/TCR gene rearrangements as targets for real-time quantitative PCR. *Methods Mol Biol,* 538, 115-150.

Van Dongen, J.J., Seriu, T., Panzer-Grumayer, E.R., Biondi, A., Pongers-Willemse, M.J., Corral, L., Stolz, F., Schrappe, M., Masera, G., Kamps, W.A., Gadner, H., Van Wering, E.R., Ludwig, W.D., Basso, G., de Bruijn, M.A., Cazzaniga, G., Hettinger, K., Van Der Does-Van Den, B., Hop, W.C., Riehm, H. & Bartram, C.R. (1998) Prognostic value of minimal residual disease in acute lymphoblastic leukaemia in childhood. *Lancet,* 352, 1731-1738.

Vardiman, J.W., Thiele, J., Arber, D.A., Brunning, R.D., Borowitz, M.J., Porwit, A., Harris, N.L., Le Beau, M.M., Hellstrom-Lindberg, E., Tefferi, A. & Bloomfield, C.D. (2009) The 2008 revision of the World Health Organization (WHO) classification of myeloid neoplasms and acute leukemia: rationale and important changes. *Blood,* 114, 937-951.

Viehmann, S., Teigler-Schlegel, A., Bruch, J., Langebrake, C., Reinhardt, D. & Harbott, J. (2003) Monitoring of minimal residual disease (MRD) by real-time quantitative reverse transcription PCR (RQ-RT-PCR) in childhood acute myeloid leukemia with AML1/ETO rearrangement. *Leukemia,* 17, 1130-1136.

von Bergh, A.R., van Drunen, E., van Wering, E.R., van Zutven, L.J., Hainmann, I., Lonnerholm, G., Meijerink, J.P., Pieters, R. & Beverloo, H.B. (2006) High incidence of t(7;12)(q36;p13) in infant AML but not in infant ALL, with a dismal outcome and ectopic expression of HLXB9. *Genes Chromosomes Cancer,* 45, 731-739.

von Neuhoff, C., Reinhardt, D., Sander, A., Zimmermann, M., Bradtke, J., Betts, D.R., Zemanova, Z., Stary, J., Bourquin, J.P., Haas, O.A., Dworzak, M.N. & Creutzig, U. (2010) Prognostic impact of specific chromosomal aberrations in a large group of pediatric patients with acute myeloid leukemia treated uniformly according to trial AML-BFM 98. *J Clin Oncol,* 28, 2682-2689.

Vormoor, J., Ritter, J., Creutzig, U., Boos, J., Heyen, P., Ludwig, W.D., Harbott, J., L"ffler, H. & Schellong, G. (1992) Acute myelogenous leukaemia in children under 2 years--

experiences of the West German AML studies BFM-78, -83 and -87. AML-BFM Study Group. *Br.J.Cancer,* 66, Suppl.18, S63-S67.

Webb, D.K., Wheatley, K., Harrison, G., Stevens, R.F., Hann, I.M. & for the, M.R.C.C.L.W.P. (1999) Outcome for children with relapsed acute myeloid leukaemia following initial therapy in the Medical Research Council (MRC) AML 10 trial. MRC Childhood Leukaemia Working Party. *Leukemia,* 13, 25-31.

Webb, D.K.H. (1999) Management of relapsed acute myeloid leukaemia. *Br.J.Haematol.,* 106, 851-859.

Weiss, B., Vora, A., Huberty, J., Hawkins, R.A. & Matthay, K.K. (2003) Secondary myelodysplastic syndrome and leukemia following 131I-metaiodobenzylguanidine therapy for relapsed neuroblastoma. *J.Pediatr Hematol.Oncol.,* 25, 543-547.

Wells, R.J., Woods, W.G., Buckley, J.D., Odom, L.F., Benjamin, D., Bernstein, I., Betcher, D., Feig, S., Kim, T., Ruymann, F., Smithson, W., Srivastava, A., Tannous, R., Buckley, C.M., Whitt, J.K., Wolff, L. & Lampkin, B.C. (1994) Treatment of newly diagnosed children and adolescents with acute myeloid leukemia: a Childrens Cancer Group study. *J.Clin.Oncol.,* 12, 2367-2377.

Wiemels, J.L., Xiao, Z., Buffler, P.A., Maia, A.T., Ma, X., Dicks, B.M., Smith, M.T., Zhang, L., Feusner, J., Wiencke, J., Pritchard-Jones, K., Kempski, H. & Greaves, M. (2002) In utero origin of t(8;21) AML1-ETO translocations in childhood acute myeloid leukemia. *Blood,* 99, 3801-3805.

Willasch, A.M., Gruhn, B., Coliva, T., Kalinova, M., Schneider, G., Kreyenberg, H., Steinbach, D., Weber, G., Hollink, I.H., Zwaan, C.M., Biondi, A., van der Velden, V.H., Reinhardt, D., Cazzaniga, G., Bader, P. & Trka, J. (2009) Standardization of WT1 mRNA quantitation for minimal residual disease monitoring in childhood AML and implications of WT1 gene mutations: a European multicenter study. *Leukemia,* 23, 1472-1479.

Woods, W.G., Kobrinsky, N., Buckley, J.D., Lee, J.W., Sanders, J., Neudorf, S., Gold, S., Barnard, D.R., DeSwarte, J., Dusenbery, K., Kalousek, D., Arthur, D.C. & Lange, B.J. (1996) Timed-sequential induction therapy improves postremission outcome in acute myeloid leukemia: a report from the Children's Cancer Group. *Blood,* 87, 4979-4989.

Woods, W.G., Neudorf, S., Gold, S., Sanders, J., Buckley, J.D., Barnard, D.R., Dusenbery, K., DeSwarte, J., Arthur, D.C., Lange, B.J. & Kobrinsky, N.L. (2001) A comparison of allogeneic bone marrow transplantation, autologous bone marrow transplantation, and aggressive chemotherapy in children with acute myeloid leukemia in remission: a report from the Children's Cancer Group. *Blood,* 97, 56-62.

Yan, X.J., Xu, J., Gu, Z.H., Pan, C.M., Lu, G., Shen, Y., Shi, J.Y., Zhu, Y.M., Tang, L., Zhang, X.W., Liang, W.X., Mi, J.Q., Song, H.D., Li, K.Q., Chen, Z. & Chen, S.J. (2011) Exome sequencing identifies somatic mutations of DNA methyltransferase gene DNMT3A in acute monocytic leukemia. *Nat Genet,* 43, 309-315.

Yang, L., Han, Y., Suarez Saiz, F. & Minden, M.D. (2007) A tumor suppressor and oncogene: the WT1 story. *Leukemia,* 21, 868-876.

Zwaan, C.M., Den Boer, M.L., Beverloo, H.B., Van der Velden, V.H., Countouriotis, A., Strauss, L., Astier, L., Apanovitch, A., Landmann-Parker, J. & Kearns, P. (2006) Dasatinib (SPRYCEL) in Children and Adolescents with Relapsed or Refractory

Leukemia: Preliminary Results of the CA180018 Phase I/II Study. *Blood, 108, abstract 2162.*

Zwaan, C.M., Kaspers, G.J.L., Pieters, R., H„hlen, K., Huismans, D.R., Zimmermann, M., Harbott, J., Slater, R., Creutzig, U. & Veerman, A.J.P. (2002a) Cellular drug resistance in childhood acute myeloid leukemia is related to chromosomal abnormalities. *Blood,* 100, 3352-3360.

Zwaan, C.M., Kaspers, G.J.L., Pieters, R., H„hlen, K., Janka-Schaub, G.E., Van Zantwijk, C.H., Huismans, D.R., De Vries, E., Rots, M.G., Peters, G.J., Jansen, G., Creutzig, U. & Veerman, A.J.P. (2002b) Different drug sensitivity profiles of acute myeloid and lymphoblastic leukemia and normal peripheral blood mononuclear cells, in children with and without Down syndrome. *Blood,* 99, 245-251.

Zwaan, C.M., Kearns, P., Caron, H., Verschuur, A., Riccardi, R., Boos, J., Doz, F., Geoerger, B., Morland, B. & Vassal, G. (2010a) The role of the 'innovative therapies for children with cancer' (ITCC) European consortium. *Cancer Treat Rev,* 36, 328-334.

Zwaan, C.M., Meshinchi, S., Radich, J.P., Veerman, A.J.P., Huismans, D.R., Munske, L., Podleschny, M., H„hlen, K., Pieters, R., Zimmermann, M., Reinhardt, D., Harbott, J., Creutzig, U., Kaspers, G.J.L. & Griesinger, F. (2003a) FLT3 internal tandem duplication in 234 children with acute myeloid leukemia (AML): prognostic significance and relation to cellular drug resistance. *Blood,* 102 2387-2394.

Zwaan, C.M., Reinhardt, D., Corbacioglu, S., Van Wering, E.R., Bökkerink, J.P., Tissing, W.J., Samuelsson, U., Feingold, J., Creutzig, U. & Kaspers, G.J. (2003b) Gemtuzumab ozogamicin: first clinical experiences in children with relapsed/refractory acute myeloid leukemia treated on compassionate use basis. *Blood,* 101, 3868-3871.

Zwaan, C.M., Reinhardt, D., Zimmerman, M., Hasle, H., Stary, J., Stark, B., Dworzak, M., Creutzig, U. & Kaspers, G.J. (2010b) Salvage treatment for children with refractory first or second relapse of acute myeloid leukaemia with gemtuzumab ozogamicin: results of a phase II study. *Br J Haematol,* 148, 768-776.

Zwaan, C.M., Reinhardt, D., Hitzler, J. & Vyas, P. (2008) Acute leukemias in children with Down syndrome. *Pediatr Clin North Am,* 55, 53-70.

12

Leukemogenesis in Down Syndrome

Lílian Barros Queiroz[1], Íris Ferrari[2],
Cezar Martins de Sá[1], Juliana Forte Mazzeu[2],
Isis Quezado Magalhães[3] and Beatriz Dolabela de Lima[1]
[1]*Departamento de Biologia Celular,*
[2]*Departamento de Genética e Morfologia,*
Instituto de Ciências Biológicas; Universidade de Brasília, Brasília, DF
[3]*Núcleo de Oncologia e Hematologia Pediátrica,*
Secretaria de Saúde do DF, Brasília, DF
Brazil

1. Introduction

Constitutional trisomy 21 or Down syndrome (DS) is the most common human genetic aneuploidy caused by the presence of all or part of an extra 21 chromosome. The incidence of DS is estimated at 1 per 700 births (Malinge et al., 2009) and is the most common genetic factor predisposing to childhood leukemia. People with DS present several clinical phenotypes, including cognitive impairment, craniofacial dysmorphy, gastrointestinal tract abnormalities, congenital heart defects, endocrine abnormalities, neuropathology leading to dementia and immunological defects. Concerning the hematopoietic system, children with DS frequently show abnormalities in platelet counts, macrocytosis and an increased prevalence of leukemia (Lange, 2000; Roizen & Amarose, 1993).

2. Manifestations of leukemia in Down Syndrome

The high frequency of leukemia in children with DS suggests that trisomy 21 is involved directly and functionally to the malignant transformation of hematopoietic cells. However, DS is not a classic genomic instability syndrome, since the overall risk of developing cancer, in particular solid tumors, including neuroblastoma and Wilms tumor, is lower in these people (Hasle, 2001; Malinge et al., 2009).

Newborns with DS have a risk 10 to 20 times higher of developing acute leukemia (AL) when compared with the incidence rates of leukemia in the general child population (Hitzler et al., 2003). The AL in children with DS presents an intriguing relationship between the age at onset of disease and the subtype of leukemia cell. DS children older than 4 years have predominantly acute lymphoblastic leukemia (ALL), whose incidence is approximately 20 times higher than in the general population. However the DS patients aged under 3 years are more likely to develop acute megakaryoblastic leukemia (AMKL), with an incidence 500 times higher than in children without DS (Hitzler et al., 2003; Issacs, 2003; Lange, 2000; Malinge et al., 2009).

The condition of patients with DS awakens, therefore, a special interest in studies on leukemogenesis not only by the high prevalence of AMKL, usually rare in the general pediatric population, but also by another form of clonal proliferation called transient myeloproliferative disorder (TMD) which affects between 5 and 10% of newborns with DS. The TMD is a clonal disease characterized by accumulation of immature megakaryoblasts in fetal liver and peripheral blood, a picture indistinguishable from AL (Hitzler et al., 2003; Malinge et al., 2009; Pine et al., 2007; Rainis et al., 2003; Zipursky, 2003). It is unclear whether all AMKLs are preceded by TMD, since several TMD cases are underdiagnosed. One study suggests that the prognosis for AMKLs preceded by TMD is better than de novo AMKL (Klusmann et al., 2008).

In contrast to AMKL, TMD usually evolves to spontaneous remission within the first three months of life and therefore is considered a pre-leukemic syndrome. This spontaneous remission can vary from 59 to 64% (Kanezaki et al., 2010; Massey et al., 2006). However, approximately 20% of children diagnosed with TMD will develop AMKL after 2 to 3 years of TMD spontaneous remission, which does not regress without chemotherapy (Malinge et al., 2009).

The biological mechanism of TMD spontaneous remission is not clear. Holt et al. (2002) showed that telomerase activity was decreased at the beginning of congenital leukemia and suggested that this deficiency could explain the spontaneous regression. Furthermore, the factors underlying the transformation of the TMD "benign" status for "evil" in AMKL are unknown (Izraeli et al., 2007; Malkin et al., 2000; Rainis et al., 2003).

In rare cases, the TMD is fatal due to poor prognostic factors such as liver fibrosis or liver dysfunction, manifested by jaundice, bleeding diathesis, fetal hydrops, cardiopulmonary failure, high white blood cell (WBC) and failure of spontaneous remission within the first 3 months (Malinge et al., 2009; Massey et al., 2006; Pine et al., 2007; Shimizu et al., 2008). Most of these variants were found in all reports. However, the risk factors for the progression to AMKL remain unclear (Kanezaki et al., 2010). Three studies in the United States, Japan and Europe reported the natural course of TMD in 264 children with DS. These studies confirmed the transient course of this disease that usually resolved spontaneously within the first 3 months of life. However, these studies revealed that the disease is not benign, since early deaths have been reported in 15 to 20% of the cases (Klusmann et al., 2008; Massey et al., 2006; Muramatsu et al., 2008). Kanezaki et al. (2010) also reported early death in 24.2% of the DS patients with TMD.

3. Mutations in *GATA1* gene and leukemogenesis in Down Syndrome

The *GATA1* (globin transcription factor 1) gene located on the X chromosome in the region Xp11.23 encodes the GATA binding protein 1 (GATA-1) belonging to the family of transcription factors with zinc finger structural motifs for DNA binding. GATA-1 is essential for survival of erythroid progenitor cells and for proper maturation of megakaryocytes, so in this way this protein has an essential rule in the erythrocytic and megakaryocytic differentiation (Wechsler et al., 2002; Yu et al., 2002).

The *GATA1* gene is 6.857 kb long with 6 exons and an open reading frame of 1,239 nucleotides starting in exon 2. The protein GATA-1 consists of 413 amino acids and 42.75 kDa with an N-terminal transactivation domain and two zinc finger domains. These two fingers are functionally distinct and cooperate to achieve specific, stable DNA binding. The first finger (NF) is necessary only for full specificity and stability of binding, whereas the second one (CF) is required for DNA binding (Martin & Orkin, 1990, Shimizu et al., 2008).

GATA1 mutations prevent the synthesis of heavy chain of GATA-1 (translated from the first ATG codon of exon 2) but not the synthesis of truncated protein, with 330 amino acids and 34.23 kDa called GATA-1s. GATA-1s is also expressed starting at codon 84 in exon 3 in consequence of an alternative translation initiation site or alternative splicing that eliminates exon 2. This truncated protein lacks the transactivation domain, but retains both zinc finger domains, as shown in figure 1. The function of GATA-1s is still quite unclear. Several experiments suggest that GATA-1s helps the megakaryocytic and erythrocyte differentiation (Weiss et al., 1997). However, studies of in vivo gene rescue indicated that only the endogenous GATA-1s expression would not be enough to restore definitive erythropoiesis unless this gene is hyper expressed (Shimizu et al., 2001). Even being detected both forms of GATA-1 in mouse embryonic tissue, their relative proportions vary during development, suggesting that the transcriptional activity of GATA1 can be modulated by the relative rate of the two forms (Calligaris et al., 1995).

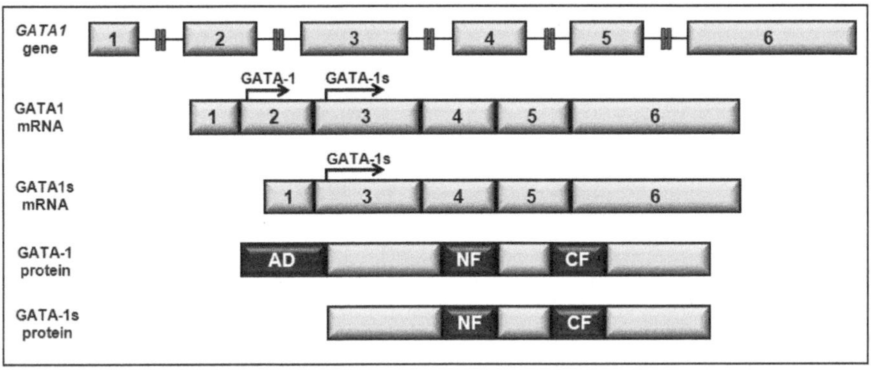

Fig. 1. Models for the expression of GATA-1 isoforms. The GATA-1 protein is translated from the GATA1 mRNA, whereas the GATA-1s protein can be translated either from the GATA-1 mRNA or from the alternative spliced GATA1s mRNA lacking exon 2.

The analysis of megakaryocyte-specific knockdown of *GATA1* in vivo has revealed a critical role for this factor in megakaryocytic development. Reduced expression (or complete absence) of GATA-1 in megakaryocytes leads to increased proliferation and deficient maturation as well as a reduced number of circulating platelets (Vyas et al., 1999; Wechsler et al., 2002). Mice harboring a heterozygous *GATA1* knockdown allele frequently develop erythroblastic leukemia (Shimizu et al., 2004).

Mutations in *GATA1* gene are described in TMD as well as in AMKL, and occur mainly in the 5′ end of the gene in exon 2, and less commonly in exon 3 (Xu et al., 2003). Mutations as insertions, duplications, deletions and point mutations, are responsible to abrogate splicing of exon 2 or to generate a stop codon prior to the alternative translational start codon at position 84. According to Rainis et al. (2003), the most frequent mutations in TMD and AMKL were deletions and insertions in exon 2 of *GATA1* corresponding to 65, 7% followed by 25.7% of point mutations and the remaining 8.6% is due to failure to identify the mutation.

Mutations in *GATA1* are frequently associated with TMD and occur in utero (Taub et al., 2004). The true frequency of TMD is unknown because it is likely that a significant proportion of these patients are not routinely diagnosed (Malinge et al., 2009; Rainis et al., 2003). Ongoing studies in Europe and North America combining screening for *GATA1* mutations and examination of neonatal blood smears will present a more precise picture of the true incidence of TMD (Malinge et al., 2009). Pine et al. (2007) examined DNA from Guthrie cards of 585 DS infants, and reported that *GATA1* mutations were detected in 3.8% of them. However, *GATA1* mutations may have been missed in patients with minor preleukemic clones, subclonal mutations, low numbers of cells on Guthrie cards, or extramedullary TMD without circulating blasts. In addition, a significant higher frequency of *GATA1* mutations in male newborns was observed. Malinge et al. (2009) presumed that it is likely that the frequency of TMD is not higher than 5% of DS newborns.

Studies have shown that *GATA1* mutations in TMD activate the proliferation of progenitor cells required to promote AMKL, featuring a multi-step disease. This process is likely to involve the participation of unidentified genes/proteins. These megakaryocytic progenitors quickly disappear after birth. Until now the molecular and cellular basis of this natural remission is unknown, but it may be related to changes in the hematopoietic microenvironment that occur during growth and neonatal development. Affected megakaryoblasts with additional genetic hits are probably subjected to clonal evolution, making them susceptible to malignant transformation to leukemic cells, leading to the development of AMKL (Shimizu et al., 2008) (figure 2).

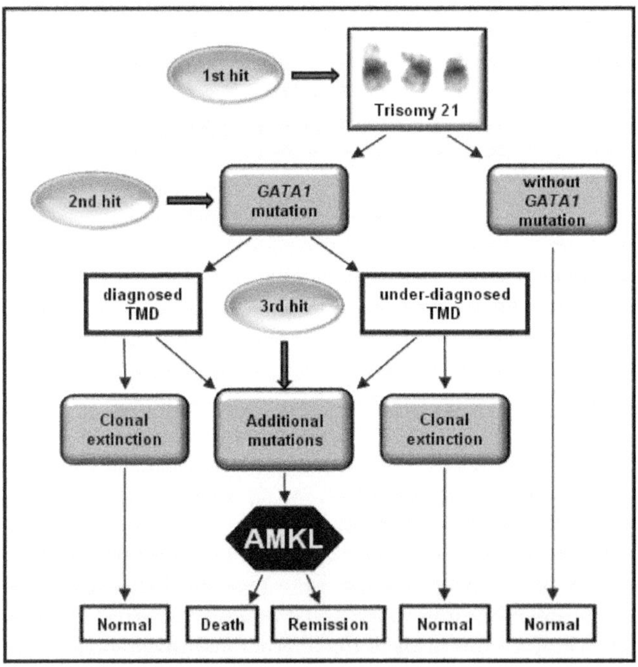

Fig. 2. A model for multi-step leukemogenesis in DS. The accumulation of hits (multiple genetic abnormalities) characterizes the evolution of TMD for AMKL.

Somatic mutations in the N-terminus activation domain of *GATA1* are found in most cases of TMD and AMKL, suggesting these mutations have a significant role in the process of leukemogenesis (Wechsler et al., 2002). *GATA1* mutations with trisomy 21 may be sufficient to promote the expansion of transient megakaryoblasts seen in TMD (Mundschau et al., 2003).

The expression levels of GATA-1 isoforms are crucial for the proper development of erythroid and megakaryocytic cells and compromised GATA-1 expression is a causal factor in leukemia (Shimizu et al., 2008). These findings strongly suggest that the qualitative deficit of GATA-1 contributes to the genesis of TMD and AMKL (Kanezaki et al., 2010). The selection of mutations that retain GATA-1s may result in disruption of normal balance between GATA-1 and GATA-1s, which probably would be involved in regulating normal development of megakaryocytes (Izraeli et al., 2007), but pass to act as an oncogene directly in the presence of trisomy 21. Alternatively, GATA-1s may be required for survival of leukemic blasts and the oncogenic effect may be purchased by the loss of the heavy chain of GATA-1. Another possibility is that this type of mutation may reflect specific mechanisms of selection or generation of this mutation in the presence of trisomy 21 (Rainis et al., 2003).
According some evidences the arising of AL is due to the cooperation between one class of mutations which interferes with differentiation (class II mutations) and another class which confers a proliferative advantage to cells (class I mutations) (Deguchi & Gilliland, 2002). It has been shown that high level expression of exogenous GATA-1 lacking the N-terminus induced differentiation rather than decreased the aberrant growth of GATA1-null megakaryocytes (Kuhl et al., 2005; Muntean & Crispino, 2005). This observation suggested that abundant GATA-1s functions like a class I mutation in TMD blasts. In contrast, reducing GATA-1 expression leads to differentiation arrest and aberrant growth of megakaryocytic cells (Vyas et al., 1999). The present data suggest that GATA-1s is expressed at very low levels in TMD blasts with GATA-1s low mutations. These levels may not be sufficient to provoke normal maturation. Together, these findings suggest that the low expression of GATA-1s might function like class II mutations in TMD blasts. Additional class I mutations or epigenetic alterations might be more effective in the development of leukemia in blast cells expressing GATA-1s at low levels (Kanezaki et al., 2010).
GATA1 mutations have not been identified in normal children, in children with DS and other types of leukemia, or in acute myeloid leukemias (AML) of children without DS. Mutations restricted to leukemic clones were not detectable in samples in remission. They were therefore selected and acquired, probably because they granted a clonal advantage (Pine et al., 2007; Wechsler et al., 2002).
Rainis et al. (2003) reported two patients with identical *GATA1* mutations in TL and subsequently in AMKL, showing that the AMKL was originated from the clone of TMD. Thus, *GATA1* is mutated in most patients with TMD, but that is not enough to generate leukemia after remission. Moreover, it has been reported that monozygotic twins that developed AMKL associated with acquired trisomy of chromosome 21 in blast cells have the same mutation that was not detected during remission. Because it was an identical mutation in the leukemic cells of twins, so it is likely that the mutation has occurred in one twin in utero and that his pre-leukemic cells have migrated to the other twin by blood embryological anastomoses.
Wechsler et al. (2002) analyzed the X chromosome inactivation in cell lysates from BM of women carrier from AMKL. Since the female leukemic cells showed the X chromosome inactivation due to monoclonality, and the mutant allele was detected only in leukemic cells, they predicted that the wild-type allele should be on the inactive X chromosome. As expected, only the truncated protein GATA-1s was observed. On the other hand Rainis et al. (2003) proposed that if there was no process of X chromosome inactivation, *GATA1* mutation would be involved in a higher frequency of patients with DS and TMD. Therefore, this inactivation of the *GATA1* mutation is considered a key event for non-occurrence of the TMD transformation to AMKL (Rainis et al., 2003).

Ahmed et al. (2004) described for the first time multiple independent *GATA1* mutations in four of 12 patients that developed AMKL, showing multiple *GATA1* mutant clones in the same individual. In these patients, analysis of mutant clones by automated sequencing allowed to confirm that each clone contained a different mutation in *GATA1.* Interestingly, at the diagnosis of AMKL only one of the three mutations was present. The presence of these multiple *GATA1* mutations suggests that mutations are a frequent event in hematopoietic cells of DS children. Using cell surface markers, Groet et al. (2005) showed the presence of several independent clonal expansions in different stages of megakaryocytic differentiation in a single patient with TMD. Probably this was due to independent clones that acquired the respective mutations in different stages of differentiation.

GATA-1s is no different from wild type in their ability to bind to DNA and interact with its co-factor friend of GATA-1 (FOG-1), but shows a reduction in their ability to transcriptional activation since it was truncated to its activation domain N-terminal (Rainis et al., 2003; Wechsler et al., 2002).

FOG-1 binds specifically to the NF zinc finger motif of GATA-1, and is expressed abundantly in erythroid and megakaryocytic cells (Crispino et al., 1999). FOG-1 is encoded by the gene *ZPFM1* as a protein of 998 amino acids which contains nine zinc finger motifs, four of them (ZFS 1, 5, 6 and 9) mediate the interaction with GATA-1 (Fox et al., 1999; Muntean & Crispino, 2005). Studies using point mutations in *GATA1* lead to a protein with a remarkable reduction of the affinity to FOG-1, but with ability of DNA binding, demonstrating that direct interaction FOG-1 and GATA-1 is required for normal erythropoiesis in vitro (Crispino et al., 1999).

A missense mutation in the *GATA1* gene was described in members without DS of a family affected with congenital dyserythropoietic anemia and thrombocytopenia. The megakaryocytes of these patients had similar changes in the megakaryocytes of mice deficient in expression of *GATA-1* suggesting that the interaction GATA-1/FOG-1 is also crucial in late stages of megakaryopoiesis (Nichols et al., 2000).

4. Other mutations associated with DS leukemia

The occurrence of mutations in exon 2 of *GATA1* in TMD suggests that there is cooperation between increased dosage of the gene or genes on chromosome 21 with the initiation of prenatal clonal proliferation of megakaryocytic precursors (Malinge et al., 2009).

Based on numerous studies with mutations in *GATA1* by several research groups, Malinge et al. (2009) concluded that the TMD and AMKL require both trisomy 21 and *GATA1* mutation but is not clear if only these alterations are enough to promote the TMD. Furthermore, the specific secondary mutations that promote the evolution of TMD to AMKL are still unknown. It has been identified cooperating mutations including *JAK3, TP53, FLT3* and *JAK2* mutations whose frequencies are shown in table 1 (Malinge et al., 2009).

The identification of activating mutations in tyrosine kinase genes in TMD and AMKL specimens has provided new insights into the evolution of AMKL. *JAK3* mutations have been detected in a small but significant fraction of DS-leukemia samples. Among the mutations found, most were considered as gain of function. JAK3 was also found in the CMK cell line (cells that do not express GATA-1 wild type and are removed from patients with AMKL) inducing a lethal biphenotypic hematopoietic disorder in mice with features of AMKL (Walters et al., 2006). Other mutations in *JAK3* have been proposed to be loss of function (De Vita et al., 2007). Additional experiments are necessary to determine how these different *JAK3* variants affect hematopoiesis and megakaryocyte development (Malinge et al., 2009).

Types of leukemia	Mutated gene	Localization	Frequencies recorded
TMD	*GATA1*	Xp11.23	97,3%
	JAK3	19p13.1	12,5%
	TP53	17p13.1	7,7%
AMKL	*GATA1*	Xp11.23	89,2%
	JAK3	19p13.1	13,2%
	FLT3	13q12.2	5,7%
	TP53	17p13.1	21,4%
	JAK2	9p24.1	6,2%

Table 1. Genetic abnormalities identified in leukemia associated SD.

5. Trisomy 21 influence on hematopoiesis

The functional contribution of the trisomy 21 in hematologic malignancies is supported by several observations such as the high incidence of leukemia in DS patients, the fact that TMD and AMKL blasts present trisomy 21 (even in children without DS), and that acquired trisomy or tetrasomy of chromosome 21 is frequently observed in blasts of different types of leukemia, including hyperdiploid ALL and de novo AML (Vyas & Crispino, 2007).

It is assumed that the cells of DS complete or partial trisomy of Hsa21, approximately 33.7 Mb, promote an overexpression of at least one of the 364 known genes, 31 antisense transcripts, and five different miRNAs (miR-99a, let-7c, miR-155, miR-125b-2, and miR-802), which could cooperate with the loss of GATA-1 in the pathogenesis of AMKL. Mutations in several genes on chromosome 21 have been identified in leukemia, and many of them recognized as encoding transcription factors acting at various stages of hematopoiesis. There should be contribution of genes present on chromosome 21 that cooperate with mutations of the *GATA1* to cause leukemogenesis (Look, 2002; Malinge et al., 2009).

The identification of the Down Syndrome Critical Region (DSCR) on the 21q22 band based in the genotype-phenotype correlations of partial trisomy in children suspected of having DS disclosed a list of genes potentially implicated in the clinical phenotype. However no specific genes have been certainly linked to the increased incidence of leukemia in DS. Few strong candidates include *ERG, ETS2,* and *RUNX1* (Lyle et al., 2009; Malinge et al., 2009).

Since the TMD is originated in a fetal liver progenitor and is restricted to children with DS (or to rare cases of acquired trisomy 21), it is presumed that trisomy 21 directly affects the development of hematopoietic cells during gestation. It has been shown that *GATA1* mutations can appear in 21-week-old embryos (Taub et al., 2004). To define the cellular context in which *GATA1* mutations occur, two groups studied hematopoiesis in trisomy 21 human fetal livers (FLs) (Chou et al., 2008; Tunstall-Pedoe et al., 2008). They found that although trisomy 21 did not alter the proportion of CD34+ and CD38- cells, trisomy 21 FLs showed a 2 to 3 fold increase of megakaryocyte erythroid progenitors (MEPs), which appeared to increase over time (35% at 16 weeks to 65% at 18 weeks).

The functional perturbations induced by trisomy 21 probably induce a highly susceptible cellular environment to additional transformations such as *GATA1* mutagenesis in TMD. The FL cell-based assay is a powerful tool to determine the specific Hsa21 genes that participate in TMD. Preliminary quantitative reverse transcription-polymerase chain reaction (qRT-PCR) studies have shown that there are no significant differences in expression of *ERG, ETS2, RUNX1,* and *SON,* top-ranked candidate leukemia oncogenes, in trisomic versus euploid FLs (Chou et al., 2008; Tunstall-Pedoe et al., 2008). However, functional studies, such as knockdown of one or more of these candidates genes in FL progenitors followed by colony assays and transplantation experiments, are necessary to determine the requirements for these genes in leukemia (Malinge et al., 2009).

6. Specific chromosome 21 genes in DS-associated leukemia

Two microarray studies comparing AMKL versus non-DS AML have recently been reported (Bourquin et al., 2006; Ge et al., 2006) and 76 genes were described that discriminate between DS AMKL and non-DS. For example, genes encoding erythroid markers, glycophorin A and CD36, were found meaningly overexpressed in AMKL, as confirmed by immunophenotypic analysis of blasts (Langebrake et al., 2005).

Analysis of the gene expression data also revealed that there is an overall increase in expression of chromosome 21 genes in AMKL, relative to non-DS AMKL. By gene set enrichment analysis, 47 Hsa21 genes, including *BACH1, SON, C21orf66,* and *GABPA,* contributed for this observed enrichment score, but the distinction between the 2 types of AMKL was not driven by differences in expression of chromosome 21 genes (Bourquin et al., 2006). By qRT-PCR and microarray analyses, Ge et al. (2006) found that 7 of 551 genes were up or down-regulated in AMKL relative to non-DS AMKL and not encoded by chromosome 21, including *BST2, DUSP6, KRT18,* and *CD36.* Differences in these two data might be explained by differences in the samples or different protocols and methods used to analyse the expression of the genes.

6.1 Candidate leukemia oncogenes encoded by chromosome 21

Of the genes on chromosome 21, several are compelling candidate leukemia oncogenes. Of these, four such candidates are *RUNX1* (AML1), which encodes the heterodimeric partner of the complex of transcription factors denominated core-binding factor β (CBFβ), cooperates with GATA-1 during megakaryocytic differentiation, and the three ETS transcription factors, which are expressed and functionally involved in megakaryocytic differentiation and sensitivity to chemotherapy (*ERG, ETS2,* and *GABPA*) (Ge et al., 2008). It has been suggested that *RUNX1* is involved in the AMKL, since mutations in the DNA-binding domain of *RUNX1* was identified in 5% of sporadic leukemia and in myeloid malignancies with acquired trisomy 21 (Osato et al., 1999; Preudhomme et al., 2000). However, despite of the loss-of-function mutations in *RUNX1* are associated with leukemia, it is not known how three copies of the chromosome 21 would promote tumorigenesis in DS (Izraeli, 2004). It is possible that cells with trisomy 21 express different levels of *RUNX1* isoforms, affecting tumor development (Levanon & Groner, 2004). Despite of the fact that the total level of RUNX1 expression was lower in AMKL compared with non-DS AML, the differential expression of RUNX1 isoforms was indeed observed in human AMKL samples (Bourquin et al., 2006). In contrast, trisomy for *Runx1* was found not to be required for the development of myeloproliferative disorder (MPD) in Ts65Dn mice (model used with partial trisomy 21) (Kirsammer et al., 2008). Furthermore, the Ts16 fetuses hematopoietic phenotype was not related with an increased ratio of *Runx1* or an altered expression of its isoforms (Gjertson et al., 1999).

Inherited hypomorphic mutations in *Runx1* cause low levels of expression in hematopoietic stem cells and result in the syndrome of thrombocytopenia with familial susceptibility to leukemia. Abnormalities in *Runx1* were not detected in AMKL (Rainis et al., 2003).

In different types of cancer, it has been shown that the *ERG* proto-oncogene is dysregulated, and its overexpression in AML samples with normal or complex karyotypes involving Hsa21 was observed (Baldus et al., 2004; Marcucci et al., 2005). An overexpression of *ERG* in human K562 cells that express both forms of GATA1 induced a switch in differentiation toward the megakaryocytic lineage and showed an increased expression of the early megakaryocytic markers, as CD41 and CD61 (Rainis et al., 2005). To confirm a role of ERG in late stages of megakaryopoiesis, Loughran et al. (2008), working with homozygous and heterozygous of mutant *Erg* mice, observed that the first one died in utero, in consequence of a defect in definitive hematopoiesis, and the second one showed thrombocytopenia with normal number of BM megakaryocytes.

Overexpression of *ETS2* has also been shown in several cancers, including AML (Baldus et al., 2004), and the amount of *ETS2* transcripts are increased in both AMKL (DS or non-DS) (Ge et al., 2008). These facts and its involvement in the regulation of megakaryocytic genes suggest that *ETS2* has an important role in TMD or AMKL. As same as for *ERG*, *ETS2* overexpression in K562 cells was found to promote a switch in differentiation from erythroid to megakaryocytic fate (Ge et al., 2008).

The ETS family member *GABPA* is not considered an oncogene and its expression in the megakyocyte suggests that the GABPA protein has a role in early stages of megakaryocytic maturation (Pang et al., 2006). Recent studies have shown that GABPA directly affects the cell cycle by regulating the expression of genes required of DNA synthesis and degradation of cell-cycle inhibitors (Yang et al., 2007). Of Hsa21 genes, *GABPA* was one of the few whose expression is elevated in AMKL versus non-DS AML (Bourquin et al., 2006).

6.2 miRNAs encoded by chromosome 21

Hsa21 encode five miRNAs and overexpression of some of these has been observed in brain and heart tissues of people with DS and has been implicated in normal and pathologic hematopoiesis (Kuhn et al., 2008). For example, miR-99a is up-regulated during megakaryocytic differentiation of CD34+ cells, whereas miR-155 and let-7c are down-regulated (Garzon et al., 2006). Notably, miR-155 has been linked to myeloproliferative and B-lymphoproliferative disorders (Garzon & Croce 2008; O'Connell et al., 2008). Studies have implicated miR-125b-2, which is overexpressed in TMD and AMKL samples compared with normal megakaryocytes, in the megakaryocytic leukemia of DS (Klusmann, 2007).

Klusmann et al. (2010) showed that miR-125b-2 is an oncogene potentially involved in the pathogenesis of trisomy 21-associated leukemia. They demonstrated in mice and human that overexpression of miR-125b-2 led to specific hyperproliferation and enhanced self-renewal capacity of megakaryocytic progenitor (MPs) and megakaryocytic/erythroid progenitors (MEPs), without affecting their normal differentiation. The miR-125b was highly expressed in AMKL blasts, whereas the identified target genes of miR-125b were down-regulated. Thus, miR-125b-2 has a role in regulating megakaryopoiesis and in the pathogenesis of trisomy 21-associated TMD and AMKL, in cooperation with GATA1s. The miR-125b-2 exerts its oncogenic potential by at least two different mechanisms: blocking post-transcriptional miRNA processing through repression of *DICER1* expression, and by inhibiting tumor suppressor genes, such as *ST18*.

7. Methods of leukemia diagnosis in DS

The diagnosis of TMD usually occurs during the first weeks after birth and is observed as hydrops fetalis. The elevated blood count associated with hepatomegaly is the common symptom in an asymptomatic neonate. Infants with TMD can also display occasionally jaundice and bleeding diatheses, respiratory distress coupled with ascites, pleural effusion, signs of heart failure, and skin infiltrates. There is megakaryocytic infiltration and liver fibrosis, likely caused by excess cytokines secreted from the megakaryoblasts. The full clinical TMD may develop only at the second or third week of life. Laboratory tests are significant for either thrombocytosis or thrombocytopenia accompanied by elevated leukocytes with excess of blasts. The blood smear may show nucleated red cells, giant platelets and megakaryocytic fragments, and, most significantly, typical deeply basophilic blasts with blebs characteristic to megakaryocytic blasts. The differential diagnosis includes leukoerythroblastic reaction associated with prematurity, sepsis, or asphyxia. However, the blasts of TMD usually persist for several weeks, and *GATA1* mutations are invariably found (Malinge et al., 2009).

AMKL is preceded in 20 to 60% of cases by an indolent prephase of myelodysplasia (MDS), characterized by thrombocytopenia and dysplastic changes, BM aspiration is often dry, and fibrosis is detected in BM biopsy (Creutzig et al., 1996; Lange et al., 1998). This MDS can last several months or years before progressing to leukemia. In contrast to MDS in non-DS children, which requires stem-cell transplantation for cure, MDS in children with DS present a highly favorable response to chemotherapy alone (Lange et al., 1998). Therefore, Hasle et al. (2003) suggested that all cases of MDS and overt myeloid leukemia in DS, children should be classified as one disease entity, and referred to as "acute myeloid leukemia of Down syndrome" or ML DS. As this is a unique disease, it should be classified separately from other cases of AML in the WHO-classification.

Immunophenotyping characterizes the hematopoietic lineage involved and their degree of maturation by monoclonal antibodies labeled with fluorochromes. Flow cytometry reveals that blasts are positive for CD34, CD33, CD41, CD61, glycophorin A, and often CD7 and CD36 (Langebrake et al., 2005, Massey et al., 2006). Savasan & Ravindranath (2003) observed that blasts of DS children with AMKL express CD36, in contrast to the low or no expression of CD36 in AML without DS. If 25% of blast cells are not detected, the diagnosis of AMKL can be given by the megakaryocytic markers CD41, CD61 and CD42a. The immunophenotype of the blasts in AMKL is generally similar to TMD, except that the percentage of CD34 cells may be lower in AMKL (Langebrake, 2005; Malinge et al., 2009).

Pine et al. (2005) demonstrate the possibility of using specific *GATA1* mutations already identified in the diagnosis of TMD or AMKL to monitor the size of the clone of leukemic cells over time with a sensitivity level (10^{-4} to 10^{-5}) beyond the microscopic detection. The study confirmed that *GATA1* mutations in TMD and AMKL can be used as clonal markers were suitable for measurement of minimal residual disease (MRD).

This approach serves as a valuable tool in monitoring the spontaneous remission of TMD and in assessing response to treatment of AMKL subcytologic level. In addition, the MRD based GATA-1s mutations has been much in demand as a prognostic parameter for newborns with TMD. One may speculate, for example, that every group of newborns showing apparent remission of TMD can be divided into two subgroups: one in which the size of the clone of blasts in TMD after morphological remission continues to decline to become undetectable versus a second group, in which a clone of blasts in the TMD remains detectable submicroscopic level. It is interesting to correlate these patterns of MRD kinetics in TMD with the probability of developing AMKL later (Hitzler & Zipursky, 2005).

Additional copies of chromosome 8 and 21 in addition to the constitutional trisomy 21 are the most frequent in AMKL, and are found in approximately 10 to 15% for each chromosome. Cytogenetic findings associated with a high rate of relapse in non-DS AML, such as monosomy 7 and deletion 5/5q- also occur in DS patients but do not seem to have a negative impact on prognosis in the rare cases (Gamis et al., 2003, 2005; Rainis et al., 2003).

The approach of molecular techniques including: PCR amplification of *GATA1* exons 2 and 3, followed by direct sequencing or analysis by denaturing high performance liquid chromatography (DHPLC), and cloning allow greater sensitivity and specificity of detection and have become essential for the identification of gene alterations in leukemias. The ability to detect mutations depends on the proportion of mutant cells in the sample. In general, for direct sequencing, approximately 20% of the sample has to have mutant cells. The sensitivity of DHPLC is higher at around 2 to 5%. Once a mutation has been identified, mutation-specific probes and primers for mutation detection by qRT-PCR can be designed that allow for more sensitive detection of mutant cells, which may be used for MRD detection (Pine et al., 2005).

Until recently, there were no reports on the expression levels of GATA-1s in TAM blasts, and the risk factors for the progression to AMKL. In 2010, Kanezaki et al. tested whether the spectrum of transcripts derived from the mutant *GATA1* genes affects the expression levels. They classified the mutations according to the types of transcripts, and investigated the modalities of expression by in vitro transfection experiments using GATA-1 expression constructs harboring mutations. They have shown that the mutations altered the amount of mutant protein. Based on the evaluation of GATA-1s expression, the mutations were classified into two groups: high and low GATA-1s expression. Phenotypic analyses of 66 TMD patients with *GATA1* mutations revealed that GATA-1s low expression mutations were significantly associated with a high risk of progression to AMKL and lower counts of both WBC and blast cells. These results suggest that quantitative differences in mutant protein levels have significant effects on the phenotype of TMD.

Nevertheless, neither mice nor humans with germline mutations expressing GATA-1s develop TMD or AMKL without trisomy 21 (Hollanda et al., 2006; Li et al., 2005). Therefore, the role of the trisomy 21 in the cellular transformation in AMKL seems to be fundamental (Klusmann et al., 2010). It remains unknown which factors on chromosome 21 cooperate with the oncogenic GATA-1s and which factors are involved in this transition from preleukemia to AMKL in only a part of these children (Kanezaki et al., 2010; Klusmann et al., 2007; Langebrake et al., 2006; Malinge et al., 2009).

8. Treatment outcome

DS children with AMKL have an excellent prognostic, with an approximately 80% cure rate, in relation to children without DS who develop AML (Arico et al.; 2008; Creutzig et al., 2005; Gamis et al., 2003; Rao et al., 2006; Taub et al., 1996). This outcome is possible on contemporary AML protocols which based in reducing treatment intensity regimens has considerably reduced the mortality rates in children with DS (Creutzig et al., 2005; Gamis et al., 2003; Whitlock et al., 2005; Zeller et al., 2005).

AMKL blasts have shown hypersensitivity to varied chemotherapeutic drugs (Zwaan et al., 2002). Probably the hypersensibility of the blasts to cytarabine (ARA-C) is due of the effect

of *GATA1* mutations and Hsa21 on the levels of cytarabine-metabolizing enzymes (Ge et al., 2005). ARA-C sensitivity is restricted to the leukemic population and may be caused by increased expression levels of the cystathionine-beta-synthase gene, which is located on Hsa21 (Taub et al., 2000). Despite of many patients respond favorably to a simple regimen including low-dose of ARA-C, this is not currently the standard of care. Since many problems have been occurred in treating of AMKL like toxic deaths, infections, and cardiac toxicity, thereby new and less-intensive protocols have been initiated in the United States and Europe (Creutzig et al., 2005; International Cooperative Pediatric AML Study Group Myeloid Leukemia DS 2006 [European Clinical Trials Database (EUDRACT) no. 2007-006219-22]; Children's Oncology Group: The Treatment of Down Syndrome Children with AML and MDS under the age of 4 Years [COG-AAML0431]; low dose cytarabine in treating infants with DS and TMD [COG-AAML0532]).
Researchs in prospective clinical trials are trying to demonstrate whether treatment of TMD by low-dose cytarabine could prevent the arise of AMKL. Another related question to be clarified is whether treatment of clinically silent disease, identified by molecular detection of *GATA1* mutations in patients who recovered from TMD, can prevent the future development of AMKL (Malinge et al., 2009).

9. Conclusion

In conclusion, many questions remain unanswered concerning the factors that contribute to the progression of TMD and AMKL in DS-patients. Progress in research to unravel these questions will improve diagnosis and treatment. Furthermore, ensuring the diagnosis of *GATA1* mutations to the DS child to monitor the progression of the disease is essential to enable better clinical decision for the treatment regimen and, consequently, better quality of life to the patients.

10. Acknowledgments

Review supported by CAPES – Project CEP-FM 34/2008 and SES-DF 339/08.

11. References

Ahmed, M.; Sternberg, A.; Hall, G.; Thomas, A.; Smith, O.; O'marcaigh, A.; Wynn, R.; Stevens, R.; Addison, M.; King, D.; Stewart, B.; Gibson, B.; Roberts, I.; Vyas, P. (2004). Natural history of GATA1 mutations in Down syndrome. *Blood*, Vol.103, No.7, pp.2480-2489, ISSN 0006-4971

Arico, M.; Ziino, O.; Valsecchi, M.G.; et al. (2008). Acute lymphoblastic leukemia and Down syndrome: presenting features and treatment outcome in the experience of the Italian Association of Pediatric Hematology and Oncology (AIEOP). *Cancer*, Vol.113, No.3, pp.515-521, ISSN 0008-543X

Baldus, C.D.; Liyanarachchi, S.; Mrozek, K.; et al. (2004). Acute myeloid leukemia with complex karyotypes and abnormal chromosome 21: amplification discloses overexpression of APP, ETS2, and ERG genes. *Proceedings of the National Academy of Sciences of the United States of America*, Vol.101, No.11, pp.3915-3920, ISSN 0027-8424

Bourquin, J.P.; Subramanian, A.; Langebrake, C.; et al. (2006). Identification of distinct molecular phenotypes in acute megakaryoblastic leukemia by gene expression profiling. *Proceedings of the National Academy of Sciences of the United States of America,* Vol.103, No.9, pp.3339-3344, ISSN 0027-8424

Calligaris, R.; Bottardi, S.; Cogoi, S.; Apezteguia, I.;Santoro, C. (1995). Alternative translation initiation site usage results in two functionally distinct forms of the GATA-1 transcription factor. *Proceedings of the National Academy of Sciences of the United States of America,* Vol.92, No.25, pp.11598-11602, ISSN 0027-8424

Chou, S.T.; Opalinska, J.B.; Yao, Y. et al. (2008). Trisomy 21 enhances human fetal erythro-megakaryocytic development. *Blood,* Vol.112, No.12, pp.4503-4506, ISSN 0006-4971

Creutzig, U.; Ritter, J.; Vormoor, J.; et al. (1996). Myelodysplasia and acute myelogenous leukemia in Down's syndrome. A report of 40 children of the AML-BFM Study Group. *Leukemia,* Vol.10, No.11, pp.1677–1686, ISSN 0887-6924

Creutzig, U.; Reinhardt, D.; Diekamp, S.; Dworzak, M.; Stary, J.; Zimmermann, M. (2005). AML patients with Down syndrome have a high cure rate with AML-BFM therapy with reduced dose intensity. *Leukemia,* Vol.19, No.8, pp.1355-1360, ISSN 0887-6924

Crispino, J.D.; Lodish, M.B.; Mackay, J.P.; Orkin, S.H. (1999). Use of altered specificity mutants to probe a specific protein-protein interaction in differentiation: the GATA-1: FOG complex. *Molecular Cell,* Vol.3, No.2, pp.219-228, ISSN 1097-2765

De Vita, S.; Mulligan, C.; McElwaine, S.; et al. (2007). Loss-of-function JAK3 mutations in TMD and AMKL of Down syndrome. *British Journal of Haematology,* Vol.137, No.4, pp.337-341, ISSN 00071048

Deguchi, K., Gilliland, D.G. (2002). Cooperativity between mutations in tyrosine kinases and in hematopoietic transcription factors in AML. *Leukemia,* Vol.16, No.4, pp.740-744, ISSN 0887-6924

Fox, A.H.; Liew, C.; Holmes, M.; Kowalski, K.; Mackay, J.; Crossley, M. (1999). Transcriptional cofactors of the FOG family interact with GATA proteins by means of multiple zinc fingers. *The EMBO Journal,* Vol.18, No.10, pp.2812-2822, ISSN 0261-4189

Gamis, A.S.; Woods, W.G.; Alonzo, T.A.; et al. (2003). Increased age at diagnosis has a significantly negative effect on outcome in children with Down syndrome and acute myeloid leukemia: a report from the Children's Cancer Group Study 2891. *Journal of Clinical Oncology,* Vol.21, No.18, pp.3415–3422, ISSN 0732-183X

Gamis, A.S. (2005). Acute myeloid leukemia and Down syndrome evolution of modern therapy—state of the art review. *Pediatric Blood & Cancer,* Vol.44, No.1, pp.13–20, ISSN 1545-5009

Garzon, R.; Pichiorri, F.; Palumbo, T.; et al. (2006). MicroRNA fingerprints during human megakaryocytopoiesis. *Proceedings of the National Academy of Sciences of the United States of America,* Vol.103, No.13, pp.5078-5083, ISSN 0027-8424

Garzon, R., Croce, C.M. (2008). MicroRNAs in normal and malignant hematopoiesis. *Current Opinion in Hematology,* Vol.15, No.4, pp.352-358, ISSN 1065-6251

Ge, Y.; Stout, M.L.; Tatman, D.A.; et al. (2005). GATA1, cytidine deaminase, and the high cure rate of Down syndrome children with acute megakaryocytic leukemia. *Journal of the National Cancer Institute,* Vol.97, No.3, pp.226-231, ISSN 0027-8874

Ge, Y.; Dombkowski, A.A.; LaFiura, K.M.; et al. (2006). Differential gene expression, GATA1 target genes, and the chemotherapy sensitivity of Down syndrome megakaryocytic leukemia. *Blood,* Vol.107, pp.1570-1581, ISSN 0006-4971

Ge, Y.; LaFiura, K.M.; Dombkowski, A.A.; et al. (2008). The role of the proto-oncogene ETS2 in acute megakaryocytic leukemia biology and therapy. *Leukemia*, Vol.22, No.3, pp.521-529, ISSN 0887-6924

Gjertson, C.; Sturm, K.S.; Berger, C.N. (1999). Hematopoietic deficiencies and core binding factor expression in murine Ts16, an animal model for Down syndrome. *Clinical Immunology*, Vol.91, No.1, pp.50-60, ISSN 1744-666X

Groet, J.; Mulligan, C.; Spinelli, M.; Serra, A.; Mcelwaine, S.; Cotter, F.E.; Dagna-Bricarelli, F.; Saglio, G.; Basso, G.; Nizetic, D. (2005). Independent clones at separable stages of differentiation, bearing different GATA1 mutations, in the same TMD patient with Down syndrome. *Blood*, Vol.106, No.5, pp.1887-1888, ISSN 0006-4971

Hasle, H. (2001). Pattern of malignant disorders in individuals with Down's syndrome. *Lancet Oncology*, Vol.2, No.7, pp.429-436, ISSN 1470-2045

Hasle, H.; Niemeyer, C.M.; Chessells, J.M.; et al. (2003). A pediatric approach to the WHO classification of myelodysplastic and myeloproliferative diseases. *Leukemia*, Vol.17, No.2, pp.277–282, ISSN 0887-6924

Hitzler, J.K.; Cheung, J.; Li, Y.; Scherer, S.W.; Zipursky, A. (2003). GATA1 mutations in transient leukemia and acute megakaryoblastic leukemia of Down syndrome. *Blood*, Vol.101, No.11, pp.4301-4304, ISSN 0006-4971

Hitzler, J.& Zipursky, A. (2005). GATA 1 mutations as clonal markers of minimal residual disease in acute megakaryoblastic leukemia of Down syndrome--a new tool with significant potential applications. Leukemia Research, Vol.29, No.11, pp.1353-1356, ISSN 0145-2126

Hollanda, L.M.; Lima, C.S.; Cunha, A.F.; Albuquerque, D.M.; Vassallo, J.; Ozelo, M.C.; Joazeiro, P.P.; Saad, S.T.; Costa, F.F. (2006) An inherited mutation leading to production of only the short isoform of GATA-1 is associated with impaired erythropoiesis. *Nature Genetics*, Vol.38, No.7, pp.807–812, ISSN 1061-4036

Holt, S.E.; Brown, E.J.; Zipursky, A. (2002). Telomerase and the benign and malignant megakaryoblastic leukemias of Down syndrome. *Journal of Pediatric Hematology/Oncology*, Vol.24, No.1, pp.14-17, ISSN 0192-8562

Issacs, H. (2003). Fetal and neonatal leukemia. *Journal of Pediatric Hematology/Oncology*, Vol.25, No.5, pp.348-361, ISSN 0192-8562

Izraeli, S. (2004). Leukemia: a developmental perspective. *British Journal of Haematology*, Vol.126, No.1, pp.3-10, ISSN 00071048

Izraeli, S.; Rainis, L.; Hertzberg, L.; Smooha, G.; Birger, Y. (2007). Trisomy of chromosome 21 in leukemogenesis. *Blood Cells Molecules and Diseases*, Vol.39, No.2, pp.156-159, ISSN 1079- 9796

Kanezaki, R.; Toki, T.; Terui, K.; Xu, G.; Wang, R.; Shimada, A.; Hama, A.; Kanegane, H.; Kawakami, K.; Endo, M.; Hasegawa, D.; Kogawa, K.; Adachi, S.; Ikeda, Y.; Iwamoto, S; Taga, T.; Kosaka, Y.; Kojima, S.; Hayashi, Y.; Ito, E. (2010). Down syndrome and GATA1 mutations in transient abnormal myeloproliferative disorder: mutation classes correlate with progression to myeloid leukemia. *Blood*, Vol.116, No.22, pp.4631-4638, ISSN 0006-4971

Kirsammer, G.; Jilani, S.; Liu, H.; et al. (2008). Highly penetrant myeloproliferative disease in the Ts65Dn mouse model of Down syndrome. *Blood*, Vol.111, No.2, pp.767-775, ISSN 0006-4971

Klusmann, J.H.; Reinhardt, D.; Hasle, H.; et al. (2007). Janus kinase mutations in the development of acute megakaryoblastic leukemia in children with and without Down's syndrome. *Leukemia,* Vol.21, No.7, pp.1584-1587, ISSN 0887-6924

Klusmann, J.H.; Creutzig, U.; Zimmermann, M.; et al. (2008). Treatment and prognostic impact of transient leukemia in neonates with Down syndrome. *Blood,* Vol.111, No.6, pp.2991-2998, ISSN 0006-4971

Klusmann, J.H.; Li, Z.; Böhmer, K.; Maroz, A.; Koch, M.L.; Emmrich, S.; Godinho, F.J.; Orkin, S.H.; Reinhardt, D. (2010). miR-125b-2 is a potential oncomiR on human chromosome 21 in megakaryoblastic leukemia. *Genes & Development,* Vol.24, No.5, pp.478-490, ISSN 0890-9369

Kuhl, C.; Atzberger, A.; Iborra, F.; Nieswandt, B.; Porcher, C.; Vyas, P. (2005). GATA1-mediated megakaryocyte differentiation and growth control can be uncoupled and mapped to different domains in GATA1. *Molecular and Cellular Biology,* Vol.25, No.19, pp.8592-8606, ISSN 1098-5549

Kuhn, D.E.; Nuovo, G.J.; Martin, M.M.; et al. (2008). Human chromosome 21-derived miRNAs are overexpressed in down syndrome brains and hearts. *Biochemical and Biophysical Research Communications,* Vol.370, No.3, pp.473-477, ISSN 0006-291X

Lange, B.J.; Kobrinsky, N.; Barnard, D.R.; et al. (1998). Distinctive demography, biology, and outcome of acute myeloid leukemia and myelodysplastic syndrome in children with Down syndrome: Children's Cancer Group Studies 2861 and 2891. *Blood,* Vol.91, No.2, pp.608–615, ISSN 0006-4971

Lange, B.J. (2000). The management of neoplastic disorders of hematopoiesis in children with Down's syndrome. *British Journal of Haematology,* Vol.110, No.3, pp.512-524, ISSN 0007- 1048

Langebrake, C.; Creutzig, U.; Reinhardt, D. (2005). Immunophenotype of Down syndrome acute myeloid leukemia and transient myeloproliferative disease differs significantly from other diseases with morphologically identical or similar blasts. *Klinische Pädiatrie,* Vol.217, No.3, pp.126-134, ISSN 0300-8630

Langebrake, C.; Klusmann, J.H.; Wortmann, K.; Kolar, M.; Puhlmann, U.; Reinhardt, D. (2006). Concomitant aberrant overexpression of RUNX1 and NCAM in regenerating bone marrow of myeloid leukemia of Down's syndrome. *Haematologica,* Vol.91, No.11, pp.1473-1480, ISSN 0390-6078

Levanon, D.; Groner, Y. (2004). Structure and regulated expression of mammalian RUNX genes. *Oncogene,* Vol.23, No.24, pp.4211-4219, ISSN 0950-9232

Li, Z.; Godinho, F.J.; Klusmann, J.H.; Garriga-Canut, M.; Yu, C.; Orkin, S.H. (2005). Developmental stage-selective effect of somatically mutated leukemogenic transcription factor GATA1. *Nature Genetics,* Vol.37, No.6, pp.613–619, ISSN 1061-4036

Look, A.T. (2002). A leukemogenic twist for GATA1. *Nature Genetics,* Vol.32, No.1, pp.83-84, ISSN 1061-4036

Loughran, S.J.; Kruse, E.A.; Hacking, D.F.; et al. (2008). The transcription factor Erg is essential for definitive hematopoiesis and the function of adult hematopoietic stem cells. *Nature Immunology,* Vol.9, No.7, pp.810-819, ISSN : 1529-2908

Lyle, R.; Bena, F.; Gagos, S.; et al. (2009). Genotype-phenotype correlations in Down syndrome identified by array CGH in 30 cases of partial trisomy and partial monosomy chromosome 21. *European Journal of Human Genetics,* Vol.17, No.4, pp. 454-466, ISSN 1018-4813

Malinge, S.; Izraeli, S.; Crispino, J.D. (2009). Insights into the manifestations, outcomes, and mechanisms of leukemogenesis in Down syndrome. *Blood,* Vol.113, No.12, pp.2619-2628, ISSN 0006-4971

Malkin, D.; Brown, E.J.; Zipursky, A. (2000). The role of p53 in megakaryocytic differentiation and the megakaryocytic leukemias of Down syndrome. *Cancer Genetics and Cytogenetics,* Vol.116, No.1, pp.1-5, ISSN 0165-4608

Marcucci, G.; Baldus, C.D.; Ruppert, A.S.; et al. (2005). Overexpression of the ETS-related gene, ERG, predicts a worse outcome in acute myeloid leukemia with normal karyotype: a Cancer and Leukemia Group B study. *Journal of Clinical Oncology,* Vol.23, pp.9234-9242, ISSN 0732-183X

Martin, D.I.; Orkin, S.H. (1990). Transcriptional activation and DNA binding by the erythroid factor GF-1/NF-E1/Eryf 1. *Genes & Development,* Vol.4, No.11, pp.1886-1898, ISSN 0890-9369

Massey, G.V.; Zipursky, A.; Chang, M.N.; et al. (2006). A prospective study of the natural history of transient leukemia (TL) in neonates with Down syndrome (DS): Children's Oncology Group (COG) study POG-9481. *Blood,* Vol.107, No.12, pp.4606-4613, ISSN 0006-4971

Mundschau, G.; Gurbuxani, S.; Gamis, A.S.; Greene, M.E.; Arceci, R.J.; Crispino, J.D. (2003). Mutagenesis of GATA1 is an initiating event in Down syndrome leukemogenesis. *Blood,* Vol.101, No.11, pp.4298–4300, ISSN 0006-4971

Muntean, A.G.; Crispino, J.D. (2005). Differential requirements for the activation domain and FOG-interaction surface of GATA-1 in megakaryocyte gene expression and development. *Blood,* Vol.106, No.4, pp.1223-1231, ISSN 0006-4971

Muramatsu, H.; Kato, K.; Watanabe, N.; et al. (2008). Risk factors for early death in neonates with Down syndrome and transient leukemia. *British Journal of Haematology,* Vol.142, No.4, pp.610-615, ISSN 00071048

Nichols, K.E.; Crispino, J.D.; Poncz, M.; White, J.G.; Orkin, S.H.; Maris, J.M.; Weiss, M.J. (2000). Familial dyserythropoietic anaemia and thrombocytopenia due to an inherited mutation in GATA1. *Nature Genetics,* Vol.24, No.3, pp.266-270, ISSN 1061-4036

O'Connell, R.M.; Rao, D.S.; Chaudhuri, A.A.; et al. (2008). Sustained expression of microRNA-155 in hematopoietic stem cells causes a myeloproliferative disorder. *Journal of Experimental Medicine,* Vol.205, No.3, pp.585-594, ISSN 0022-1007

Osato, M.; Asou, N.; Abdalla, E.; et al. (1999). Biallelic and heterozygous point mutations in the runt domain of the AML1 gene associated with myeloblastic leukemias. *Blood,* Vol.93, No.6, pp.1817-1824, ISSN 0006-4971

Pang, L.; Xue, H.H.; Szalai, G.; et al. (2006). Maturation stage-specific regulation of megakaryopoiesis by pointed-domain Ets proteins. *Blood,* Vol.108, No.7, pp.2198-2206, ISSN 0006-4971

Pine, S.R.; Guo, Q.; Yin, C.; et al. (2005). GATA1 as a new target to detect minimal residual disease in both transient leukemia and megakaryoblastic leukemia of Down syndrome. *Leukemia Research,* Vol.29, No.11, pp.1353–1356, ISSN 0145-2126

Pine, S.R.; Guo, Q.; Yin, C.; Jayabose, S.; Druschel, C.M.; Sandoval, C. (2007). Incidence and clinical implications of GATA1 mutations in newborns with Down syndrome. *Blood,* Vol.110, No.6, pp.2128-2131, ISSN 0006-4971

Preudhomme, C.; Warot-Loze, D.; Roumier, C.; et al. (2000). High incidence of biallelic point mutations in the Runt domain of the AML1/PEBP2 alpha B gene in Mo acute myeloid leukemia and in myeloid malignancies with acquired trisomy 21. *Blood,* Vol.96, No.8, pp.2862-2869, ISSN 0006-4971

Rainis, L.; Bercovich, D.; Strehl, S.; et al. (2003). Mutations in exon 2 of GATA1 are early events in megakaryocytic malignancies associated with trisomy 21. *Blood,* Vol.102, No.3, pp.981-986, ISSN 0006-4971

Rainis, L.; Toki, T.; Pimanda, J.E.; et al. (2005). The protooncogene ERG in megakaryoblastic leukemias. *Cancer Research,* Vol.65, No.17, pp.7596-7602, ISSN 0008-5472

Rao, A.; Hills, R.K.; Stiller, C.; et al. (2006). Treatment for myeloid leukemia of Down syndrome: population based experience in the UK and results from the Medical Research Council AML 10 and AML 12 trials. *British Journal of Haematology,* Vol.132, No.5, pp.576-583, ISSN 00071048

Roizen, N.J.; Amarose, A.P. (1993). Hematologic abnormalities in children with Down syndrome. *American Journal of Medical Genetics,* Vol.46, No.5, pp.510-512, ISSN 1552-4868

Savasan, S.B.S.; Ravindranath, Y. (2003). Cd36 Expression Is Associated With Superior In Vitro Ara-C Sensitivity In Acute Megakaryocytic Leukemia With And Without Down Syndrome. *Medical and Pediatric Oncology,* Vol.41, No.10, pp.274-275, ISSN 1096-911X

Shimizu, R.; Takahashi, S.; Ohneda, K.; Engel, J. D.; Yamamoto, M. (2001). In vivo requirements for GATA-1 functional domains during primitive and definitive erythropoiesis. *Embo Journal,* Vol.20, No.18, pp.5250-5260.

Shimizu, R.; Kuroha, T.; Ohneda, O.; et al. (2004). Leukemogenesis caused by incapacitated GATA-1 function. *Molecular and Cellular Biology,* Vol.24, No.24, pp.10814-10825, ISSN 1098-5549

Shimizu, R.; Engel, JD, Yamamoto, M. (2008). GATA1-related leukaemias. *Nature Reviews Cancer,* Vol.8, No.4, pp.279-287, ISSN 1474-175X

Taub, J.W.; Matherly, L.H.; Stout, M.L.; Buck, S.A.; Gurney, J.G.; Ravindranath, Y. (1996). Enhanced metabolism of 1-beta-D-arabinofuranosylcytosine in Down syndrome cells: a contributing factor to the superior event free survival of Down syndrome children with acute myeloid leukemia. *Blood,* Vol.87, No.8, pp.3395-3403, ISSN 0006-4971

Taub, J.W.; Huang, X.; Ge, Y.; et al. (2000). Cystathionine-beta-synthase cDNA transfection alters the sensitivity and metabolism of 1-beta-D-arabinofuranosylcytosine in CCRF-CEM leukemia cells in vitro and in vivo: a model of leukemia in Down syndrome. *Cancer Research,* Vol.60, No.22, pp.6421–6426, ISSN 0008-5472

Taub, J.W.; Mundschau, G.; Ge, Y.; et al. (2004). Prenatal origin of GATA1 mutations may be an initiating step in the development of megakaryocytic leukemia in Down syndrome. *Blood,* Vol.104, No.5, pp.1588-1589, ISSN 0006-4971

Tunstall-Pedoe, O.; Roy, A.; Karadimitris, A.; et al. (2008). Abnormalities in the myeloid progenitor compartment in Down syndrome fetal liver precede acquisition of GATA1 mutations. *Blood,* Vol.112, No.12, pp.4507-4511, ISSN 0006-4971

Vyas, P.; Ault, K.; Jackson, C.W.; Orkin, S.H.; Shivdasani, R.A. (1999). Consequences of GATA-1 deficiency in megakaryocytes and platelets. *Blood,* Vol.93, No.9, pp.2867-2875, ISSN 0006-4971

Vyas, P.; Crispino, J.D. (2007). Molecular insights into Down syndrome-associated leukemia. *Current Opinion in Pediatrics,* Vol.19, No.1, pp.9-14, ISSN 1040-8703

Walters, D.K.; Mercher, T.; Gu, T.L.; et al. (2006). Activating alleles of JAK3 in acute megakaryoblastic leukemia. *Cancer Cell,* Vol.10, No.1, pp.65-75, ISSN 1535-6108

Wang, Z.; Burge, C.B. (2008). Splicing regulation: from a parts list of regulatory elements to an integrated splicing code. *RNA,* Vol.14, No.5, pp.802-813, ISSN 1355-8382

Wechsler, J.; Greene, M.; McDevitt, M.A.; Anastasi, J.; Karp, J.E.; Le Beau, M.M.; Crispino, J.D. (2002). Acquired mutations in GATA1 in the megakaryoblastic leukemia of Down syndrome. *Nature Genetics,* Vol.32, No.1, pp.148–152, ISSN 1061-4036

Weiss, M. J.; Yu, C.; Orkin, S. H. (1997). Erythroid-cell-specific properties of transcription factor GATA-1 revealed by phenotypic rescue of a gene-targeted cell line. *Molecular and Cellular Biology,* Vol.17, No.3, pp.1642-1651, ISSN 1098-5549

Whitlock, J.A.; Sather, H.N.; Gaynon, P.; et al. (2005). Clinical characteristics and outcome of children with Down syndrome and acute lymphoblastic leukemia: a Children's Cancer Group study. *Blood,* Vol.106, No.13, pp.4043-4049, ISSN 0006-4971

Xu, G.; Nagano, M.; Kanezaki, R.; et al. (2003). Frequent mutations in the GATA-1 gene in the transient myeloproliferative disorder of Down syndrome. *Blood,* Vol;102, No.8, pp.2960-2968, ISSN 0006-4971

Yang, Z.F.; Mott, S.; Rosmarin, A.G. (2007). The Ets transcription factor GABP is required for cell-cycle progression. *Nature Cell Biology,* Vol.9, No.3, pp.339-346, ISSN 1097 -6256

Yu, C.; Niakan, K.K.; Matsushita, M.; Stamatoyannopoulos, G. Orkin, S.H.; Raskind, W.H. (2002). X-linked thrombocytopenia with thalassemia from a mutation in the amino finger of GATA-1 affecting DNAbinding rather than FOG-1 interaction. *Blood,* Vol.100, No.6, pp.2040-2045, ISSN 0006-4971

Zeller, B.; Gustafsson, G.; Forestier, E.; et al. (2005). Acute leukaemia in children with Down syndrome: a population-based Nordic study. *British Journal of Haematology,* Vol.128, No.6, pp.797–804, ISSN 0007-1048

Zipursky, A. (2003). Transient leukemia: a benign form of leukemia in newborn infants with trisomy 21. *British Journal of Haematology,* Vol.120, No.6, pp.930-938, ISSN 0007-1048

Zwaan, C.M.; Kaspers, G.J.; Pieters, R.; et al. (2002). Different drug sensitivity profiles of acute myeloid and lymphoblastic leukemia and normal peripheral blood mononuclear cells in children with and without Down syndrome. *Blood,* Vol.99, No.1, pp.245-251, ISSN 0006-4971

Part 4

Treatment and Future Prospects

13

Hematologic Malignancies in Pregnancy

C. Vandenbriele[1], A. Vassou[2], G. Pentheroudakis[3],
K. Van Calsteren[4] and F. Amant[5]
[1]Internal medicine, University Hospitals Gasthuisberg,
[2]Hematology Department,
[3]Oncology Department, University Hospital of Ioannina, Hellas
[4]Obstetrics, University Hospitals Gasthuisberg,
[5]Leuven Cancer Institute, Gynecologic Oncology, University Hospitals Gasthuisberg,
Belgium

1. Introduction

Cancer and especially hematological cancer during pregnancy is infrequent and its management is difficult for patients and their families, but also for their physicians since two lives with different priorities have to be considered. Treatment should adhere the standard treatment for the specific type and stage of cancer. Small adaptations can be considered in order to avoid adverse effects on fetal development. This chapter reviews the available data regarding the different aspects of diagnosis and - especially chemotherapeutical - treatment of hematological cancer during pregnancy.
First we will discuss the general approach of a woman diagnosed with cancer during pregnancy. Second we will give a quick overview of chronic leukemia, Hodgkin and non-Hodgkin disease during pregnancy and a more extended overview of acute leukemia during pregnancy.

2. Diagnosis

2.1 Physical examination and routine blood tests

The rare occurrence and subtle presentation of these malignancies in pregnancy often results in a delay in diagnosis, which may worsen the prognosis. In addition, the physiological changes associated with pregnancy can mask certain laboratory abnormalities that are typically present in patients with hematological disorders (simple anemia of pregnancy, leukocytosis or gestational thrombocytopenia may temporarily hide a more serious hematological process such as leukemia) (Sadural and Smith, 1995; Doll et al., 1988).

2.2 Histopathological examination

The diagnosis of an hematological malignancy requires a lymph node biopsy or bone marrow aspirate and/or biopsy for diagnosis. Biopsies can safely be performed under local anesthesia during pregnancy. Overall, it appears that with modern surgical and anesthetic techniques, elective surgery - under general anesthesia - in a pregnant woman is safe even during the first trimester. The risk of spontaneous abortion is comparable with that of normal miscarriage and there is no significant increase in the risk of maternal death, birth defects or late neurodevelopmental delays (Cohen-Kerem et al., 2005; Doll et al., 1988).

2.3 Diagnostic medical imaging

The available information on radiation-induced embryonic damage is derived from animal studies, follow-up of individuals exposed to atomic bomb explosions in Japan (Jablon and Kato, 1970; Miller and Mulvihill, 1976), and statistical analyses (Fenig et al., 2001).

The possible embryonic or fetal damage from radiation may be classified into two principal types. Firstly, the deterministic radiation effects, such as mental retardation and organ malformations, which arise above a threshold dose of 0.1 - 0.2 Gy (Kal and Struikmans, 2005). Teratogenic effects mainly occur after exposure to radiation in the first 12 weeks of pregnancy, when the embryo is in the stage of organogenesis and the CNS is especially sensitive to radiation (Kal and Struikmans, 2005).

Secondly, there are stochastic effects. They generally manifest many years later (so-called *"late"* effects) and cannot definitively be associated to the radiation exposure. Examples of these effects include cancer induction and genetic effects (in the offspring of irradiated individuals). These effects do not occur in relation to a certain threshold, but it is the probability of the effect that increases with administered dose.

Several studies have shown no increase in abortion, growth retardation or congenital malformation from diagnostic exposures below 10cGy (at any time during gestation)(Doll et al., 1988; Nuyttens et al., 2002). The estimated fetal dose from routine radiologic diagnostic procedures is less than 10 cGy. The probability of developmental damage or childhood cancer due to embryonic-fetal irradiation of 1cGy does not exceed one in 1000, and may be only one in 10 000 or even less. These figures are very low when compared to the overall 4-6% rate of birth defects in the general population (Fenig et al., 2001). However, abdominal and pelvic CT are associated with high exposures and should therefore be avoided during pregnancy (Doll et al., 1988; Pereg D. et al., 2008; Pereg D. et al., 2007). The more because ultrasonography or magnetic resonance imaging (MRI) may provide the desired diagnostic information without increasing the risk of fetal malformations. Iodinated contrast seems safe to use in pregnancy (Chen et al., 2008). Gadolinium adds to sensitivity and specificity but crosses the placenta resulting in high fetal concentrations. Gadolinium is associated with nephrogenic systemic fibrosis in adults with an impaired kidney function. Children under 1 year are considered at low-risk to develop nephrogenic systemic fibrosis, because of their immature renal function. If needed, preference should be given to Gadobenate dimeglumine (Multihance®) and Gadoterate meglumine (Dotarem®) contrast media since no unconfounded cases of nephrogenic systemic fibrosis have been reported with these agents (Bellin et al., 2005). In contrast to previous belief, gadolinium-enhanced magnetic resonance imaging is thus possible during pregnancy (Webb et al., 2005). PET-CT has been increasingly used for both staging and treatment follow-up in patients with lymphoma. FDG (fluor-2-deoxy-D-glucose) can cross the placenta and reach the fetus. It may involve higher radiation exposure than regular CT and its use cannot be recommended during pregnancy. It should be performed for (re)evaluation after delivery (Doll et al., 1988). Positron emission tomography scan (^{18}F-PET) is a highly sensitive technique for the detection of tumoral lesions. Since PET-technology is based on positron-electron annihilation and the detection of rather high energy photons, the biological effect of the used radiopharmaceuticals is more significant. Optimization of the scanning protocol is therefore even more crucial, which should also include an evaluation of the protocol and necessity of the concurrent CT-scan in case of a combined PET/CT examination. A standard ^{18}F-FDG-PET examination results in a dose exposure of a 6-month old fetus of 5-6 mSv, which is still acceptable in many indications in view of the important information PET can add to the staging of e.g. lymphoma. In any case, consultation of the nuclear medicine physician and medical physicist before the pregnant patient presents herself to the nuclear department, allows to take some simple measures which can significantly limit the fetal exposure by limiting the dose of the radiopharmaceutical, supplementary maternal hydration and the use of a bladder catheter.

3. Obstetrical and placental issues

3.1 General follow-up

Prenatal care in women diagnosed with cancer during pregnancy should be performed in a high-risk obstetric unit. As treatment options will be dependent on the gestational age, it is very important to have a correct dating of the pregnancy. Before oncological treatment is started, we advise to perform a careful fetal examination by ultrasonographic screening, to ensure there are no pre-existing fetal anomalies. Further ultrasound scans should be performed every 2-3 weeks to evaluate the fetal growth, development and well-being. In case of abnormal findings, more stringent monitoring of the fetus or even preterm delivery might be necessary. Pregnancy-related complications should be treated according to the standard obstetrical care.

3.2 Monitoring around treatment

Before every cycle of cytotoxic treatment, an evaluation of fetal morphology, growth and well-being must be carried out by ultrasound screening. After treatment, it is important to consider fetal well-being and counsel patients to be alert when contractions occur, since an increased incidence in preterm contractions was reported after cytotoxic treatment during pregnancy (Van Calsteren et al., 2010). Furthermore, since cases have been described of neonatal pancytopenia, the possibility of fetal anemia has to be considered and checked before and after chemotherapy in pregnancy (Doppler measurement of peak systolic velocity of the middle cerebral artery).

3.3 The delivery

Delivery should take place in a hospital with a neonatal care unit. The timing of delivery needs to be determined according to the oncological treatment schedule and the maturation of the fetus. As in non cancer patients, a (near-) term delivery (> 35-37 weeks) should be aimed for (Van Calsteren et al., 2010). Prematurity and low birth weight associated with preterm delivery have been identified as negative contributing factors in the neurological and emotional development of children (Wood et al., 2000; Doyle, 2004; Mikkola et al., 1997; Ancel et al., 2006). When delivery before 34 weeks is inevitable, fetal lung maturation by corticosteroids should be considered and managed according to local policy (Crowley et al., 1990). The mode of delivery is determined based on obstetrical indications. To allow the bone marrow to recover and to minimize the risk of maternal and fetal neutropenia/thrombocytopenia/anemia, delivery should be planned 3 weeks after the last dose of anthracycline-based chemotherapy (Loibl et al. 2006). Chemotherapy should not be administered after 35 weeks since spontaneous labor becomes more likely. Furthermore, neonates - especially preterm babies - have limited capacity to metabolize and eliminate drugs due to liver and renal immaturity. The delay of delivery after chemotherapy will allow fetal drug excretion via the placenta (Sorosky et al., 1997). Chemotherapy can be restarted when needed after delivery. An interval of one week after an uncomplicated caesarean section is required.

3.4 Postpartum

Although placental metastases are rare, the placenta should be analysed histopathologically after delivery (Alexander et al., 2003). In the absence of safety data, breastfeeding during or shortly after chemotherapy is contraindicated. Primary inhibition of milk production is needed because especially lipophylic agents can accumulate in the milk.

Cancer type	Cases placental M+	Cases fetal M+	Cases fetal and placental M+	Total
Melanoma	21	3	3	27
Breast cancer	15	0	0	15
Lung cancer	8	1	1	10
Leukemia	6	3	0	9
Lymphoma	3	2	1	6

Table 1. Case reports of placental/fetal metastasis (Alexander et al., 2003)

3.5 Transplacental transfer of chemotherapy during pregnancy

Chemotherapy during pregnancy has been associated with congenital malformations and neonatal bone marrow suppression, suggesting that at least a fraction of these drugs is passing the placenta (Cardonick E and Iacobucci A, 2004.). Transfer mainly occurs by passive diffusion, but also active transporters like P-glycoprotein, Multidrug Resistance Proteins and Breast Cancer Resistance Protein have an important role in the regulation of the placental drug transfer (Syme et al., 2004.). In humans only a few case reports are available, however results are not conclusive (Gaillard et al., 1995; Grohard et al., 1989; Roboz et al., 1979, D'Incalci et al., 1983; Karp et al., 1983; Koc et al., 1994). Results in a baboon model showed that transplacental transfer of chemotherapeutics varies substantially among different drugs. Significant levels of platinum (57.5+14.2% of maternal plasma levels (n=7)) after intravenous carboplatinum administration were detected in fetal plasma samples, but lower levels of doxorubicin (7.5+3.2%, (n=6)), epirubicin (4.0+1.6%, (n=8)), docetaxel (not detectable in fetal samples, (n=9)), paclitaxel (1.4+0.8%, (n=7)), vinblastine (18.5+15.5%, (n=9)) and 4-OH-cyclophosphamide (25.1+6.3%, (n=3)) were measured (Van Calsteren et al., 2010a, 2010b, 2011)

3.6 Short and long term effect of prenatal exposure to chemotherapy on children

The potential fetal effects depend on the gestational age at exposure. During the implantation period (first 10 days after conception) the number of surviving omnipotent stem cells will determine whether a miscarriage occurs, or a normal embryo will develop. Between 10 days and 8 weeks after the conception organogenesis occurs and therefore, this period is at risk for congenital malformations. For foetal protection, the administration of chemotherapy is considered contraindicated until a gestational age of 10 weeks. If a 'safety period' of 4 weeks is respected, chemotherapy may start from a gestational age of 14 weeks (Amant et al., 2009). During the second and third trimester of pregnancy, no major malformations are expected to be caused by cytotoxic treatment. However, cases of growth restriction, prematurity, intra-uterine and neonatal death, and hematopoietic suppression have been reported (Cardonick and Iacobucci, 2004).

Data on the long term of children after prenatal exposure to chemotherapy are scarce. Based on theoretical assumptions, potential problems of neurodevelopmental delay, sterility, carcinogenesis and genetic defects have to be considered, but up till now available data do not suggest these problems. A study that includes 84 children who were born to mothers who received chemotherapy during pregnancy for haematological malignancies and with a median follow-up of 19 years, did not show any congenital, neurological, immunological and psychological abnormalities including normal learning and educational behaviour (Aviles et al., 2001). Hahn et al. surveyed 57 parents/guardians regarding outcomes of children exposed to chemotherapy in utero for breast cancer treatment. At ages ranging from 2 to 157 months, most children had a normal development. Only 2 children required special attention in school: 1 had attention deficit disorder, whereas the other was the child with Down syndrome (Hahn et al., 2006). In a small study, 10 children were between 2 months and 66 months of age when a full neurologic and cardiologic examination was performed. Whether the occurrence of a cortical malformation in a twin whose fraternal twin was normal, was related to cytotoxic drugs remains unclear. Otherwise, we encountered no development problems (Van Calsteren et al., 2006).

The few studies that looked at the cardiac effect of chemotherapy in the foetus showed that acute myocardial dysfunction can appear during pregnancy with anthracyclines. (Cardonick and Lacobucci, 2004; Germann et al., 2004). However, follow-up with cardiac ultrasound in 81 children who received anthracycline treatment in utero (age 9 - 29 years, mean 17 year) was reassuring (Aviles et al., 2006).

4. Supportive treatment

4.1 Antiemetics

Up to 70% of cancer patients may suffer from nausea or emesis following chemotherapy. No association was found between treatment with metoclopramide, anti-histamines or ondansetron-based anti-emetics and fetal malformations in both animal models and humans (Tincello and Johnstone, 1996; Siu et al., 2002; Guikontes et al., 1992; World, 1993).

4.2 Antibiotics

As pregnant women with malignancy might be treated with antibiotics - especially due to neutropenic fever - their effects on the mother and fetus must be addressed. There is large data regarding fetal safety of penicillins, cephalosporins and erythromycin. Aminoglycosides seem to be safe in first trimester on limited data. A higher rate of cardiovascular malformations was found after treatment with trimethoprim-sulfamethazine in the second-third months of pregnancy. Quinolones that cause arthropathy and tetracyclines that affect bone and teeth should be avoided during pregnancy. Sulfonamides, similar to other folate antagonists have been associated with neural tube defects and cardiac malformations and should be avoided as well (Pereg et al., 2008; Werler et al.2005).

4.3 Pain control

Paracetamol has been reported to be used by up to 65% of pregnant women. It can be administered safely throughout pregnancy. NSAID's are preferably not used during pregnancy, but if needed can be considered during the first and second trimester of pregnancy. In the third trimester (> 32 weeks) NSAID's are contraindicated because they are associated with premature closure of the ductus arteriosus, oligohydramnion and prolonged gestation and labor (Pereg et al., 2008; Cardonick and Lacobucci, 2004).

4.4 Growth factors

Erythropoietin does not cross the placenta and its use is felt to be safe in pregnancy (Briggs and Yaffee, 2005). Granulocyte colony-stimulating factor use in pregnancy has been reported in a registry series of 20 patients with severe chronic neutropenia with a median dose of 2.7 mcg/kg/day administered daily or every other day during all three trimesters with an average duration of three trimesters. These data, although limited, did not reveal an increase in adverse congenital abnormalities or fetal death compared to pregnant patients that did not receive the drug (Dale et al., 2003).

4.5 Bisphosphonates

Animal studies with bisphosphonates have displayed maternal toxicity, foetal underdevelopment, embryolethality, hypocalcaemia and skeletal retardation during pregnancy. Bisphosphonates are therefore contra-indicated in pregnancy and have a FDA category C pregnancy risk. A recent literature search including 51 patients exposed to bisphosphonates shortly prior to conception or during pregnancy did not find evidence of skeletal abnormalities or malformations in the foetuses of the exposed mothers (Djokanovic et al., 2008). If bisphosphonates are indicated in a pregnant patient hypocalcemia affecting the contractility of the uterus must be avoided.

4.6 Leukapheresis

Leukapheresis has been used in both acute and chronic leukemia to rapidly reduce high whiteblood cell counts in patients with impending vascular occlusion. Experience with leukapheresis during pregnancy is limited to only a handful of cases used to treat both chronic and acute leukemias (Ali et al., 2004a, 2004b; Bazarbashi et al, 1991; Broccia et al., 1984; Fitzgerald et al., 1993, 1986; Nolan et al., 1988). In general, the therapy was tolerated well by the mother and the fetus. Although experience is limited, leukapheresis may be used as a short-term temporizing measure when no other options exist or in patients refusing other therapies during pregnancy.

4.7 Corticoids

Regarding the use of corticoids, methylprednisolone and hydrocortisone are extensively metabolized in the placenta. They are therefore preferred over dexa- or betamethasone (Amant et al., 2009).

5. Leukemia in pregnancy

The diagnosis of leukemia in a pregnant woman is a dramatic event that generates complex ethical and therapeutic dilemmas. Leukemia often presents as a medical emergency and induction of appropriate therapy must be initiated promptly. The therapeutic decisions should involve a multidisciplinary team including at least an haematologist, an obstetrician, a neonatologist, a psychologist and a social worker. Hypothetically the treatment decision must be based on data from prospective clinical trials but unfortunately the available data in the literature derives from retrospective case reports and case series.

Leukemia occurring during pregnancy is very rare with an estimated incidence of one per 100.000 pregnancies annually (Pavlidis, 2002). This frequency is 3.5 times lower than the incidence of leukemia in the general population in Western world. This is explained by the fact that acute lymphoblastic leukemia occurs mainly in childhood, while acute myeloid leukemia occurs usually in late adulthood, thus relatively sparing the childbearing ages.

The majority of cases of leukemia during pregnancy are acute leukemias, of which two-thirds are acute myeloid leukemias and one-third acute lymphoblastic leukemias (Pentheroudakis and Pavlidis, 2006). The main chronic leukemia during pregnancy is chronic myeloid leukemia and accounts for about 10% of all pregnancy-associated leukemias, since chronic lymphocytic leukemia is extremely rare (Caligiuri and Mayer, 1989).

5.1 Acute leukemia in pregnancy

Since Virchow's first description in 1856 of leukemia in pregnant woman, more than 500 cases have been reported (Sadural and Smith, 1995). Acute leukemias are diagnosed more frequently during the later stages of pregnancy. It is estimated that 23% of acute leukemias diagnosed during pregnancy were detected in the first trimester, 37% in the second and 40% in the third trimester respectively (Caliguiri, 1992).

The initial diagnosis of acute leukemia is often challenging and sometimes can be delayed because pregnant women frequently describe various non-specific symptoms like fatigue. Anemia, as already mentioned, is accompanied by marked thrombocytopenia and neutropenia. Recurrent infections and bleeding reflect bone marrow failure. The diagnostic approach is the same as in the general population. Bone marrow aspiration for morphologic examination and biopsy, detailed immunophenotyping, cytogenetics and molecular studies are essentials.

No prospective studies comparing outcome in nonpregnant and pregnant women with acute leukemia are available. Case control series and historical control comparisons offer no evidence to suggest that pregnancy has an impact on the course and prognosis of acute leukemia provided that therapy is not delayed (Fey and Surbek, 2008).

Vertical transmission of leukemia in the fetus is exceptionally rare due to placental barrier and fetal immune system. Nevertheless the placenta is not an absolute barrier and single maternal leukemic cells can pass from mother to fetus and few cases of leukemic placenta infiltration and leukemia dissemination to the fetus have been described (Dildy et al., 1989; Osada et al., 1990; Van der Velden et al., 2001).

Cytotoxic agents have a relatively low molecular weight; most of them can cross the placenta and reach the fetus. When treating a pregnant woman with chemotherapy it is crucial to consider that many physiologic changes occur in gestation, which can potentially alter the effectiveness of antineoplastic agents by changing their metabolism or clearance (Redmond, 1985). Plasma volume is increased up to 50%, the amniotic fluid creates a pharmacologic third space and renal clearance and hepatic oxidation of drugs are enhanced (Williams and Schilsky, 2000; Muchlow, 1986). For different drugs, among which chemotherapy, changes in pharmacokinetic characteristics have been shown. Recently we described a lower plasma drug exposure for doxorubicin, epirubicin, paclitaxel and carboplatin during pregnancy (Van Calsteren et al., 2010)). However these findings could not be related to different outcomes, and therefore it is currently advised to administer the same drug regimens/dosages to pregnant and nonpregnant women (Cardonick and Iacobucci, 2004).

5.1.1 Acute Myeloid Leukemia (AML)

Treatment protocols for AML consist of a combination of cytarabine with an anthracycline as an induction course in order to achieve complete remission. Afterwards various intensive chemotherapy combinations are administered as consolidation therapy.

Cytarabine as an antimetabolite carries a significant risk to the fetus. A review of 93 cases of pregnant women exposed to cytarabine alone or in combination with other chemotherapeutic agents reported 4 cases of limb malformations associated with first trimester exposure. The administration in the second and third trimester was associated with transient neonatal cytopenias in 5 cases, intrauterine fetal death in 6 cases, intrauterine growth retardation in 12 cases and 2 cases of neonatal deaths from severe infections (Cardonick and Iacobucci, 2004). Cytarabine use in the first trimester is not advocated and termination of pregnancy is strongly preferred.

Idarubicin and daunorubicin are the anthracyclines in the treatment regimens for AML. Idarudicin is more lipophilic compared to other anthracyclines and so placenta transfer is more likely to occur. Therefore it may be associated with higher rates of fetal complications and should be avoided during pregnancy (Cardonick and Iacobucci, 2004).

The experience with the administration of anthracyclines during pregnancy is limited mostly to doxorubicin and daunorubicin. Of 28 pregnancies after the first trimester, exposed to doxorubicin and daunorubicin for the treatment of various hematologic malignancies, 21 pregnancies were delivered without any complications (Turchi and Villasis, 1988). The results of daunorubicin are worrying especially the combination with cytarabine which is associated with serious fetal morbidity and mortality (Azim et al., 2010). A stillborn fetus was reported in one case after exposure to daunorubicin. Congenital anomalies including limb deformities, ventral septal defect and cardiomyopathy were also reported (Azim et al., 2010).

Doxorubicin has been extensively studied in gestational breast cancer and results are rather reassuring (Hahn et al., 2006). 162 Pregnancies with malignancies, including 25 in the first trimester, were exposed to doxorubicin and reported complications were pre-eclampsia, midtrimester miscarriage, transient neonatal neutropenia with sepsis, intrauterine growth retardation and intrauterine fetal death in 18 cases (Cardonick and Iacobucci, 2004). Since doxorubicin seems to be as effective as the other anthracyclines for the treatment of leukemia, it is the preferred anthracycline during pregnancy (Shapira et al., 2008). Six pregnant patiens with AML were treated with a doxorubicin-based regimen with normal outcomes except from one premature delivery (Greenlund et al., 2001; Fassas et al., 1984). Doxorubicin is considered relatively safe throughout pregnancy and is not associated with an increased risk for severe congenital malformations (Azim et al., 2010). Whether in utero exposure to anthracyclines is cardiotoxic to the developing fetus is unknown (Cardonick and Iacobucci, 2004; Avilés et al., 2006).

In relapsed AML termination of pregnancy is recommended, because therapy requires high-dose chemotherapy, stem cell transplantation or experimental drugs, which cannot be delivered during pregnancy (Shapira et al., 2008).

In summary when a pregnant woman is diagnosed with AML during the 1st trimester a strong recommendation for pregnancy termination must be given. In 2nd and 3rd trimesters treatment with cytarabine and doxorubicin should be instituted promptly. Delivery should be planned after the 32nd week of gestation and 2-3 weeks following treatment to allow bone marrow recovery.

5.1.2 Acute Promyelocytic Leukemia (APL)

APL is a unique type of AML characterized by the reciprocal chromosomal translocation t(15;17) (q22;q21) and its molecular equivalent the PML/RARα fusion gene. APL has been reported in approximately 10% of cases of leukemia in pregnancy, similar to the percentage in non-pregnant women (Carradice et al., 2002). It is frequently associated with disseminated intravascular coagulation, which may severely complicate the management of pregnancy, labor and delivery.

As in other types of leukemia, management of APL in pregnancy cannot be based on evidence from clinical trials and relies on data from historical cases. A novel treatment strategy of APL was the introduction of All-Trans-Retinoic-Acid (ATRA). ATRA targets the fusion product of t(15;17). Pharmacological levels of ATRA lead to remission by differentiation of cells of the leukemic clone. By combining ATRA with induction and consolidation chemotherapy, APL has one of the more favorable outcomes (Sanz and Lo-Coco, 2011).

As with other vitamin A derivatives, ATRA exposure during the 1st trimester carries an 85% risk of teratogenicity, including severe neurological and cardiovascular malformations (Fadilah et al., 2001). ATRA appears to be reasonably safe and well tolerated if given outside the first trimester (Fadilah et al., 2001). A review of 15 cases of APL in pregnancy treated with ATRA did not reveal any fetal malformations that could be attributed to ATRA (Carradice et al., 2002; Fadilah et al., 2001; Giagounidis et al., 2006). However, close monitoring for fetal cardiac complications is mandatory throughout pregnancy (Yang and Hladnik, 2009). The most important maternal adverse effect of ATRA is the potentially lethal retinoic acid syndrome, which may be reversed with early administation of dexamethasone.

The combination of ATRA with an anthracycline during the 2nd and 3rd trimesters has been reported in several case reports (Shapira et al., 2008). This regimen appears reasonably safe and is not associated with increased toxicity for either the pregnant woman or the fetus. Among 15 women receiving this regimen, 13 were diagnosed in late pregnancy and yielded live newborns, whereas 2 patients in 6th and 10th week of gestation at time of APL diagnosis had an abortion (Breccia et al., 2002).

The confirmation of diagnosis of APL in the 2nd and 3rd trimester should be followed by the initiation of ATRA with an anthracycline if the leukocyte count is less than 10,000/mm3. If the leukocyte count is greater than 10,000/mm3 an anthracycline alone is recommended to decrease the risk of ATRA syndrome. Arsenic trioxide is teratogenic and contraindicated in pregnancy (Rizack et al., 2009).

5.1.3 Acute Lymphoblastic Leukemia (ALL)

ALL is relatively rare among adults and only 21 cases of pregnant patients with ALL have been reported (Rizack et al., 2009). Because ALL is a highly aggressive disease, it is critical that multiagent chemotherapy is administered immediately after the diagnosis. It has been shown that survival is significantly longer in patients whose induction therapy is started before delivery, than in those treated after delivery.

Methotrexate (a folate antagonist), a crucial component of most intensification protocols of ALL, is highly teratogenic and abortifacient when administered during the first trimester. Also the exposure to high dose methotrexate after the 1st trimester was associated with cranial dysostosis, delayed ossification, hypertelorism, wide nasal bridge, micrognatia, anomalies of external ears and cleft palate (aminopterin syndrome)(Ebert et al., 1997). The risk of fetal malformations diminishes as pregnancy advances (Ebert et al., 1997). Thereafter, termination of pregnancy is recommended for patients prior to the 20th week of gestation followed by the standard intensification chemotherapeutic ALL protocol. After the 20th week a modified anti ALL regimen that does not include methotrexate, may be used until the 3rd trimester (Rizack et al., 2009). Cyclophosphamide, vinca alkaloids, L-asparaginase, anthracyclines, cytarabine and steroids have been used in these regimens (Ali et al., 2009). However, all modified ALL protocols must be considered as " bridging treatment" until the 3rd trimester. In the 3rd trimester treatment protocols as in non-pregnant women must be followed (Molkenboer et al., 2005). Close obstetric care and monitoring of the mother and fetus are essential to ensure the best possible outcome (Matsouka et al., 2008). Delivery after 32 weeks is suggested, simultaneous to a non-cytopenic period.

5.2 Chronic leukemia in pregnancy

5.2.1 Chronic Myelogenous Leukemia (CML)

The incidence of CML associated with pregnancy is estimated to be 1/75000 pregnancies (Celiloglu et al., 2000). The diagnostic approach is identical as in non-pregnant patients. The cytogenetic study reveals the Philadelphia chromosome and possibly additional chromosomal abnormalities of the clonal evolution. The disease is characterized by the presence of the bcr/abl fusion gene.

The introduction of imatinib mesylate, a tyrosine kinase inhibitor, has revolutionized the treatment of this disease. Pre-clinical models have suggested that imatinib may be teratogenic and therefore the present recommendation for women treated with imatinib is to use contraception (Azim et al., 2010). It has been reported that the concentration of imatinib and its active metabolite were higher in the placenta than in the maternal blood, while they were low or undetected in the umbilical cord. These findings suggest limited placental transfer of imatinib in late pregnancy (Russell et al., 2007).

It seems that administering imatinib during the first trimester is associated with a considerable risk of congenital anomalies and spontaneous abortions, while late exposure does not have the same impact. Nevertheless in patients diagnosed with CML during pregnancy, imatinib should not be the treatment of choice due to the limited experience (Shapira et al., 2008). Very limited data are available about the safety of second-generation oral tyrosine kinase inhibitors (dastinib, nilotinib) during pregnancy and it is recommended that patients on these drugs should avoid pregnancy (Conchon et al., 2010).

Interferon-alpha (INFα), an immune modulator, does not cross the placenta to a great extent due to its high molecular weight (19kDa) and does not inhibit DNA synthesis. All reported cases of pregnant women with CML, treated with interferon, resulted in healthy babies and normal maternal outcomes. Given the available pre-clinical and clinical data, interferon can be safely administered throughout pregnancy and it is the treatment of choice for patients diagnosed with CML in pregnancy. Patients in the 2nd or 3rd trimester - who cannot tolerate or fail interferon therapy - may be treated with hydroxyurea or imatinib (Rizack et al., 2009).

Hydroxyurea is a cytotoxic drug, which inhibits DNA synthesis, and is capable of crossing the placenta. Several cases of hydroxyurea administration during pregnancy have been reported. Hydroxyurea treatment should be avoid in 1st trimester and could be given to patients who cannot tolerate interferon therapy during the 2nd or 3rd trimesters (Thauvin-Robinet et al., 2001).

5.2.2 Chronic Lymphocytic Leukemia (CLL)

CLL, a predominantly disease of the elderly, is very rarely associated with the reproductive period. Only five cases of CLL in pregnancy have been reported in literature (Chrisomalis and al., 1996; Baynes et al., 1996; Welsh and al., 2000; Gurman, 2002; Ali et al., 2004). In two of these cases placental infiltration has been described but with no impact on the fetus. Because CLL has an indolent clinical course, therapy of pregnant patients with CLL can usually be delayed until post partum. If intervention is required leukapheresis could be an option. Chlorambucil is contraindicated during the 1st trimester because of its teratogenicity and there are not enough data to recommend its use during late pregnancy. Fludarabine must be avoided in pregnancy. Autoimmune complications should be managed with corticosteroids as in non-pregnant patients (Rizack et al., 2009).

5.2.3 Hairy Cell Leukemia (HCL)

HCL is a type of chronic leukemia of late age at presentation with male predominance. Therefore it is extremely rare during pregnancy. Six cases of pregnancy-associated HCL have been reported and all pregnancies came to term without complications, resulting in delivery of healthy neonates (Shapira et al., 2008). When therapy is indicated in HCL during pregnancy, interferon-alpha is the treatment of choice (Baer et al., 1992).

5.2.4 Summary recommendations for the management of leukemia's in pregnancy

	1st trimester	2nd trimester	3rd trimester
AML	pregnancy termination	Cytarabine-doxorubicin	cytarabine-doxorubicin
APL	pregnancy termination	ATRA & anthracycline	ATRA & anthracycline
ALL	pregnancy termination	>20w modified protocols	Standard protocols
CML	Interferon-alpha	Interferon-alpha	Interferon-alpha

Table 2. Recommendations for the management of leukemia's in pregnancy

6. Hodgkin disease in pregnancy

Hodgkin's disease (HD) is a unique malignant disorder, usually arising in lymph nodes and defined by the presence of the pathognomonic Reed-Sternberggiant cell (Sadural and Smith, 1995). HD is a neoplasia with a peak incidence between the ages of 20-30 and another peak incidence after the age of 55. The illness affects male patients more than female patients. Although it represents only 0.5% of all cancers, it is not rare to diagnose HD in pregnant women, due to the peak incidence among young people. In these cases the incidence varies between 1:1,000 and 1:6,000 deliveries (Anselmo et al., 1999). It is curable even in advanced stages and ABVD (doxorubicin, bleomycin, vinblastin and dacarbazine) is considered the standard of care chemotherapy regimen in this disease (Connors, 2005).

6.1 Chemotherapy and Hodgkin disease in pregnancy

Based on the results of an extended literature review, we suggest that patients diagnosed with HD in pregnancy should be treated with the ABVD-regimen rather than with M-/COPP-regimen. ABVD outside the first trimester seems feasible and safe. Patients with early stage HD diagnosed in the first trimester should be followed-up at short intervals for signs of disease progression without any treatment until the second trimester (Fisher et al.,1996; Pereg et al., 2007). Offering single agent vinblastine along with steroids is another option (Nisce et al., 1986), yet congenital anomalies and spontaneous abortions have been described with this approach. Patients diagnosed close to term could be good candidates for delivery anticipation to avoid any potential hazards to the fetus.
If advanced HD is diagnosed during the first trimester, termination of the pregnancy should be considered followed by appropriate staging and adequate doses of combination chemotherapy (Cannellos et al, 1992).
Treatment should not be delayed during pregnancy if patient presents with symptomatic (i.e. B symptoms), Bulky, subdiaphragmatic, or progressive HD after the first trimester.
Relapsed HL during pregnancy can be treated with chemotherapy, if the patient has been previously treated only with radiotherapy (Cannellos et al., 1992). Data in these cases are very rare.

6.2 Radiotherapy and Hodgkin Disease in pregnancy

Patients with HD stage I and II are treated mainly with polychemotherapy followed by radiotherapy (RT) given only to the originally involved sites (involved-field radiotherapy). In these cases, the average fetal exposure should not exceed 0.1–0.2 Gy, which is the threshold dose at which deterministic effects (e.g. mental retardation, organ malformation) can be expected (Kal and Struikmans,2005). In stage III-IV disease, RT seems to be of no benefit if given routinely in patients who show a complete remission after chemotherapy: RT could benefit patients with partial responses after chemotherapy in these cases (Fenig et al., 2001; Kal and Struikmans,2005).

6.3 Possible decision tree for treatment of Hodgkin Disease in pregnancy

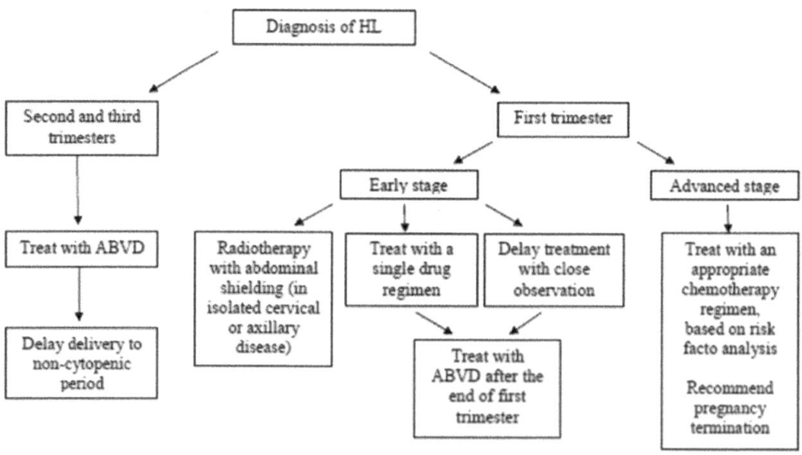

Fig. 1. Proposal of a possible algorithm for the treatment of pregnancy associated HD (Pereg, 2007)

7. Non-Hodgkin disease in pregnancy

Non-Hodgkin-lymphoma (NHL) forms a heterogeneous group of hematologic malignancies. According to the WHO-classification, we can divide them in three groups: indolent, aggressive and very aggressive. This disease is extremely rare in pregnancy, but the occurrence of NHL during pregnancy is expected to increase due not only to the currenttrend to postpone pregnancy, but the increasing incidence of HIV-associated lymphoma in developing countries (Pereg et al., 2007). NHL has an age dependent incidence pattern with a sharp increase in frequency starting in middle life (in contrast to HD). These differences in age distributions together with the higher incidence of NHL in young males compared to women, probably explains the scarcity of reports of NHL associated with pregnancy (Lishner et al., 1994). However, NHL in pregnancy is most commonly associated with more aggressive histology and disseminated disease. (Mavrommatis et al., 1998). Management of NHL varies significantly depending on the pathological subtype.

7.1 Indolent Non-Hodgkin Lymphoma

Indolent lymphomas are diseases of the elderly and have been rarely described during pregnancy. The exact incidence remains unknown as a significant proportion of the available reports lack a detailed pathological description. A large fraction of these tumors have an indolent course and thus could be safely watched during the course of pregnancy. In patients requiring active therapy, they could be offered regimens that have been shown to be safe in aggressive lymphomas (Nisce et al., 1986; Pereg et al., 2007).

7.2 Aggressive Non-Hodgkin Lymphoma

Treatment during the first trimester is complex and patients with aggressive disease should be counselled regarding therapeutic abortion, taking into consideration the fetal risk of staging and chemotherapy (Koren et al., 1990). Close observation or radiation therapy (Spitzer et al., 1991) during the first trimester could be considered in those patients presenting with early stage disease, low-volume disease, no B symptoms, and low international prognostic index (IPI) score. Patients with bulky disease or poorer prognostic indicators, such as high IPI score, B symptoms, or high Ki-67 in their biopsies should be treated immediately after pregnancy termination. Beyond the first trimester, standard chemotherapy should be instituted due to the poor prognosis of aggressive NHL without therapy.

Evidence regarding the fetal safety of CHOP during the first trimester is extremely limited. CHOP is considered to be safe in second and third trimester, however only seven case reports have been published. No reviewed data is available about the safety of M-/VACOP-exposition during pregnancy.

Literature suggests that anti-metabolites (such as 6-MP) in first trimester should be avoided (as mentioned by several previous review-rapports, although large data is lacking). Rituximab seems safe and without significant consequences for the foetus (Decker et al.,2006; Friedrichs et al., 2006; Rey et al., 2008).

Overall it seems that offering standard regimens like CHOP or CHOP-like regimens (e.g. R-CHOP) is safe and feasible, certainly in 2nd and 3rd trimester.

7.3 Possible decision tree for treatment of Non-Hodgkin Disease in first trimester of pregnancy

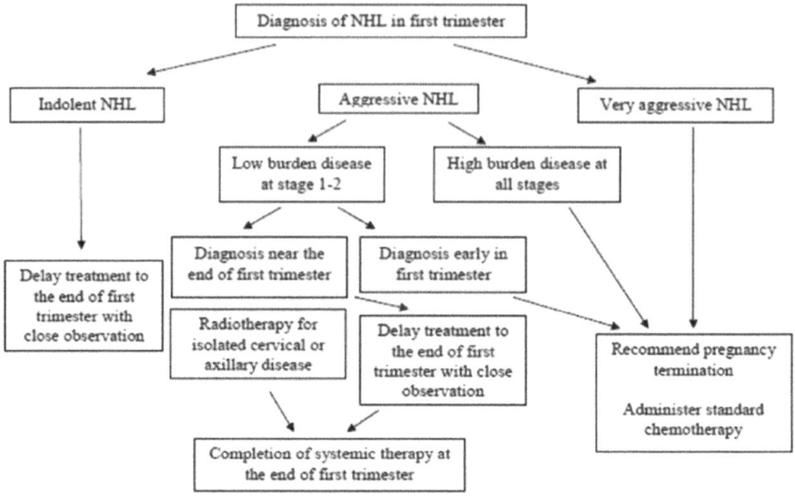

Fig. 2. Shows a possible algorithm for the treatment of first-trimester-associated NHL. Systemic therapy outside the first trimester (R-CHOP) seems to be safe for all forms of NHL (Pereg, 2007).

8. Summary and conclusion

Hematological malignancies are uncommon during pregnancy. Nevertheless, it includes a very complex medical, but also ethical and psychological problem. Delay in diagnosis and treatment will influence the prognosis for acute leukemia and aggressive/advanced lymphomas. Delay in treatment and even diagnostic delay may influence the prognosis for chronic leukemia and indolent non-Hodgkin lymphomas. In selected cases with limited disease of early stage Hodgkin's disease, treatment may be safely postponed until after delivery.The decision to use chemotherapy during pregnancy must be carefully weighed against the effect of treatment delay on maternal survival. If possible, chemotherapy should be avoided during the first trimester or abortion should be taken in consideration. If the mother decides to continue the pregnancy and multidrug treatment in first trimester is required, anthracycline antibiotics, vinca alkaloids or single-agent treatment followed by multi-agent therapy after first trimester should be considered. Use of chemotherapy in the second and third trimesters seems to be relatively safe. Radiotherapy during pregnancy is possible, if the fetal exposure does not exceed the threshold dose of 10cGy. Seen the complexity of the decisions in treatment of pregnancy-associated cancer, this should be approached interdisciplinary and should be individually for each patient. Every decision should be made together with the patient, after careful balancing of both the risks and benefits.

9. References

A predictive model for aggressive non-Hodgkin's lymphoma. The International Non-Hodgkin's Lymphoma Prognostic Factors Project. *N Engl J Med*1993;329:987–994.

Alexander A, Samlowski WE, Grossman D, et al. Metastatic melanoma in pregnancy: risk of transplacental metastases in the infant. *J Clin Oncol* 2003;21: 2179-86.

Ali R, Ozkalemkas F, Kimya Y, Koksal N, Ozkan H, Ozkocaman V, Hoyrazli A, Cetinkaya M, Tunali A. Acute leukemia and pregnancy. *Leuk Res.* 2009 Mar;33(3):e26-28.

Ali R, Ozkalemkas F, Ozkocaman V, et al. Successful labor in the course of chronic lymphocytic leukemia (CLL) and management of CLL during pregnancy with leukapheresis. *Ann Hematol* 2004;83:61–63

Ali R, Ozkalemkas F, Ozkocaman V, et al. Successful pregnancy and delivery in a patient with chronic myelogenous leukemia (CML), and management of CML with leukapheresis during pregnancy: A case report and review of the literature. *Jpn J Clin Oncol* 2004;34:215–217.

Amant et al. Gynecologic cancers in pregnancy: guidelines of an international consensus meeting. *Int J Gynecol Cancer* 2009;19 Suppl 1: S1-12).

Amant F, Brepoels L, Halaska MJ, Gziri MM &Calsteren KV. Gynaecologic cancer complicatine pregnancy: an overview. *Best Pract Res Clin Obstet Gynaecol.* 2010 Feb;24(1):61-79. Epub 2009 Sep 8. Review.

Ancel PY, Livinec F, Larroque B, et al. Cerebral palsy among very preterm children in relation to gestational age and neonatal ultrasound abnormalities: the EPIPAGE cohort study. *Pediatrics* 2006;117: 828-35.

Anselmo AP et al. Hodgkin's disease during pregnancy: diagnostic and therapeutic management. *Fetal Diagn Ther.* 1999 Mar-Apr;14(2):102-5

Avilés A, Neri N, Nambo MJ. Long-term evaluation of cardiac function in children who received anthracyclines during pregnancy. *Ann Oncol.* 2006 Feb;17(2):286-288.

Aviles A, Neri N. Hematological malignancies and pregnancy: a final report of 84 children who receive chemotherapy in utero. *Clin Lymphoma* 2001;2:173-177.

Aviles A, Niz J. Long term-term follow-up of children born to mothers with acute leukemia during pregnancy. *Med Pediatr Oncol* 1998;16:3-6

Azim HA Jr, Pavlidis N, Peccatori FA. Treatment of the pregnant mother with cancer: a systematic review on the use of cytotoxic, endocrine, targeted agents and immunotherapy during pregnancy. Part II: Hematological tumors. *Cancer Treat Rev.* 2010;36(2):110-121

Baer MR, Ozer H, Foon KA. Interferon-alpha therapy during pregnancy in chronic myelogenous leukaemia and hairy cell leukaemia. *Br J Hematol* 1992;81:167-169.

Baynes TL, Crickmay GF, Jones RV. Pregnancy in a case of CLL. *J Obstet Gynecol Br Comm* 1996;75:1165-1168.

Bazarbashi MS, Smith MR, Karanes C, et al. Successful management of Ph chromosome chronic myelogenous leukemia with leukapheresis during pregnancy. *Am J Hematol* 1991;38:235–237.

Bellin MF, Webb JA, Van Der Molen AJ, et al. Safety of MR liver specific contrast media. *Eur Radiol* 2005;15(8): 1607-14.

Breccia M, Cimino G, Alimena G, De Carolis S, Lo Coco F, Mandelli F. AIDA treatment for high-risk acute promyelocytic leukemia in a pregnant woman at 21 weeks of gestation. *Haematologica.* 2002;87(2):ELT12

Briggs GC FR, Yaffee SJ. A Reference Guide to Fetal and Neonatal Risk: Drugs in Pregnancy and Lactation. *Philadelphia: Lippincott, Williams and Wilkins*; 2005.

Broccia G, Casula P, Andria M. Chronic myelocytic leukemia in pregnancy: Report of a case treated with leukapheresis. *Tumori* 1984;70:371-374.

Caligiuri MA. Leukemia and pregnancy: effects of treatment on mother and child. *Advanc Oncol* 1992;8:10-17.

Caliguiri MA, Mayer RJ. Pregnancy and leukemia. *Semin Oncol*1989;16:388-396.

Canellos GP, Anderson JR, Propert KJ, et al. Chemotherapy of advanced Hodgkin's disease with MOPP, ABVD, or MOPP alternating with ABVD. *N. Engl J Med* 1992;327:1478-1484.

Cardonick E, Lacobucci A. Use of chemotherapy during human pregnancy. *Lancet Oncol* 2004;5:283-91.

Carradice D, Austin N, Bayston K, Ganly PS Successful treatment of acute promyelocytic leukaemia during pregnancy. *Clin Lab Haematol.* 2002 Oct;24(5):307-11.

Celiloglu M, Altunyurt S, Undar B. Hydroxyurea treatment for chronic myeloid leukemia during pregnancy. *Acta Obstet Gynecol Scand.* 2000;79(9):803-804.

Chen MM, Coakley FV, Kaimal A & Laros RK Jr.Guidelines for computed tomography and magnetic resonance imaging use during pregnancy and lactation.*Obstet Gynecol.* 2008 Aug;112(2 Pt 1):333-40.

Chrisomalis L, Baxi LV, Heller D. Chronic lymphocytic leukemia in pregnancy. *Am J Obstet Gynecol* 1996;175:1381-1382.

Cohen-Kerem et al. ,Pregnancy outcome following non-obstetric surgical intervention. *Am J Surg.* 2005 Sep;190(3):467-73

Conchon M, Sanabani SS, Serpa M, Novaes MM, Nardinelli L, Ferreira PB, Dorliac-Llacer PE, Bendit I. Successful Pregnancy and Delivery in a Patient with Chronic Myeloid Leukemia while on Dasatinib Therapy. *Adv Hematol.*;2010:136252 Epub 2010 Mar 7.

Connors JM. State-of-the-art therapeutics:Hodgkin's lymphoma.*J Clin Oncol* 2005;23:640-840.

Crowley P, Chalmers I, Keirse MJ. The effects of corticosteroid administration before preterm delivery: an overview of the evidence from controlled trials. *Br J Obstet Gynaecol* 1990;97: 11-25.

D'Incalci M, Broggini M, Buscaglia M, Pardi G. Transplacental passage of doxorubicin. *Lancet* 1983; 1: 75.

Dale DC, Cottle TE, Fier CJ, et al. Severe chronic neutropenia: Treatment and follow-up of patients in the Severe Chronic Neutropenia International Registry. *Am J Hematol* 2003;72:82-93

Decker M et al. Rituximab plus CHOP for treatment of diffuse large B-cell lymphoma during second trimester of pregnancy. *Lancet Oncol.* 2006 Aug;7(8):693-4.

Dildy GA, Moise KJ, Carpenter RJ, et al. Maternal malignancy metastatic to the products of conception: A review. *Obstet Gynacol Surv* 1989;44:535-540.

Djokanovic N, Klieger-Grossmann C, Koren G. Does treatment with bisphosphonates endanger the human pregnancy? J Obstet Gynaecol Can 2008;30:1146-1148.

Doll DC, Ringenberg QS & Yarbro JW. Management of cancer during pregnancy. Arch Intern Med. 1988;148(9):2058-64.

Doyle LW. Neonatal intensive care at borderline viability--is it worth it? Early Hum Dev 2004;80: 103-13.

Ebert U, Löffler H, Kirch W. Cytotoxic therapy and pregnancy. *Pharmacol Ther* 1997;74(2):207-220.

Fadilah SA, Hatta AZ, Keng CS, Jamil MA, Singh S. Successful treatment of acute promyelocytic leukemia in pregnancy with all-trans retinoic acid. *Leukemia* 2001;15(10):1665-1666.

Fassas A, Kartalis G, Klearchou N, Tsatalas K, Sinacos Z, Mantalenakis S. Chemotherapy for acute leukemia during pregnancy. Five case reports. *Nouv Rev Fr Hematol.* 1984;26(1):19-24.

Fenig E et al. Pregnancy and radiation. *Cancer Treat Rev.* 2001 Feb;27(1):1-7.

Fey MF, Surbek D. Leukemia and pregnancy. *Recent Results Cancer Res* 2008;178:97-110.

Fisher PM, Hancock BW. Hogdkin's disease in the pregnant patient. *Br J Hosp Med.* 1996 Nov 20-Dec 10;56(10): 529-32

Fitzgerald D, Rowe JM, Heal J. Leukapheresis for control of chronic myelogenous leukemia during pregnancy. *Am J Hematol* 1986;22:213–218

Fitzgerald JM, McCann SR. The combination of hydroxyurea and leucapheresis in the treatment of chronic myeloid leukemia in pregnancy.*Clin Lab Haematol* 1993;15:63–65.

Friedrichs B et al. The effects of rituximab treatment during pregnancy on a neonate. *Haematologica.* 2006 Oct;91(10):1426-7. Epub 2006 Sep 7.

Gaillard B, Leng JJ, Grellet J, Ducint D, Saux MC. Transplacental passage of epirubicin. *J Gynecol Obstet Biol Reprod (Paris)* 1995; 24: 63-8.

Germann N, Goffinet F, Goldwasser F. Anthracyclines during pregnancy: embryo-fetal outcome in 160 patients. *Ann Oncol* 2004;**15**(1): 146-50

Giagounidis AA, Beckmann MW, Giagounidis AS, Aivado M, Emde T, Germing U, Riehs T, Heyll A, Aul C. Acute promyelocytic leukemia and pregnancy. *Eur J Haematol.* 2000;64(4):267-271.

Gilman EA, Kneale GW, Knox EG, Steward AM. Pregnancy, x-rays and childhood cancers: effect of exposure, age and radiation dose. *J Radiol Prot.* 1988; **8**: 3–8.

Greenlund LJ, Letendre L, Tefferi A. Acute leukemia during pregnancy: a single institutional experience with 17 cases. *Leuk Lymphoma.* 2001 May;41(5-6):571-7.

Grohard P, Akbaraly JP, Saux MC, Gimenez S, Robert J, Brachet-Liermain A et al. Transplacental passage of doxorubicin. *J Gynecol Obstet Biol Reprod (Paris)* 1989; 18: 595-600.

Guikontes E, Spantideas A & Diakakis J. Ondansetron and hyperemesis gravidarum. *Lancet* 1992;340:1223.

Gurman G. Pregnancy and successful labor in the course of chronic lymphocytic leukemia. *Am J Hematol* 2002;71:208-210.

Hahn KM, Johnson PH, Gordon N, Kuerer H, Middleton L, Ramirez M, Yang W, Perkins G, Hortobagyi GN, Theriault RL. Treatment of pregnant breast cancer patients and outcomes of children exposed to chemotherapy in utero. *Cancer.* 2006 Sep 15;107(6):1219-26.

Jablon S, Kato H. Childhood cancer in relation to prenatal exposure to atomic-bomb radiation. *Lancet.* 1970 Nov 14;2(7681):1000-3.

Kal HB, Struikmans H., Radiotherapy during pregnancy: fact and fiction. Lancet Oncol. 2005 May;6(5): 328-33

Karp GI, von Oeyen P, Valone F, Khetarpal VK, Israel M, Mayer RJ et al. Doxorubicin in pregnancy: possible transplacental passage. *Cancer Treat Rep* 1983; 67: 773-7.

Koc ON, McFee M, Reed E, Gerson SL. Detection of platinum-DNA adducts in cord blood lymphocytes following in utero platinum exposure. *Eur J Cancer* 1994; 30A: 716-7.)

Koren G et al. The Motherisk guide to cancer in pregnancy and lactation. 2nd ed. Toronto, Canada: Motherisk Program; 2005

Lishner M et al. Non-Hodgkin's lymphoma and pregnancy. *Leuk Lymphoma*. 1994 Aug;14(5-6):411-3.

Loibl S, von Minckwitz G, Gwyn K, et al. Breast carcinoma during pregnancy. International recommendations from an expert meeting. *Cancer* 2006;106: 237-46.

Matsouka C, Marinopoulos S, Barbaroussi D, Antsaklis A. Acute lymphoblastic leukemia during gestation. *Med Oncol*. 2008;25(2):190-193

Mavrommatis CG et al. Non-Hodgkin's lymphoma during pregnancy--case report. *Eur J Obstet Gynecol Reprod Biol*. 1998 Jul;79(1):95-7.

Mikkola K, Ritari N, Tommiska V, et al. Neurodevelopmental outcome at 5 years of age of a national cohort of extremely low birth weight infants who were born in 1996-1997. *Pediatrics* 2005;116: 1391-400.

Miller RW, Mulvihill JJ. Small head size after atomic irradiation. *Teratology*. 1976 Dec;14(3):355-7.

Molkenboer JF, Vos AH, Schouten HC, Vos MC. Acute lymphoblastic leukaemia in pregnancy. *Neth J Med*. 2005;63(9):361-3.

Muchlow IC. The fate of drugs in pregnancy. *Clin Obstet Gynaecol* 1986; 13:161-175.

Nisce LZ, Tome MA, He S, Lee 3rd BJ, Kutcher GJ. Management of coexisting Hodgkin's disease and pregnancy. *Am J Clin Oncol* 1986;9:146–51.

Nolan TE, Ross WB, Caldwell C. Chronic granulocytic leukemia in pregnancy. A case report. *J Reprod Med* 1988;33:661–663.

Nuyttens JJ et al. Fetal dose during radiotherapy: clinical implementation and review of the literature. *Cancer Radiother*. 2002 Dec;6(6):352-7.

Osada S, Horibe K, Oiwa K, et al. A case of infantile acute monocytic leukemia caused by vertical transmission of the mother's leukemic cells. *Cancer*1990;65:1146-1149.

Pavlidis N. Coexistence of pregnancy and Malignancy. *The Oncologist* 2002; 7:279-287.

Pentheroudakis G, Pavlidis N. Cancer and pregnancy: poema magna, not anymore. *Eur J Cancer* 2006;42:126-40.

Pereg D et al. Cancer in pregnancy: gaps, challenges and solutions. *Cancer Treat Rev*. 2008 Jun;34(4):302-12. Epub 2008 Mar 4.

Pereg D, Koren G, Lishner M. The treatment of Hodgkin's and non-Hodgkin's lymphoma in pregnancy. *Haematologica* 2007;92:1230–7.

Redmond GP. Physiologic changes during pregnancy and their implications for pharmacologic treatment. *Clin Invest Med* 1985; 8:317-32

Rey J et al. Rituximab combined with chemotherapy for lymphoma during pregnancy. *Leuk Res*. 2009 Mar;33(3):e8-9. Epub 2008 May 19.

Rizack T, Mega A, Legare R, Castillo J. Management of hematological malignancies during pregnancy. *Am J Hematol*. 2009;84(12):830-841.

Roboz J, Gleicher N, Wu K, Chanihian P, Kerenyi T, Holland J. Does doxorubicin cross the placenta? *Lancet* 1979; 2: 1382-3.

Russell MA, Carpenter MW, Akhtar MS, Lagattuta TF, Egorin MJ. Imatinib mesylate and metabolite concentrations in maternal blood, umbilical cord blood, placenta and breast milk. *J Perinatol*. 2007;27(4):241-243.

Sadural E, Smith LG. Hematologic Malignancies during pregnancy. *Clin Obstet Gynecol* 1995;38: 535-546.

Sanz MA, Lo-Coco F. Modern approaches to treating acute promyelocytic leukemia. *J Clin Oncol*. 2011 Feb 10;29(5):495-503.

Shapira T Pereg D &Lishner M How I treat acute and chronic leukemia in pregnancy.*Blood Rev* 2008;247-259.

Siu SS, Yip SK, Cheung CW, et al. Treatment of intractable hyperemesis gravidarum by ondansetron. *Eur J Obstet Gynecol Reprod Biol* 2002;105:73–74.

Sorosky JI, Sood AK, Buekers TE. The use of chemotherapeutic agents during pregnancy. *Obstet Gynecol Clin North Am* 1997;24: 591-9.

Spitzer M et al. Non-Hodgkin's lymphoma during pregnancy. *Gynecol Oncol.* 1991 Dec;43(3):309-12.

Syme MR, Paxton JW, Keelan JA. Drug transfer and metabolism by the human placenta. *Clin Pharmacokinet* 2004;43(8): 487-514

Thauvin-Robinet C, Maingueneau C, Robert E, Elefant E, Guy H, Caillot D, Casasnovas RO, Douvier S, Nivelon-Chevallier A. Exposure to hydroxyurea during pregnancy: a case series. *Leukemia*. 2001;15(8):1309-1311.

Tincello DG, Johnstone MJ. Treatment of hyperemesis gravidarum with the 5-HT3 antagonist ondansetron (Zofran). *Postgrad Med J* 1996;72:688–689.

Turchi JJ, Villasis C. Antracyclines in the treatment of malignancy in pregnancy. *Cancer* 1988; 61:425-440.

Van Calsteren K, Berteloot P, Hanssens M, et al. In utero exposure to chemotherapy: effect on cardiac and neurologic outcome. *J Clin Oncol* 2006;24(12): e16-e17

Van Calsteren K, Heyns L, De Smet F, et al. Cancer during pregnancy: an analysis of 215 patients emphasizing the obstetrical and the neonatal outcomes. *J Clin Oncol* 2010;28: 683-9.

Van Calsteren K, Verbesselt R, Beijnen J, et al. Transplacental transfer of anthracyclines, vinblastine and 4-hydroxy-cyclophosphamide in a baboon model. *Gynecol Oncol* 2010;119(3):594-600. Epub 2010 Sep 17).

Van Calsteren K, Verbesselt R, Devlieger R, et al. Transplacental transfer of paclitaxel, docetaxel, carboplatin and trastuzumab in a baboon model. *Int J Gynecol Cancer* 2010; Dec;20(9):1456-64

Van Calsteren K, Verbesselt R, Ottevanger N, et al.Pharmacokinetics of chemotherapeutic agents in pregnancy: a preclinical and clinical study.Acta Obstet Gynecol Scand. 2010 Oct;89:1338-45

Van Calsteren, K, Verbesselt R, Van Bree R, et al. Substantial variation in transplacental transfer of chemotherapeutic agents in a mouse model. *Reprod Sci* 2011 Jan;18(1):57-63. Epub 2010 Sep 8

Van der Velden VHJ, Willemse MJ, Mulder MF, et al. Clearance of maternal leukemic cells in neonate. *Br J Haematol* 2001;114:104-106.

Webb JA, Thomsen HS & Morcos SK; Members of Contrast Media Safety Committee of European Society of Urogenital Radiology (ESUR). The use of iodinated and gadiolinium contrast media during pregnancy and lactation. *Eur Radiol.* 2005 Jun;15(6):1234-40. Epub 2004 Dec 18

Welsh TM, Thompson J, Lim S. Chronic lymphocytic leukemia in pregnancy. *Leukemia* 2000;14:1155-1156.

Werler MM et al. Use of over-the-counter medications during pregnancy. *Am J Obstet Gynecol*. 2005 Sep;193(3 Pt 1):771-7.

Williams S, Schilsky R. Antineoplastic drugs administered during pregnancy *Semin Oncol* 2000; 27(6):618-622.

Wood NS, Marlow N, Costeloe K, Gibson AT, Wilkinson AR. Neurologic and developmental disability after extremely preterm birth. EPICure Study Group. *N Engl J Med* 2000;343: 378-84

World MJ. Ondansetron and hyperemesis gravidarum. *Lancet* 1993;341:185

Yang D, Hladnik L. Treatment of acute promyelocytic leukemia during pregnancy. *Pharmacotherapy*. 2009;29(6):709-724.

14

Cord Blood Transplantation in Adults with Acute Leukemia

Takaaki Konuma[1] and Satoshi Takahashi[2]
[1]*Department of Cellular and Molecular Medicine, Graduate School of Medicine, Chiba University, Chiba,*
[2]*Division of Molecular Therapy, Advanced Clinical Research Center, Institute of Medical Science, University of Tokyo, Tokyo, Japan*

1. Introduction

Allogeneic hematopoietic stem cell transplantation (HSCT) with some graft sources such as bone marrow (BM), mobilized peripheral blood (PB) and cord blood (CB) offers the only curative potential for many patients with high risk hematological malignancies, particularly acute leukemia. Although BM from human leukocyte antigen (HLA)-identical related donors within immediate families is a frontline graft source for this treatment, an alternative stem cell source has increasingly provided for patients lacking HLA-identical related donors. Recently, CB has been considered an acceptable alternative to source of stem cells in unrelated allogeneic HSCT for pediatric and adult patients without HLA-identical related or unrelated donors. This review focuses on clinical results of cord blood transplantation (CBT) including factors associated with transplantation outcomes and clinical comparison studies of CBT and other sources of allogeneic HSCT in adults with acute leukemia. Several strategies including a reduced intensity regimen and double CB units from different donors have been developed to overcome the limited cell dose in CBT for adults. Moreover, to reflect the current encouraging reports and potential starategies, the possibility of CB for immune therapy in the setting of allogeneic HSCT is also discussed.

More than 50 years ago in 1957, Thomas et al. reported the first experience with allogeneic bone marrow transplantation (BMT) in patients with advanced leukemia (Thomas et al., 1957) and since then allogeneic HSCT has been a curative treatment for patients with both malignant and non-malignant hematologic diseases (Appelbaum, 2007). The initial purpose of infusion of BM was rescue of the BM function against myeloablaitive dose of radiation and/or chemotherapy, which generates killing of leukemia cells. Thereafter, the evidence of a graft-versus-leukemia (GVL) effect, which is mediated by both host histocompatibility antigen-specific T cells, tumor antigen-specific T cells and Natural killer (NK) cells against leukemia cells, confirmed that allogeneic HSCT is also the only form of cancer immune therapy for leukemia refractory to chemotherapy (Jenq & van den Brink, 2010).

Although allogeneic HSCT was initially limited to the approximately two-thirds of patients with a suitably HLA-identical related donor, an alternative stem cell source has increasingly provided for patients lacking HLA-identical related donors. After Broxmeyer et al.

demonstrated that CB included a number of hematopoietic stem/progenitor cells that would be capable of hematopoietic reconstitution in humans (Broxmeyer et al., 1989), the first CBT was reported by Gluckman et al. in a child with Fanconi anemia using CB from his HLA-matched sister in 1988 (Gluckman et al., 1989). Since the first success of CBT, Rubinstein et al. established the first unrelated CB bank at the New York Blood Center in 1992 (Rubinstein et al., 1993, 1995). Since then, CB banks have been developed worldwide for not only related but also unrelated CBT with more than 3000 CB transplants performed annually around the world (Foeken et al., 2010). In 1996, Laporte et al. reported a first adult patient with chronic myelogenous leukemia (CML) who underwent the transplantation of CB from unrelated donor (Laporte et al., 1996). Earlier, most patients were pediatric (Kurtzberg et al., 1996; Wagner et al., 1996; Rubinstein et al., 1998) because of the relatively lower cell doses in CB grafts, followed by an increased number of adult CBT (Laughlin et al., 2001; Sanz et al., 2001), showing that CB could effectively restore hematopoiesis with acceptable incidence of severe graft-versus-host disease (GVHD). Recently, CB has been considered an acceptable alternative to source of hematopoietic stem cells (HSCs) in unrelated allogeneic HSCT for pediatric and adult patients without HLA-identical related or unrelated donors.

In comparison with other sources of allogeneic HSCT, CBT has several clinical advantages, including rapid and convenient availability because of the stored CB units in the CB bank, less stringent criteria for HLA matching for donor-recipient selection, lower incidence of GVHD without compromising GVL effects, low risk of viral transmitting and the absence of risk for donors, whereas limited cell dose remains the main disadvantage in CBT. The limited cell dose might contribute to higher incidence of graft failure and delayed neutrophil recovery, which are mostly due to higher risk of bacterial and fungal infections in the early phase after CBT (Narimatsu et al., 2005; Parody et al., 2006; Tomonari et al., 2007; Yazaki et al., 2009; Miyakoshi et al., 2007; van Burik & Brunstein, 2007; Delaney et al., 2009). Moreover, viral infections may be more common after CBT than after BMT/PBSCT, essentially attributable to delayed immune reconstitutions after CBT (Tomonari et al., 2003a, 2003b, 2004, 2005; Parody et al., 2006; van Burik & Brunstein, 2007; Delaney et al., 2009). The advantages and disadvantages of CB as a source of allogeneic HSCT are shown in Table1.

2. Clinical results in adults with acute leukemia

2.1 Factors associated with clinical outcomes in CBT

It is known that larger total nucleated cell (TNC) dose improve faster hematopoietic recovery, decrease treatment-related mortality (TRM) and survival of CBT recipients (Rubinstein et al., 1998; Laughlin et al., 2001; Gluckman et al., 2004; Arcese et al., 2006; Barker et al., 2010). Recent New York Blood Center analysis of 1061 recipients of single-unit myeloablative CBT for leukemia or myelodysplastic syndrome (MDS) demonstrated that TNC dose and HLA-match each affected survival via their effect on TRM (Barker et al., 2010). These analysis recommended the best transplantation outcomes were in recipients of 6 of 6 units regardless of precryopreservation TNC dose (median, 4.0×10^7cells/kg), indicating that HLA match at HLA-A and -B antigens and -DRB1 alleles, rather than high TNC dose, was the more favorable graft characteristic. Further, recipients of 4 of 6 units required a precryopreservation TNC $\geq 5.0\times10^7$cells/kg to achieve comparable TRM and disease-free survival (DFS) to that of recipients of 5 of 6 units with a TNC $\geq 2.5\times10^7$cells/kg. In contrast, the minimum cell dose is not clear for adults who have indications for CBT. In a

	CB	BM/ mobilized PB
Advantages		
Availability of grafts	Rapid (less than one month)	Prolonged (a few months)
Requirement of HLA matching	4/6 or higher	6/6
Risk of severe GVHD	Lower risk	Higher risk
Risk of viral transmission	Very low risk	Low Risk
Risk of donor	No risk	Low Risk
Disadvantages		
Number of infused nucleated cells	Limited cell dose	Higher cell dose
Speed of hematopoietic recovery	Delay	Faster than CB
Risk of infection after HSCT	Higher risk than BM/PB	High risk
Possibility of donor lymphocyte infusion or second HSCT from same donor	Impossible	Possible
Potential of congenital disease transmission	Low potential	Few potential

CB indicates cord blood; BM, bone marrow; PB, peripheral blood; HLA, human leukocyte antigen; GVHD, graft-versus-host disease; HSCT, hematopoietic stem cell transplantation.

Table 1. Advantages and disadvantages of CB as a source of hematopoietic stem cell compared with BM or mobilized PB

Japanease study, patients receiving CB grafts containing 1-2×10^7cells/kg were observed and four of seven low-cell-dose recipients survived with longer follow-up (Takahashi et al., 2006). Those results indicated that CB grafts containing fewer than 2×10^7cells/kg may be useful for cases for which no grafts with higher cell doses or other stem cell sources are available. On the other hands, Wagner et al. demonstrated that a correlation between higher CD34+ cell dose and rate of engraftment in pediatric patients (Wagner et al., 2002). However, CD34+ cell measurement is not standardized between CB banks.

HLA compatibility was thought to be another key factor in CBT outcome, as with other stem cell sources. Several studies have shown that HLA mismatch at HLA-A, -B antigens and -DRB1 alleles leads to delayed engraftment, increased severity of acute GVHD, increased TRM and decreased survival (Rubinstein et al., 1998; Gluckman et al., 2004; Barker et al., 2010; Delaney & Ballen, 2010). Although increasing the number of HLA mismatching might be associated with decreased relapse risk in patients with leukemia, suggested GVL effect increased in HLA-mismatched CBT, HLA-mismatch does not offer any benefit in DFS (Barker et al., 2010). In general, recommended CB unit is ≥ 4 of 6 HLA-A, -B antigen and -DRB1 allele matched with the patient.

The role of anti-HLA antibodies in graft rejection of organ transplantations has been analyzed extensively. The majority of CBTs have HLA disparities. Takanashi et al. reported the impact that patients' pretransplantation anti-HLA antibodies have on the outcome of myeloablative CBT using single unit (Takanashi et al., 2010). Of 386 cases tested, 89 (23.1%) were anti-HLA antibody-positive. Of the 89 antibody-positive cases, 20 patients had specificity against the CB HLA. Cumulative incidence (CI) of neutrophil recovery 60 days after transplantation was 83% for the antibody-negative group, 73% for antibody-positive, but only 32% for the positive against CB ($p<0.0001$). These data suggested that patients' pretransplantation anti-HLA antibodies should be tested and considered in the selection of CB.

The logistics of the selection of CB grafts, including how to select double-unit grafts, for transplantation are as practiced by each centers (Shaw et al., 2009; Rocha & Gluckman, 2009; Barker et al., 2011).

2.2 Comparisons of unrelated donor cord blood and other stem cell sources

After Laughlin et al. initially reported the feasibility in adult patients receiving myeloablative CBT (Laughlin et al., 2001), two registration-based and one single-institution studies comparing both CBT and BMT from unrelated donor in adult patients with acute leukemia after myeloablative conditioning were published (Laughlin et al., 2004; Rocha et al., 2004; Takahashi et al., 2004). Selected studies are detailed in Table 2. These studies demonstrated that hematological recovery after CBT was slower when compared to unrelated BMT and that the incidence of severe acute and chronic GVHD was significantly lower after CBT than after BMT. However, the DFS rate and relapse incidence in CB recipients were not inferior to those in BM recipients. In a two meta-analysis using pooled comparative data from the above three reports, Hwang et al. reported that TRM (pooled estimate 1.04, 95% confidence interval [CI]=0.52-2.08; p=0.91) and DFS (pooled estimate 0.59, 95%CI=0.18-1.96; p=0.39) were not statistically different in adults (Hwang et al., 2007), whereas Wang et al. reported overall survival (OS) after CBT (hazard ratio [HR] 1.26, 95%CI=1.13-1.40) was statistically inferior in adults (Wang et al., 2010). Recently, Eapen et al. reported a comparative analysis of CBT from unrelated donor with BMT or peripheral blood stem cell transplantation (PBSCT) from unrelated donors in 1525 adult patients with acute leukemia after myeloablative conditioning (Eapen et al., 2010). 165 received CBT, 888 received PBSCT, and 472 received BMT. Leukaemia-free survival (LFS) in patients after CBT was comparable with that after 8/8 and 7/8 allele-matched PBSCT or BMT. However, TRM was higher after CBT than after 8/8 allele-matched PBSCT (HR 1.62, 95%CI=1.18-2.23; p=0.003) or BMT (HR 1.69, 95%CI=1.19-2.39; p=0.003). Grades II to IV acute and chronic GVHD were lower in CBT recipients compared with allele-matched PBSCT (HR 0.57, 95%=0.42-0.77; p=0.002 and HR 0.38, 95%CI=0.27-0.53; p=0.003, respectively), while the incidence of chronic, but not acute GVHD, was lower after CBT than after 8/8 allele-matched BMT (HR 0.63, 95%CI=0.44-0.90; p=0.01).

Data comparing both CBT and BMT or PBSCT from related donors in adult patients is equally encouraging. We studied the outcomes of 171 adults with hematological malignancies who received unrelated CBT as a primary unrelated stem cell source (n=100), or BMT or PBSCT from related donors (n=71;55 BMT and 16 PBSCT) followed by myeloablative regimens (Takahashi et al., 2007). Significant delays in engraftment occurred after CBT. The CIs of grades III to IV acute and extensive type chronic GVHD among CBT recipients were significantly lower than those among BMT/PBSCT recipients. Multivariate analysis demonstrated no apparent differences in TRM (9% in CBT and 13% in BMT/PBSCT), relapse (17% in CBT and 26% in BMT/PBSCT) and DFS (70% in CBT and 60% in BMT/PBSCT). Unrelated CB could be as safe and effective a stem cell source as related BM or mobilized PB for adult patients when it is used as a primary unrelated stem cell source.

Reference	Disease	HSC source: number of patients	Median age (years)	Median time to ANC≥500/µl (days)	Incidence of grade II-IV acute GVHD (%)	Incidence of TRM (year)	Relapse rate (year)	Probablity of DFS (year)
Laughlin et al.,2004	AML ALL CML MDS	CB:150	16-60	27	41	63%	17%	23% (3)
		uBM:367		20	48	46%	23%	33% (3)
		MuBM:83		18	51	65%	14%	19% (3)
Roche et al.,2004	AML	CB:98	25	26	26	44% (2)	23% (2)	33% (2)
	ALL	uBM:584	32	19	39	38% (2)	23% (2)	38% (2)
Takahashi et al.,2004	AML ALL Other	CB:68	36	22	30	9% (1)	16% (2)	74% (2)
		uBM:39	26	18	30	29% (1)	25% (2)	44% (2)
Takahashi et al.,2007	AML ALL Other	CB:100	37	22	52	9% (1)	17% (3)	70% (3)
		rBM/PB:71	40	17	52	13% (1)	26% (3)	60% (3)
Kumar et al.,2008	ALL138	CB:19	19	NA	32*	34% (3)	5% (3)	61% (3)
		rBM:90	90	NA	20*	44% (3)	26% (3)	27% (3)
		uBM:15	15	NA	10*	53% (3)	20% (3)	13% (3)
		MuBM:14	14	NA	7*	86% (3)	0% (3)	14% (3)
Atsuta et al.,2009	AML:484	CB:173	38	NA	32	30% (1)	31% (2)	36% (2)
		uBM:311	38	NA	35	19% (1)	24% (2)	54% (2)
	ALL:336	CB:114	34	NA	28	21% (1)	31% (2)	45% (2)
		uBM:222	32	NA	42	23% (1)	24% (2)	51% (2)
Eapen et al.,2010	AML ALL	CB:165	28	24	30	37% (2)	1.00**	1.00**
		uBM:332	39	19	39	22% (2)	0.85**	1.15**
		MuBM:140			46	34% (2)	0.84**	0.93**
		uPB:632	33	14	48	24% (2)	0.85**	1.12**
		MuPB:256			52	38% (2)	0.91**	0.91**

CBT indicates cord blood transplantation; AML, acute myeloid leukemia; ALL, acute lymphoblastic leukemia; CML, chronic myelogenous leukemia; MDS, myelodysplastic syndrome; HSC, hematopoietic stem cell; CB, cord blood; uBM, unrelated bone marrow; MuBM, mismatched unrelated bone marrow; rBM/PB, related bone marrow/ peripheral blood; uPB, unrelated peripheral blood; MuPB, mismatched unrelated peripheral blood; ANC, absolute neutrophil count; NA, information not available; GVHD, graft-versus-host disease; TRM, treatment-related mortality; DFS, disease-free survival.
* The incidence of grade III-IV acute GVHD was shown in this study.
**Results were expressed as hazard ratios (the relative rate of occurrence of the event with CB as compared with another).

Table 2. Published comparative reports of CBT and other stem cell sources in adults with acute leukemia

Another alternative option for patients lacking an HLA-matched related and unrelated donor is allogeneic HSCT from haploidentical related donors. Almost all patients will have available to them a haploidentical family member donor. However, randomized study has never been published the comparison of outcomes of haploidentical HSCT and CBT for adult patients with leukemia (Ballen & Spitzer, 2011). Clinical study comparing haploidentical HSCT to CBT are warranted.

Reports of disease-specific outcomes for adult patients with acute myeloid leukemia (AML) or acute lymphoblastic leukemia (ALL) after CBT are still limited (Ooi et al., 2004, 2008, 2009; Konuma et al, 2009a). Kumar et al. studied the relative impact of donor source on outcomes following myeloablative HSCT for 138 adult patients with ALL (Kumar et al., 2008). When compared with unrelated BMT, OS with CBT was better (relative risk [RR] 0.3, 95%CI=0.1-0.7; p=0.01). Recently, Atsuta et al. reported a disease-specific comparison of CBT and HLA allele-matched unrelated BMT among 484 patients with AML (AML; 173 CB and 311 BM) and 336 patients with ALL (ALL; 114 CB and 222 BM) who received myeloablative transplantations (Atsuta et al., 2009). In multivariate analyses, among AML cases, lower OS (HR 1.5, 95%CI=1.0-2.0; p=0.028) and LFS (HR 1.5, 95%CI=1.1-2.0; p=0.012) were observed in CB recipients. The relapse rate did not differ between the 2 groups of AML (HR 1.2, 95%CI=0.8-1.9; p=0.38). However, the TRM rate showed higher trend in CB recipients (HR 1.5, 95%CI=1.0-2.3; p=0.085). In ALL, there was no significant difference between the groups for relapse (HR 1.4, 95%CI=0.8-2.4; p=0.19) and TRM (HR 1.0, 95%CI=0.6-1.7; p=0.98), which contributed to similar OS (HR 1.1, 95%CI=0.7-1.6; p=0.78) and LFS (HR 1.2, 95%CI=0.9-1.8; p=0.28).

Taken together, their results showed that CBT is feasible in adults when a CB unit contains a higher number of cells and when a transplant is needed urgently, and should be considered an option as an allogeneic stem cell source for patients lacking an HLA-matched unrelated donor. The results also showed that despite increased HLA disparity, CBT from unrelated donors is promising in adults with acute leukemia.

3. Improvement methods of engraftment and delay hematopoietic recovery

The relatively low number of HSCs and progenitors per one unit is a main limitation of CB instead of BM or mobilized PB as a stem cell source for HSCT, especially in adults. The low cell dose available for HSCT might contribute to higher incidence of graft failure, delayed hematopoietic recovery and delayed immune reconstitution. As a consequence, it is well known that transplanted cell dose is associated with TRM and survival after CBT. There have been several developing strategies to overcome the obstacle of low number of cell dose using CB as a stem cell source for transplantation, especially in adults.

3.1 Ex vivo expansion of cord blood

To improve limited cell dose contained in CB grafts, one attractive option is ex vivo expansion of CB which has been shown to have greater proliferative and self-renewal capacity when compared to the other sources of HSCs (Broxmeyer et al., 1992; Hows et al., 1992). Initial CB expansion attempts have used a variety of cytokines, such as stem cell factor (SCF), fms-like tyrosine kinase 3 (flt-3) ligand, thrombopoietin (TPO) and G-CSF (granulocyte colony-stimulating factor), reagents, such as polyamine copper chelator, tetraethylenepentamine (TEPA), and mesenchymal stem cells (MSCs), to cell culture. Several clinical studies were investigated, but have not achieved clinically relevant effects (Shpall et al., 2002; de Lima et al., 2008, 2010; Jaroscak et al., 2003; Delaney et al., 2010; Kelly et al., 2009) (Table 3). Delancy et al. report the development of a clinically relevant Notch-mediated ex vivo expansion system for CB CD34+ cells and the phase I study involving transplantation of a non-manipulated unit along with CB progenitors from a second CB unit that have undergone Notch-mediated ex vivo expansion in 10 patients with acute leukemia (Delaney et al., 2010). After ex vivo expansion, there was an average fold expansion of CD34+ cells of 164 and an average fold expansion of total cell numbers of 562. The infused CD34+ cell dose derived from the expanded CB graft averaged 6×10^6 CD34+cells/kg versus 0.24×10^6 CD34+cells/kg (p=0.0004) from the non-manipulated CB graft. Time to absolute neutrophil count (ANC) ≥500/µl was shortened significantly with a median time of 16 days (range, 7-34 days) compared with cohort of 20 patients undergoing double CBT with a median time of 26 days (range, 16–48 days; p= 0.002), despite loss of contribution to engraftment from the expanded cell graft. This is highly suggestive of a facilitating effect of the cultured cells in promoting engraftment from the non-manipulated CB unit. This is the first instance of rapid engraftment derived from ex vivo expanded CB stem/progenitor cells in humans.

Expansion type	Reference	Number of patients	Cytokines	Days in culture	TNC fold expansion (folds)	CD34+ fold expansion (folds)	Median time to ANC≥500 /µl (days)	Median time to PLT≥20000/µl (days)	Incidence of each grade acute GVHD (%)	Survival (duration of follow up)
Liquid culture	Shpall et al.,2002	37	SCF,G-CSF,TPO	10	56	4	28	106	II to IV:67% III to IV:40%	32% (30 months)
	de Lima et al.,2008	10	SCF,Flt3L, G-CSF,TPO,IL-6+TEPA	21	219	6	30	48	II to IV:44% III to IV:0%	30% (180 days)
	Delany et al.,2010	10	Notch ligand,SCF, Flt3L,TPO,IL-6,IL-3	16	562	164	16	NA	II to IV:9/9 III to IV:1/9	7/10 alive (1 year)
Stromal co-culture	de Lima et al.,2010	32	SCF,Flt3L, G-CSF,TPO+ MSCs	14	40	14	15	40	II to IV:50% III to IV:16%	40% (1 year)
Continuous perfusion system	Jaroscak et al.,2003	27	PIXY321,Flt3L,EPO	12	2.4	0.5	22	71	II to IV:36% III to IV:22%	39% (41 months)

CBT indicates cord blood transplantation; CB, cord blood; SCF, stem cell factor; G-CSF, granulocyte colony-stimulating factor; TPO, thrombopoietin; Flt3L, fms-like tyrosine kinase 3 ligand; IL, interleukin; TEPA, tetraethylenepentamine; MSCs, mesenchymal stem cells; PIXY321, granulocyte-macrophage colony-stimulating factor/interleukin-3 fusion protein; EPO, erythropoietin; TNC, total nucleated cell; ANC, absolute neutrophil count; PLT, platelet; NA, information not available; GVHD, graft-versus-host disease.

Table 3. Published clinical trials of CBT using ex vivo expanded CB

3.2 Reduced-intensity conditioning regimen

Myeloablative conditioning (MAC) regimens for allogeneic HSCT have been restricted to younger patients without comorbidities, because TRM occurs more frequently among elderly patients and those with serious comorbidities. Reduced-intensity conditioning (RIC) regimens have emerged as a novel transplantation modality for those patients with the expectation of reducing TRM and increasing survival after allogeneic HSCT. This strategy was recently expanded for quick use with stem cell sources not only from BM or mobilized PB, but also from CB (Barker et al., 2003; Miyakoshi et al., 2004; Chao et al., 2004; Misawa et al., 2006; Brunstein et al., 2007; Komatsu et al., 2007; Majhail et al., 2008; Uchida et al., 2008; Cutler & Ballen, 2009; Horwitz & Chao, 2010). Several studies have reported on CBT using RIC for adult patients with leukemia, and selected studies using mainly single CB unit are detailed in Table 4. The University of Minnesota group initially reported unrelated CBT for adults after RIC, demonstrating that 0-2 antigen mismatched CBT was sufficient to engraft most adults after RIC and was associated with low incidence of severe acute GVHD (Barker et al., 2003). They reported the updated results of this strategy in 110 adult patients with hematological disease to confirm the suitability of this strategy (Brunstein et al., 2007). Neutrophil recovery was achieved in 92% at the median of 12 days. The incidence of grades III to IV acute GVHD was 22%. However, these studies included the results of transplantation of both single and double CB grafts, because the target cell dose for the CB graft was $3x10^7$cells/kg. Recenly, same group reported the comparative efficacy of CBT after RIC relative to MAC in 119 adult patients with AML in CR (complete remission) (Oran et al., 2011). The incidence of neutrophil recovery at day +42 was higher with RIC (RIC:94% vs MAC:82%; p<0.1). Incidence of grades II to IV acute GVHD was decreased (RIC:47% vs MAC:67%; p<0.01). Using RIC, 3-year LFS was decreased (RIC:31% vs MAC:55%; p=0.02) and 3-year relapse incidence was increased (RIC:43% vs MAC:9%; p<0.01). Two-year TRM was similar (RIC:19% vs MAC:27%; p=0.55). In multivariate analysis, RIC recipients and those in CR2 with CR1 duration <1 year had higher risk of relapse and poorer LFS with no independent predictors of TRM. Further studies are warranted to establish criteria for eligible patients and optimal RIC regimens for CBT.

Reference	Number of patients	Conditining regimen	Median TNC cell dose (/kg)	Median CD34+ cell dose (/kg)	Median time to ANC≥500 /μl (days)	Incidence of grade II-IV acute GVHD (%)	Incidence of TRM (year)	Relapse rate (year)	Probablity of OS (year)
Miyakoshi et al.,2004	30	Flu/Mel/TBI4 Gy	3.1	0.7	17.5	27	27% (100 days)	10%[3/30pt]	33% (1)
Chao et al.,2004	13	Flu/CY/ATG	2.1	1.3	12	40%[2/5pt]	31%[4/13pt]	46%[6/13pt]	22% (4)
Misawa et al.,2006	12	Flu/CY/TBI3 Gy	2.5	0.9	17	62.5	50%[6/12pt]	8%[1/12pt]	42% (1)
Brustein et al.,2007*	110 (2CB:93) (1CB:17)	CY/Flu/TBI2 Gy	3.7(2CB) 3.3(1CB)	4.9(2CB) 3.8(1CB)	12	59	26% (3)	31% (3)	45% (3)
Komatsu et al.,2007	17	Flu/BU	2.6	0.7	18	0	24%[4/17pt]	41%[7/17pt]	35%[6/17pt] (13months)
Majhail et al.,2008	43	CY/Flu/TBI2 Gy	4.0	0.4	NA	49	28%(180 days)	NA	34% (3)
Uchida et al.,2008	70	Flu/Mel/TBI4 Gy	2.8	0.8	18	61	53%[37/70pt]	26%[18/70pt]	23% (2)

CBT indicates cord blood transplantation; Flu, fludarabine; Mel, melphalan; TBI, total body irradiation; CY, cyclophosphamide; ATG, antithymocyte globulin; BU, busulfan; TNC, total nucleated cell; ANC, absolute neutrophil count; NA, information not available; GVHD, graft-versus-host disease; pt, patients; TRM, treatment-related mortality; OS, overall survival.
*Some results included CBT using double unit cord blood.

Table 4. Published reports of CBT using reduced-intensity conditioning in adults

3.3 Transplantation using multiple grafts of cord blood

Double CBT (dCBT) was initially developed as a strategy to overcome the cell dose limitation preventing the number of adults transplanted with single unit CB, and has been widely used in United States and Europe. Several studies have reported on double CBT for adult patients with acute leukemia (Barker et al., 2005; Ballen et al., 2007; Rodrigues et al., 2009; MacMillan et al., 2009a; Gutman et al., 2009; Verneris et al., 2009; Cutler et al., 2010; Rocha et al., 2010a, 2010b; Brunstein et al., 2010; Delaney et al., 2009; Stanevsky et al., 2010), and representative studies are detailed in Table 5. Several studies showed that double CBT is associated with a higher incidence of acute GVHD compared with single CBT (sCBT). Interestingly,the risk of relapse after double CBT is significantly lower compared with single CBT for patients with leukemia in remission, suggesting that a greater GVL effect due to HLA disparity for the double CB recipient (Brunstein et al., 2007, 2010; Rodrigues et al., 2009; Verneris et al., 2009). On the other hand, neutrophil engraftment and LFS were similar for recipients of single or double CB units. Recently, Roche et al. also reported the results of single (n=377) and double (n=230) CBT in adult patients with AML or ALL in remission (Rocha et al., 2010a). In patients transplanted in CR 1, there were no statistical differences in CI of neutrophil recovery (dCBT 78% vs sCBT 82%; p=0.11). Acute GVHD was higher after dCBT compared with sCBT (45% vs 27%; p<0.001). At 3 years, relapse incidence was 15% after dCBT and 25% after sCBT (p=0.03). Estimated 3 years LFS was 53% after dCBT and

Reference	Number of patients	Conditioning regimen	Median time to ANC≥500/μl (days)	Incidence of grade II-IV acute GVHD (%)	Incidence of TRM (year)	Relapse rate (year)	Probablity of DFS (year)
Barker et al.,2005	23	CY/TBI13.2Gy	23	65	22%(6months)	NA	57% (1)
Brunstein et al.,2007	93	Flu/CY/TBI2Gy	12*	62	26%(3)*	31%(3) *	39% (3)
Ballen et al., 2007	21	Flu/Mel/ATG	20	40	19%(6months)	14% [3/21pt]	67% (1)
Rodrigues et al.,2009	26	MAC,RIC	17	32	31% (1)	13% (1)	57% (1)
MacMillan et al.,2009a	185	MAC42%,RIC 58%	NA	58%	24%(1)	NA	NA
Gutman et al.,2009**	31	CY/TBI12Gy/Flu	NA	81	21% (2)	3% (2)	76% (2)
Verneris et al.,2009	93	CY/TBI13.2Gy	25	48	29%(1)	19%(5)	51% (5)
Cutler et al.,2010	32	Flu/Mel/ATG	21	9	34%(2)	34%(2)	31%(2)
Rocha et al.,2010a	230	RIC53%	CR1:78%*** CR2<:85%***	CR1:45 CR2<:33	CR1:32%(3) CR2<:34%(3)	CR1:15%(3) CR2<:31%(3)	CR1:53%(3) CR2<:35%(3)
Brunstein et al.2010	128	CY/TBI12Gy/Flu	26	60	34 % (5)	15% (5)	51% (3)

CBT indicates cord blood transplantation; CB, cord blood; CY, cyclophosphamide; TBI, total body irradiation; Flu, fludarabine; Mel, melphalan; ATG, antithymocyte globulin; MAC, myeloablative conditioning; RIC, reduced-intensity conditioning; ANC, absolute neutrophil count; NA, information not available; CR, complete remission; GVHD, graft-versus-host disease; TRM, treatment-related mortality; pt, patients; DFS, disease-free survival.
*Some results included CBT using single unit cord blood.
** This study included 27 patients received two units (six of whom had one of the two units CD34+ selected and ex vivo expanded) and four received single units.
***Results were expressed as cumulative incidence of neutrophil recovery.

Table 5. Published reports of CBT using double units CB in adults

39% after sCBT (p=0.09). However, in patients transplanted in CR2 and CR3, estimated 3 years LFS was 35% after dCBT and 31% after sCBT (p=0.48). These data concluded double CBT has extended the use of CBT for patients otherwise not eligible for single CBT and importantly is associated with better outcomes in adults with acute leukemia transplanted in early phase of the disease. Brunstein et al. reported 536 patients with leukemia who underwent transplantation with an HLA allele-matched related donor (MRD, n=204), HLA allele-matched unrelated donor (MUD, n=152) or 1-antigen-mismatched unrelated adult donor (MMUD, n=52) or 4-6/6 HLA matched double CB (dCB, n=128) graft after myeloablative conditioning (Brunstein et al., 2010). All patients received MAC with cyclophosphamide (CY) 120 mg/kg and total body irradiation (TBI) 12 to 13.2 Gy with the addition of fludarabine (Flu) 75 mg/m^2 in recipients of dCBT. LFS at 5 years was similar for each donor type (dCB 51%, MRD 33%, MUD 48%, MMUD 38%). The risk of relapse was lower in recipients of dCB (15%) compared with MRD (43%), MUD (37%) and MMUD (35%), yet nonrelapse mortality was higher for dCB (34%), MRD (24%), and MUD (14%). They conclude that LFS after double CBT is comparable with that observed after MRD and MUD transplantation. Although clinical experience using double CBT is progressing as described above, 1 CB unit ultimately dominates and confers durable engraftment, but little is known about the mechanism of the determinants of durable engraftment by 1 CB unit after double CBT. More recently, Avery et al. demonstrated that indicators of CB unit potency including TNC dose, colony-forming unit (CFU), CD3+, and viable CD34+ cell content, predict the dominating unit, but HLA matching does not appear to play a role in unit dominance (Avery et al., 2011).

3.4 Co-transplantation with third party donor

Fernandez et al. have developed the strategy of single unit CBT with co-infusion of a limited number of mobilized HSC (MHSC) from an HLA-mismached third party donor (TPD) (Fernández et al., 2003; Magro et al., 2006; Bautista et al., 2009). They reported the updated results of this strategy in 55 adult patients with high-risk hematological malignancies (Bautista et al., 2009). The median CB cell dose of 2.37x10^{7}cells/kg (the median CB CD34+ cells of 0.11x10^{6}cells/kg) and the median TPD-MHSC CD34+ cells of 2.4x10^{6}cells/kg were transplanted. The median time to recovery of neutophils and CB derived neutophils as well as to complete CB chimerism was 10, 21 and 44 days. Finally, TPD-MHSC derived hematopoiesis disappeared completely. The 5 years OS and DFS were 56 % and 47%, respectively. This strategies suggested that transient hematopoiesis from TPD-MHSC might reduce the incidence of neutropenia-related serious infection, thus leading to the possibility of decreased TRM early after CBT in adult patients.

3.5 Intrabone transplantation

To improve efficient engraftment possibly due to better stem cell homing to the bone marrow, Frassoni et al. reported the phase I/II study of direct intrabone transplantation of single unit CB in 32 patients with acute leukemia (Frassoni et al., 2008). Although the median transplanted cell dose was 2.6x10^{7}cells/kg (range, 1.4-4.2), the median time to recovery of neutrophils in 28 patients and platelets in 27 patients was 23 days (range, 14-44) and 36 days (range 16-64), respectively. All patients with hematopoietic recovery showed complete donor engraftment from 30 days after CBT. No patient developed grades III to IV acute GVHD. This preliminary data suggest that direct intrabone CBT overcomes the problem of graft failure even when low numbers of single unit unrelated HLA-mismatched CB are transplanted in adults and need to be confirmed in a larger number of adult patients.

3.6 Improvement of homing capacity

The interaction of stromal-derived factor-1 (SDF-1)/CXCL12 with CXCR4 mediates the homing of HSCs to the BM. CD26, a surface serine dipeptidylpeptidase IV (DPPIV), cleaves the amino-terminal dipeptide from some chemokines, including SDF-1. Diprotin A, which is inhibitor of CD26 peptidase activity, enhances engraftment of HSCs from CB into nonobese diabetic/severe combined immunodeficiency (NOD/SCID) mice (Campbell et al., 2007). Based on these data, the clinical trial to look the efficiency of CB engraftment using Diprotin A is now warranted. Moreover, several clinical trials should be investigated to answer the efficacy of co-infusion of haploidentical MSCs for the enhancement of engraftment and prevention of graft failure in CBT (Macmillan et al., 2009b; Gonzalo-Daganzo et al., 2009; Bernardo et al., 2011).

4. Immune therapy using cord blood

4.1 Immune reconstitution after CBT

Infection-related mortality is the primary cause of death early after CBT, with most deaths occurring in the first 3-6 months after transplant. Komanduri et al. reported prolonged T lymphopenia, impaired T cell functional responses to superantigens and cytomegalovirus (CMV), thymopoietic failure were important causes of delayed immune reconstitution after CBT in adult (Komanduri et al., 2007). For several months, until recovery of the thymus is restored to support de-novo T cell generation, protective antiviral immunity depends on the activity of postthymic T cells infused within the CB grafts. However, almost all T cells in CB grafts are naïve lymphocytes that have been functionally altered by placental factors to provide a protective environment during pregnancy. T cells in CB grafts need to undergo in-vivo priming, T helper (Th)1/T cytotoxic (Tc)1 maturation, and peripheral expansion before they can afford immunologic protection. Remarkable immunophenotypic changes are notable already in the first 2-3 weeks after CBT. These changes result from apparent 'homeostatic' peripheral T cell expansion in the lymphopenic environment (Szabolcs & Niedzwiecki, 2007; Szabolcs & Cairo, 2010).

4.2 Cellular therapy for viral infection or leukemia after CBT

One of the major limitations of CBT is the lack of donor cells available for posttransplantation donor leukocyte infusions (DLI) to boost immunity for severe viral infection or induce GVL activity for leukemia relapse, because the initial donor is unavailable. Although there was no obvious available source for adoptive cell therapy in the setting of CBT, several researches suggest that adoptive immune therapy using CB immune cells have the potential to improve the outcomes after CBT (Hanley et al., 2010).

4.2.1 Cytotoxic T lymphocytes

Ex vivo generation of T cells from CB naïve T cells has been achieved in several methods using CD3/CD28 costimulation, interleukin (IL)-2, and IL-7 (Mazur et al., 2008; Davis et al., 2010). Moreover, several researchers successfully have generated antigens-specific cytotoxic T lymphocytes (CTLs) from CB. Park et al. developed a protocol to in-vitro-prime and expand CMV-specific CTLs from CB (Park et al., 2006). Recently, Hanley et al. reported the generation of single cultures of CTLs from CB that are specific for CMV, Epstein-Barr virus (EBV) and adenovirus (Adv) (Hanley et al., 2009). The CB CTLs recognized multiple viral epitopes, including CD4-restricted Adv-hexon epitopes and immunosubdominant CD4- and CD8-restricted CMVpp65 epitopes. A clinical trial using CB derived multivirus specific CTLs for prevention and treatment of these virus infection in CB transplant is now underway. To generate CB derived T cells recognizing B-lineage ALL because GVT effects are largely mediated by CTLs, several researchers developed CB derived T cells are expanded and genetically modified to express CD19 chimeric antigen receptors (Serrano et al., 2006; Micklethwaite et al., 2010). The genetically modified T-cell clones revealed an ability to lyse CD19+ leukemic cells specifically and repetitively.

4.2.2 NK cell

NK cells are a subset of lymphocytes with functions associated with innate immunity. NK cells also have been found to substantially contribute to GVT effects. Adoptive immune therapy with NK cells to treat malignancy is actively being investigated in early phase clinical trials. Ruggeri et al. reported the PB derived NK cell alloreactively is capable of preventing relapse of AML in the setting of killer immunoglobulin-like receptor (KIR) ligand-mismatched haploidentical HSCT (Ruggeri et al., 2002). Two retrospective studies on the effects of KIR ligand-mismatching in CBT for leukemia have result in conflicting results. Willemze et al. reported that a favourable effect of KIR ligand-mismatching on relapse rate and survival (Willemze et al., 2009), whereas Brunstein et al. reported no effect on relapse (Brunstein et al., 2009). The impact of KIR ligand-mismatching on relapse after CBT remains to be determined. NK cells are present at the similar percentages in both CB and PB. However, CB NK cells express a relatively higher percentage of inhibitory receptors, such as CD94/NKG2A and KIR (Verneris & Miller, 2009). The expanded CB NK cells exhibit anti leukemic activity in mouse model (Xing et al., 2010). Based on these data, the efficiency of CB NK cells to treat leukemia relapse is now underway.

4.2.3 Regulatory T cell

Regulatory T cells (Tregs) are a suppressive subset of the naturally occurring T cells characterized by their constitutive expression of CD4 and the IL-2 receptor α chain (CD25). Tregs are also characterized by high levels of the forkhead box protein 3 (FoxP3). Tregs can abrogate GVHD in murine models of major histocompatibility complex (MHC) mismatched allogeneic HSCT through suppression of alloreactive effector T cells. In contrast to Tregs from PB, Tregs are readily purified from CB. CB Tregs have greater expansion potential when compared to PB Tregs (Tolar et al., 2009). Brunstein et al. reported that infusion of ex vivo expanded Tregs from CB reduced the incidence of grades II to IV acute GVHD in CBT recipients compared with historical controls without Tregs (Brunstein et al., 2011).

4.2.4 MSCs

MSCs were initially described as a BM-derived mononuclear cell population adhered to plastic with a fibroblast-like morphology, when cultured ex vivo. Thereafter, MSCs can also be isolated from CB (Tolar et al., 2009). These cells are capable of differentiation into multiple lineages, including bone, cartilage and adipocyte cells in particular. The functional aspects of MSCs include tissue repair, hematopoietic engraftment support, immune modulation. Clinical trial studying the effects of BM derived MSCs for the treatment of standard therapy-resistant severe GVHD has been initiated recently with promising results (Le Blanc et al., 2008). However, whether CB derived MSCs have similar beneficial effects for the treatment of severe GVHD is unknown.

5. Problem of donor cell leukemia

Donor cell-derived hematological malignancy is a rare complication after allogeneic HSCT. Previous studies reported that 0.12-5% of patients developed donor cell leukemia (DCL) after allogeneic HSCT (Hertenstein et al., 2005; Flynn & Kaufman, 2007; Wiseman, 2010). Several reports demonstrated that donor cell-derived hematological malignancy occurred in patients after CBT (Matsunaga et al., 2005; Fraser et al., 2005; Ando et al., 2006; Sevilla et al., 2006; Mitsui et al., 2007; Nagamura-Inoue et al., 2007; Hamaki et al., 2008; Konuma et al., 2009b; Crow et al., 2010; Castleton et al., 2010; Ballen et al., 2010; Wang et al., 2011). Ballen et al. reported the occurrence of donor-derived hematological malignancies after double CBT (Ballen et al., 2010). Sixteen patients developed a second hematological malignancy (both cases of MDS/myeloproliferative diseases (MPD) and 14 of the lymphomas) at a median of 134 days after double CBT. The mechanism for causing DCL after allogeneic HSCT is not well understood. The presence of preleukemic clones found only rarely in CB samples might contribute to the development of DCL after CBT (Mori et al., 2002). Moreover, various factors including impaired tumor surveillance, chronic antigenic stimulation by differences between donor and recipient cells, perturbations within the host BM microenvironment, premature aging of the donor cells, and the associated chromosomal instability might contribute to the development of DCL after allogeneic HSCT (Flynn & Kaufman, 2007; Wiseman, 2010). It has been hypothesized that donor cell-derived hematological malignancy may be substantially more frequent with a CB source of stem cells (Greaves, 2006). Further research and the increasing number of reports will improve understanding of the clinical implications of the donor cell-derived hematological malignancies after CBT.

6. Conclusion

Clinical results of CBT for acute leukemia have improved recently in adult patients. In addition to the potent HSCs in CB, multiple populations of stem cells with stem cell properties have been identified from CB and have led to the idea that CB can be used for regenerative therapies. In fact, clinical trials are now underway in type 1 diabetes, cerebral palsy and peripheral vascular disease. Moreover, recent studies demonstrated that it is possible to generate induced pluripotent stem (iPS) cells from human CB (Giorgetti et al., 2009; Haase et al., 2009; Hu et al., 2011; Broxmeyer et al., 2011). These data offer CB derived iPS cells are also considered an ideal source for future regenerative therapies.

7. Acknowledgments

The authors thank all of the physicians and staff at the hospitals and the 11 cord blood banks in Japan on this study and thank Maki Monna-Oiwa for her secretarial assistance. This work was supported in part by The Kobayashi Foundation. The authors apologize to those whose important contributions to the field could not be cited in the list of references.

8. References

Ando T, Yujiri T, Mitani N, Takeuchi H, Nomiyama J, Suguchi M, Matsubara A, & Tanizawa Y. (2006). Donor cell-derived acute myeloid leukemia after unrelated umbilical cord blood transplantation. *Leukemia* 20(4):744-745.

Appelbaum FR. (2007). Hematopoietic-cell transplantation at 50. *N Engl J Med* 357(15):1472-1475.

Arcese W, Rocha V, Labopin M, Sanz G, Iori AP, de Lima M, Sirvent A, Busca A, Asano S, Ionescu I, Wernet P, & Gluckman E; Eurocord-Netcord Transplant group. (2006). Unrelated cord blood transplants in adults with hematologic malignancies. *Haematologica* 91(2):223-230.

Atsuta Y, Suzuki R, Nagamura-Inoue T, Taniguchi S, Takahashi S, Kai S, Sakamaki H, Kouzai Y, Kasai M, Fukuda T, Azuma H, Takanashi M, Okamoto S, Tsuchida M, Kawa K, Morishima Y, Kodera Y, & Kato S; Japan Cord Blood Bank Network. (2009). Disease-specific analyses of unrelated cord blood transplantation compared with unrelated bone marrow transplantation in adult patients with acute leukemia. *Blood* 113(8):1631-1638.

Avery S, Shi W, Lubin M, Gonzales AM, Heller G, Castro-Malaspina H, Giralt S, Kernan NA, Scaradavou A, & Barker JN. (2011). Influence of infused cell dose and HLA match on engraftment after double-unit cord blood allografts. *Blood* 117(12):3277-3285.

Ballen KK, Spitzer TR, Yeap BY, McAfee S, Dey BR, Attar E, Haspel R, Kao G, Liney D, Alyea E, Lee S, Cutler C, Ho V, Soiffer R, & Antin JH. (2007). Double unrelated reduced-intensity umbilical cord blood transplantation in adults. *Biol Blood Marrow Transplant* 13(1):82-89.

Ballen KK, Cutler C, Yeap BY, McAfee SL, Dey BR, Attar EC, Chen YB, Haspel RL, Liney D, Koreth J, Ho V, Alyea EP, Soiffer RJ, Spitzer TR, & Antin JH. (2010). Donor-derived second hematologic malignancies after cord blood transplantation. *Biol Blood Marrow Transplant* 16(7):1025-1031.

Ballen KK, & Spitzer TR. (2011). The great debate: haploidentical or cord blood transplant. *Bone Marrow Transplant* 46(3):323-329.

Barker JN, Weisdorf DJ, DeFor TE, Blazar BR, Miller JS, & Wagner JE. (2003). Rapid and complete donor chimerism in adult recipients of unrelated donor umbilical cord blood transplantation after reduced-intensity conditioning. *Blood* 102(5):1915-1919.

Barker JN, Weisdorf DJ, DeFor TE, Blazar BR, McGlave PB, Miller JS, Verfaillie CM, & Wagner JE. (2005). Transplantation of 2 partially HLA-matched umbilical cord blood units to enhance engraftment in adults with hematologic malignancy. *Blood* 105(3):1343-1347.

Barker JN, Scaradavou A, & Stevens CE. (2010). Combined effect of total nucleated cell dose and HLA match on transplantation outcome in 1061 cord blood recipients with hematologic malignancies. *Blood* 115(9):1843-1849.

Barker JN, Byam C, & Scaradavou A. (2011). How I treat: the selection and acquisition of unrelated cord blood grafts. *Blood* 117(8):2332-2339.

Bautista G, Cabrera JR, Regidor C, Forés R, García-Marco JA, Ojeda E, Sanjuán I, Ruiz E, Krsnik I, Navarro B, Gil S, Magro E, de Laiglesia A, Gonzalo-Daganzo R, Martín-Donaire T, Rico M, Millán I, & Fernández MN. (2009). Cord blood transplants supported by co-infusion of mobilized hematopoietic stem cells from a third-party donor. *Bone Marrow Transplant* 43(5):365-373.

Bernardo ME, Ball LM, Cometa AM, Roelofs H, Zecca M, Avanzini MA, Bertaina A, Vinti L, Lankester A, Maccario R, Ringden O, Le Blanc K, Egeler RM, Fibbe WE, & Locatelli F. (2011). Co-infusion of ex vivo-expanded, parental MSCs prevents life-threatening acute GVHD, but does not reduce the risk of graft failure in pediatric patients undergoing allogeneic umbilical cord blood transplantation. *Bone Marrow Transplant* 46(2):200-207.

Broxmeyer HE, Douglas GW, Hangoc G, Cooper S, Bard J, English D, Arny M, Thomas L, & Boyse EA. (1989). Human umbilical cord blood as a potential source of transplantable hematopoietic stem/progenitor cells. *Proc Natl Acad Sci U S A* 86(10):3828-3832.

Broxmeyer HE, Hangoc G, Cooper S, Ribeiro RC, Graves V, Yoder M, Wagner J, Vadhan-Raj S, Benninger L, Rubinstein P, et al. (1992). Growth characteristics and expansion of human umbilical cord blood and estimation of its potential for transplantation in adults. *Proc Natl Acad Sci U S A* 89(9):4109-4113.

Broxmeyer HE, Lee MR, Hangoc G, Cooper S, Prasain N, Kim YJ, Mallett C, Ye Z, Witting S, Cornetta K, Cheng L, & Yoder MC. (2011). Hematopoietic stem/progenitor cells, generation of induced pluripotent stem cells, and isolation of endothelial progenitors from 21-23.5 year cryopreserved cord blood. *Blood* 117(18):4773-4777.

Brunstein CG, Barker JN, Weisdorf DJ, DeFor TE, Miller JS, Blazar BR, McGlave PB, & Wagner JE. (2007). Umbilical cord blood transplantation after nonmyeloablative conditioning: impact on transplantation outcomes in 110 adults with hematologic disease. *Blood* 110(8):3064-3070.

Brunstein CG, Wagner JE, Weisdorf DJ, Cooley S, Noreen H, Barker JN, DeFor T, Verneris MR, Blazar BR, & Miller JS. (2009). Negative effect of KIR alloreactivity in recipients of umbilical cord blood transplant depends on transplantation conditioning intensity. *Blood* 113(22):5628-5634.

Brunstein CG, Gutman JA, Weisdorf DJ, Woolfrey AE, Defor TE, Gooley TA, Verneris MR, Appelbaum FR, Wagner JE, & Delaney C. (2010). Allogeneic hematopoietic cell transplantation for hematologic malignancy: relative risks and benefits of double umbilical cord blood. *Blood* 116(22):4693-4699.

Brunstein CG, Miller JS, Cao Q, McKenna DH, Hippen KL, Curtsinger J, Defor T, Levine BL, June CH, Rubinstein P, McGlave PB, Blazar BR, & Wagner JE. (2011). Infusion of ex vivo expanded T regulatory cells in adults transplanted with umbilical cord blood: safety profile and detection kinetics. *Blood* 117(3):1061-1070.

Campbell TB, Hangoc G, Liu Y, Pollok K, & Broxmeyer HE. (2007). Inhibition of CD26 in human cord blood CD34+ cells enhances their engraftment of nonobese diabetic/severe combined immunodeficiency mice. *Stem Cells Dev* 16(3):347-354.

Castleton AZ, Brazma D, Howard-Reeves J, Chanalaris A, Glanville J, Nizetic D, Chakraverty R, & Nacheva EP. (2010). Genome gains at chromosome 21q21/22 segment leads to co-amplification of Down Syndrome Critical Regions and known oncogenes in a case of donor cell-derived acute myeloid leukaemia following allogeneic sex mismatched umbilical cord blood transplantation for chronic myeloid leukaemia. *Br J Haematol* 151(3):285-288.

Chao NJ, Koh LP, Long GD, Gasparetto C, Horwitz M, Morris A, Lassiter M, Sullivan KM, & Rizzieri DA. (2004). Adult recipients of umbilical cord blood transplants after nonmyeloablative preparative regimens. *Biol Blood Marrow Transplant* 10(8):569-575.

Crow J, Youens K, Michalowski S, Perrine G, Emhart C, Johnson F, Gerling A, Kurtzberg J, Goodman BK, Sebastian S, Rehder CW, & Datto MB. (2010). Donor cell leukemia in umbilical cord blood transplant patients: a case study and literature review highlighting the importance of molecular engraftment analysis. *J Mol Diagn* 12(4):530-537.

Cutler C, & Ballen K. (2009). Reduced-intensity conditioning and umbilical cord blood transplantation in adults. *Bone Marrow Transplant* 44(10):667-671.

Cutler C, Stevenson K, Kim HT, Brown J, McDonough S, Herrera M, Reynolds C, Liney D, Kao G, Ho V, Armand P, Koreth J, Alyea E, Dey BR, Attar E, Spitzer T, Boussiotis VA, Ritz J, Soiffer R, Antin JH, & Ballen K. (2011). Double umbilical cord blood transplantation with reduced intensity conditioning and sirolimus-based GVHD prophylaxis. *Bone Marrow Transplant* 46(5):659-667.

Davis CC, Marti LC, Sempowski GD, Jeyaraj DA, & Szabolcs P. (2010). Interleukin-7 permits Th1/Tc1 maturation and promotes ex vivo expansion of cord blood T cells: a critical step toward adoptive immunotherapy after cord blood transplantation. *Cancer Res* 70(13):5249-5258.

Delaney C, Gutman JA, & Appelbaum FR. (2009). Cord blood transplantation for haematological malignancies: conditioning regimens, double cord transplant and infectious complications. *Br J Haematol* 147(2):207-216.

Delaney C, (2010). Heimfeld S, Brashem-Stein C, Voorhies H, Manger RL, & Bernstein ID. Notch-mediated expansion of human cord blood progenitor cells capable of rapid myeloid reconstitution. *Nat Med* 16(2):232-236.

Delaney M, & Ballen KK. (2010). The role of HLA in umbilical cord blood transplantation. *Best Pract Res Clin Haematol* 23(2):179-187.

de Lima M, McMannis J, Gee A, Komanduri K, Couriel D, Andersson BS, Hosing C, Khouri I, Jones R, Champlin R, Karandish S, Sadeghi T, Peled T, Grynspan F, Daniely Y, Nagler A, & Shpall EJ. (2008). Transplantation of ex vivo expanded cord blood cells using the copper chelator tetraethylenepentamine: a phase I/II clinical trial. *Bone Marrow Transplant* 41(9):771-778.

de Lima M, Robinson S, McMannis J, Alousi AM, Saliba RM, Munsell M, Kebriaei P, Hosing C, Parmar S, Cooper L, Shah N, Kelly SS, Rondon G, Fernandez-Vina M, Maewall I, Bosque D, Bollard CM, Chen JJ, McNiece IK, Komanduri KV, Nieto Y, Jones R, Andersson BS, Popat U, Champlin RE, Simmons PJ, & Shpall EJ. (2010). Mesenchymal Stem Cell (MSC) Based Cord Blood (CB) Expansion (Exp) Leads to Rapid Engraftment of Platelets and Neutrophils. *ASH Annual Meeting Abstracts* 116: abstract362.

Eapen M, Rocha V, Sanz G, Scaradavou A, Zhang MJ, Arcese W, Sirvent A, Champlin RE, Chao N, Gee AP, Isola L, Laughlin MJ, Marks DI, Nabhan S, Ruggeri A, Soiffer R, Horowitz MM, Gluckman E, & Wagner JE; Center for International Blood and Marrow Transplant Research; Acute Leukemia Working Party Eurocord (the European Group for Blood Marrow Transplantation); National Cord Blood Program of the New York Blood Center. (2010). Effect of graft source on unrelated donor haemopoietic stem-cell transplantation in adults with acute leukaemia: a retrospective analysis. *Lancet Oncol* 11(7):653-660.

Fernández MN, Regidor C, Cabrera R, García-Marco JA, Forés R, Sanjuán I, Gayoso J, Gil S, Ruíz E, Little AM, McWhinnie A, & Madrigal A. (2003). Unrelated umbilical cord blood transplants in adults: Early recovery of neutrophils by supportive co-transplantation of a low number of highly purified peripheral blood CD34+ cells from an HLA-haploidentical donor. *Exp Hematol* 31(6):535-544.

Flynn CM, & Kaufman DS. (2007). Donor cell leukemia: insight into cancer stem cells and the stem cell niche. *Blood* 109(7):2688-2692.

Foeken LM, Green A, Hurley CK, Marry E, Wiegand T, & Oudshoorn M; Donor Registries Working Group of the World Marrow Donor Association (WMDA). (2010). Monitoring the international use of unrelated donors for transplantation: the WMDA annual reports. *Bone Marrow Transplant* 45(5):811-818.

Fraser CJ, Hirsch BA, Dayton V, Creer MH, Neglia JP, Wagner JE, & Baker KS. (2005). First report of donor cell-derived acute leukemia as a complication of umbilical cord blood transplantation. *Blood* 106(13):4377-4380.

Frassoni F, Gualandi F, Podestà M, Raiola AM, Ibatici A, Piaggio G, Sessarego M, Sessarego N, Gobbi M, Sacchi N, Labopin M, & Bacigalupo A. (2008). Direct intrabone transplant of unrelated cord-blood cells in acute leukaemia: a phase I/II study. *Lancet Oncol* 9(9):831-839.

Giorgetti A, Montserrat N, Aasen T, Gonzalez F, Rodríguez-Pizà I, Vassena R, Raya A, Boué S, Barrero MJ, Corbella BA, Torrabadella M, Veiga A, Izpisua & Belmonte JC. (2009). Generation of induced pluripotent stem cells from human cord blood using OCT4 and SOX2. *Cell Stem Cell* 5(4):353-357.

Gluckman E, Broxmeyer HA, Auerbach AD, Friedman HS, Douglas GW, Devergie A, Esperou H, Thierry D, Socie G, Lehn P, et al. (1989). Hematopoietic reconstitution in a patient with Fanconi's anemia by means of umbilical-cord blood from an HLA-identical sibling. *N Engl J Med* 321(17):1174-1178.

Gluckman E, Rocha V, Boyer-Chammard A, Locatelli F, Arcese W, Pasquini R, Ortega J, Souillet G, Ferreira E, Laporte JP, Fernandez M, & Chastang C. (1997). Outcome of cord-blood transplantation from related and unrelated donors. Eurocord Transplant Group and the European Blood and Marrow Transplantation Group. *N Engl J Med* 337(6):373-381.

Gluckman E, Rocha V, Arcese W, Michel G, Sanz G, Chan KW, Takahashi TA, Ortega J, Filipovich A, Locatelli F, Asano S, Fagioli F, Vowels M, Sirvent A, Laporte JP, Tiedemann K, Amadori S, Abecassis M, Bordigoni P, Diez B, Shaw PJ, Vora A, Caniglia M, Garnier F, Ionescu I, Garcia J, Koegler G, Rebulla P, & Chevret S; Eurocord Group. (2004). Factors associated with outcomes of unrelated cord blood transplant: guidelines for donor choice. *Exp Hematol* 32(4):397-407.

Gonzalo-Daganzo R, Regidor C, Martín-Donaire T, Rico MA, Bautista G, Krsnik I, Forés R, Ojeda E, Sanjuán I, García-Marco JA, Navarro B, Gil S, Sánchez R, Panadero N, Gutiérrez Y, García-Berciano M, Pérez N, Millán I, Cabrera R, & Fernández MN. (2009). Results of a pilot study on the use of third-party donor mesenchymal stromal cells in cord blood transplantation in adults. *Cytotherapy* 11(3):278-288.

Greaves MF. (2006). Cord blood donor cell leukemia in recipients. *Leukemia* 20(9):1633-1634.

Gutman JA, Leisenring W, Appelbaum FR, Woolfrey AE, & Delaney C. (2009). Low relapse without excessive transplant-related mortality following myeloablative cord blood transplantation for acute leukemia in complete remission: a matched cohort analysis. *Biol Blood Marrow Transplant* 15(9):1122-1129.

Haase A, Olmer R, Schwanke K, Wunderlich S, Merkert S, Hess C, Zweigerdt R, Gruh I, Meyer J, Wagner S, Maier LS, Han DW, Glage S, Miller K, Fischer P, Schöler HR, &

Martin U. (2009). Generation of induced pluripotent stem cells from human cord blood. *Cell Stem Cell* 5(4):434-441.

Hamaki T, Kajiwara K, Kami M, Murashige N, Funaki M, Harima A, Kogure K, Yamada K, Kodo H, & Kouzai Y. (2008). Donor cell-derived acute monoblastic leukemia involving MLL gene translocation in an adult patient who received umbilical cord blood transplantation. *Bone Marrow Transplant* 41(1):91-92.

Hanley PJ, Cruz CR, Savoldo B, Leen AM, Stanojevic M, Khalil M, Decker W, Molldrem JJ, Liu H, Gee AP, Rooney CM, Heslop HE, Dotti G, Brenner MK, Shpall EJ, & Bollard CM. (2009). Functionally active virus-specific T cells that target CMV, adenovirus, and EBV can be expanded from naive T-cell populations in cord blood and will target a range of viral epitopes. *Blood* 114(9):1958-1967.

Hanley PJ, Cruz CR, Shpall EJ, & Bollard CM. (2010). Improving clinical outcomes using adoptively transferred immune cells from umbilical cord blood. *Cytotherapy* 12:713-720.

Hertenstein B, Hambach L, Bacigalupo A, Schmitz N, McCann S, Slavin S, Gratwohl A, Ferrant A, Elmaagacli A, Schwertfeger R, Locasciulli A, Zander A, Bornhäuser M, Niederwieser D, & Ruutu T; Chronic Leukaemia Working Party of the European Group for Blood and Marrow Transplantation. (2005). Development of leukemia in donor cells after allogeneic stem cell transplantation--a survey of the European Group for Blood and Marrow Transplantation (EBMT). *Haematologica* 90(7):969-975.

Horwitz ME, & Chao N. (2010). Non-myeloablative umbilical cord blood transplantation. *Best Pract Res Clin Haematol* 23(2):231-236.

Hows JM, Bradley BA, Marsh JC, Luft T, Coutinho L, Testa NG, & Dexter TM. (1992). Growth of human umbilical-cord blood in longterm haemopoietic cultures. *Lancet* 340(8811):73-76.

Hu K, Yu J, Suknuntha K, Tian S, Montgomery K, Choi KD, Stewart R, Thomson JA, & Slukvin II. (2011). Efficient generation of transgene-free induced pluripotent stem cells from normal and neoplastic bone marrow and cord blood mononuclear cells. *Blood* 117(14):e109-119.

Hwang WY, Samuel M, Tan D, Koh LP, Lim W, & Linn YC. (2007). A meta-analysis of unrelated donor umbilical cord blood transplantation versus unrelated donor bone marrow transplantation in adult and pediatric patients. *Biol Blood Marrow Transplant* 13(4):444-453.

Jaroscak J, Goltry K, Smith A, Waters-Pick B, Martin PL, Driscoll TA, Howrey R, Chao N, Douville J, Burhop S, Fu P, & Kurtzberg J. (2003). Augmentation of umbilical cord blood (UCB) transplantation with ex vivo-expanded UCB cells: results of a phase 1 trial using the AastromReplicell System. *Blood* 101(12):5061-5067.

Jenq RR, & van den Brink MR. (2010). Allogeneic haematopoietic stem cell transplantation: individualized stem cell and immune therapy of cancer. *Nat Rev Cancer* 10(3):213-221.

Kelly SS, Sola CB, de Lima M, & Shpall E. (2009). Ex vivo expansion of cord blood. *Bone Marrow Transplant* 44(10):673-681.

Komanduri KV, St John LS, de Lima M, McMannis J, Rosinski S, McNiece I, Bryan SG, Kaur I, Martin S, Wieder ED, Worth L, Cooper LJ, Petropoulos D, Molldrem JJ, Champlin RE, & Shpall EJ. (2007). Delayed immune reconstitution after cord blood transplantation is characterized by impaired thymopoiesis and late memory T-cell skewing. *Blood* 110(13):4543-4551.

Komatsu T, Narimatsu H, Yoshimi A, Kurita N, Kusakabe M, Hori A, Murashige N, Matsumura T, Kobayashi K, Yuji K, Tanaka Y, & Kami M. (2007). Successful engraftment of mismatched unrelated cord blood transplantation following reduced intensity preparative regimen using fludarabine and busulfan. *Ann Hematol* 86(1):49-54.

Konuma T, Takahashi S, Ooi J, Tomonari A, Tsukada N, Kato S, Sato A, Monma F, Kasahara S, Nagamura-Inoue T, Uchimaru K, Iseki T, Tojo A, Yamaguchi T, & Asano S. (2009a). Myeloablative unrelated cord blood transplantation for acute leukemia patients between 50 and 55 years of age: single institutional retrospective comparison with patients younger than 50 years of age. *Ann Hematol* 88(6):581-588.

Konuma T, Ooi J, Takahashi S, Tomonari A, Tsukada N, Kato S, Sato A, Monma F, Hongo E, Uchimaru K, Tojo A, & Asano S. (2009b). Donor cell-derived myelodysplastic syndrome after cord blood transplantation. *Bone Marrow Transplant* 43(5):429-431.

Kumar P, Defor TE, Brunstein C, Barker JN, Wagner JE, Weisdorf DJ, & Burns LJ. (2008). Allogeneic hematopoietic stem cell transplantation in adult acute lymphocytic leukemia: impact of donor source on survival. *Biol Blood Marrow Transplant* 14(12):1394-1400.

Kurtzberg J, Laughlin M, Graham ML, Smith C, Olson JF, Halperin EC, Ciocci G, Carrier C, Stevens CE, & Rubinstein P. (1996). Placental blood as a source of hematopoietic stem cells for transplantation into unrelated recipients. *N Engl J Med* 335(3):157-166.

Laporte JP, Gorin NC, Rubinstein P, Lesage S, Portnoi MF, Barbu V, Lopez M, Douay L, & Najman A. (1996). Cord-blood transplantation from an unrelated donor in an adult with chronic myelogenous leukemia. *N Engl J Med* 335(3):167-170.

Laughlin MJ, Barker J, Bambach B, Koc ON, Rizzieri DA, Wagner JE, Gerson SL, Lazarus HM, Cairo M, Stevens CE, Rubinstein P, & Kurtzberg J. (2001). Hematopoietic engraftment and survival in adult recipients of umbilical-cord blood from unrelated donors. *N Engl J Med* 344(24):1815-1822.

Laughlin MJ, Eapen M, Rubinstein P, Wagner JE, Zhang MJ, Champlin RE, Stevens C, Barker JN, Gale RP, Lazarus HM, Marks DI, van Rood JJ, Scaradavou A, & Horowitz MM. (2004). Outcomes after transplantation of cord blood or bone marrow from unrelated donors in adults with leukemia. *N Engl J Med* 351(22):2265-2275.

Le Blanc K, Frassoni F, Ball L, Locatelli F, Roelofs H, Lewis I, Lanino E, Sundberg B, Bernardo ME, Remberger M, Dini G, Egeler RM, Bacigalupo A, Fibbe W, & Ringdén O; Developmental Committee of the European Group for Blood and Marrow Transplantation. (2008). Mesenchymal stem cells for treatment of steroid-resistant, severe, acute graft-versus-host disease: a phase II study. *Lancet* 371(9624):1579-1586.

MacMillan ML, Weisdorf DJ, Brunstein CG, Cao Q, DeFor TE, Verneris MR, Blazar BR, & Wagner JE. (2009a). Acute graft-versus-host disease after unrelated donor umbilical cord blood transplantation: analysis of risk factors. *Blood* 113(11):2410-2415.

Macmillan ML, Blazar BR, DeFor TE, & Wagner JE. (2009b). Transplantation of ex-vivo culture-expanded parental haploidentical mesenchymal stem cells to promote engraftment in pediatric recipients of unrelated donor umbilical cord blood: results of a phase I-II clinical trial. *Bone Marrow Transplant* 43(6):447-454.

Magro E, Regidor C, Cabrera R, Sanjuán I, Forès R, Garcia-Marco JA, Ruiz E, Gil S, Bautista G, Millán I, Madrigal A, & Fernandez MN. (2006). Early hematopoietic recovery after single unit unrelated cord blood transplantation in adults supported by co-infusion of mobilized stem cells from a third party donor. *Haematologica* 91(5):640-648.

Majhail NS, Brunstein CG, Tomblyn M, Thomas AJ, Miller JS, Arora M, Kaufman DS, Burns LJ, Slungaard A, McGlave PB, Wagner JE, & Weisdorf DJ. (2008). Reduced-intensity allogeneic transplant in patients older than 55 years: unrelated umbilical cord blood is safe and effective for patients without a matched related donor. *Biol Blood Marrow Transplant* 14(3):282-289.

Matsunaga T, Murase K, Yoshida M, Fujimi A, Iyama S, Kuribayashi K, Sato T, Kogawa K, Hirayama Y, Sakamaki S, Kohda K, & Niitsu Y. (2005). Donor cell derived acute myeloid leukemia after allogeneic cord blood transplantation in a patient with adult T-cell lymphoma. *Am J Hematol* 79(4):294-298.

Mazur MA, Davis CC, & Szabolcs P. (2008). Ex vivo expansion and Th1/Tc1 maturation of umbilical cord blood T cells by CD3/CD28 costimulation. *Biol Blood Marrow Transplant* 14(10):1190-1196.

Micklethwaite KP, Savoldo B, Hanley PJ, Leen AM, Demmler-Harrison GJ, Cooper LJ, Liu H, Gee AP, Shpall EJ, Rooney CM, Heslop HE, Brenner MK, Bollard CM, & Dotti G. (2010). Derivation of human T lymphocytes from cord blood and peripheral blood with antiviral and antileukemic specificity from a single culture as protection against infection and relapse after stem cell transplantation. *Blood* 115(13):2695-2703.

Misawa M, Kai S, Okada M, Nakajima T, Nomura K, Wakae T, Toda A, Itoi H, Takatsuka H, Itsukuma T, Nishioka K, Fujimori Y, Ogawa H, & Hara H. (2006). Reduced-intensity conditioning followed by unrelated umbilical cord blood transplantation for advanced hematologic malignancies: rapid engraftment in bone marrow. *Int J Hematol* 83(1):74-79.

Mitsui H, Nakazawa T, Tanimura A, Karasuno T, & Hiraoka A. (2007). Donor cell-derived chronic myeloproliferative disease with t(7;11)(p15;p15) after cord blood transplantation in a patient with Philadelphia chromosome-positive acute lymphoblastic leukemia. *Int J Hematol* 86(2):192-195.

Miyakoshi S, Yuji K, Kami M, Kusumi E, Kishi Y, Kobayashi K, Murashige N, Hamaki T, Kim SW, Ueyama J, Mori S, Morinaga S, Muto Y, Masuo S, Kanemaru M, Hayashi T, Takaue Y, & Taniguchi S. (2004). Successful engraftment after reduced-intensity umbilical cord blood transplantation for adult patients with advanced hematological diseases. *Clin Cancer Res* 10(11):3586-3592.

Miyakoshi S, Kusumi E, Matsumura T, Hori A, Murashige N, Hamaki T, Yuji K, Uchida N, Masuoka K, Wake A, Kanda Y, Kami M, Tanaka Y, & Taniguchi S. (2007). Invasive fungal infection following reduced-intensity cord blood transplantation for adult patients with hematologic diseases. *Biol Blood Marrow Transplant* 13(7):771-777.

Mori H, Colman SM, Xiao Z, Ford AM, Healy LE, Donaldson C, Hows JM, Navarrete C, & Greaves M. (2002). Chromosome translocations and covert leukemic clones are generated during normal fetal development. *Proc Natl Acad Sci U S A* 99(12):8242-8247.

Nagamura-Inoue T, Kodo H, Takahashi TA, Mugishima H, Tojo A, & Asano S. (2007). Four cases of donor cell-derived AML following unrelated cord blood transplantation for adult patients: experiences of the Tokyo Cord Blood Bank. *Cytotherapy* 9(8):727-728.

Narimatsu H, Matsumura T, Kami M, Miyakoshi S, Kusumi E, Takagi S, Miura Y, Kato D, Inokuchi C, Myojo T, Kishi Y, Murashige N, Yuji K, Masuoka K, Yoneyama A, Wake

A, Morinaga S, Kanda Y, & Taniguchi S. (2005). Bloodstream infection after umbilical cord blood transplantation using reduced-intensity stem cell transplantation for adult patients. *Biol Blood Marrow Transplant* 11(6):429-436.

Ooi J, Iseki T, Takahashi S, Tomonari A, Takasugi K, Shimohakamada Y, Yamada T, Ishii K, Ohno N, Nagamura F, Uchimaru K, Tojo A, & Asano S. (2004). Unrelated cord blood transplantation for adult patients with de novo acute myeloid leukemia. *Blood* 103(2):489-491.

Ooi J, Takahashi S, Tomonari A, Tsukada N, Konuma T, Kato S, Kasahara S, Sato A, Monma F, Nagamura F, Iseki T, Tojo A, & Asano S. (2008). Unrelated cord blood transplantation after myeloablative conditioning in adults with acute myelogenous leukemia. *Biol Blood Marrow Transplant* 14(12):1341-1347.

Ooi J, Takahashi S, Tomonari A, Tsukada N, Konuma T, Kato S, Kasahara S, Sato A, Monma F, Nagamura F, Iseki T, Tojo A, & Asano S. (2009). Unrelated cord blood transplantation after myeloablative conditioning in adults with ALL. *Bone Marrow Transplant* 43(6):455-459.

Oran B, Wagner JE, Defor TE, Weisdorf DJ, & Brunstein CG. (2011). Effect of Conditioning Regimen Intensity on Acute Myeloid Leukemia Outcomes after Umbilical Cord Blood Transplantation. *Biol Blood Marrow Transplant* 2011 Jan 11. [Epub ahead of print]

Park KD, Marti L, Kurtzberg J, & Szabolcs P. (2006). In vitro priming and expansion of cytomegalovirus-specific Th1 and Tc1 T cells from naive cord blood lymphocytes. *Blood* 108(5):1770-1773.

Parody R, Martino R, Rovira M, Vazquez L, Vázquez MJ, de la Cámara R, Blazquez C, Fernández-Avilés F, Carreras E, Salavert M, Jarque I, Martín C, Martínez F, López J, Torres A, Sierra J, & Sanz GF; Infectious/Non-infectious Complications Subcommittee of the Grupo Español de Trasplante Hematopoyético (GETH). (2006). Severe infections after unrelated donor allogeneic hematopoietic stem cell transplantation in adults: comparison of cord blood transplantation with peripheral blood and bone marrow transplantation. *Biol Blood Marrow Transplant* 12(7):734-748.

Rocha V, Labopin M, Sanz G, Arcese W, Schwerdtfeger R, Bosi A, Jacobsen N, Ruutu T, de Lima M, Finke J, Frassoni F, & Gluckman E; Acute Leukemia Working Party of European Blood and Marrow Transplant Group; Eurocord-Netcord Registry. (2004). Transplants of umbilical-cord blood or bone marrow from unrelated donors in adults with acute leukemia. *N Engl J Med* 351(22):2276-2285.

Rocha V, & Gluckman E; Eurocord-Netcord registry and European Blood and Marrow Transplant group. (2009). Improving outcomes of cord blood transplantation: HLA matching, cell dose and other graft- and transplantation-related factors. *Br J Haematol* 147(2):262-274.

Rocha V, Labopin M, Mohty M, Sanz GF, Rio B, Furst S, Sirvent A, Socié G, Tabrizzi R, Yakoubagha I, Deconinck E, Cornelissen JJ, Arcese W, Ribera JM, Nikiforakis E, Michallet M, Crotta A, Ruggeri A, & Gluckman E. (2010a). Outcomes After Double Unit Unrelated Cord Blood Transplantation (UCBT) Compared with Single UCBT In Adults with Acute Leukemia In Remission. An Eurocord and ALWP Collaboration Study. *ASH Annual Meeting Abstracts* 116: abstract910.

Rocha V, Crotta A, Ruggeri A, Purtill D, Boudjedir K, Herr AL, Ionescu I, & Gluckman E; Eurocord Registry. (2010b). Double cord blood transplantation: extending the use of unrelated umbilical cord blood cells for patients with hematological diseases. *Best Pract Res Clin Haematol* 23(2):223-229.

Rodrigues CA, Sanz G, Brunstein CG, Sanz J, Wagner JE, Renaud M, de Lima M, Cairo MS, Fürst S, Rio B, Dalley C, Carreras E, Harousseau JL, Mohty M, Taveira D, Dreger P, Sureda A, Gluckman E, & Rocha V. (2009). Analysis of risk factors for outcomes after unrelated cord blood transplantation in adults with lymphoid malignancies: a study by the Eurocord-Netcord and lymphoma working party of the European group for blood and marrow transplantation. *J Clin Oncol* 27(2):256-263.

Rubinstein P, Rosenfield RE, Adamson JW, & Stevens CE. (1993). Stored placental blood for unrelated bone marrow reconstitution. *Blood* 81(7):1679-1690.

Rubinstein P, Dobrila L, Rosenfield RE, Adamson JW, Migliaccio G, Migliaccio AR, Taylor PE, & Stevens CE. (1995). Processing and cryopreservation of placental/umbilical cord blood for unrelated bone marrow reconstitution. *Proc Natl Acad Sci U S A* 92(22):10119-10122.

Rubinstein P, Carrier C, Scaradavou A, Kurtzberg J, Adamson J, Migliaccio AR, Berkowitz RL, Cabbad M, Dobrila NL, Taylor PE, Rosenfield RE, & Stevens CE. (1998). Outcomes among 562 recipients of placental-blood transplants from unrelated donors. *N Engl J Med* 339(22):1565-1577.

Ruggeri L, Capanni M, Urbani E, Perruccio K, Shlomchik WD, Tosti A, Posati S, Rogaia D, Frassoni F, Aversa F, Martelli MF, & Velardi A. (2002). Effectiveness of donor natural killer cell alloreactivity in mismatched hematopoietic transplants. *Science* 295(5562):2097-2100.

Sanz GF, Saavedra S, Planelles D, Senent L, Cervera J, Barragán E, Jiménez C, Larrea L, Martín G, Martínez J, Jarque I, Moscardó F, Plumé G, Andreu R, Regadera AI, García I, Mollá S, Solves P, de La Rubia J, Bolufer P, Benlloch L, Soler MA, Marty ML, & Sanz MA. (2001). Standardized, unrelated donor cord blood transplantation in adults with hematologic malignancies. *Blood* 98(8):2332-2338.

Serrano LM, Pfeiffer T, Olivares S, Numbenjapon T, Bennitt J, Kim D, Smith D, McNamara G, Al-Kadhimi Z, Rosenthal J, Forman SJ, Jensen MC, & Cooper LJ. (2006). Differentiation of naive cord-blood T cells into CD19-specific cytolytic effectors for posttransplantation adoptive immunotherapy. *Blood* 107(7):2643-2652.

Sevilla J, Querol S, Molines A, González-Vicent M, Balas A, Carrió A, Estella J, Angel Díaz M, & Madero L. (2006). Transient donor cell-derived myelodysplastic syndrome with monosomy 7 after unrelated cord blood transplantation. *Eur J Haematol* 77(3):259-263.

Shaw BE, Veys P, Pagliuca A, Addada J, Cook G, Craddock CF, Gennery AR, Goldman J, Mackinnon S, Madrigal JA, Marks DI, Navarrete C, Potter MN, Querol S, Regan F, Russell NH, & Hough RE. (2009). Recommendations for a standard UK approach to incorporating umbilical cord blood into clinical transplantation practice: conditioning protocols and donor selection algorithms. *Bone Marrow Transplant* 44(1):7-12.

Shpall EJ, Quinones R, Giller R, Zeng C, Baron AE, Jones RB, Bearman SI, Nieto Y, Freed B, Madinger N, Hogan CJ, Slat-Vasquez V, Russell P, Blunk B, Schissel D, Hild E, Malcolm J, Ward W, & McNiece IK. (2002). Transplantation of ex vivo expanded cord blood. *Biol Blood Marrow Transplant* 8(7):368-376.

Stanevsky A, Shimoni A, Yerushalmi R, & Nagler A. (2010). Double umbilical cord blood transplant: more than a cell dose? *Leuk Lymphoma* 51(6):975-982.

Szabolcs P, & Niedzwiecki D. (2007). Immune reconstitution after unrelated cord blood transplantation. *Cytotherapy* 9(2):111-122.

Szabolcs P, & Cairo MS. (2010). Unrelated umbilical cord blood transplantation and immune reconstitution. *Semin Hematol* 47(1):22-36.

Takahashi S, Iseki T, Ooi J, Tomonari A, Takasugi K, Shimohakamada Y, Yamada T, Uchimaru K, Tojo A, Shirafuji N, Kodo H, Tani K, Takahashi T, Yamaguchi T, & Asano S. (2004). Single-institute comparative analysis of unrelated bone marrow transplantation and cord blood transplantation for adult patients with hematologic malignancies. *Blood* 104(12):3813-3820.

Takahashi S, Ooi J, Tomonari A, Konuma T, Tsukada N, Tojo A, Yamaguchi T, & Asano S. (2006). Posttransplantation engraftment and safety of cord blood transplantation with grafts containing relatively low cell doses in adults. *Int J Hematol* 84(4):359-362.

Takahashi S, Ooi J, Tomonari A, Konuma T, Tsukada N, Oiwa-Monna M, Fukuno K, Uchiyama M, Takasugi K, Iseki T, Tojo A, Yamaguchi T, & Asano S. (2007). Comparative single-institute analysis of cord blood transplantation from unrelated donors with bone marrow or peripheral blood stem-cell transplants from related donors in adult patients with hematologic malignancies after myeloablative conditioning regimen. *Blood* 109(3):1322-1330.

Takanashi M, Atsuta Y, Fujiwara K, Kodo H, Kai S, Sato H, Kohsaki M, Azuma H, Tanaka H, Ogawa A, Nakajima K, & Kato S. (2010). The impact of anti-HLA antibodies on unrelated cord blood transplantations. *Blood* 116(15):2839-2846.

Thomas ED, Lochte HL Jr, Lu WC, & Ferrebee JW. (1957). Intravenous infusion of bone marrow in patients receiving radiation and chemotherapy. *N Engl J Med* 257(11):491-496.

Tolar J, Hippen KL, & Blazar BR. (2009). Immune regulatory cells in umbilical cord blood: T regulatory cells and mesenchymal stromal cells. *Br J Haematol* 147(2):200-206.

Tomonari A, Iseki T, Ooi J, Takahashi S, Shindo M, Ishii K, Nagamura F, Uchimaru K, Tani K, Tojo A, & Asano S. (2003a). Cytomegalovirus infection following unrelated cord blood transplantation for adult patients: a single institute experience in Japan. *Br J Haematol* 121(2):304-311.

Tomonari A, Iseki T, Takahashi S, Ooi J, Takasugi K, Shimohakamada Y, Ohno N, Nagamura F, Uchimaru K, Tani K, Tojo A, & Asano S. (2003b). Varicella-zoster virus infection in adult patients after unrelated cord blood transplantation: a single institute experience in Japan. *Br J Haematol* 122(5):802-805.

Tomonari A, Takahashi S, Iseki T, Ooi J, Yamada T, Takasugi K, Shimohakamada Y, Ohno N, Nagamura F, Uchimaru K, Tani K, Tojo A, & Asano S. (2004). Herpes simplex virus infection in adult patients after unrelated cord blood transplantation: a single-institute experience in Japan. *Bone Marrow Transplant* 33(3):317-320.

Tomonari A, Takahashi S, Ooi J, Iseki T, Takasugi K, Uchiyama M, Konuma T, Futami M, Ohno N, Uchimaru K, Tojo A, & Asano S. (2005). Human herpesvirus 6 variant B infection in adult patients after unrelated cord blood transplantation. *Int J Hematol* 81(4):352-355.

Tomonari A, Takahashi S, Ooi J, Tsukada N, Konuma T, Kobayashi T, Sato A, Takasugi K, Iseki T, Tojo A, & Asano S. (2007). Bacterial bloodstream infection in neutropenic adult patients after myeloablative cord blood transplantation: experience of a single institution in Japan. *Int J Hematol* 85(3):238-241.

Uchida N, Wake A, Takagi S, Yamamoto H, Kato D, Matsuhashi Y, Matsumura T, Seo S, Matsuno N, Masuoka K, Kusumi E, Yuji K, Miyakoshi S, Matsuzaki M, Yoneyama A, & Taniguchi S. (2008). Umbilical cord blood transplantation after reduced-intensity conditioning for elderly patients with hematologic diseases. *Biol Blood Marrow Transplant* 14(5):583-590.

van Burik JA, & Brunstein CG. (2007). Infectious complications following unrelated cord blood transplantation. *Vox Sang* 92(4):289-296.

Verneris MR, Brunstein CG, Barker J, MacMillan ML, DeFor T, McKenna DH, Burke MJ, Blazar BR, Miller JS, McGlave PB, Weisdorf DJ, & Wagner JE. (2009). Relapse risk after umbilical cord blood transplantation: enhanced graft-versus-leukemia effect in recipients of 2 units. *Blood* 114(19):4293-4299.

Verneris MR, & Miller JS. (2009). The phenotypic and functional characteristics of umbilical cord blood and peripheral blood natural killer cells. *Br J Haematol* 147:185-191.

Wagner JE, Rosenthal J, Sweetman R, Shu XO, Davies SM, Ramsay NK, McGlave PB, Sender L, & Cairo MS. (1996). Successful transplantation of HLA-matched and HLA-mismatched umbilical cord blood from unrelated donors: analysis of engraftment and acute graft-versus-host disease. *Blood* 88(3):795-802.

Wagner JE, Barker JN, DeFor TE, Baker KS, Blazar BR, Eide C, Goldman A, Kersey J, Krivit W, MacMillan ML, Orchard PJ, Peters C, Weisdorf DJ, Ramsay NK, & Davies SM. (2002). Transplantation of unrelated donor umbilical cord blood in 102 patients with malignant and nonmalignant diseases: influence of CD34 cell dose and HLA disparity on treatment-related mortality and survival. *Blood* 100(5):1611-1618.

Wang E, Hutchinson CB, Huang Q, Lu CM, Crow J, Wang FF, Sebastian S, Rehder C, Lagoo A, Horwitz M, Rizzieri D, Yu J, Goodman B, Datto M, & Buckley P. (2011). Donor cell-derived leukemias/myelodysplastic neoplasms in allogeneic hematopoietic stem cell transplant recipients: a clinicopathologic study of 10 cases and a comprehensive review of the literature. *Am J Clin Pathol* 135(4):525-540.

Wang J, Zhan P, Ouyang J, Chen B, Zhou R, & Yang Y. (2010). Unrelated donor umbilical cord blood transplantation versus unrelated donor bone marrow transplantation in adult and pediatric patients: A meta-analysis. *Leuk Res* 34(8):1018-1022.

Willemze R, Rodrigues CA, Labopin M, Sanz G, Michel G, Socié G, Rio B, Sirvent A, Renaud M, Madero L, Mohty M, Ferra C, Garnier F, Loiseau P, Garcia J, Lecchi L, Kögler G, Beguin Y, Navarrete C, Devos T, Ionescu I, Boudjedir K, Herr AL, Gluckman E, & Rocha V; Eurocord-Netcord and Acute Leukaemia Working Party of the EBMT. (2009). KIR-ligand incompatibility in the graft-versus-host direction improves outcomes after umbilical cord blood transplantation for acute leukemia. *Leukemia* 23(3):492-500.

Wiseman DH. (2011). Donor Cell Leukemia: A Review. *Bone Marrow Transplant* 17(6):771-789.

Xing D, Ramsay AG, Gribben JG, Decker WK, Burks JK, Munsell M, Li S, Robinson SN, Yang H, Steiner D, Shah N, McMannis JD, Champlin RE, Hosing C, Zweidler-McKay PA, Shpall EJ, & Bollard CM. (2010). Cord blood natural killer cells exhibit impaired lytic immunological synapse formation that is reversed with IL-2 exvivo expansion. *J Immunother* 33(7):684-696.

Yazaki M, Atsuta Y, Kato K, Kato S, Taniguchi S, Takahashi S, Ogawa H, Kouzai Y, Kobayashi T, Inoue M, Kobayashi R, Nagamura-Inoue T, Azuma H, Takanashi M, Kai S, Nakabayashi M, & Saito H; Japan Cord Blood Bank Network. (2009). Incidence and risk factors of early bacterial infections after unrelated cord blood transplantation. *Biol Blood Marrow Transplant* 15(4):439-446.

15

Evidence-Based Guided Interventions in Acute Leukemia

Ron Ram, Liat Vidal, Ronit Gurion, Pia Raanani and Ofer Shpilberg
Institute of Hematology, Davidoff Cancer Center, Beilinson Hospital,
Rabin Medical Center and Sackler School of Medicine, Tel- Aviv University
Israel

1. Introduction

Evidence based medicine (EBM) is becoming a cornerstone in the establishment of practical guidelines and is nowadays part of the process of decision making in medicine (Woolf 2000). In evidence based medicine, decision making is based on relevant clinical trials ranked by their relevance and validity according to established criteria. Indeed, well designed randomized controlled trials (RCTs) are considered the "gold standard". However, since hematological disorders such as acute leukemia are rare, RCTs with a large enough sample size are difficult to conduct.

Systematic reviews use a preplanned, explicit methodology to answer a predefined question and evaluate the benefit and harm of healthcare interventions. Meta-analyses quantitatively assemble results from RCTs to increase power when individual studies are too small to detect a statistically significant effect (Gale and Lazarus 2011). The quality of a systematic review reflects the quality of its included studies. Potential sources of bias are heterogeneity between the RCTs included, publication bias and difficulties in accessing data from the original clinical trials.

In this chapter we attempted to assemble the evidence on the available meta-analyses analyzing the data in acute myeloid leukemia (AML) and acute lymphoblastic leukemia (ALL) patients. In certain domains, when no meta-analyses were identified, a literature search was performed and, if applicable, suggestions for future studies were made.

2. Methods

We searched The Cochrane and MEDLINE databases for systematic reviews. In Pubmed we crossed MeSH terms for 'acute myeloid leukemia' or 'acute lymphoblastic leukemia' with Clinical Queries to limit the search for systematic reviews.

We included systematic reviews of RCTs (with or without meta-analyses) assessing the effect of different chemotherapy regimens and supportive care on overall survival of patients with acute leukemia. We included the use of these treatment options in the following clinical settings: remission induction, post remission (consolidation) including autologous and allogeneic stem cell transplantation and maintenance.

We assessed the risk of bias in the systematic reviews by the following domains: use of explicit inclusion/exclusion criteria and a predefined protocol; comprehensive search;

whether selection bias was avoided; assessment of risk of bias of original trials; correct statistical methods to pool the data. Assessment of risk of bias in each of the systematic reviews based on the AMSTAR protocol is summarized in tables 1-2 and 4 (Liberati, *et al* 2009, Oxman and Guyatt 1991, Shea, *et al* 2007, Shea, *et al* 2009).
For the evaluation of prospective comparative trials in the transplantation field, we searched for meta-analyses including genetically randomized trials. These trials were defined by patient allocation to an intervention on the basis of sibling donor availability (donor group versus no-donor group) and were evaluated for potential bias as previously discussed (Ram, *et al* 2011).

3. An overview of systematic reviews in acute myeloid leukemia

Survival of AML patients has constantly been increasing from about 5-10% in 1975 to about 25% of diagnosed patients according to SEER data (1975-2007) in US population. This progress is the result of the progress in supportive care enabling treatment with intensive chemotherapy to induce remission and the use of allogeneic hematopoietic cell transplantation (HCT), as well as the use of prognostic factors in clinical decision making. For the majority of patients with AML this disease still has grave consequences. Our understanding of cytogenetic and molecular factors in the pathogenesis and the prognosis of patients with AML has evolved tremendously during the last decade. Still our ability to cure has remained unsatisfactory.
Treatment of AML with curative intent is generally divided into remission induction and post remission (also referred to as consolidation) courses (Dohner, *et al* 2010). Management of patients with AML depends mainly on their age, their response to therapy and the cytogenetic and molecular factors of the leukemic clone, stratifying patients into favorable, standard and unfavorable risk groups.
We herein reviewed the results of systematic reviews assessing chemotherapy for patients with AML. For each systematic review we evaluated the methodological quality using the AMSTAR assessment tool (Table 1).

3.1 Induction therapy

For more than 3 decades remission induction treatment consists of anthracyclines administered for 3 days and cytarabine given at a dose of 100-200 mg/m^2 in continuous infusion for 7 days. Efforts to improve response rate and survival of patients with AML included the addition of other chemotherapeutic drugs to the standard induction regimen, using different types and doses of anthracyclines, as well as different doses of cytarabine.

3.1.1 Does the type of anthracycline affect overall survival of adult patients with AML?

A systematic collaborative overview of individual patient data of RCTs that compared an idarubicin-based induction regimen with a different anthracycline-based regimen included trials from 1984 to 1993 including 1898 patients (AML Collaborative Group, 1998). Compared to daunorubicin, idarubicin improved remission rate (53% *vs.* 62%, respectively, $p = 0.002$) and overall survival (14% odds reduction, $p = 0.03$), however disease free survival (DFS) did not differ significantly (15% odds reduction, $p=0.07$). This overview fulfilled 4 of 11 criteria of the AMSTAR tool.
Since the publication of this systematic review new data has accumulated (Mandelli, *et al* 2009, Rowe, *et al* 2004).

3.1.2 Does the dose of anthracyclines during induction have an effect on survival?

Historically, the conventional induction anthracycline dose was the equivalent of daunorubicin 45-50 mg/m^2 daily given for 3 days. Large case series and observational studies supported a dose escalation to 60 mg/m^2. It remained questionable if the dose response curve has reached a plateau and whether the dose amplification benefit can be confirmed in RCTs. A few RCTs evaluated various dosages of anthracyclines. No published systematic review has summarized their findings so far.

Two RCTs evaluated dose intensification of anthracyclines (Fernandez, *et al* 2009, Lowenberg, *et al* 2009). Patients <60 years old treated with 90 mg/m^2 of daunorubicin, as compared with the standard 45 mg/m^2, achieved a higher rate of complete remission (CR) (70.6% *vs.* 57.3%; P<0.001) and a better overall survival (P=0.003) (Lowenberg, *et al* 2009). In another trial, >60 year-old patients treated with higher doses of daunorubicin, i.e. 90 mg/m^2 as compared to 45 mg/m^2 daily, for 3 days, had higher CR rates (64% for the high dose *vs.* 54% for the standard dose; P=0.002) (Pautas, *et al* 2010). There was no significant difference between the two groups in the incidence of hematological adverse events, 30-day mortality (11% and 12% in the 2 groups, respectively), or the incidence of adverse events (P=0.08). An overall survival benefit was demonstrated only in 2 subgroups: patients aged 60 to 65 years, and those with favorable cytogenetics. Paustas et al. compared 3-days of daunorubicin 80 $mg/m^2/day$ with 3 or 4-days of idarubicin 12 $mg/m^2/day$ in 468 patients aged 50 to 70 years. While a statistically significant higher rate of CR was demonstrated in patients treated with idarubicin (P = .04), there were no significant differences in the other outcomes.

Thus, conventional dose for remission induction in adult patients < 60 years with AML should be between 60 to 90 $mg/m^2/day$. There is no clear benefit for higher doses (90 $mg/m^2/day$) of daunorubicin compared to 45 mg/m^2 daily in adults >65 years.

3.1.3 Do higher doses of cytarabine during remission induction treatment improve survival?

Kern and Estey reviewed the literature to examine the effect of high dose cytarabine (≥1000 $mg/m^2/dose$) in induction therapy compared with standard dose (100-200 $mg/m^2/day$) cytarabine (Kern and Estey 2006). The search yielded 3 trials, evaluating 1691 adult AML patients < 60 years. There was no difference between high dose and standard dose cytarabine with regard to CR rate (relative risk 1.00; 95% CI 0.92 to 1.10) or early death rate (RR 1.53; 95% CI 0.84 to 2.78, random-effects model). However, 4-year overall survival was better in patients given high dose cytarabine (weighted mean difference, 6.211; 95% CI, 2.701 to 9.721). In this meta-analysis time to event data was analyzed as continuous data, the assumptions made for converting median to mean and their variance to standard deviation were not described, and weighted mean difference was used to pool results. This review fulfilled 7 of 11 criteria of the AMSTAR criteria.

3.2 Post remission therapy

3.2.1 What is the role of transplantation in patients with AML?

3.2.1.1 Autologous hematopoietic cell transplantation

Four systematic reviews evaluated the effect of autologous hematopoietic cell transplantation (HCT) in first CR (Ashfaq, *et al* 2010, Levi, *et al* 2004, Nathan, *et al* 2004, Wang, *et al* 2010).

Nathan et al. compared the efficacy of autologous HCT with chemotherapy (or no further treatment) in patients aged 15 to 55 years (Nathan, *et al* 2004). Their search yielded 6 trials including 1044 patients. Patients who underwent autologous HCT had a better DFS (probabilities ratio of 1.24, 95% CI 1.06 to 1.44) with similar long term mortality rate (RR 1.01, 95% CI 0.89 to 1.15). This review fulfilled 9 of 11 criteria of the AMSTAR tool. Levi et al performed a systematic review on the same question with similar findings (Levi, *et al* 2004). A more recent systematic review included 12 RCTs (Wang, *et al* 2010). Patients treated with autologous HCT had lower relapse rate,better DFS, but no overall survival benefit probably because of higher treatment related mortality. Of note, at present, transplant related mortality is lower than the estimated 4% reported in these systematic reviews.

3.2.1.2 Allogeneic hematopoietic cell transplantation

Eight reviews and meta-analyses were identified but only three of them were systematic and comprehensive (Ashfaq, *et al* 2010, Hubel, *et al* 2011, Koreth, *et al* 2009). Koreth et al. performed a systematic review comparing allogeneic HCT with conventional consolidation chemotherapy or autologous HCT (Koreth, *et al* 2009). Patients allocated to the allogeneic HCT arm had an overall survival benefit (HR 0.90 95% CI 0.82 to 0.97, 15 trials), and relapse free survival (HR 0.80 95% CI, 0.74 to 0.86, 18 trials). In an analysis stratified according to the cytogenetic risk groups, only intermediate and poor risk AML patients allocated to the allogeneic HCT arm had improved overall survival, while favorable risk patients had similar overall survival in both allocated arms. This review fulfilled 10 of 11 criteria of the AMSTAR tool.
Another comprehensive systematic review (without a quantitative summary) was done through the National Institute for Health Research Health Technology Assessment (HTA) program in UK (Ashfaq, *et al* 2010). The results and conclusions of this very detailed review were consistent with those of the previous ones. Other systematic reviews were published earlier and were not as comprehensive (Oliansky, *et al* 2008, Schlenk, *et al* 2004, Visani, *et al* 2006, Yanada, *et al* 2005).

3.3 Consolidation – dose intensity of cytarabine

A systematic overview without a quantitative analysis of chemotherapy for patients with AML was conducted by The Swedish Council of Technology Assessment in Health Care (Kimby, *et al* 2001). In one trial consolidation was compared to no further treatment. This trial was closed early due to inferior remission duration in the latter group. In all the trials comparing high dose cytarabine to standard dose or maintenance therapy, high dose cytarabine was shown to be superior to the comparator, though overall survival advantage was not consistently shown. Consolidation with high dose cytarabine seemed to be of value mainly for patients with core binding factor AML and in younger patients, due to a high mortality rate in patients older than 60 years. This overview fulfilled 1 of 10 criteria of the AMSTAR tool.

3.4 Maintenance therapy instead of consolidation chemotherapy

This question was reviewed by Kimby et al. who found limited data to indicate that post-remission maintenance therapy with long-term attenuated chemotherapy can prolong remission duration compared to no further therapy (Kimby, *et al* 2001). However, the data in support of these conclusions are sparse and effect on survival was not shown.

3.5 Role of azacitidine

Azacitidine was not exclusively assessed in AML patients but rather analyzed in a pooled myelodysplasia/AML group of patients (20%- 30% blasts, defined by the WHO as AML)

AMSTAR criterion / Study ID by author year	The AML collaborative group 1998	Kern 2006	Nathan 2004	Levi 2004	Yanada 2005	Koreth 2009	Ashfaq 2010	Kimby 2001
Was an 'a priori' design provided?	Yes	Yes	Yes	Yes	Yes	Yes	Yes	Not reported
Was there duplicate study selection and data extraction?	Not reported	Yes	Yes	Yes	No	Yes	Yes	Not reported
Was a comprehensive literature search performed?	No	Yes	Yes	No	No	Yes	No	Not reported
Was the status of publication used as an inclusion criterion? (i.e. grey literature was included)	Yes	Yes	No	No	No	Yes	Yes	No
Was a list of studies (included and excluded) provided?	No	No	Yes	No	Yes	Yes	Yes	No
Were the characteristics of the included studies provided?	Yes	Yes	Yes	Yes	Yes	Yes	Yes	Yes
Was the scientific quality of the included studies assessed and documented?	Yes	Yes	Yes	Yes	Not reported	Yes	Yes	No
Was the scientific quality of the included studies used appropriately in formulating conclusions?	No	No	No	Yes	No	No	No	No
Were the methods used to combine the findings of studies appropriate?	Yes	No, analyzed survival data as a continuous variable	Unclear	Yes	Yes	Yes	Not applicable	Not applicable
Was the likelihood of publication bias assessed?	No	No	Yes	No	Yes	Yes	No	No
Were potential conflicts of interest included?	No	No	Yes	No	No	Yes	No	No
Total	5	6	8-9	6	5	10	6	1

Table 1. Assessment of risk of bias using AMSTAR criteria in systematic reviews in the field of AML

(Edlin, *et al* 2010). This RCT shows an overall survival benefit for azacytidine compared to best supportive care, low dose cytarabine, or intensive chemotherapy. Two RCTs that evaluated the effect of azacytidine in patients with high risk MDS (including patients with 20%- 30% blasts) showed improved time to transformation or death in patients given azacytidine (Fenaux, *et al* 2009, Silverman, *et al* 2002).

Azacytidine was also given as part of post remission chemotherapy: in the MRC AML 9 trial, patients given the azacitidine-chemotherapy arm as consolidation had fewer relapses comparedto patients given only chemotherapy ($p = 0.003$), but a higher treatment related mortality (4.5% vs. 0%), without a statistically significant improved long term survival (Rees, *et al* 1996).

In another trial, patients were randomized to post remission consolidation with different chemotherapy regimens: standard dose cytarabine-daunorubicin *vs.* the same treatment followed by amsacrine and azacytidine vs. thioguanine and standard dose cytarabine-daunorubicin (Volger, *et al* 1995). The 5-year DFS was 38%, 31%, and 27% ($p<0.05$), respectively.

4. Acute promyelocytic leukemia

Acute promyelocytic leukemia (APL) is usually characterized by a specific gene rearrangement and the generation of the PML-RARα fusion transcript which results from a translocation between chromosomes 15 and 17. Targeted therapy with all-trans retinoic acid (ATRA) and anthracycline-based chemotherapy results in cure in 70-80% of patients.

Two systematic reviews evaluated the first line treatment of patients with APL (Xu, *et al* 2009a, Xu, *et al* 2009b).

The first one includes 7 RCTs (392 patients) comparing ATRA plus arsenic trioxide to other treatments. Compared with arsenic trioxide monotherapy, arsenic trioxide plus ATRA affected neither CR or DFS rates nor mortality of relapsed APL patients. Arsenic trioxide plus ATRA improved CR rate, DFS, mortality rate and adverse reactions compared to the same regimen including also chemotherapy. The review fulfilled 6 of 11 criteria of the AMSTAR tool.

A systematic review and meta-analysis including 5 randomized controlled trials (328 patients) compared ATRA plus arsenic trioxide regimen with ATRA monotherapy in patients with APL showed an improved 2-year DFS rate in the group treated with ATRA arsenic trioxide.

5. An overview of systematic reviews in acute lymphoblastic leukemia

Acute lymphoblastic leukemia (ALL) is the most common acute leukemia in children, while the incidence is much lower in adults (National Cancer Institute. SEER Cancer Statistics Review Available at: http://seer.cancer.gov/csr/1975_2006). The outcome of pediatric ALL patients has evolved from an overall survival of less than 10% in the 1960s to approximately 80% at present (Pui, *et al* 2008). However, adult patients have a less optimistic prognosis. While the remission rate reaches 90%, the survival rate is only 40%-50% (Fielding 2008). ALL patients are stratified and treated according to algorithms that integrate the presenting features, leukemia features and early response to therapy (Faderl, *et al* 2003); However the classification to standard and poor risk disease varies among the major studies conducted in adult ALL patients (Hoelzer, *et al* 1988, Kantarjian, *et al* 2004, Lazarus, *et al* 2006, Le, *et al* 2006, Rowe, *et al* 2005, Ram, *et al 2010*).

Treatment of adult ALL patients usually consists of remission induction and consolidation/intensification phases followed by either HCT or maintenance therapy.
As stated above, because the disease is relatively rare in adults, much of the knowledge and protocols have been adopted from pediatric regimens. Although we aim to focus on adult population, a portion of the data is based on evidence from pediatric trials.
For each systematic review we evaluated the methodological quality using the AMSTAR assessment tool (table 2).

5.1 Is there a specific induction regimen which is better?

Different groups use various induction regimens, which have not been compared head to head (Gokbuget and Hoelzer 2009, Kantarjian, *et al* 2004, Larson, *et al* 1995, Linker, *et al* 2002, Thomas, *et al* 2004b). In adult patients, the use of growth factors such as granulocyte colony-stimulating factor that accelerate hematopoietic recovery has greatly improved the success rate of ALL therapy (Kantarjian, *et al* 2004) and will be reviewed in a different part of this chapter.
One individual patient data meta-analysis examined the role of incorporating different types of anthracycines into pediatric induction regimens (CALLCG, 2009) and identified 4 trials recruiting 958 patients. They found that there was a borderline significant reduction in bone marrow leukemia relapse rate (OR 0.77, 95% CI 0.60 to 1.00; p=0.05) among patients treated with anthracyclines compared to those not, though there was no difference in non-bone marrow leukemia relapse rate (OR 0.88, 95% CI 0.63 to 1.25; p=0.5). The reduction in relapse rate translated into improved relapse free survival (OR 0.81; 95% CI, 0.66 to 1.00; p=0.05). However, event free survival (EFS) and overall survival were similar between the two groups. No significant differences in outcomes were demonstrated when different anthracyclines or when different adninistration schedules were compared. As this meta-analysis has been solely conducted in a pediatric population, results might not be applicable for adult patients. This systematic review fulfilled 5 of 11 criteria of the AMSTAR tool.

5.2 What is the role of pediatric inspired regimens for adult patients, mainly for the group of adolescents and young adults?

Several recent studies comparing the outcome of adolescents and young adults (AYAs) up to the age of 45 years, treated with pediatric versus adult protocols, demonstrated improved survival for AYAs who were treated by pediatric groups (Boissel, *et al* 2003, Ramanujachar, *et al* 2007, Stock, *et al* 2008). All are non-randomized trials and are therefore prone to significant bias. Thus, these trials are difficult to interpret because of the wide spectrum of patients' age, the small number of patients, the variations in the regimens utilized and the varying application of HCT in different studies. Recently our group completed a systematic review and meta analysis of all published comparative studies. We showed that up to the age of 20 years, pediatric inspired regimens are superior to conveintional afults chemotherapy (Ram, *et al* 2011). Currently there are several groups conducting prospective trials (e.g., US AALL0232) to further elucidate which is the best treatment for AYAs. Only then, solid conclusions to tailor the best treatment for AYAs should be drawn.

5.3 What is the role of thyrosine kinase inhibitors in the treatment of Philadelphia positive ALL?

Philadelphia positive ALL is a disease with a historically dismal prognosis in which HCT provided the only chance for cure (Fielding and Goldstone 2008). Recently, the introduction of tyrosine kinase inhibitors (TKIs) has opened wide new perspectives of how to treat these patients (Thomas, *et al* 2004a). We were not able to identify systematic reviews assessing the

	Induction Regimens	Role of post remission HCT					Maintenance Regimes			CNS prophylaxis
Study ID by author / AMSTAR criterion	CALLCG, BJH 2009	Ram, Cancer 2010	Yanada, Cancer 2006	Orsi, BMT 2007	Hahn, BBMT 2006	Ashfaq, Health Teq Asses 2010	CALLCG, Lancet 1996	CALLCG, BJH 2010	Escherich, Leukemia 2011	Clarke, JCO 2003
Was an 'a priori' design provided?	Yes	Yes	Yes	Yes	Yes	Yes	Yes	Yes	Yes	Yes
Was there duplicate study selection and data extraction?	No	No	Yes	Yes	No	No	No	No	No	No
Was a comprehensive literature search performed?	Yes	Yes	Yes	Yes	Yes	Yes	Yes	Yes	No	Yes
Was the status of publication used as an inclusion criterion? (i.e. gray literature was included)	No	Yes	Yes	No	No	No	No	No	No	No
Was a list of studies (included and excluded) provided?	No	Yes	No	Yes	No	Yes	No	No	Yes	No
Were the characteristics of the included studies provided?	Yes	Yes	Yes	Yes	Yes	Yes	No	Yes	Yes	Yes
Was the scientific quality of the included studies assessed and documented?	No	Yes	Yes	Yes	Yes	No	No	Yes	No	No
Was the scientific quality of the included studies used appropriately in formulating conclusions?	No	Yes	Yes	Yes	Yes	No	No	No	No	No
Were the methods used to combine the findings of studies appropriate?	Yes	Yes	Yes	Yes	Yes	Yes	Yes	Yes	Yes	Yes
Was the likelihood of publication bias assessed?	No	Yes	No	Yes	No	No	No	Yes	No	No
Were potential conflicts of interest included?	Yes	Yes	No	No	No	Yes	No	Yes	Yes	No
Overall grading	5	10	8	9	6	6	3	7	5	4

Table 2. Assessment of risk of bias using AMSTAR criteria in systematic reviews in the field of ALL

role of the different tyrosine kinase inhibitors. Prospective comparison, for example, by using genetic randomization based on donor availability along with intention-to-treat analysis, is necessary to draw conclusions on the clinical utility of allogeneic HCT for these patients.

5.4 What is the role of allogeneic HCT in first CR?

Allogeneic HCT provides a potential curative approach for patients with ALL, mainly through the anti-leukemic effect of the graft. Nonetheless, the relatively high non-relapse mortality compared to other treatment options limits the widespread use of this approach (Hahn, *et al* 2006, Ram, *et al* 2011).

As stated in the Methods section, the preferred way to assess the role of allogeneic HCT is to use a genetic randomization design, allocating patients with a matched sibling donor and those lacking sibling donor to the donor/transplantation arm and the no-donor/alternative treatment arm, respectively (Ram, *et al* 2011).

Five systematic reviews were conducted (Ashfaq, *et al* 2010, Hahn, *et al* 2006, Orsi *et al* 2007, Ram, *et al* 2010, Yanada *et al* 2006), 3 out of which included also a meta analysis (Orsi *et al* 2007, Ram, *et al* 2010, Yanada *et al* 2006). All three meta-analyses showed that overall, for ALL patients achieving first CR, allogeneic HCT carries a survival benefit compared to the other options. While all 3 meta-analyses used similar search criteria, the strict intention to treat (ITT) inclusion criteria were different. Moreover, the two largest trials in the field (Cornelissen *et al* 2009, Goldstone *et al* 2008) were included only in the most recently published meta-analysis only (Ram, *et al* 2010). This meta-analysis included 10 genetically trials, randomizing 2,600 patients for the main comparison of allogeneic HCT vs. other treatments, with only seven trials, randomizing 1,863 patients, following strict ITT criteria (table 2). In this meta-analysis, survival benefit was statistically significant for the standard-risk patients (RR for all-cause mortality 0.80, 95% CI 0.68–0.94), while for the high-risk it it was not (RR 0.88, 95% CI 0.76–1.01) (Ram, *et al* 2010). As expected, there was a significant increase in non-relapse mortality in the allogeneic HCT arm (RR 2.99; 95% CI, 1.37-6.53) and a significant decrease in the relapse rate (RR 0.52; 95% CI, 0.33-0.83). This systematic review fulfilled 10 of 11 criteria of the AMSTAR tool.

Although a systematic review published by Yanada et al showed a similar survival advantage in favor of the donor group (HR 1.29, 95% CI 1.02 to 1.63, $p = 0.037$), superiority could be demonstrated for the high-risk patients subgroup only (HR 1.42, 95% CI 1.06 to 1.90; $p = 0.019$). This systematic review fulfilled 8 of 11 criteria of the AMSTAR tool.

The difference between the two meta-analyses might stem from two main causes: The first is the inclusion of the two recent large trials in the last meta-analysis only (Cornelissen *et al* 2009, Goldstone *et al* 2008) and the second from the different methodologies and inclusion criteria used in the various studies (with more emphasis on strict ITT methodology in the recently published meta-analysis).

Orsi et al. conducted an individual patient meta-analysis of four trials (Hunault *et al.*, 2004, Labar *et al* 2004, Ribera *et al* 2005, Thomas, *et al* 2004b). They also showed survival benefit for the donor group (mean EFS was 5.88 years in the donor group and 4.88 years in the no-donor group) with survival rate of 44.2% (± 2.9%) at 7 years in the donor group and 31.6% (± 2.2%) in the non-donor group, log-rank test p = 0.011. Performance of allogeneic HCT in first CR was found to be cost effective. This systematic review fulfilled 9 of 11 criteria of the AMSTAR tool.

To summarize, all meta-analyses suggest overall survival benefit for patients undergoing a matched donor allogeneic HCT in first CR when compared to other modalities. By drawing firm conclusions based on strict ITT trials it is suggested that allogeneic HCT may be more effective for the standard risk group.

5.5 Is there a role for autologous HCT in first CR?

We identified three systematic reviews that reported on the comparison between post remission autologous HCT and maintenance chemotherapy (Ashfaq, *et al* 2010, Hahn, *et al* 2006, Ram, *et al* 2010). One of them also performed a meta-analysis of the available RCTs. Both Hahn et al. and Ashfaq et al. concluded that both autologous HCT and maintenance chemotherapy yield a similar outcome (Ashfaq, *et al* 2010, Hahn, *et al* 2006). They also suggested that autologous HCT might be a superior option for high risk patients. In the meta-analysis performed by our group (Ram, *et al* 2010), five conventionally randomized trials enrolling 963 patients were identified. Similar to previous systematic reviews, survival was comparable between the two arms (RR 1.02, 95%CI, 0.88 to 1.19) for both standard and high risk patients. However there was a significant increase in non-relapse mortality in the autologous HCT arm (RR 1.77; 95% CI, 1.12 to 2.8), though no statistically significant difference was demonstrated in the relapse risk (RR 0.92; 95% CI, 0.73-1.15).

	Yanada, Cancer 2006	Orsi, BMT 2007	Ram, Cancer 2010
*Bernasconi 1992**			+
*Sebban 1994**	+	+	+
*Attal 1995**			+
*Takeuchi 2002**	+		+
*Dombret 2002,Thomas 2004**	+	+	+
Labar 2004#	+		+
Hunault 2004#	+	+	+
*Ribera 2005**	+	+	+
*Vey 2006**			+
Cornelissen 2008#			+
*Goldstone 2008**			+
*Fielding, 2009**			+

*True ITT trial #Not strictly ITT trial – Reasons for the inability to perform ITT analysis: Labar,2004- inclusion of patients with no siblings in the non-donor arm; Hunault, 2004- inclusion of patients>50 years in the non-donor group ; Cornelissen,2008- inclusion of patients who underwent matched unrelated donor transplantation in the nondonor study arm

Table 3. Comparisons between 3 meta-analyses assessing the role of allogeneic hematopoietic cell transplantation in first complete remission

5.6 Which is the best maintenance therapy?

The post remission high relapse rate of adult ALL patients has encouraged the exploration of various post-remission modalities. The optimal type and duration of maintenance therapy and the value of further intensification are still debated.

We identified 3 relevant systematic reviews (CALLCG *et al* 1996, Eden, *et al* 2010, Escherich, *et al* 2011), reporting on pediatric patients.

The first, evaluating the impact of duration and intensity of the different maintenance regimens, included 16 trials, randomizing 746 patients (CALLCG et al., 1996) showed that maintenance treatment administered for up to 3 years was associated with a significantly lower relapse rate albeit a similar rate of death from leukemia. Of note, maintenance duration beyond 3 years did not yield any superiority . More intensive regimens were associated with significantly fewer relapse events and with prolonged survival (absolute difference in survival of about 3% at 5 years and of 4% at 8 years). This systematic review fulfilled 3 of 11 criteria of the AMSTAR tool.

The second systematic review evaluated the addition of steroids plus vincristine pulses during the maintenance period (Eden, *et al*). In an individual patient meta-analysis vincristine-prednisone pulses were shown to improves EFS (70.1% vs. 62% at 5 years; OR 0.71, 95% CI 0.61 to 0.84; p = 0.00004), while vincristine - dexamethasone pulses did not have this effect (80.9% vs. 79.9% at 5 year; OR 0.94; 95% CI, 0.8 to 1.11;p = 0.5) Overall survival was not affected by both combinations. (Bostrom, *et al* 2003). Results of this meta-analysis should be taken with caution as they might be significantly biased by different pre-maintenance induction regimens. This systematic review fulfilled 7 of 11 criteria of the AMSTAR tool.

The third systematic review compared between the various thiopurines (mainly thioguanine and metcaptopurine) as maintenance (Escherich, *et al*). In a meta-analysis of 3 trials, event-free survival was similar for the two agents (OR 0.89, 95% CI, 0.78 to 1.03). However in a subgroup analysis of males aged<10 years there was a significant benefit for thiogouanine in terms of EFS (OR 0.70, 95% CI, 0.58 to 0.84), although this did not result in a significant difference in overall survival (OR 0.83, 95% CI, 0.62 to 1.10). It was concluded that mercaptopurine, and not thiogouanine, should be the thiopurine drug of choice for maintenance. Although this conclusion is valid for pediatric patients, in the absence of data in adults this may also be applicable for them. This systematic review fulfilled 5 of 11 criteria of the AMSTAR tool.

5.7 What is the role of CNS prophylaxis and is there a "gold-standard" regimen?

CNS involvement at presentation in adult ALL patients is estimated as 5% (Lazarus, *et al* 2006). Nevertheless, without prophylaxis administration, CNS recurrence occurs in approximately 30% of adult patients in complete response (Omura, *et al* 1980). There are several options to administer CNS prophylaxis therapy. These include cranial radiotherapy and intrathecal or intraventricular chemotherapy.

One pediatric systematic review with individual patient meta-analysis (Clarke, *et al* 2003) reported that prophylactic radiotherapy reduced CNS relapse slightly more than long-term intrathecal therapy, however no survival benefit was shown. Also, higher than 21 Gy radiation dose did not correlate with lower relapse risk and, the addition of intravenous methotrexate to regimens containing either radiation and intrathecal therapy led to a better EFS. This systematic review fulfilled 4 of 11 criteria of the AMSTAR tool.

6. An overview of systematic reviews in supportive care for patients with acute leukemia

Supportive care in acute leukemia has improved dramatically during the last decades and contributed to the improved overall survival of AL patients.

7. Myeloid growth factors

The use of G-CSF and GM-CSF results in a dose dependent increase in the levels of circulating neutrophils, mainly as a result of shortening the transit time from stem cell to mature cells (Griffin 2001). During intensive chemotherapy, acute leukemia patients experience prolonged and profound neutropenia, which is a risk factor for bacterial and fungal infections, for increased mortality. Patients with acute leukemia can be treated with myeloid growth factors as primary or secondary prophylaxis (before or after the development of neutropenia, respectively) or for priming (before or concurrent with chemotherapy) with the aim of sensitizing blast cells and recruiting them into cell-cycle, thus enhancing their susceptibility to cytotxic agents like cytarabine.

Five systematic reviews assessed the effect of myeloid growth factors in acute leukemia patients.

The first one is a comprehensive systematic review and meta-analysis, published in 2007 by Sung et al and comprises 148 RCTs, randomizing 16,839 patients with all types of cancer. Patients were randomly assigned to receive chemotherapy with or without prophylaxis with myeloid growth factors (Sung, *et al* 2007). There was no difference between the two groups in short term all cause mortality and in infection related mortality. However, the use of myeloid-growth factors was associated with reduction of clinically and microbiologically documented infections (RR 0.75, 95% CI 0.62 to 0.92, and RR 0.86, 95% CI, 0.77-0.96, respectively). Subgroup analysis of acute leukemia patients did not show any difference in short term all cause mortality and infection related mortality, as well (Sung, *et al* 2007). This systematic review fulfilled 9 of 11 criteria of the AMSTAR tool.

The second systematic review and meta-analysis compared the prophylactic use of G-CSF in patients with AML receiving chemotherapy, to placebo/no treatment (control group) (Wang, *et al* 2009a, Wang, *et al* 2009b). This review included seven trials with almost 2000 participants, and did not show difference in overall survival between the G-CSF group and the control group (Wang, *et al* 2009a) This systematic review fulfilled 5 of 11 criteria of the AMSTAR tool.

In a systematic review and meta-analysis recently conducted by our group, we questioned the role of myeloid growth factors administrated to AML patients concurrent with or post chemotherapy (Gurion, *et al.*, 2011). There was no difference in short term and long term all cause mortality, CR rate, DFS and relapse rate between the arm receiving growth factors and the control arm. Furthermore, the use of myeloid growth factors was not associated with a reduction in the incidence of infections. This systematic review fulfilled 10 of the 11 criteria of the AMSTAR tool.

Another recently published systematic review compared the administration of myeloid growth factors in AML patients receiving chemotherapy to control/placebo (Heuser, *et al* 2011). Among patients receiving primary prophylaxis, time to neutrophil recovery and hospitalization stay were shorter, yet no difference was shown in CR, event and DFS and overall survival, compared to no prophylaxis. Among patients receiving growth factors for priming, there was also no difference in CR, event free and disease free survival overall survival. This review fulfilled 7 of 11 criteria of the AMSTAR tool.

In another meta-analysis, the use of myeloid growth factors for priming did not affect CR rate, DFS or overall survival (Sung, *et al* 2009). Subgroup analyses according to type of myeloid growth factors, the timing of administration and patients' age did not affect

outcomes. The main limitation of these meta-analyses is their heterogeneity in terms of patients' characteristics, chemotherapy regimens and trial designs.
To conclude, the main beneficial effects of growth factors are acceleration of neutrophil recovery by 2 to 5 days and a reduction in the length of hospitalization.(Griffin 2001, Inoue, *et al* 1990, Lemoli, *et al* 1991, Lowenberg, *et al* 1988, Park, *et al* 1989). With regard to priming with growth factors in AML, 2 meta-analyses did not demonstrate a statistical significant effect on remission rate and overall survival and therefore do not support their regular use.

7.2 Prophylactic anti-infectious treatment

Two systematic review and meta-analyses assessed the effect of antibacterial and antifungal prophylaxis in neutropenic patients receiving chemotherapy.
Gafter-Gvili et al. evaluated the use of antibacterial prophylaxis for afebrile neuropenic patients (Gafter-Gvili, *et al* 2005). The administration of antibacterial prophylaxis reduced all-cause mortality by 33% (95% CI 0.55 to 0.81) in neutropenic patients who received any antibiotic prophylaxis and by 48% (95% CI 0.35 to 0.77) in patients who received quinolones for prophylaxis compared to placebo or no intervention. Also, the occurrence of febrile episodes and bacterial infections decreased significantly. This review fulfilled 10 of 11 criteria of the AMSTAR tool.
Robenshtock et al. evaluated antifungal agents for prophylaxis in neutropenic patients following chemotherapy or after allogeneic HCT (Robenshtok, *et al* 2007). All-cause mortality was reduced significantly in patients receiving antifungal prophylaxis compared with placebo, no treatment, or non-systemic antifungals (RR 0.84, 95% CI, 0.74 to 0.95). In a subgroup analysis of patients with acute leukemia there was a significant reduction in fungal-related mortality and documented invasive fungal infections, yet there was no difference in mortality. This review fulfilled 10 of 11 criteria of the AMSTAR tool.

7.3 Transfusion support

One systematic review and meta-analysis evaluated the prophylactic use of platelets in patients with hematological malignancies(Stanworth, *et al* 2004). Three studies compared prophylactic with therapeutic use of platelets. There was no difference in all-cause mortality, or mortality due to hemorrhagic cause. Of note, studies were conducted between 1974-1982 and were small with marked heterogeneity, thus the results of this meta-analysis should be taken with caution. Three prospective studies compared the platelet transfusion thresholds of 10 *vs.* 20×10^9 /L. There were no statistically significant differences between the groups with regards to mortality, remission rates, number of participants with severe bleeding events or red cell transfusion requirements.
The main limitation of this review is the inclusion of a limited number of small studies in different three meta-analyses, carrying a potential risk for bias, though no publication bias was reported. This review fulfilled 8 of 11 criteria of the AMSTAR tool.
Recently, two published RCTs compared low dose to high dose prophylactic platelets transfusion (Heddle, *et al* 2009, Slichter, *et al*). Both showed no difference in grade 2-4 bleeding incidence between patients allocated to low threshold of platelets administration and no difference between different doses of platelet transfusion. However, one of the studies was prematurely stopped because of 5.2% grade 4 bleeding in the lower dose platelets compared to none in the high dose (Heddle, *et al* 2009).

AMSTAR / Study ID by author	Sung et al	Wang et al	Gurion et al	Heuser et al	Sung et al	Gafter et al	Robenshtock et al	Stanworth et al
Was an 'a priori' design provided?	Yes	Yes	Yes	Yes	Yes	Yes	Yes	Yes
Was there duplicate study selection and data extraction?	Yes	No, not reported	Yes	Yes	Yes	Yes	Yes	Yes
Was a comprehensive literature search performed?	Yes No search in conference proceedings and in databases of ongoing trials	Yes No search in databases of ongoing trials	Yes	Yes No search in conference proceedings and in databases of ongoing trials	Yes No search in databases of ongoing trialV	Yes No search in databases of ongoing trials	Yes No search in databases of ongoing trials	Yes No search in conference proceedings except for ASH 2002
Was the status of publication used as an inclusion criterion? (i.e. grey literature was included)	No	No	No	Yes Unpublished trials were excluded	No	No	No	No
Was a list of studies (included and excluded) provided?	No, only a list of included studies was provided	No, only a list of included studies was provided	Yes	No, only a list of included studies was provide	No, only a list of included studies was provide	Yes	Yes	Yes
Were the characteristics of the included studies provided?	Yes	Yes	Yes	Yes	Yes	Yes	Yes	Yes
Was the scientific quality of the included studies assessed and documented?	Yes	No	Yes	No, only blindness was reported.	Yes, used Jadad scale for assessing quality	No	Yes	Yes
Was the scientific quality of the included studies used appropriately in formulating conclusions?	Yes	Yes	Yes	Not applicable	Yes	Yes	Yes	Yes
Were the methods used to combine the findings of studies appropriate?	Yes	Yes	Yes	Yes	Yes	Yes	Yes	Yes
Was the likelihood of publication bias assessed?	Yes	R1	Yes	No	Yes	Yes	Yes	No
Were potential conflicts of interest included?	Yes	R1	Yes	Yes	No	Yes	Yes	No

Table 4. Assessment of risk of bias using AMSTAR criteria in systematic reviews of supportive care in acute leukemia

8. Conclusions

The progress made in the last 4 decades in the treatment of patients with acute leukemia is the consequence of a constant process of testing, data compilation and re-testing. Data gathering on a specific question using explicit, preplanned scientific methods to identify select and synthesize all relevant studies is the process of systematic review, which provides the clinician with the best evidence, and should form the basis for rational medical decision-making.

In this chapter we examined the evidence accumulated in various aspects of leukemia management, based on RCTs and systematic reviews and meta-analyses. While in certain areas such as the role of tyrosine kinase inhibitors in Philadelphia positive ALL or allogeneic transplant in adult patients with ALL a consensus could be reached according to the data published so far, many questions are still open in the field of leukemia which warrant conduction of further clinical trials.

9. References

(1998) A systematic collaborative overview of randomized trials comparing idarubicin with daunorubicin (or other anthracyclines) as induction therapy for acute myeloid leukaemia. AML Collaborative Group, 1998. *Br J Haematol,* 103, 100-109.

Ashfaq, K., Yahaya, I., Hyde, C., Andronis, L., Barton, P., Bayliss, S. & Chen, Y.F. (2010) Clinical effectiveness and cost-effectiveness of stem cell transplantation in the management of acute leukaemia: a systematic review. *Health Technol Assess,* 14, iii-iv, ix-xi, 1-141.

Boissel, N., Auclerc, M.F., Lheritier, V., Perel, Y., Thomas, X., Leblanc, T., Rousselot, P., Cayuela, J.M., Gabert, J., Fegueux, N., Piguet, C., Huguet-Rigal, F., Berthou, C., Boiron, J.M., Pautas, C., Michel, G., Fiere, D., Leverger, G., Dombret, H. & Baruchel, A. (2003) Should adolescents with acute lymphoblastic leukemia be treated as old children or young adults? Comparison of the French FRALLE-93 and LALA-94 trials. *J Clin Oncol,* 21, 774-780.

Bostrom, B.C., Sensel, M.R., Sather, H.N., Gaynon, P.S., La, M.K., Johnston, K., Erdmann, G.R., Gold, S., Heerema, N.A., Hutchinson, R.J., Provisor, A.J. & Trigg, M.E. (2003) Dexamethasone versus prednisone and daily oral versus weekly intravenous mercaptopurine for patients with standard-risk acute lymphoblastic leukemia: a report from the Children's Cancer Group. *Blood,* 101, 3809-3817.

Br J Haematol. 2009 May;145(3):376-88. Beneficial and harmful effects of anthracyclines in the treatment of childhood acute lymphoblastic leukaemia: a systematic review and meta-analysis. Childhood Acute Lymphoblastic Leukaemia Collaborative Group (CALLCG).

Childhood ALL Collaborative Group (1996). Duration and intensity of maintenance chemotherapy in acute lymphoblastic leukaemia: overview of 42 trials involving 12 000 randomised children. *Lancet,* 347, 1783-1788.

Childhood ALL Collaborative Group (2009). Beneficial and harmful effects of anthracyclines in the treatment of childhood acute lymphoblastic leukaemia: a systematic review and meta-analysis. *Br J Haematol,* 145, 376-388.

Clarke, M., Gaynon, P., Hann, I., Harrison, G., Masera, G., Peto, R. & Richards, S. (2003) CNS-directed therapy for childhood acute lymphoblastic leukemia: Childhood ALL Collaborative Group overview of 43 randomized trials. *J Clin Oncol,* 21, 1798-1809.

Cornelissen JJ, van der Holt B, Verhoef GE, van't Veer MB, van Oers MH, Schouten HC, Ossenkoppele G, Sonneveld P, Maertens J, van Marwijk Kooy M, Schaafsma MR, Wijermans PW, Biesma DH, Wittebol S, Voogt PJ, Baars JW, Zachée P, Verdonck LF, Löwenberg B, Dekker AW (2009) Myeloablative allogeneic versus autologous stem cell transplantation in adult patients with acute lymphoblastic leukemia in first remission: a prospective sibling donor versus no-donor comparison. *Blood,* 113, 1375-1382.

Dohner, H., Estey, E.H., Amadori, S., Appelbaum, F.R., Buchner, T., Burnett, A.K., Dombret, H., Fenaux, P., Grimwade, D., Larson, R.A., Lo-Coco, F., Naoe, T., Niederwieser, D., Ossenkoppele, G.J., Sanz, M.A., Sierra, J., Tallman, M.S., Lowenberg, B. & Bloomfield, C.D. (2010) Diagnosis and management of acute myeloid leukemia in adults: recommendations from an international expert panel, on behalf of the European LeukemiaNet. *Blood,* 115, 453-474.

Duration and intensity of maintenance chemotherapy in acute lymphoblastic leukaemia: overview of 42 trials involving 12 000 randomised children. Childhood ALL Collaborative Group. Lancet 1996;347(9018):1783-8

Eden, T.O., Pieters, R. & Richards, S. (2010) Systematic review of the addition of vincristine plus steroid pulses in maintenance treatment for childhood acute lymphoblastic leukaemia - an individual patient data meta-analysis involving 5,659 children. *Br J Haematol,* 149, 722-733.

Edlin, R., Connock, M., Tubeuf, S., Round, J., Fry-Smith, A., Hyde, C. & Greenheld, W. Azacitidine for the treatment of myelodysplastic syndrome, chronic myelomonocytic leukaemia and acute myeloid leukaemia. *Health Technol Assess,* 14 Suppl 1, 69-74.

Escherich, G.M., Richards, S., Stork, L.C. & Vora, A.J. Meta-analysis of randomised trials comparing thiopurines in childhood acute lymphoblastic leukaemia. *Leukemia.*

Faderl, S., Jeha, S. & Kantarjian, H.M. (2003) The biology and therapy of adult acute lymphoblastic leukemia. *Cancer,* 98, 1337-1354.

Fenaux, P., Mufti, G.J., Hellstrom-Lindberg, E., Santini, V., Finelli, C., Giagounidis, A., Schoch, R., Gattermann, N., Sanz, G., List, A., Gore, S.D., Seymour, J.F., Bennett, J.M., Byrd, J., Backstrom, J., Zimmerman, L., McKenzie, D., Beach, C. & Silverman, L.R. (2009) Efficacy of azacitidine compared with that of conventional care regimens in the treatment of higher-risk myelodysplastic syndromes: a randomised, open-label, phase III study. *Lancet Oncol,* 10, 223-232.

Fernandez, H.F., Sun, Z., Yao, X., Litzow, M.R., Luger, S.M., Paietta, E.M., Racevskis, J., Dewald, G.W., Ketterling, R.P., Bennett, J.M., Rowe, J.M., Lazarus, H.M. & Tallman, M.S. (2009) Anthracycline dose intensification in acute myeloid leukemia. *N Engl J Med,* 361, 1249-1259.

Fielding, A. (2008) The treatment of adults with acute lymphoblastic leukemia. *Hematology Am Soc Hematol Educ Program,* 381-389.

Fielding, A.K. & Goldstone, A.H. (2008) Allogeneic haematopoietic stem cell transplant in Philadelphia-positive acute lymphoblastic leukaemia. *Bone Marrow Transplant,* 41, 447-453.

Gafter-Gvili, A., Fraser, A., Paul, M., van de Wetering, M., Kremer, L. & Leibovici, L. (2005) Antibiotic prophylaxis for bacterial infections in afebrile neutropenic patients following chemotherapy. *Cochrane database of systematic reviews,* CD004386.

Gale, R.P. & Lazarus, H.M. (2011) How helpful are meta-analyses in determining the best therapy of blood diseases? *Acta Haematol,* 125, 91-101.

Gokbuget, N. & Hoelzer, D. (2009) Treatment of adult acute lymphoblastic leukemia. *Semin Hematol,* 46, 64-75.

Goldstone AH, Richards SM, Lazarus HM, Tallman MS, Buck G, Fielding AK, Burnett AK, Chopra R, Wiernik PH, Foroni L, Paietta E, Litzow MR, Marks DI, Durrant J, McMillan A, Franklin IM, Luger S, Ciobanu N, Rowe JM (2008) n adults with standard-risk acute lymphoblastic leukemia, the greatest benefit is achieved from a matched sibling allogeneic transplantation in first complete remission, and an autologous transplantation is less effective than conventional consolidation/maintenance chemotherapy in all patients: final results of the International ALL Trial (MRC UKALL XII/ECOG E2993). *Blood,* 111, 1827-1833.

Gurion R, Belnik-Plitman Y, Gafter-Gvili A, Paul M, Vidal L, Ben-Bassat I, 32 Shpilberg O, Raanani P. (2011) Colony-stimulating factors for prevention and treatment of infectious complications in patients with acute myelogenous leukemia. Cochrane Database 34 Syst Rev. 2011 Sep 7;9:CD008238.

Griffin, J.D. (ed.) (2001) *Hematopoietic growth factor.* Lippincott Wiliams & Wilkins, Philadelphia.

Hahn, T., Wall, D., Camitta, B., Davies, S., Dillon, H., Gaynon, P., Larson, R.A., Parsons, S., Seidenfeld, J., Weisdorf, D. & McCarthy, P.L., Jr. (2006) The role of cytotoxic therapy with hematopoietic stem cell transplantation in the therapy of acute lymphoblastic leukemia in adults: an evidence-based review. *Biol Blood Marrow Transplant,* 12, 1-30.

Heddle, N.M., Cook, R.J., Tinmouth, A., Kouroukis, C.T., Hervig, T., Klapper, E., Brandwein, J.M., Szczepiorkowski, Z.M., AuBuchon, J.P., Barty, R.L. & Lee, K.A. (2009) A randomized controlled trial comparing standard- and low-dose strategies for transfusion of platelets (SToP) to patients with thrombocytopenia. *Blood,* 113, 1564-1573.

Heuser, M., Zapf, A., Morgan, M., Krauter, J. & Ganser, A. (2011) Myeloid growth factors in acute myeloid leukemia: systematic review of randomized controlled trials. *Annals of hematology,* 90, 273-281.

Hoelzer, D., Thiel, E., Loffler, H., Buchner, T., Ganser, A., Heil, G., Koch, P., Freund, M., Diedrich, H., Ruhl, H. & et al. (1988) Prognostic factors in a multicenter study for treatment of acute lymphoblastic leukemia in adults. *Blood,* 71, 123-131.

Hubel, K., Weingart, O., Naumann, F., Bohlius, J., Fresen, M.M., Engert, A. & Wheatley, K. (2011) Allogeneic stem cell transplant in adult patients with acute myelogenous leukemia: a systematic analysis of international guidelines and recommendations. *Leuk Lymphoma,* 52, 444-457.

Hunault M, Harousseau JL, Delain M, Truchan-Graczyk M, Cahn JY, Witz F, Lamy T, Pignon B, Jouet JP, Garidi R, Caillot D, Berthou C, Guyotat D, Sadoun A, Sotto JJ, Lioure B, Casassus P, Solal-Celigny P, Stalnikiewicz L, Audhuy B, Blanchet O, Baranger L, Béné MC, Ifrah NBlood (2004) Better outcome of adult acute lymphoblastic leukemia after early genoidentical allogeneic bone marrow transplantation (BMT) than after late high-dose therapy and autologous BMT: a GOELAMS trial. *104,* 10, 3028-3037.

Inoue, C., Murate, T., Hotta, T. & Saito, H. (1990) Response of leukemic cells to the sequential combination of GM-CSF and G-CSF. *International journal of cell cloning,* 8, 54-62.

Kantarjian, H., Thomas, D., O'Brien, S., Cortes, J., Giles, F., Jeha, S., Bueso-Ramos, C.E., Pierce, S., Shan, J., Koller, C., Beran, M., Keating, M. & Freireich, E.J. (2004) Long-term follow-up results of hyperfractionated cyclophosphamide, vincristine, doxorubicin, and dexamethasone (Hyper-CVAD), a dose-intensive regimen, in adult acute lymphocytic leukemia. *Cancer,* 101, 2788-2801.

Kern, W. & Estey, E.H. (2006) High-dose cytosine arabinoside in the treatment of acute myeloid leukemia: Review of three randomized trials. *Cancer,* 107, 116-124.

Kimby, E., Nygren, P. & Glimelius, B. (2001) A systematic overview of chemotherapy effects in acute myeloid leukaemia. *Acta Oncol,* 40, 231-252.

Koreth, J., Schlenk, R., Kopecky, K.J., Honda, S., Sierra, J., Djulbegovic, B.J., Wadleigh, M., DeAngelo, D.J., Stone, R.M., Sakamaki, H., Appelbaum, F.R., Dohner, H., Antin, J.H., Soiffer, R.J. & Cutler, C. (2009) Allogeneic stem cell transplantation for acute myeloid leukemia in first complete remission: systematic review and meta-analysis of prospective clinical trials. *Jama,* 301, 2349-2361.

Labar B, Suciu S, Zittoun R, Muus P, Marie JP, Fillet G, Peetermans M, Stryckmans P, Willemze R, Feremans W, Jaksic B, Bourhis JH, Burghouts JP, de Witte T (2004) Allogeneic stem cell transplantation in acute lymphoblastic leukemia and non-Hodgkin's lymphoma for patients <or=50 years old in first complete remission: results of the EORTC ALL-3 trial. *Haematologica,* 89, 809-817.

Larson, R.A., Dodge, R.K., Burns, C.P., Lee, E.J., Stone, R.M., Schulman, P., Duggan, D., Davey, F.R., Sobol, R.E., Frankel, S.R. & et al. (1995) A five-drug remission induction regimen with intensive consolidation for adults with acute lymphoblastic leukemia: cancer and leukemia group B study 8811. *Blood,* 85, 2025-2037.

Lazarus, H.M., Richards, S.M., Chopra, R., Litzow, M.R., Burnett, A.K., Wiernik, P.H., Franklin, I.M., Tallman, M.S., Cook, L., Buck, G., Durrant, I.J., Rowe, J.M. & Goldstone, A.H. (2006) Central nervous system involvement in adult acute lymphoblastic leukemia at diagnosis: results from the international ALL trial MRC UKALL XII/ECOG E2993. *Blood,* 108, 465-472.

Le, Q.H., Thomas, X., Ecochard, R., Iwaz, J., Lheritier, V., Michallet, M. & Fiere, D. (2006) Initial and late prognostic factors to predict survival in adult acute lymphoblastic leukaemia. *Eur J Haematol,* 77, 471-479.

Lemoli, R.M., Gulati, S.C., Strife, A., Lambek, C., Perez, A. & Clarkson, B.D. (1991) Proliferative response of human acute myeloid leukemia cells and normal marrow enriched progenitor cells to human recombinant growth factors IL-3, GM-CSF and G-CSF alone and in combination. *Leukemia : official journal of the Leukemia Society of America, Leukemia Research Fund, U.K,* 5, 386-391.

Levi, I., Grotto, I., Yerushalmi, R., Ben-Bassat, I. & Shpilberg, O. (2004) Meta-analysis of autologous bone marrow transplantation versus chemotherapy in adult patients with acute myeloid leukemia in first remission. *Leuk Res,* 28, 605-612.

Liberati, A., Altman, D.G., Tetzlaff, J., Mulrow, C., Gotzsche, P.C., Ioannidis, J.P., Clarke, M., Devereaux, P.J., Kleijnen, J. & Moher, D. (2009) The PRISMA statement for reporting systematic reviews and meta-analyses of studies that evaluate health care interventions: explanation and elaboration. *PLoS Med,* 6, e1000100.

Linker, C., Damon, L., Ries, C. & Navarro, W. (2002) Intensified and shortened cyclical chemotherapy for adult acute lymphoblastic leukemia. *J Clin Oncol,* 20, 2464-2471.

Lowenberg, B., Ossenkoppele, G.J., van Putten, W., Schouten, H.C., Graux, C., Ferrant, A., Sonneveld, P., Maertens, J., Jongen-Lavrencic, M., von Lilienfeld-Toal, M., Biemond, B.J., Vellenga, E., van Marwijk Kooy, M., Verdonck, L.F., Beck, J., Dohner, H., Gratwohl, A., Pabst, T. & Verhoef, G. (2009) High-dose daunorubicin in older patients with acute myeloid leukemia. *N Engl J Med,* 361, 1235-1248.

Lowenberg, B., Salem, M. & Delwel, R. (1988) Effects of recombinant multi-CSF, GM-CSF, G-CSF and M-CSF on the proliferation and maturation of human AML in vitro. *Blood cells,* 14, 539-549.

Mandelli, F., Vignetti, M., Suciu, S., Stasi, R., Petti, M.C., Meloni, G., Muus, P., Marmont, F., Marie, J.P., Labar, B., Thomas, X., Di Raimondo, F., Willemze, R., Liso, V., Ferrara, F., Baila, L., Fazi, P., Zittoun, R., Amadori, S. & de Witte, T. (2009) Daunorubicin versus mitoxantrone versus idarubicin as induction and consolidation chemotherapy for adults with acute myeloid leukemia: the EORTC and GIMEMA Groups Study AML-10. *J Clin Oncol,* 27, 5397-5403.

Nathan, P.C., Sung, L., Crump, M. & Beyene, J. (2004) Consolidation therapy with autologous bone marrow transplantation in adults with acute myeloid leukemia: a meta-analysis. *J Natl Cancer Inst,* 96, 38-45.

National Cancer Institute. SEER Cancer Statistics Review (Available at: http://seer.cancer.gov/csr/1975_2006).

Oliansky, D.M., Appelbaum, F., Cassileth, P.A., Keating, A., Kerr, J., Nieto, Y., Stewart, S., Stone, R.M., Tallman, M.S., McCarthy, P.L., Jr. & Hahn, T. (2008) The role of cytotoxic therapy with hematopoietic stem cell transplantation in the therapy of acute myelogenous leukemia in adults: an evidence-based review. *Biol Blood Marrow Transplant,* 14, 137-180.

Omura, G.A., Moffitt, S., Vogler, W.R. & Salter, M.M. (1980) Combination chemotherapy of adult acute lymphoblastic leukemia with randomized central nervous system prophylaxis. *Blood,* 55, 199-204.

Orsi C, Bartolozzi B, Messori A, Bosi A (2007) Event-free survival and cost-effectiveness in adult acute lymphoblastic leukaemia in first remission treated with allogeneic transplantation. *Bone Marrow Transplant,* 40, 643-649.

Oxman, A.D. & Guyatt, G.H. (1991) Validation of an index of the quality of review articles. *J Clin Epidemiol,* 44, 1271-1278.

Park, L.S., Waldron, P.E., Friend, D., Sassenfeld, H.M., Price, V., Anderson, D., Cosman, D., Andrews, R.G., Bernstein, I.D. & Urdal, D.L. (1989) Interleukin-3, GM-CSF, and G-CSF receptor expression on cell lines and primary leukemia cells: receptor heterogeneity and relationship to growth factor responsiveness. *Blood,* 74, 56-65.

Pautas, C., Merabet, F., Thomas, X., Raffoux, E., Gardin, C., Corm, S., Bourhis, J.H., Reman, O., Turlure, P., Contentin, N., de Revel, T., Rousselot, P., Preudhomme, C., Bordessoule, D., Fenaux, P., Terre, C., Michallet, M., Dombret, H., Chevret, S. & Castaigne, S. (2010) Randomized study of intensified anthracycline doses for induction and recombinant interleukin-2 for maintenance in patients with acute myeloid leukemia age 50 to 70 years: results of the ALFA-9801 study. *J Clin Oncol,* 28, 808-814.

Pui, C.H., Robison, L.L. & Look, A.T. (2008) Acute lymphoblastic leukaemia. *Lancet,* 371, 1030-1043.

Ram, R., Gafter-Gvili, A., Shpilberg, O. & Raanani, P. (2011) Allogeneic hematopoietic cell transplantation for adult patients with acute leukemia: the role of meta-analyses. *Acta Haematol,* 125, 39-46.

Ram, R., Gafter-Gvili, A., Vidal, L., Paul, M., Ben-Bassat, I., Shpilberg, O. & Raanani, P. (2010) Management of adult patients with acute lymphoblastic leukemia in first complete remission: systematic review and meta-analysis. *Cancer,* 116, 3447-3457.

Ram R., Wolach O., Vidal L., Gafter-Gvili A., Shpilberg O., Raanani P.: Adolescents and Young Adults with Acute Lymphoblastic Leukemia Have Better Outcomes When Treated with Pediatric-Inspired Regimens - Systematic Review and Meta-Analysis of Comparative Trials. American Society of Hematology, 2011 Abstract number 2591

Ramanujachar, R., Richards, S., Hann, I., Goldstone, A., Mitchell, C., Vora, A., Rowe, J. & Webb, D. (2007) Adolescents with acute lymphoblastic leukaemia: outcome on UK national paediatric (ALL97) and adult (UKALLXII/E2993) trials. *Pediatr Blood Cancer,* 48, 254-261.

Rees, J.K., Gray, R.G. & Wheatley, K. (1996) Dose intensification in acute myeloid leukaemia: greater effectiveness at lower cost. Principal report of the Medical Research Council's AML9 study. MRC Leukaemia in Adults Working Party. *Br J Haematol,* 94, 89-98.

Ribera JM, Oriol A, Bethencourt C, Parody R, Hernández-Rivas JM, Moreno MJ, del Potro E, Torm M, Rivas C, Besalduch J, Sanz MA, Ortega JJ (2005) Comparison of intensive chemotherapy, allogeneic or autologous stem cell transplantation as post-remission treatment for adult patients with high-risk acute lymphoblastic leukemia. Results of the PETHEMA ALL-93 trial. *Haematologica,* 90, 1346-1356.

Robenshtok, E., Gafter-Gvili, A., Goldberg, E., Weinberger, M., Yeshurun, M., Leibovici, L. & Paul, M. (2007) Antifungal prophylaxis in cancer patients after chemotherapy or hematopoietic stem-cell transplantation: systematic review and meta-analysis. *Journal of clinical oncology : official journal of the American Society of Clinical Oncology,* 25, 5471-5489.

Rowe, J.M., Buck, G., Burnett, A.K., Chopra, R., Wiernik, P.H., Richards, S.M., Lazarus, H.M., Franklin, I.M., Litzow, M.R., Ciobanu, N., Prentice, H.G., Durrant, J., Tallman, M.S. & Goldstone, A.H. (2005) Induction therapy for adults with acute lymphoblastic leukemia: results of more than 1500 patients from the international ALL trial: MRC UKALL XII/ECOG E2993. *Blood,* 106, 3760-3767.

Rowe, J.M., Neuberg, D., Friedenberg, W., Bennett, J.M., Paietta, E., Makary, A.Z., Liesveld, J.L., Abboud, C.N., Dewald, G., Hayes, F.A., Tallman, M.S. & Wiernik, P.H. (2004) A phase 3 study of three induction regimens and of priming with GM-CSF in older adults with acute myeloid leukemia: a trial by the Eastern Cooperative Oncology Group. *Blood,* 103, 479-485.

Schlenk, R.F., Benner, A., Krauter, J., Buchner, T., Sauerland, C., Ehninger, G., Schaich, M., Mohr, B., Niederwieser, D., Krahl, R., Pasold, R., Dohner, K., Ganser, A., Dohner, H. & Heil, G. (2004) Individual patient data-based meta-analysis of patients aged 16 to 60 years with core binding factor acute myeloid leukemia: a survey of the German Acute Myeloid Leukemia Intergroup. *J Clin Oncol,* 22, 3741-3750.

Shea, B.J., Bouter, L.M., Peterson, J., Boers, M., Andersson, N., Ortiz, Z., Ramsay, T., Bai, A., Shukla, V.K. & Grimshaw, J.M. (2007) External validation of a measurement tool to assess systematic reviews (AMSTAR). *PLoS One,* 2, e1350.

Shea, B.J., Hamel, C., Wells, G.A., Bouter, L.M., Kristjansson, E., Grimshaw, J., Henry, D.A. & Boers, M. (2009) AMSTAR is a reliable and valid measurement tool to assess the methodological quality of systematic reviews. *J Clin Epidemiol,* 62, 1013-1020.

Silverman, L.R., Demakos, E.P., Peterson, B.L., Kornblith, A.B., Holland, J.C., Odchimar-Reissig, R., Stone, R.M., Nelson, D., Powell, B.L., DeCastro, C.M., Ellerton, J., Larson, R.A., Schiffer, C.A. & Holland, J.F. (2002) Randomized controlled trial of azacitidine in patients with the myelodysplastic syndrome: a study of the cancer and leukemia group B. *J Clin Oncol,* 20, 2429-2440.

Slichter, S.J., Kaufman, R.M., Assmann, S.F., McCullough, J., Triulzi, D.J., Strauss, R.G., Gernsheimer, T.B., Ness, P.M., Brecher, M.E., Josephson, C.D., Konkle, B.A., Woodson, R.D., Ortel, T.L., Hillyer, C.D., Skerrett, D.L., McCrae, K.R., Sloan, S.R., Uhl, L., George, J.N., Aquino, V.M., Manno, C.S., McFarland, J.G., Hess, J.R., Leissinger, C. & Granger, S. Dose of prophylactic platelet transfusions and prevention of hemorrhage. *N Engl J Med,* 362, 600-613.

Stanworth, S.J., Hyde, C., Heddle, N., Rebulla, P., Brunskill, S. & Murphy, M.F. (2004) Prophylactic platelet transfusion for haemorrhage after chemotherapy and stem cell transplantation. *Cochrane database of systematic reviews,* CD004269.

Stock, W., La, M., Sanford, B., Bloomfield, C.D., Vardiman, J.W., Gaynon, P., Larson, R.A. & Nachman, J. (2008) What determines the outcomes for adolescents and young adults with acute lymphoblastic leukemia treated on cooperative group protocols? A comparison of Children's Cancer Group and Cancer and Leukemia Group B studies. *Blood,* 112, 1646-1654.

Sung, L., Alibhai, S.M., Beyene, J., Gamis, A., Almeida, R., Smith, S. & Aplenc, R. (2009) Hematopoietic colony-stimulating factor priming does not influence survival in acute myeloid leukemia: a meta-analysis of randomized trials. *Leukemia : official journal of the Leukemia Society of America, Leukemia Research Fund, U.K,* 23, 811-813.

Sung, L., Nathan, P.C., Alibhai, S.M., Tomlinson, G.A. & Beyene, J. (2007) Meta-analysis: effect of prophylactic hematopoietic colony-stimulating factors on mortality and outcomes of infection. *Annals of internal medicine,* 147, 400-411.

Thomas, D.A., Faderl, S., Cortes, J., O'Brien, S., Giles, F.J., Kornblau, S.M., Garcia-Manero, G., Keating, M.J., Andreeff, M., Jeha, S., Beran, M., Verstovsek, S., Pierce, S., Letvak, L., Salvado, A., Champlin, R., Talpaz, M. & Kantarjian, H. (2004a) Treatment of Philadelphia chromosome-positive acute lymphocytic leukemia with hyper-CVAD and imatinib mesylate. *Blood,* 103, 4396-4407.

Thomas, X., Boiron, J.M., Huguet, F., Dombret, H., Bradstock, K., Vey, N., Kovacsovics, T., Delannoy, A., Fegueux, N., Fenaux, P., Stamatoullas, A., Vernant, J.P., Tournilhac, O., Buzyn, A., Reman, O., Charrin, C., Boucheix, C., Gabert, J., Lheritier, V. & Fiere, D. (2004b) Outcome of treatment in adults with acute lymphoblastic leukemia: analysis of the LALA-94 trial. *J Clin Oncol,* 22, 4075-4086.

Visani, G., Olivieri, A., Malagola, M., Brunori, M., Piccaluga, P.P., Capelli, D., Pomponio, G., Martinelli, G., Isidori, A., Sparaventi, G. & Leoni, P. (2006) Consolidation therapy for adult acute myeloid leukemia: a systematic analysis according to evidence based medicine. *Leuk Lymphoma,* 47, 1091-1102.

Volger, W.R., Weiner, R.S., Moore, J.O., Omura, G.A., Bartolucci, A.A. & Stagg, M. (1995) Long-term follow-up of a randomized post-induction therapy trial in acute myelogenous leukemia (a Southeastern Cancer Study Group trial). *Leukemia,* 9, 1456-1460.

Wang, J., An, L., Chen, S., Ouyang, J., Zhou, R., Chen, B. & Yang, Y. (2009a) Prophylactic use of granulocyte colony-stimulating factor after chemotherapy does not affect survival rate in acute myeloid leukemia: a meta-analysis. *Acta haematologica,* 121, 223-226.

Wang, J., Ouyang, J., Zhou, R., Chen, B. & Yang, Y. (2010) Autologous hematopoietic stem cell transplantation for acute myeloid leukemia in first complete remission: a meta-analysis of randomized trials. *Acta Haematol,* 124, 61-71.

Wang, J., Zhan, P., Ouyang, J., Chen, B. & Zhou, R. (2009b) Prophylactic use of granulocyte colony-stimulating factor after induction chemotherapy in patients with newly diagnosed acute myeloid leukemia may increase the complete remission rate: a meta-analysis of five randomised controlled trials. *Leukemia & lymphoma,* 50, 457-459.

Woolf, S.H. (2000) Evidence-based medicine and practice guidelines: an overview. *Cancer Control,* 7, 362-367.

Xu, S.N., Chen, J.P., Liu, J.P. & Xia, Y. (2009a) [Arsenic trioxide in combination with all-trans retinoic acid for acute promyelocytic leukemia: a systematic review and meta-analysis]. *Zhong Xi Yi Jie He Xue Bao,* 7, 1024-1034.

Xu, S.N., Chen, J.P., Liu, J.P. & Xia, Y. (2009b) [Efficacy of arsenic trioxide for acute promyelocytic leukemia: a systematic review and meta-analysis]. *Zhong Xi Yi Jie He Xue Bao,* 7, 801-808.

Yanada M, Matsuo K, Suzuki T, Naoe T (2006) Allogeneic hematopoietic stem cell transplantation as part of postremission therapy improves survival for adult patients with high-risk acute lymphoblastic leukemia: a metaanalysis. *Cancer,* 106, 2657-2663.

Yanada, M., Matsuo, K., Emi, N. & Naoe, T. (2005) Efficacy of allogeneic hematopoietic stem cell transplantation depends on cytogenetic risk for acute myeloid leukemia in first disease remission: a metaanalysis. *Cancer,* 103, 1652-1658.

16

Acute Lymphoblastic Leukemia in Adolescents and Young Adults

Josep-Maria Ribera
Clinical Hematology Department
Institut Català d'Oncologia
Hospital Universitari Germans Trias i Pujol
Institut de Recerca contra la Leucemia Josep Carreras
Universitat Autònoma de Barcelona
Spain

1. Introduction

The development of effective therapy for children with acute lymphoblastic leukemia (ALL) is one of the greatest successes of clinical oncology, with long-term survival achieved in about 90% of children 1-10 years of age (Pui et al 2008, Pulte et al 2008). However, cure rates for adults with ALL remain relatively low, at only 40%-50% (Gokbuget et al 2009, Larson et al 2008). In the last two decades significant improvements in survival for older adolescent and adults (aged 15-59 years) with ALL have been observed, being especially evident in patients aged 15-19 yr.

Age is a continuous prognostic variable in ALL with no single age at which prognosis deteriorates markedly. Within childhood ALL populations, older children have shown inferior outcomes (Pulte et al 2009, Smith et al 2010) while younger adults have shown superior outcomes among adult ALL patients (Moorman et al 2010, Juliusson et al 2010). The definition of the age range that encompasses the adolescent and young adults (AYA) patient is controversial, ranging from 15 to 21 yr in some studies, from 15-30 yr in others or even from 15 to 40-45 yr in others. This chapter will focus on the results of treatment of AYA with ALL.

2. Clinical and biologic characteristics in adolescents and young adults

The incidence of ALL decreases with age, ranging from 9-10 cases/100,000 persons/year in childhood (representing 30% of all cancers) to 1-2 cases/100,000 persons/year in adults. In adolescents the incidence is 3 cases/100,000 persons/year and represents 6% of all cancers at that age (Bleyer et al 2006).

Several clinical and biologic characteristics of ALL are age-dependent. In this sense, T-ALL is more frequent in AYA (25%) than in children (10-15%) or in older adults (Pullen et al 1999). However, the most important differences lie in cytogenetic and molecular characteristics. For example, there is a lower frequency of hyperdiploidy >50 chromosomes or *ETV6/RUNX1* (previously *TEL/AML1*) in AYAs (20%) compared to children 1 to 9 years of age (>30%) (Moorman et al 2010). In addition, the frequency of *MLL* (myeloid-lymphoid leukemia or mixed lineage leukemia gene, usually associated with 11q23) rearrangements in non-infant ALL increases with age, being infrequent in children 1-9 yr of age and about 6% in adults (Moorman et al 2010). Regarding structural changes, there is a progressive increase in the frequency of t(9;22)(q34;q11) or *BCR-ABL* rearrangements, ranging from less than 3% in children under 18 yr. to 6% at ages 18-25 and to 15-20% at ages 25-35 yr, and to more than 30% over the age of 35 yr (Secker-Walker et al 1991). Finally, in recent studies, adolescents were more likely to have detectable minimal residual disease (MRD) during or at the end of remission induction (Pui et al 2011).

In summary, with increasing age there is a progressive increase in the frequency of subsets of ALL patients with genetic abnormalities associated with poor prognosis and these changes have already become evident in AYA patients.

As far as host factors are concerned, several features are observed in less young patients, being responsible for increased treatment toxicity. They include differences in the metabolism of chemotherapeutic agents, depleted marrow reserve and increased extramedullary toxicity. All these issues increase the frequency of life-threatening infections, organ failure, and treatment delays and dose reductions in planned chemotherapy.

3. Which is the best treatment strategy? Pediatric-based vs. adult-based treatments

3.1 Retrospective comparative studies

A number of comparisons of the clinical outcome of adolescents enrolled in adult and pediatric clinical trials have resulted in interesting observations about the appropriate treatment strategy for prospective studies in AYA. Several retrospective reports have shown that adolescents (15- 20 yr.) and young adults treated by adult oncologists or hematologists with adult ALL protocols have poorer outcomes than similarly aged patients treated by pediatricians with pediatric protocols, despite having similar biologic characteristics of the disease (Boissel et al 2003, de Bont et al 2004, Testi et al 2004, Hallbook et al 2006, Schroeder et al 2006, Ramanujachar et al 2007, Lopez-Hernandez et al 2008, Stock et al 2008, Al-Khabori et al 2010).

The first study in which such different outcomes were reported was performed in France (Boissel et al 2003). A comparison of AYA aged 15-20 yr. treated with the pediatric-based protocol FRALLE-93 (n=77) with patients of the same age and comparable clinical and biologic characteristics of ALL who received the adult-based protocol LALA-94 (n=100) showed a complete remission (CR) rate of 94% vs. 83%. After a median follow-up of 3.5 yr, the event-free survival (EFS) probabilities were 67% vs. 41% at 5 years. Multivariate analysis showed an independent influence of the protocol on the outcome. The differences in the drugs employed and, especially in the dose-intensity, could explain the better results of the FRALLE-93 protocol. In this protocol the cumulated dose of prednisone was five-fold higher, the vinca alkaloids three-fold and the asparaginase 20-fold higher than in the LALA-94 study. In addition, in the FRALLE-93 study the dose of prednisone in induction was higher and asparaginase was also given in this period, in contrast with the LALA-94 trial. Moreover, the time interval between CR and post-remission therapy was 2 days in FRALLE-93 vs. 7 days in the LALA-94 study.

The North-American Cancer and Acute Leukemia Group B (CALGB) and the Children's Cancer Group (CCG) performed a retrospective comparison of presenting features, planned treatment, CR rate, and outcome of 321 AYA aged 16 to 20 years who were treated on consecutive trials in either the CCG or the CALGB from 1988 to 2001 (Stock et al 2008). Both cohorts were comparable for the main clinical and biologic characteristics, although the median age of the patients in the CALGB studies was 19 yr. compared to 16 yr. for the CCG patients. CR rates were identical (90%) for both the CALGB and CCG AYA. The CCG AYA had a 63% EFS and 67% overall survival (OS) probabilities at 7 years in contrast to the CALGB AYA, in whom the 7-year EFS was only 34% and the OS was 46%. While the CALGB AYA aged 16 to 17 years achieved similar outcomes to all the CCG AYA with a 7-year EFS of 55%, the EFS for 18- to 20-year-old CALGB patients was only 29%. CALGB AYAs had a significant increase in CNS relapse (11%) compared to CCG AYAs (1.5%). Comparison of the regimens showed that the CCG AYA received earlier and more intensive and prolonged CNS prophylaxis and higher cumulative doses of nonmyelosuppressive agents (vinca alkaloid, steroids and asparaginase), as well as longer duration of maintenance therapy than CALGB AYAs. There were no differences in outcomes in those who reached maintenance therapy on time compared with those who were delayed.

A similar Dutch study in patients aged 15-21 yr yielded similar results (de Bont et al 2004), with a 5-yr EFS of 69% for comparable patients treated with the more dose-intensive pediatric protocol DCOG vs. 34% for those treated with adult protocols ALL-5 and ALL-18 from the HOVON Group. Likewise, comparative retrospective studies from Italy also showed a poorer prognosis for patients aged 14-18 yr treated with adult-type protocols (Testi et al 2004). In turn, a Swedish study compared patients aged 10-40 yr treated with the pediatric trial NOPHO-92 (n=144) vs. a similar group of patients included in the Swedish Adult ALL Group (n=99) (Hallbook et al 2006). A significantly higher CR rate (99% vs. 90%) and EFS were observed in patients treated with the pediatric protocol, with the type of treatment being an independent prognostic variable on multivariate analysis. However, it is of note that adults aged 26-40 yr had a significantly poorer prognosis than AYA (15-25 yr.). Another study from Denmark yielded similar results (Schroeder et al 2006). In a retrospective study from the British Medical Research Council (MRC) performed only in adolescents (15-17 yr) included in the ALL97/revised99 (pediatric, n=61) or UKALLXII/E2993 (adult, n = 67) trials between 1997 and 2002 (Ramanujachar et al 2007), the EFS (65% vs. 49%) was higher and the rate of death in remission was lower in the former group of patients. In a retrospective study from the Princess Margaret Hospital from Toronto restricted to AYA with T-ALL 40 patients (median age 30 yr, range 17-69) were treated with several adult type protocols and were compared with 32 patients (median age 32 yr, range 17-64) treated with a DFCI protocol (Al-Khabori et al 2010). Although there were no differences in CR attainment (93% vs. 84%), the OS and relapse-free survival (RFS) probabilities were significantly higher in patients treated with the DFCI trial (83% vs .56% and 88% vs. 23%, respectively). On multivariate analysis the treatment group (DFCI vs. non-DFCI) was the major prognostic factor influencing both RFS and OS. Other studies from different countries (Lopez-Hernandez et al 2008) have shown similar results (Table 1).

Only one population-based study from Finland showed that the outcome of AYA with ALL treated with pediatric or adult protocols was comparable (Usvasalo et al 2008). One hundred and twenty-eight patients (10-16 yr, median age 12.9 yr) were treated with the pediatric Nordic (NOPHO) protocols and 97 patients (17-25 yr, median age 18.9 yr) with Finnish Leukemia Group National protocols. All patients were centrally referred and treated in five academic centers. The 5-year EFS was 67% for the pediatric treatment group and 60% for the adult treatment group. There were no significant differences in the cumulative doses of corticosteroids, vincristine and asparaginase between pediatric and adult protocols, although pediatric protocols used a higher cumulative dose of methotrexate and lower

Country (reference)	Protocol	Age (yr)	N	CR (%)	EFS (%)
USA (32)	CCG(P)	16-20	197	90	63
	CALGB(A)		124	90	34
France (12)	FRALLE93(P)	15-20	77	94	67
	LALA94 (A)		100	83	41
Holland (13)	DCOG (P)	15-18	47	98	69
	HOVON (A)		44	91	34
Italy (35)	AIEOP (P)	14-18	150	94	80
	GIMEMA (A)		95	89	71
Sweden (11)	NOPHO-92(P)	10-40	144	99	65
	Adult (A)		99	90	48
UK (25)	ALL97 (P)	15-17	61	98	65
	UKALLXII(A)		67	94	49
Canada (1)	DFCI (P)	17-64	32	84	83*
	Adult (A)	17-69	40	93	56*
Mexico (16)	LALIN (P)	15-25	20	90	70
	LALA (A)		20	80	40
Finland (38)	NOPHO (P)	10-25	128	96	67
	ALL (A)		97	97	60

N: number of patients; CR: complete remission. EFS: event-free survival.
* Overall survival

Table 1. Retrospective comparative studies in adolescents and young adults with acute lymphoblastic leukemia treated with pediatric-based (P) vs. adult-based (A) protocols.

doses of anthracyclines than adult protocols; epipodophyllotoxins and mitoxantrone were not included in the pediatric protocols. The authors attributed the similar results to the similarity of the pediatric and adult protocols and to the centralized care of the patients in five academic centers, ensuring good compliance and adherence to the protocols. Finally, the retrospective data from the MD Anderson Cancer Center using the Hyper-CVAD regimen (not including asparaginase) have also reported favorable results in 102 AYA (median age 19 yr), with CR 97% and OS 65% (Thomas et al 2008). Preliminary reports from 60 AYA patients aged 12-40 yr treated at the MD Anderson Cancer Center with modified augmented Berlin-Frankfurt-Münster (BFM) therapy showed very promising results (2-yr DFS and OS probabilities of 85% and 91%, respectively) in the subset of patients younger than 25 yr (Rytting et al 2010), stressing the importance of treating these patients in large referral centers.

In summary, the 5- to 6-yr EFS rate for AYA treated with pediatric regimens ranges from 65% to 70% vs. 35% to 50% for adult regimens in almost but not all retrospective comparative studies. However, it is of note that these studies have mainly focused on patients aged 15-21 years, but few have evaluated the results in young adults up to 30 years or more, in whom the frequency of adverse prognostic factors is progressively increasing.

The reasons for the better results of pediatric protocols are multiple (Stock 2010). The first and probably the most important reason lay in the protocol itself. The dose-intensity and the dose-density of the key chemotherapeutic agents for ALL are clearly higher in pediatric protocols. This is especially relevant for drugs such as vincristine (usually capped to 2 mg in adult protocols), glucocorticoids, asparaginase and methotrexate. Conversely, pediatric-based protocols include lower doses of alkylating agents, high-dose cytarabine and antracyclines than adult trials. In addition CNS prophylaxis is more intense and prolonged in pediatric regimens than in adult trials. Most of the pediatric protocols include delayed intensifications and an extended maintenance chemotherapy phase, the former being omitted in many adult trials. The use of allogeneic stem cell transplantation (SCT) as part of first line therapy (associated with a transplant-related mortality [TRM] of 20%), is restricted to patients with very high-risk features in pediatric trials, whereas it is more widely used in adult trials, even in standard-risk patients in first CR.

The second reason is the tolerability to essential drugs such as asparaginase, steroids and vincristine, which is poorer in AYA compared to children, being a reflection of changes in the metabolism of these drugs during late adolescence. The incidences of diabetes mellitus, pancreatitis, thrombosis and osteonecrosis are more frequent in the former group. The increased toxicity influences adherence to treatment, which is critical for the outcome of ALL patients.

The third reason is the disparity in the practice patterns of the pediatric and adult hematologists/oncologists and patient compliance. Adherence to treatment is usually higher in pediatric than in adult-derived studies, probably due both to a highly skilled supportive staff, the better tolerability of pediatric protocols and a stricter control of time points of chemotherapy delivery in pediatric than in adult hematology units (Burke et al 2007) However, in the U.S. and Canada most children and adolescents with ALL treated with pediatric protocols are managed in institutions and academic centers participating in national-sponsored clinical trials, whilst most AYA treated with adult protocols are managed throughout study groups by community-based medical oncologists. The fact that the most striking differences are observed in the 18 to 20-years-old group could be explained by the emancipation of some of these patients from parental control and support and the possible need to face significantly more challenges in access to health care due to insurance issues (Kantarjian et al 2009).

3.2 Prospective trials

3.2.1 Results of the treatment of adolescents in pediatric trials

Barry et al reported the outcome of adolescents treated in the Dana-Farber Cancer Institute (DFCI) ALL Consortium Protocols conducted between 1991 and 2000 (Barry et al 2007). A total of 844 patients aged 1 to 18 years, with newly diagnosed ALL were enrolled into two consecutive DFCI-ALL Consortium Protocols. Outcomes were compared in three age groups: children aged 1 to 10 years (n = 685), young adolescents aged 10 to 15 years (n = 108), and older adolescents aged 15 to 18 years (n = 51). With a median follow-up of 6.5 years, the 5-year EFS for those aged 1 to 10 years was 85%, compared with 77% for those aged 10 to 15 years, and 78% for those aged 15 to 18 years. There was no difference in the rate of treatment-related complications between the 10- to 15-year and 15- to 18-year age groups.

Nachman et al reported the results of the CCG1961 trial including AYA up to 21 yr (Nachman et al 2009). The EFS and overall survival (OS) rates were 71.5% and 77.5%, respectively. Rapid responder patients randomly assigned to augmented therapy had 5-year EFS 81.8% vs 66.8% for patients receiving standard therapy, but 1 versus 2 interim maintenance and delayed intensification courses had no significant impact on EFS. WBC count over $50x10^9/L$ was an adverse prognostic factor. Given the excellent outcome with this chemotherapy there seems to be no role for the routine use of stem cell transplantation in first remission

In turn, the results of the total therapy studies XIIIA, XIIIB, XIV and XV from St Jude Children's Research Hospital including 963 pediatric patients, 89 of whom were older adolescents (aged 15 to 18 yr.), have recently been published (Pui et al 2011). In the first three studies the 44 older adolescents had significantly poorer EFS and OS than the 403 younger patients. On the contrary, in study XV (incorporing the level of MRD to guide treatment, with featured intensive methotrexate, vincristine, glucocorticoid and asparaginase and early triple intrathecal chemotherapy for higher risk ALL) the EFS of 45 older adolescents was 86.4%, similar to 87.4% for the 453 younger children. The OS was also comparable (87.9% vs. 94.1%, respectively). The authors concluded that most older adolescents with ALL can be cured with risk-adjusted intensive chemotherapy without SCT. In summary, with modern approaches of treatment of ALL with pediatric-based protocols the unfavorable prognosis of adolescents is disappearing and hopefully, this improvement could be translated to young adults.

3.2.2 Results of prospective studies in adolescent and young adults

Some studies have evaluated or are currently evaluating the feasibility and results of the pediatric-based protocols administered to adults up to 30 or even up to 50 or 60 years of age (table 2). The Spanish PETHEMA group compared the results of the pediatric protocol ALL96 in adolescents (15-18yr, n=35) and young adults (18-30 yr, n=46) with standard-risk (SR) ALL (Ribera et al 2008). Both groups were comparable for the main clinical and biologic characteristics of ALL. The CR rate was 98% and after a median follow-up of 4.2 yr., 6-year EFS and OS were 61% and 69%, with no differences between adolescents and young adults. No significant differences were observed in the timing of treatment delivery, although the hematologic toxicity in consolidation and reinforcement cycles was higher in young adults than in adolescents. These results suggest that pediatric protocols can be effectively and safely employed in adult patients with SR ALL, at least up to the age of 30 yr.

Country (reference)	Protocol	Age (yr)	N	CR (%)	EFS (%)
Spain (26)	PETHEMA ALL-96	15-18	35	94	60
		19-30	46	100	63
France (32)	GRAALL-2003	15-45	172	95	58
USA (6)	DFCI	18-50	74	82	72.5**
Canada (34)	Modified DFCI	17-71	68	85	65***
France (10)	FRALLE2000	18-55	40	90	72***

* Results restricted to adolescents; **Estimated at 2 years; *** Overall survival.
N: number of patients; CR: complete remission. EFS: event-free survival.

Table 2. Prospective studies in adolescents and young adults with acute lymphoblastic leukemia treated with pediatric-based or inspired protocols

The French GRAALL group has reported the results of the pediatric-inspired GRAALL-2003 study including 215 patients aged 15-60 yr (Huguet et al 2009). In this study there was an 8.6-fold, 3.7-fold and 16-fold increase in cumulative doses of prednisone, vincristine and asparaginase, respectively, compared with the previous adult-based LALA-94 protocol, although the GRAALL-2003 trial retained some adult options, such as allogeneic SCT for patients with high-risk ALL. The CR rate was 93.5% and at 42 months the EFS and overall survival (OS) rates were 55% and 60%, respectively. The CR rate, EFS and OS compared favorably with the previous LALA-94 experience. It is of note, however, that in patients over 45 yr there was a higher cumulative incidence of chemotherapy-related deaths (23% vs. 5%) and deaths in first CR (22% vs. 5%), although the incidence of relapse remained stable (30 vs. 32%). The results of this study suggest that pediatric-inspired therapy is feasible in young adults with ALL at least until the age of 45 yr, in whom the outcome clearly improves.

Based on the promising results obtained in adolescents with ALL, the DFCI Combined Adult/Pediatric ALL Consortium has applied a true pediatric protocol to adults aged 18-50 yr (DeAngelo et al 2006). Specifically, the investigators used an extended course of asparaginase for 30 weeks. The preliminary results in 94 patients, with a median age of 28 yr have shown a CR in 79 patients (84%). With a median follow-up of 45 months, the estimated DFS rate was 66% and the OS rate was 68%. This study proved that extended asparaginase treatment was feasible in adults and the drug-related toxicity was manageable, although the incidence of pancreatitis (13%) and thrombosis/embolism (19%) was a matter of concern. In turn, the Princess Margaret Hospital used a modified Dana Farber Cancer Institute pediatric protocol in 68 adult patients (17 to 71 yr), with a CR rate of 85% and 3-yr OS and DFS of 65% and 77%, respectively (Storring et al 2009). The University of South California group (Srivastava et al 2008) used an augmented BFM pediatric regimen with eight doses of pegylated asparaginase to treat adults with ALL aged 19-57 yr (median 33), with a 3-yr projected EFS of 65%. Toxicity attributable to asparaginase was frequent but manageable. However, older patients had significantly less tolerance to asparaginase, vincristine and steroids compared to children or adolescents. In the FRALLE group from France 28 Philadelphia chromosome-negative adult ALL patients 16 to 57 years of age were treated in the FRALLE 2000 protocol consisting of a prednisone pre-phase and a four-drug induction including asparaginase, consolidation, delayed intensification and maintenance chemotherapy. The 4-yr DFS was 90% vs. 47% seen in matched historical controls (Haiat et al 2011).

The largest prospective phase II trial to evaluate the feasibility of the use of a true pediatric regimen in AYA is currently ongoing in the US (C-10403 trial) (available at www.clinicaltrials.gov. NCT00558519) AYAs from 16 to 39 yr are treated by adult oncologists/hematologists with one treatment arm of the current AALL0232 trial from the pediatric COG group. More than half of the 300 planned patients have been currently enrolled. This study will prospectively analyze the genetic characteristics, MRD, treatment adherence, tolerability and psycho-social and socio-economic conditions that likely influence treatment outcomes.

The results from these prospective studies demonstrate the feasibility and tolerability of pediatric-based regimens in AYA with SR ALL, at least until 30-50 yr. All these trials have the increased cumulative dosages of the most important drugs for ALL therapy, the cautious observance of dose-intensity and the reduction of the delays between the different phases of the therapy in common. If these results can be confirmed with a longer follow-up, they will have an impact on the clinical management of AYA patients in the future. Finally, few specific data are available on long-term complications of successful treatment of AYA (see www.survivorshipguidelines.org by the COG group) and a comprehensive approach to the follow-up for this significant group of patients with ALL is lacking. The next generation of studies, incorporating biological, pharmacological and psychosocial issues will further improve the cure rate and quality of life of these patients.

4. Acknowledgment

Supported in part by grants RD06/0020/1056 from RTICC, Instituto Carlos III, PI051490 from Fondo de Investigaciones Sanitarias and FIJC P/EF-10 from Jose Carreras Leukemia Foundation.

5. References

[1] Al-Khabori M, Minden MD, Yee KWL, et al. Improved survival using an intensive, pediatric-based chemotherapy regimen in adults with T-cell acute lymphoblastic leukemia. Leuk & Lymphoma. 2010; 51: 61-65.

[2] Barry E, DeAngelo DJ, Neuberg D, et al. Favorable outcome for adolescents with acute lymphoblastic leukemia treated on Dana Farber Cancer Institute ALL Consortium protocols. J Clin Oncol. 2007; 25: 813-819.

[3] Bleyer A, O'Leary M, Barr R, Ries LAG (eds). Cancer Epidemiology in Older Adolescents and Young Adults 15 to 29 years of Age, including SEER Incidence and Survival: 1975–2000. National Cancer Institute, NIH Pub. No. 06–5767. Bethesda, MD 2006.

[4] Boissel N, Auclerc M-F, Lheritier V, et al. Should adolescents with acute lymphoblastic leukemia be treated as old children or young adults? Comparison of the French FRALLE-93 and LALA-94 trials. J Clin Oncol. 2003;21:774–780.

[5] Burke ME, Albriton K, Marina N. Challenges in the recruitment of adolescents and young adults to cancer clinical trials. Cancer. 2007; 110: 2385-93.

[6] DeAngelo DJ, Silverman LB, Couban S, et al. A multicenter phase II study using a dose intensified pediatric regimen in adults with untreated acute lymphoblastic leukaemia. Blood. 2006; 108: 526a

[7] De Bont JM, van der Holt B, Dekker AW, van der Does-van den Berg A, Sonneveld P, Pieters R. Significant difference in outcome for adolescents with acute lymphoblastic leukemia treated on pediatric vs adult protocols in the Netherlands. Leukemia. 2004;18: 2032–2035.

[8] Gokbuget N, Hoelzer D. Treatment of adult acute lymphoblastic leukemia. Semin Hematol. 2009; 46: 64-75.

[9] Haiat S, Marjanovic Z, Lapusan S, et al. Outcome of 40 adults aged from 18 to 55 years with acute lymphoblastic leukemia treated with double delayed intensification pediatric protocol. Leuk Res. 2011;35: 66-72.

[10] Hallbook H, Gustafsson G, Smedmyr B, Soderhall S, Heyman M; Swedish Adult Acute Lymphocytic Leukemia Group; Swedish Childhood Leukemia Group. Treatment outcome in young adults and children >10 years of age with acute lymphoblastic leukemia in Sweden: a comparison between a pediatric protocol and an adult protocol. Cancer. 2006;107:1551-61.

[11] Huguet F, Raffoux E, Thomas X, et al. Pediatric inspired therapy in adults with Philadelphia chromosome-negative acute lymphoblastic leukemia: the GRAALL/2003 study. J Clin Oncol. 2009; 27: 911-8.
[12] Juliusson, G, Karlsson K, Hallböök H. Population-based analyses in adult acute lymphoblastic leukemia. Blood. 2010;116:1011.
[13] Kantarjian HM, O'Brien S. Insurance policies in the United States may explain part of the outcome differences of adolescents and young adults with acute lymphoblastic leukemia treated on adult versus pediatric regimens. Blood. 2009; 113: 1861.
[14] Larson R, Stock W. Progress in the treatment of adults with acute lymphoblastic leukemia. Curr Opin Hematol .2008; 15: 400-7.
[15] Lopez-Hernandez MA, Alvarado-Ibarra M, Jiménez-Alvarado RM, De Diego-Flores JE, González-Avante CM. Adolescents with de novo acute lymphoblastic leukemia: efficacy and safety of a pediatric vs. adult treatment protocol. Gac Med Mex. 2008; 144: 485-9.
[16] Moorman AV, Chilton L, Wilkinson J, et al. A population-based cytogenetic study of adults with acute lymphoblastic leukemia. Blood. 2010;115:206-214.
[17] Moorman AV, Ensor HM, Richards SM, et al. Prognostic effect of chromosomal abnormalities in childhood B-precursor acute lymphoblastic leukaemia: results from the UK Medical Research Council ALL 97/99 randomised trial. Lancet Oncol. 2010; 11: 429-438.
[18] Nachman JB, La MK, Hunger SP, et al. Young Adults With Acute Lymphoblastic Leukemia Have an Excellent Outcome With Chemotherapy Alone and Benefit From Intensive Postinduction Treatment: A Report From the Children's Oncology Group. J Clin Oncol.2009; 27:5189-5194
[19] Pui CH, Robison LL, Look AT. Acute lymphoblastic leukaemia. Lancet. 2008; 371:1030-43.
[20] Pui CH, Pei D, Campana D, et al. Improved prognosis for older adolescents with acute lymphoblastic leukemia. J Clin Oncol. 2011; 29: 386-391.
[21] Pullen J, Shuster JJ, Link M, et al. Significance of commonly used prognostic factors differs for children with T cell acute lymphocytic leukemia (ALL), as compared to those with B-precursor ALL. A Pediatric Oncology Group (POG) study. Leukemia. 1999; 13:1696–1707.
[22] Pulte D, Gondos A, Brenner H. Trends in 5-and 10-year survival after diagnosis with childhood hematologic malignancies in the United States 1990-2004. J Natl Cancer Inst. 2008; 100: 1271-3.
[23] Pulte D, Gondos A, Brenner H. Trends in survival after diagnosis with hematologic malignancy in adolescence and young adulthood in the United States, 1981-2005. Cancer. 2009; 115: 4973-4979.
[24] Ramanujachar R, Richards S, Hann I, Webb DD. Adolescents with acute lymphoblastic leukaemia: outcome on UK national paediatric (ALL97) and adult (UKALLXII/E2993) trials. Pediatr Blood Cancer. 2007;48:254-61.
[25] Ribera JM, Oriol A, Sanz MA, et al. Comparison of the results of the treatment of adolescents and young adults with standard-risk acute lymphoblastic leukemia with the pediatric-based protocol PETHEMA ALL-96. J Clin Oncol. 2008; 26:1843-9.

[26] Rytting ME, Kantarjian HM, Thomas ED, et al. Adolescent and Young Adult Patients Treated with Modified Augmented Berlin-Frankfurt-Muenster Therapy [abstract]. Blood. 2010; 114

[27] Schroder H, Kjeldahl M, Boesen AM, et al. Acute lymphoblastic leukemia in adolescents between 10 and 19 years of age in Denmark. Dan Med Bull. 2006;53:76-9.

[28] Secker-Walker LM, Craig JM, Hawkins JM, Hoffbrand AV. Philadelphia positive acute lymphoblastic leukemia in adults: age distribution, BCR breakpoint and prognostic significance. Leukemia. 1991;5:196–199.

[29] Smith MA, Siebel NL, Altefruse SF, et al. Outcomes of children and adolescents with cancer: challenges for the twenty-first century. J Clin Oncol. 2010; 28:2625-2634.

[30] Srivastava P, Watkins K, Mark L, et al. Treatment of adults with newly diagnosed acute lymphoblastic leukemia with multiple doses of intravenous pegylated asparaginase in an intensified pediatric regimen. Haematologica. 2008; 93 (s1): 366.

[31] Stock W, La M, Sanford B, et al. What determines the outcomes for adolescents and young adults with acute lymphoblastic leukemia treated on cooperative protocols? A comparison of Children's Cancer Group and Cancer and Leukemia Group B studies. Blood. 2008;112:1646-74.

[32] Stock W. Adolescents and young adults with acute lymphoblastic leukemia. Hematology 2010. American Society of Hematology Education Program Book. 2010; 21-29.

[33] Storring JM, Minden MD, Kao S, et al. Treatment of adults with BCR-ABL negative acute lymphoblastic leukaemia with a modified paediatric regimen. Br J Haematol. 2009; 146: 76-85.

[34] Testi AM, Valsecchi MG, Conter V, et al. Difference in outcome of adolescents with acute lymphoblastic leukemia (ALL) enrolled in pediatric (AIEOP) and adult (GIMEMA) protocols. Blood. 2004;104:1954a

[35] Thomas DA, O'Brien S, Rytting M, et al. Acute lymphoblastic leukemia (ALL) or lymphoblastic lymphoma (LL) after frontline therapy with hyper-CVAD regimens [abstract]. Blood. 2008; 112: 674.

[36] Usvasalo A, Räty R, Knuutila S, et al. Acute lymphoblastic leukemia in adolescents and Young adults in Finland. Haematologica. 2008; 93: 1161-8.

[37] Available at www.clinicaltrials.gov NCT00558519.

Vitamin D and Acute Myeloid Leukemia

Hun Ju Lee[1], Candace S. Johnson[2],
Donald Trump[3] and Meir Wetzler[1]
[1]*Leukemia Section, Department of Medicine,*
[2]*Department of Pharmacology and Therapeutics and*
[3]*Department of Medicine, Roswell Park Cancer Institute, Buffalo, NY*
USA

1. Introduction

The clearest role for vitamin D in human is in bone health as a regulator of serum calcium and skeletal homeostasis. Additional roles of vitamin D have been suggested, which include differentiation, apoptosis, angiogenesis and immunoregulation. Prevalence of vitamin D level

Vitamin D analogue	Chemical description	Comments
Vitamin D_1	Compound of ergocalciferol with lumisterol (stereoisomer of ergosterol) 1:1 ratio	
Vitamin D_2	Ergocalciferol (made from ergosterol)	
Vitamin D_3	Cholecalciferol (made from 7-dehydrocholesterol in the skin)	
Vitamin D_4	22-dihydroergocalciferol	
Vitamin D_5	Sitocalciferol (made from 7-dehydrositosterol)	
Vitamin D_6	Calciferol	
25-(OH) Vitamin D	Calcidiol or calcifediol; indicates no distinction between D_2 and D_3 forms. When relevant, forms are distinguished as $25(OH)D_2$ and $25(OH)D_3$	Vitamin D with one hydroxyl group added equivalent to liver activation.
Ercalcitriol	$1,25(OH)_2\ D_2$	
Calcitriol	$1,25(OH)_2\ D_3$	Vitamin D with two hydroxyl groups added equivalent to renal activation.
Doxercalciferol	$1\alpha(OH)D_2$	
Alfacalcidiol	$1\alpha(OH)D_3$	Vitamin D with one hydroxyl group added equivalent to renal activation

Table 1. Vitamin D Analogues

monitoring has significantly increased as the awareness of its potential importance to health has increased. Also, the readily available supply of vitamin D allows for intervention.

Vitamin D is generated in the skin from the non-enzymatic conversion of pro-vitamin D_3 to pre-vitamin D_3. Dietary intake of vitamin D is usually limited to selective foods, with the exception of certain kinds of fish which contain sizable amounts; supplements are commonly used. Vitamin D is either stored in adipose tissue or converted in the liver by the enzyme 25-hydoxylase to 25(OH) vitamin D_3, the most stable metabolite of vitamin D that reflects solar and dietary exposure (Binkley, Ramamurthy et al. 2010). There are many different analogues of vitamin D as shown in table 1.

Vitamin D body stores are reflected in the measurement of the serum level of the relatively stable (half-life approximately 3 weeks) surrogate marker 25 (OH) vitamin D_3 [25(OH)D_3]. Enzyme-linked immunosorbant assay (ELISA) is the most commonly used methodology in the United States (Hollis 2007); however, there are more sensitive and costly methods to measure vitamin D levels, e.g. mass spectroscopy (Yuan, Kosewick et al. 2011). Currently, the Institute of Medicine (2011) has put forth a guideline on recommended daily allowance and appropriate levels but this issue still remains controversial (Toner, Davis et al. 2010). In this paper, we will use the following definitions for vitamin D levels (Ross, Manson et al. 2011): Vitamin D deficiency as <10ng/ml (<25nmol/L) of 25(OH)D_3 in the serum. Vitamin D insufficiency as serum 25(OH)D_3 between 10-32ng/ml (25-75 nmol/L) (Rosen 2011). Subnormal vitamin D levels as less than 32 ng/ml of 25(OH)D_3 (Lee, HJ 2010). There are currently no standards of measurement or methods to measure vitamin D levels in the clinical setting. There have been numerous publications regarding vitamin D, but no consensus has yet been reached as illustrated in Table 2.

Author	*Year*	*Normal*	*Insufficient*	*Deficient*
Holick (Holick 2007)	2007	≥ 30 mg/ml	21-29 ng/ml	< 20 mg/ml
Lee (Lee, Eisman et al. 2009)	2009	> 25 ng/ml	12-24 ng/ml	< 12 ng/ml
Vashi (Vashi, Trukova et al. 2010)	2010	≥ 32 ng/ml	< 32 ng/ml (suboptimal)	N/R
Napoli (Napoli, Vattikuti et al. 2010)	2010	≥ 30 ng/ml	20-29 ng/ml	< 20 ng/ml
Drake (Drake, Maurer et al. 2010)	2010	≥ 25 ng/ml	< 25 ng/ml	N/R
Fedirko (Fedirko, Bostick et al. 2010)	2010	≥ 32 ng/ml	20-31.9 ng/ml	< 20 ng/ml
Rosen (Rosen 2011)	2011	> 30 ng/ml	10-30 ng/ml	< 10 ng/ml
Choo (Choo, Mamedov et al. 2011)	2011	≥ 30 ng/ml	< 30 ng/ml	N/R
Shanafelt (Shanafelt, Drake et al. 2011)	2011	≥25 ng/ml	< 25 ng/ml	N/R
Fiscella (Fiscella, Winters et al. 2011)	2011	N/R	N/R	< 20 ng/ml
Chadha (Chadha, Fakih et al. 2011)	2011	N/R	N/R	< 20 ng/ml

Abbreviations: N/R, not reported

Table 2. Various Definitions of Vitamin D Levels (25-Hydroxy Vitamin D_3)

1.1 Initial observation

An epidemiologic study estimated that one billion people worldwide have subnormal vitamin D levels due to decreased exposure to sunlight or dietary inadequacy (Holick 2011). Many studies suggest the detrimental effect of vitamin D insufficiency on heart, kidney, dermatologic, endocrine, and autoimmune diseases (Gueli, Verrusio et al. 2011). The well-established target organs of vitamin D are the intestines, kidney and bone, but several other

tissues also express vitamin D receptors (VDR), including normal and neoplastic hematopoietic cells (Haussler, Whitfield et al. 1998). In the early 1980s, *in vitro* data showed the ability of 1α,25-dihydroxy vitamin D_3 to differentiate acute myeloid leukemia (AML) [HL-60] into mature myeloid cells (Miyaura, Abe et al. 1981).
Vitamin D is a potentially exciting therapy for AML investigators due to its promising *in vitro* data and its safety (Trump, Deeb et al. 2010). The appropriate patient population selection and the development of optimum dosing and delivery schedule will maximize its clinical effect.

2. Epidemiologic evidence for vitamin D and leukemia

The epidemiology of vitamin D levels have not been extensively studied in AML as it has in other solid tumors (Toner, Davis et al. 2010). However, a study in northern Finland, where colder temperatures discourage extensive outdoor activities and minimize UV exposure during the winter months, found that majority of acute leukemia cases were diagnosed during the winter months of the year, rather than during the summer months (Timonen 1999). A possible explanation for this increase may be seasonal variation in levels of 25(OH)D_3. It is estimated that 25(OH)D_3 levels can vary by 8 to 12 ng/ml from the mean population during different seasons. Therefore, winter months can significantly increase the percentage of the population with low levels of 25(OH)D_3, possibly increasing the risk of leukemia (Bolland, Grey et al. 2007). In addition, a large epidemiological study (Boscoe and Schymura 2006) using data from the North American Association of Central Cancer Registries and the National Cancer Institute's Surveillance, Epidemiology and End Results database found an inverse relationship between ultraviolet-B exposure and the incidence of leukemia; however, this study did not examine vitamin D levels and would make it difficult to conclude that vitamin D played a role in increased incidence of leukemia.
Similarly, a study in the United Arab Emirates (UAE) found that acute leukemia was more common among adult females than among adult males, despite the fact that the population of the UAE consists of more males than females, and acute leukemia is widely known to be more common in males. The authors' hypothesis was that the women's deprived sunlight exposure, due to their conservative clothing, may have contributed to their higher incidence of acute leukemia (Hassan, Islam et al. 2009). It would be difficult to conclude that vitamin D played a role in the increased incidence due to lack of dietary information on the populations.
However, these observations lend credibility to the association between AML and vitamin D.

2.1 Vitamin D and solid tumors

Initial observation by Garland et al. (Garland, Comstock et al. 1989) demonstrated higher mortality rates of colon cancer in the northeast when compared to the south and southwest United States, which suggested an association between sunlight exposure and cancer outcome. This finding led to several epidemiologic observations linking subnormal vitamin D levels to increased risk of breast (Garland, Garland et al. 1990), colorectal (Jenab, Bueno-de-Mesquita et al. 2010) and prostate cancers (Barnett, Nielson et al. 2010).
Giovannucci et al. performed a large prospective observational cohort study composed of 51,529 U.S. male healthcare providers and illustrated that low levels 25(OH) D_3 (<25nmol/L) were associated with increased cancer incidence and mortality in men. Strongest association was seen with gastrointestinal cancers (Giovannucci, Liu et al. 2006).
On the contrary, a large randomized double blind controlled trial of 2,686 men and women aged 65 to 85 years of age from Oxford, England showed that supplementation of vitamin

D3 100,000 IU every 4 months versus placebo had a preventive benefit of reduced fracture in the vitamin D3 group after follow-up of five years. However, the cancer incidence was not statistically significant with relative risk (95% CI) 1.09 (0.86-1.36) (Trivedi, Doll et al. 2003). On the other hand, a study from Creighton University (Lappe, Travers-Gustafson et al. 2007) where they performed a population based, double blind, randomized placebo-controlled trial showed the opposite. Eligible subjects were >55 years and free of known cancer prior to entering study. Subjects were randomly assigned to take daily dosages of 1,400-1,500 mg supplemental calcium, 1,400-1,500 mg supplemental calcium plus 1,100 IU of vitamin D3, or placebo. Patients were prospectively followed for 4 years and the study showed that the calcium plus vitamin D group had a 60% reduction in cancer risk compared to placebo. The reasons for these differences are not clear but may be related to the supplementation offered and the subjects' pre-treatment vitamin D levels.

Further, the Nurses' Health Study, consisting of 32,826 participants, showed that the odds ratios for colorectal cancer were inversely associated with the 25(OH) D_3 serum levels (Feskanich, Ma et al. 2004). Similarly, Garland et al. (Garland, Garland et al. 2006) showed, in a meta-analysis of 980 women, that high dietary vitamin D intake was associated with significant reduction in developing breast cancer when compared with low vitamin D intake.

Various VDAs have been extensively tried as cancer therapeutic agents, but so far no ideal agent or delivery schedule has been clearly delineated. The most promising data was calcitriol in combination with docetaxel in prostate cancer; however, the phase III trial was halted by the data safety monitoring board because the survival rate in the vitamin D group was lower than the placebo group (Trump, Deeb et al. 2010). Among the concerns about the trial were that it included two different variables between the two arms; the control arm used docetaxel every three weeks, while the experimental arm, which included the addition of vitamin D, used docetaxel weekly. Second, there was limited rationale for calcitriol dose, which was probably inadequate, and the dose used was well below the calcitriol human maximally tolerated dose. This trial further highlights the need for continued exploration to define the appropriate dose and schedule to study in therapeutic and preventative trials.

2.2 Vitamin D and hematologic malignancies (NHL, CLL)

A prospective Mayo Clinic study of 983 newly diagnosed NHL patients found that vitamin D insufficiency (<25 ng/ml, as determined by liquid chromatography-tandem mass spectrometry) was associated with inferior event free survival (EFS) and overall survival (OS) in diffuse large B- and T-cell lymphoma patients (Drake, Maurer et al. 2010). Similarly, the Mayo Clinic also examined 543 newly diagnosed CLL patients and found vitamin D insufficiency at diagnosis to be associated with decreased time until initiation of treatment (Shanafelt, Drake et al. 2011). These results lend credence to the possible correlation of adverse clinical effect of vitamin D insufficiency in newly diagnosed hematological malignancies.

These studies illustrate observations that low vitamin D levels are associated with poorer clinical outcomes. Therefore, supplementation and corollary studies are needed to understand the effect of vitamin D on hematologic malignancies.

2.3 Vitamin D and AML

Lee et al. (Lee, HJ 2010) have recently reported 25(OH)D_3 levels at the time of diagnosis of AML and their association with survival. A cohort of 97 newly diagnosed AML patients treated on similar protocols showed that patients with subnormal 25(OH)D_3 (<32ng/ml) had significantly worse progression free survival (PFS) and OS when compared to those with normal 25(OH)D_3 levels (≥32ng/ml) (Figure 1).

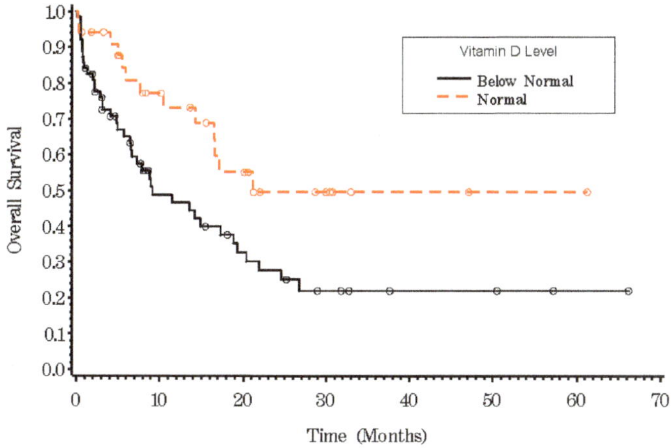

(A)

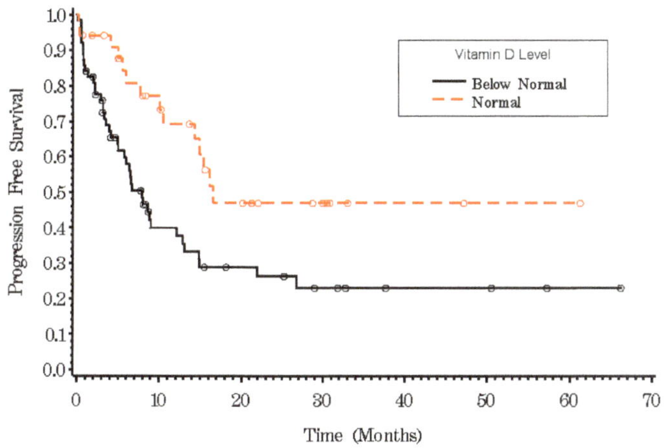

(B)

Fig. 1. A: Overall Survival; B: Progression Free Survival

Therefore, one may hypothesize the benefit of supplementing AML patients with subnormal $25(OH)D_3$ levels to see if they would benefit from $25(OH)D_3$ normalization. There are several reports (Drake, Maurer et al. 2010; Lee HJ 2010; Shanafelt, Drake et al. 2011) indicating that low levels of vitamin D have been shown to be associated with worse clinical outcome; however, there are no prospective studies evaluating whether supplementation would improve outcome. It would be worthwhile to conduct a trial studying the effect of vitamin D supplementation in newly diagnosed AML patients.

2.4 Clinical trials with VDA in myelodysplastic syndrome and AML

Exploration of vitamin D as a possible therapeutic intervention for AML was propelled by the success of all-trans-retinoic acid (ATRA) treatment as a differentiating agent for AML blasts (James, Williams et al. 1999). Vitamin D differentiates myeloid blasts to monocytes in vitro (Miyaura, Abe et al. 1981) and ex vivo (Lee, Kim et al. 1996), which prompted early clinical trials to investigate the anti-leukemic effects of VDAs in myelodysplastic syndromes (MDS) and AML (Table 3).

Author	Dx	#N	Median Age	Vitamin D	Chemotherapy	RR	CR
Petrich (Petrich, Kahl et al. 2008)	MDS	15	77	12.5 μg/d x 12 wks of doxercalciferol	Single agent	0%	0%
Siitonen (Siitonen, Timonen et al. 2007)	MDS	19	73	1 μg/d $1,25(OH)D_3$	Valproic acid and 13 cRA	16%	0%
Mellibovsky (Mellibovsky, Diez et al. 1998)	MDS	19	75	266 μg 3xwk (calcifediol) 5 pts and 0.25-0.75 μg/d calcitriol 14 pts	None	58%	NA
Ferrero (Ferrero, Bruno et al. 1996)	MDS	53	74	1-1.5 μg/d calcitriol	cRA and intermittent	52%	NR
Slapak (Slapak, Desforges et al. 1992)	AML	29	73	0.25 μg oral Q12hrs Calcitriol	Cytarabine, hydroxyurea	79%	45%
Petrini (Petrini, Dastoli et al. 1991)	AML	21	67.5	20 mg BID AraC x 7d Q3w, 1 μg $1(OH)D_3$	low dose ARA-C	62%	17%
Hellstrom (Hellstrom, Robert et al. 1990)	MDS, AML	69	NR	1 μg/d of $1\alpha(OH)D_3$	Low dose ARA-C	26%	NR

Abbreviations: NR: Not Reported, AraC: Cytosine Arabinoside, wk: Weeks, pts: patients, cRA: cis-retinoic acid, RR: Response Rate, CR: Complete Response

Table 3. Vitamin D Trials in Myelodysplastic Syndrome / Acute Myeloid Leukemia

Seven studies examined the effects of various VDAs in AML and MDS, either single agent or combined with other chemotherapy, including low-dose cytarabine, hydroxyurea, and valproic acid. All studies were small, ranging from 15 to 69 patients, and median age, when reported, ranged from 67.5 to 77. Overall response rates ranged from 0% to 79%, and complete response (CR) rates ranged from 0% to 45% when reported. Early results were mixed, as single agent VDA induced partial differentiation of myeloid blast cells in a few patients with a paucity of clinical improvements (Mellibovsky, Diez et al. 1998). Combination trials with VDA and chemotherapy resulted in mixed results in MDS/AML (Hellstrom, Robert et al. 1990; Petrini, Caracciolo et al. 1991; Petrini, Dastoli et al. 1991; Slapak, Desforges et al. 1992; Ferrero, Bruno et al. 1996; Siitonen, Timonen et al. 2007).

Slapak et al. (Slapak, Desforges et al. 1992) showed promising results in a study of 29 AML patients, who were treated with a regimen of low-dose cytarabine, hydroxyurea, and calcitriol (0.25μg, oral every 12 hours) begun on day 1 of cytarabine and continued until relapse or the patient went off study. Three patients died within 60 days, and of the remainder, the overall response rate was 79%; 45% achieved CR and 34% achieved partial remission (PR). The median overall survival was 14 months for those who responded and 12 months overall. Although all patients developed transient thrombocytopenia and granulocytopenia and 20 patients required platelet transfusions transiently, the study nonetheless showed promise due to its high overall response rate and low induction death rate. Two patients experienced asymptomatic hypercalcemia (11.2mg/dl and 11.5mg/dl) but did not require treatment. The authors proposed that the favorable results might be due to the synergistic effects of cytarabine, hydroxyurea, and calcitriol, although they did not propose a specific mechanism (Slapak, Desforges et al. 1992)(Trump, Deeb et al. 2010).

Vitamin D was studied in 19 low-risk MDS patients with a median age of 75 years (Mellibovsky, Diez et al. 1998). Five patients received 266 mcg of calcifediol three times per week, and 14 patients received 0.25-0.75 micrograms per day of calcitriol. Of the patients treated with calcifediol, one responded, one progressed, and the other three patients did not respond. Of the 14 patients treated with calcitriol, 10 responded while the other four did not. The authors concluded that vitamin D_3 metabolites could be used to induce hematological responses in patients with low or intermediate risk MDS without the risk of hypercalcemia (Mellibovsky, Diez et al. 1998).

Petrich et al. (Petrich, Kahl et al. 2008) conducted a phase II trial of doxercalciferol (12.5 μg daily for 12 weeks) in 15 MDS patients. Only 9 of the 15 patients completed the whole 12 weeks, and no one responded. Stable disease was observed in six patients, and eight patients had disease progression, including two chronic myelomonocytic leukemia patients, who developed an increase in their monocyte count. Doxercalciferol was well tolerated; one patient experienced grade 3 rash, and one patient had grade 3 hypercalcemia and needed to be removed from the study. All toxicities resolved upon discontinuation of doxercalciferol. The authors therefore concluded that the study dose and scheduling of doxercalciferol appeared to have no efficacy in MDS patients (Petrich, Kahl et al. 2008).

All the clinical trials were conducted with very low doses of VDA. Also, there have been no pharmacokinetic studies examining whether supplementation was sufficient to observe clinical responses. In the future, studies of pharmacokinetic and novel markers (e.g. miRNA, methylation pattern of vitamin D responsive elements) may be used to select and properly dose populations that may benefit from VDA.

3. Molecular mechanism of vitamin D in AML

Cardinal features of AML are the inability to differentiate and the clonal expansion of myeloid blasts. Intensive biological research and clinical trials to eradicate AML cells with cytotoxic chemotherapy have yielded minimal improvements and have rarely led to cures, especially in those 60 years or older (Burnett, Wetzler et al. 2011). Vitamin D predominantly exerts its effects through binding to the cognate nuclear VDR; ligand bound VDR heterodimerizes with the retinoic X receptor (RXR) and binds to vitamin D responsive elements in the promoter regions of target genes, such as *CYP24A1*, *BGLAP* (osteocalcin) and cyclin dependent kinase inhibitor 1A (*CDKN1A*, $p21^{Waf1/Cip1}$), several protein kinase C (*PKC*) isoforms (Shimizu, Taira et al. 2002), the p42 extracellular regulated kinase (p42 *ERK*), p38-ERK and c-Jun N-terminal kinases (*JNK*) families of mitogen activated protein kinases (*MAPKs*) which are important in differentiation, metabolism and cell cycle (Wang and Studzinski 2001; Ji, Kutner et al. 2002; Hughes and Brown 2006; Marcinkowska, Garay et al. 2006; Studzinski, Garay et al. 2006). One of the main anti-proliferative and differentiating actions of vitamin D is the induction of cell cycle arrest by up-regulating anti-proliferative genes, such as p21, CCAAT/enhancer-binding protein α (*C/EBPA*) and interferon α-inducible protein 27 (*IFI27*, p27). Further, non-genomic actions of vitamin D through increased activation of voltage gated calcium channels can alter the actions of Ras/Raf/mitogen-activated protein kinase (ERK) pathway as well as phosphoinositidine-3-kinase catalytic, alpha polypeptide (PI3K)/Akt pathway which have been shown to be activated in AML (Trump, Deeb et al. 2010). VDR is essential for vitamin D function. VDR is a highly conserved gene found in primitive organisms such as the sea squirt (*Ciona intestinalis*), a chordate invertebrate, showing that VDR was important even early in evolution (Reschly and Krasowski 2006). Calcium regulation is a key component to regulation of life itself, and vitamin D therefore is crucial to any system that relies on calcium for signaling. The VDR gene has been sequenced and compared among many different species, and now VDR polymorphism is an active area of research (Reschly and Krasowski 2006). VDR polymorphisms have been extensively studied in solid tumors and have been shown to have predictive value in cancer prognosis and recurrence (Kostner, Denzer et al. 2009). There are a limited number of studies of VDR polymorphisms in AML. In a French study (Rocha, Porcher et al. 2009), the investigators looked at VDR polymorphism (*Apa*I, *Taq*I and *Bsm*I), and demonstrated worse toxicity and survival after allogeneic transplantation in leukemia patients with VDR *Taq*I polymorphism. Binding affinity would be greatly affected by different VDR polymorphisms, given the structural variations induced by the polymorphism; hence, understanding structural and functional variations will allow for rational therapy design. Functional activity of VDR has been shown to be impaired by AML associated chromosomal translocations *PLZF-RAR* α, *PML-RAR* α and *AML-ETO1*; these fusion proteins interfere with VDR nuclear localization by binding to VDR (Puccetti, Obradovic et al. 2002).

3.1 Leukemia, vitamin D and the effect on apoptosis

Programmed cell death may be aberrant in AML cells as they continue to proliferate uncontrollably without activating the apoptotic pathway. AML has been known to be deregulated in the FAS induced apoptosis as a means of avoiding death (Testa and Riccioni 2007). VDAs have been shown to increase the expression of the FAS ligand and activate caspase-2,-3,-6 and -9 (Chen, Huang et al. 2008). Further, Vitamin D has been shown to down-regulate telomerase activity in ovarian cancers, which are known to have the highest level of telomerase activity in solid cancers (Jiang, Bao et al. 2004). Vitamin D was reported to disrupt telomerase reverse transcriptase (*TERT*) mRNA, therefore inducing apoptosis through telomere shortening and ultimately resulting in down regulation of telomerase activity(Jiang, Bao et al. 2004). Since AML has been reported to have high telomerase activity (Capraro, Zane et al. 2011), it would suggest that vitamin D may have a similar effect in this disease as well. Indeed, *in vitro* exposure of the leukemic cell line, HL-60, known to have high telomerase activity (Capraro, Zane et al. 2011), to vitamin D, led to down-regulation of the telomerase activity. This down regulation was associated with induction of p21, PI3K/AKT/mTOR pathways which play a key role in differentiation (Seol, Kim et al. 1998; Yamada, Ozaki et al. 2008). In summary, vitamin D, can modulate several pathways that will lead to AML apoptosis and should be exploited in AML treatment.

3.2 Leukemia, vitamin D and the effect on proliferative signaling

The FMS-like tyrosine kinase 3 (*FLT-3*) is mutated (internal tandem duplication, ITD) in cells of approximately 25-30% of AML patients (Burnett, Wetzler et al. 2011), providing such cells with a proliferative advantage. FLT-3 exerts its proliferative effect through the activation of many different pathways, e.g., PI3K/AKT/mTOR, RAS/RAF/ERK and signal transducer and activator of transcription (STAT). Ultimately, these signaling pathways will down-regulate pro-apoptotic signals, such as the B-cell chronic lymphocytic leukemia/lymphoma 2 (BCL2)-family of proteins, and repress tumor suppressive genes, such as p21 and breast cancer 1 (BRCA1) (Stirewalt and Radich 2003). Of note, AML cells with chromosome 7 deletion were extremely sensitive to VDA but FLT-3 positive AML cells did not differentiate in the presence of VDA (Gocek, Kielbinski et al. 2010). This raises the question as to whether a FLT-3 inhibitor would restore the ability of FLT-3-ITD positive AML cells to differentiate in response to VDA. The data also emphasizes potential importance of detailed molecular characteristics of patients' AML cells and VDA use only in certain AML subgroups.

3.3 Leukemia, vitamin D and the effect on tumor suppressor genes

Leukemia cells must avoid or turn off negative regulators in order to proliferate. One example is the tumor suppressor transcription factor p53, whose inactivation, rather than mutation, is observed in many cancer types (Bohlig and Rother 2011); p53 is negatively regulated by murine double minute 2 (MDM2). It was recently shown that vitamin D alone induced monocytic differentiation of two wild-type p53 AML cell lines as well as a p53-null AML cells. Combination of a small molecule inhibitor (nutlin-3a) of p53-MDM2 interaction and vitamin D accelerated programmed cell death (Thompson, Andreeff et al. 2010). Interestingly, MDM2 levels dropped significantly in the presence of vitamin D_3, possibly contributing to the apoptotic effect. Additional factors were found to contribute to the sensitization of the wild-type p53 cells to apoptosis when exposed to combinations such as BCL2, ERK and others. The authors suggested that vitamin D_3 recruits its co-activators to enable p53 to become more effective in inducing cell death. This illustrates only a small amount of the complexities of cellular cross-talk seen in the vitamin D signaling pathway.

3.4 Leukemia, vitamin D and the effect on the tumor microenvironment

The bone marrow microenvironment is known to provide a nurturing environment for the hematopoietic stem cells. Leukemic stem cells also start to exploit the bone marrow microenvironment for survival advantage from conventional chemotherapy. Conventional chemotherapy induction is able to clear peripheral blood of leukemic cells, but patients ultimately relapse due to leukemic stem cells in the protected bone marrow microenvironment. Clinical trials (Harousseau, Witz et al. 2000; von Lilienfeld-Toal, Hahn-Ast et al. 2007; Borthakur, Kantarjian et al. 2008) have attempted to use granulocyte colony-stimulating factor (G-CSF) in order to bring out leukemic stem cells from the bone marrow. However, this method has not been shown to be widely effective. The mechanism by which G-CSF mediates mobilization is by sympathetic nervous system suppression of osteoblasts and modulation of serum calcium in the endosteal proximity of the bone marrow (Metcalf 1985). A recent report by Kawamori et al. (Kawamori, Katayama et al. 2010) demonstrated the regulatory role of VDR on mobilization of hematopoietic cells by using VDR knockout mice; lack of VDR caused inability to mobilize hematopoietic cells. The authors demonstrated that VDR is important for calcium regulation in the endosteal proximity of the bone marrow. *RANK ligand,* a gene downstream of VDR, is also stimulated by the sympathetic nervous system and aids in the stabilization of VDR. Jeanson and Scadden (Jeanson and Scadden 2010) reported that VDR knockout mice had marked accumulation of hematopoietic stem cells in the spleen, which was reversed by dietary calcium supplementation, thus adding credence to the importance of calcium/VDR regulation of stem cell trafficking. These data suggest that low

vitamin D levels can cause leukemic stem cells to hide in the protective layers of the bone marrow to avoid cytotoxic chemotherapy agents.
Further, anemia, bone marrow hypocellularity, and extramedullary hematopoiesis have been observed in vitamin D deficient rickets and have disappeared following vitamin D treatment. In two case reports, myelofibrosis and marrow dysfunction have been described secondary to vitamin D deficiency, and both improved following vitamin D supplementation (Balasubramanian, Varadharajan et al. 2005; Bhakhri and Debata 2010).
These results suggest that the interaction between the bone marrow microenvironment and the leukemia cells may be mediated, at least partially, by vitamin D.

4. Future directions

Three studies have shown the prognostic significance of vitamin D deficiency in hematologic malignancies, including CLL (Shanafelt, Drake et al. 2011), NHL (Drake, Maurer et al. 2010) and AML (Lee HJ 2010). There have been no studies evaluating the clinical significance of vitamin D supplementation on raising the 25(OH)D_3 levels of patients with hematologic malignancies to normal. It would be worthwhile to carefully design a pharmacokinetic study to evaluate supplementation of vitamin D in AML patients. Following the pharmacokinetic study, the next question of whether vitamin D supplementation affects outcome will need to be separately evaluated in a large phase III clinical trial. At least two possibilities exist, either that the mere supplementation of vitamin D, with its multitude effects on bone and other tissues, is causing better outcomes or that vitamin D has a specific differentiation effect. The support for the latter is the preclinical finding that AML cells with chromosome 7 deletion are extremely sensitive to the VDA calcitriol, while FLT3-ITD positive cells are resistant to this differentiation therapy (Gocek, Kielbinski et al. 2010). There are other in vitro studies showing anti-proliferative, pro-apoptotic and differentiating properties of vitamin D on AML (Nowak, Stewart et al. 2009). Finally, the search for an ideal VDA that will not cause hypercalcemia is still on-going. A group from South Korea recently tested 11 VDAs and found that one compound had significant anti-leukemic activity with low proclivity toward hypercalcemia (Yoon, Kim et al. 2008). These new findings in the biology and improvements in VDAs will hopefully lead to an improved treatment option for AML patients.

5. Acknowledgments

Supported partially by grant from the National Cancer Institute Grant CA16056 (HJL, CSJ, DT, MW).

6. References

(2011). "Dietary reference intake for calcium and vitamin D." Institute of Medicine.
Balasubramanian, S., R. Varadharajan, et al. (2005). "Myelofibrosis and vitamin D deficient rickets--a rare association." Indian Pediatr 42(5): 482-484.
Barnett, C. M., C. M. Nielson, et al. (2010). "Serum 25-OH vitamin D levels and risk of developing prostate cancer in older men." Cancer Causes Control 21(8): 1297-1303.
Bhakhri, B. K. and P. K. Debata (2010). "Nutritional rickets presenting with myelofibrosis." Indian J Pediatr 77(12): 1437-1439.

Binkley, N., R. Ramamurthy, et al. (2010). "Low vitamin D status: definition, prevalence, consequences, and correction." Endocrinol Metab Clin North Am 39(2): 287-301, table of contents.

Bohlig, L. and K. Rother (2011). "One Function-Multiple Mechanisms: The Manifold Activities of p53 as a Transcriptional Repressor." J Biomed Biotechnol 2011: 464916.

Bolland, M. J., A. B. Grey, et al. (2007). "The effects of seasonal variation of 25-hydroxyvitamin D and fat mass on a diagnosis of vitamin D sufficiency." Am J Clin Nutr 86(4): 959-964.

Borthakur, G., H. Kantarjian, et al. (2008). "Treatment of core-binding-factor in acute myelogenous leukemia with fludarabine, cytarabine, and granulocyte colony-stimulating factor results in improved event-free survival." Cancer 113(11): 3181-3185.

Boscoe, F. P. and M. J. Schymura (2006). "Solar ultraviolet-B exposure and cancer incidence and mortality in the United States, 1993-2002." BMC Cancer 6: 264.

Burnett, A., M. Wetzler, et al. (2011). "Therapeutic advances in acute myeloid leukemia." J Clin Oncol 29(5): 487-494.

Capraro, V., L. Zane, et al. (2011). "Telomere deregulations possess cytogenetic, phenotype, and prognostic specificities in acute leukemias." Exp Hematol 39(2): 195-202 e192.

Chadha, M. K., M. Fakih, et al. (2011). "Effect of 25-hydroxyvitamin D status on serological response to influenza vaccine in prostate cancer patients." Prostate 71(4): 368-372.

Chen, W. J., Y. T. Huang, et al. (2008). "Induction of apoptosis by vitamin D2, ergocalciferol, via reactive oxygen species generation, glutathione depletion, and caspase activation in human leukemia Cells." J Agric Food Chem 56(9): 2996-3005.

Choo, C. S., A. Mamedov, et al. (2011). "Vitamin D insufficiency is common in patients with nonmetastatic prostate cancer." Nutr Res 31(1): 21-26.

Drake, M. T., M. J. Maurer, et al. (2010). "Vitamin D insufficiency and prognosis in non-Hodgkin's lymphoma." J Clin Oncol 28(27): 4191-4198.

Fedirko, V., R. M. Bostick, et al. (2010). "Blood 25-hydroxyvitamin D3 concentrations and incident sporadic colorectal adenoma risk: a pooled case-control study." Am J Epidemiol 172(5): 489-500.

Ferrero, D., B. Bruno, et al. (1996). "Combined differentiating therapy for myelodysplastic syndromes: a phase II study." Leuk Res 20(10): 867-876.

Feskanich, D., J. Ma, et al. (2004). "Plasma vitamin D metabolites and risk of colorectal cancer in women." Cancer Epidemiol Biomarkers Prev 13(9): 1502-1508.

Fiscella, K., P. Winters, et al. (2011). "Racial disparity in death from colorectal cancer: does vitamin D deficiency contribute?" Cancer 117(5): 1061-1069.

Garland, C. F., G. W. Comstock, et al. (1989). "Serum 25-hydroxyvitamin D and colon cancer: eight-year prospective study." Lancet 2(8673): 1176-1178.

Garland, C. F., F. C. Garland, et al. (2006). "The role of vitamin D in cancer prevention." Am J Public Health 96(2): 252-261.

Garland, F. C., C. F. Garland, et al. (1990). "Geographic variation in breast cancer mortality in the United States: a hypothesis involving exposure to solar radiation." Prev Med 19(6): 614-622.

Giovannucci, E., Y. Liu, et al. (2006). "Prospective study of predictors of vitamin D status and cancer incidence and mortality in men." J Natl Cancer Inst 98(7): 451-459.

Gocek, E., M. Kielbinski, et al. (2010). "Different susceptibilities to 1,25-dihydroxyvitamin D3-induced differentiation of AML cells carrying various mutations." Leuk Res 34(5): 649-657.

Gocek, E. and G. P. Studzinski (2009). "Vitamin D and differentiation in cancer." Crit Rev Clin Lab Sci 46(4): 190-209.

Gueli, N., W. Verrusio, et al. (2011). "Vitamin D: drug of the future. A new therapeutic approach." Arch Gerontol Geriatr.

Harousseau, J. L., B. Witz, et al. (2000). "Granulocyte colony-stimulating factor after intensive consolidation chemotherapy in acute myeloid leukemia: results of a randomized trial of the Groupe Ouest-Est Leucemies Aigues Myeloblastiques." J Clin Oncol 18(4): 780-787.

Hassan, I. B., S. I. Islam, et al. (2009). "Acute leukemia among the adult population of United Arab Emirates: an epidemiological study." Leuk Lymphoma 50(7): 1138-1147.

Haussler, M. R., G. K. Whitfield, et al. (1998). "The nuclear vitamin D receptor: biological and molecular regulatory properties revealed." J Bone Miner Res 13(3): 325-349.

Hellstrom, E., K. H. Robert, et al. (1990). "Treatment of myelodysplastic syndromes with retinoic acid and 1 alpha-hydroxy-vitamin D3 in combination with low-dose ara-C is not superior to ara-C alone. Results from a randomized study. The Scandinavian Myelodysplasia Group (SMG)." Eur J Haematol 45(5): 255-261.

Holick, M. F. (2007). "Vitamin D deficiency." N Engl J Med 357(3): 266-281.

Holick, M. F. (2011). "Vitamin D: evolutionary, physiological and health perspectives." Curr Drug Targets 12(1): 4-18.

Hollis, B. W. (2007). "Assessment of circulating 25(OH)D and 1,25(OH)2D: emergence as clinically important diagnostic tools." Nutr Rev 65(8 Pt 2): S87-90.

Hughes, P. J. and G. Brown (2006). "1Alpha,25-dihydroxyvitamin D3-mediated stimulation of steroid sulphatase activity in myeloid leukaemic cell lines requires VDRnuc-mediated activation of the RAS/RAF/ERK-MAP kinase signalling pathway." J Cell Biochem 98(3): 590-617.

James, S. Y., M. A. Williams, et al. (1999). "Leukemia cell differentiation: cellular and molecular interactions of retinoids and vitamin D." Gen Pharmacol 32(1): 143-154.

Jeanson, N. T. and D. T. Scadden (2010). "Vitamin D receptor deletion leads to increased hematopoietic stem and progenitor cells residing in the spleen." Blood 116(20): 4126-4129.

Jenab, M., H. B. Bueno-de-Mesquita, et al. (2010). "Association between pre-diagnostic circulating vitamin D concentration and risk of colorectal cancer in European populations:a nested case-control study." BMJ 340: b5500.

Ji, Y., A. Kutner, et al. (2002). "Derivatives of vitamins D2 and D3 activate three MAPK pathways and upregulate pRb expression in differentiating HL60 cells." Cell Cycle 1(6): 410-415.

Jiang, F., J. Bao, et al. (2004). "Induction of ovarian cancer cell apoptosis by 1,25-dihydroxyvitamin D3 through the down-regulation of telomerase." J Biol Chem 279(51): 53213-53221.

Kawamori, Y., Y. Katayama, et al. (2010). "Role for vitamin D receptor in the neuronal control of the hematopoietic stem cell niche." Blood 116(25): 5528-5535.

Kostner, K., N. Denzer, et al. (2009). "The relevance of vitamin D receptor (VDR) gene polymorphisms for cancer: a review of the literature." Anticancer Res 29(9): 3511-3536.

Lappe, J. M., D. Travers-Gustafson, et al. (2007). "Vitamin D and calcium supplementation reduces cancer risk: results of a randomized trial." Am J Clin Nutr 85(6): 1586-1591.

Lee, HJ, M. J., Tan W, Wilding G, Ford LA, Sait S, Block AW, Barcos M, Vigil CE, Griffiths EA, Thompson JE, Wang ES, Johnson CS, Trump D, Wetzler W. (2010) "Subnormal

Vitamin D Levels Are Associated with Adverse Outcome In Newly-Diagnosed Similarly-Treated Adult Acute Myeloid Leukemia (AML) Patients." American Society of Hematology Annual Meeting.
Lee, P., J. A. Eisman, et al. (2009). "Vitamin D deficiency in critically ill patients." N Engl J Med 360(18): 1912-1914.
Lee, Y. Y., E. S. Kim, et al. (1996). "Effect of a vitamin D3 analog, EB1089, on hematopoietic stem cells from normal and myeloid leukemic blasts." Leukemia 10(11): 1751-1757.
Marcinkowska, E., E. Garay, et al. (2006). "Regulation of C/EBPbeta isoforms by MAPK pathways in HL60 cells induced to differentiate by 1,25-dihydroxyvitamin D3." Exp Cell Res 312(11): 2054-2065.
Mellibovsky, L., A. Diez, et al. (1998). "Vitamin D treatment in myelodysplastic syndromes." Br J Haematol 100(3): 516-520.
Metcalf, D. (1985). "The granulocyte-macrophage colony-stimulating factors." Science 229(4708): 16-22.
Miyaura, C., E. Abe, et al. (1981). "1 alpha,25-Dihydroxyvitamin D3 induces differentiation of human myeloid leukemia cells." Biochem Biophys Res Commun 102(3): 937-943.
Napoli, N., S. Vattikuti, et al. (2010). "High prevalence of low vitamin D and musculoskeletal complaints in women with breast cancer." Breast J 16(6): 609-616.
Nowak, D., D. Stewart, et al. (2009). "Differentiation therapy of leukemia: 3 decades of development." Blood 113(16): 3655-3665.
Petrich, A., B. Kahl, et al. (2008). "Phase II study of doxercalciferol for the treatment of myelodysplastic syndrome." Leuk Lymphoma 49(1): 57-61.
Petrini, M., F. Caracciolo, et al. (1991). "Low-dose ARA-C and 1(OH) D3 administration in acute non lymphoid leukemia: pilot study." Haematologica 76(3): 200-203.
Petrini, M., G. Dastoli, et al. (1991). "Synergistic effects of alpha interferon and 1,25 dihydroxyvitamin D3: preliminary evidence suggesting that interferon induces expression of the vitamin receptor." Haematologica 76(6): 467-471.
Puccetti, E., D. Obradovic, et al. (2002). "AML-associated translocation products block vitamin D(3)-induced differentiation by sequestering the vitamin D(3) receptor." Cancer Res 62(23): 7050-7058.
Reschly, E. J. and M. D. Krasowski (2006). "Evolution and function of the NR1I nuclear hormone receptor subfamily (VDR, PXR, and CAR) with respect to metabolism of xenobiotics and endogenous compounds." Curr Drug Metab 7(4): 349-365.
Rocha, V., R. Porcher, et al. (2009). "Association of drug metabolism gene polymorphisms with toxicities, graft-versus-host disease and survival after HLA-identical sibling hematopoietic stem cell transplantation for patients with leukemia." Leukemia 23(3): 545-556.
Rosen, C. J. (2011). "Clinical practice. Vitamin D insufficiency." N Engl J Med 364(3): 248-254.
Ross, A. C., J. E. Manson, et al. (2011). "The 2011 report on dietary reference intakes for calcium and vitamin D from the Institute of Medicine: what clinicians need to know." J Clin Endocrinol Metab 96(1): 53-58.
Seol, J. G., E. S. Kim, et al. (1998). "Telomerase activity in acute myelogenous leukaemia: clinical and biological implications." Br J Haematol 100(1): 156-165.
Shanafelt, T. D., M. T. Drake, et al. (2011). "Vitamin D insufficiency and prognosis in chronic lymphocytic leukemia." Blood 117(5): 1492-1498.
Shimizu, T., N. Taira, et al. (2002). "Involvement of diverse protein kinase C isoforms in the differentiation of ML-1 human myeloblastic leukemia cells induced by the vitamin D3 analogue KH1060 and the phorbol ester TPA." Cancer Lett 186(1): 67-74.

Siitonen, T., T. Timonen, et al. (2007). "Valproic acid combined with 13-cis retinoic acid and 1,25-dihydroxyvitamin D3 in the treatment of patients with myelodysplastic syndromes." Haematologica 92(8): 1119-1122.

Slapak, C. A., J. F. Desforges, et al. (1992). "Treatment of acute myeloid leukemia in the elderly with low-dose cytarabine, hydroxyurea, and calcitriol." Am J Hematol 41(3): 178-183.

Stirewalt, D. L. and J. P. Radich (2003). "The role of FLT3 in haematopoietic malignancies." Nat Rev Cancer 3(9): 650-665.

Studzinski, G. P., E. Garay, et al. (2006). "Vitamin D receptor signaling of monocytic differentiation in human leukemia cells: role of MAPK pathways in transcription factor activation." Curr Top Med Chem 6(12): 1267-1271.

Testa, U. and R. Riccioni (2007). "Deregulation of apoptosis in acute myeloid leukemia." Haematologica 92(1): 81-94.

Thompson, T., M. Andreeff, et al. (2010). "1,25-dihydroxyvitamin D3 enhances the apoptotic activity of MDM2 antagonist nutlin-3a in acute myeloid leukemia cells expressing wild-type p53." Mol Cancer Ther 9(5): 1158-1168.

Timonen, T. T. (1999). "A hypothesis concerning deficiency of sunlight, cold temperature, and influenza epidemics associated with the onset of acute lymphoblastic leukemia in northern Finland." Ann Hematol 78(9): 408-414.

Toner, C. D., C. D. Davis, et al. (2010). "The vitamin D and cancer conundrum: aiming at a moving target." J Am Diet Assoc 110(10): 1492-1500.

Trivedi, D. P., R. Doll, et al. (2003). "Effect of four monthly oral vitamin D3 (cholecalciferol) supplementation on fractures and mortality in men and women living in the community: randomised double blind controlled trial." BMJ 326(7387): 469.

Trump, D. L., K. K. Deeb, et al. (2010). "Vitamin D: considerations in the continued development as an agent for cancer prevention and therapy." Cancer J 16(1): 1-9.

Vashi, P. G., K. Trukova, et al. (2010). "Impact of oral vitamin D supplementation on serum 25-hydroxyvitamin D levels in oncology." Nutr J 9: 60.

von Lilienfeld-Toal, M., C. Hahn-Ast, et al. (2007). "A randomized comparison of immediate versus delayed application of G-CSF in induction therapy for patients with acute myeloid leukemia unfit for intensive chemotherapy." Haematologica 92(12): 1719-1720.

Wang, X. and G. P. Studzinski (2001). "Activation of extracellular signal-regulated kinases (ERKs) defines the first phase of 1,25-dihydroxyvitamin D3-induced differentiation of HL60 cells." J Cell Biochem 80(4): 471-482.

Yamada, O., K. Ozaki, et al. (2008). "Multistep regulation of telomerase during differentiation of HL60 cells." J Leukoc Biol 83(5): 1240-1248.

Yoon, J. S., J. Y. Kim, et al. (2008). "Antileukemic effect of a synthetic vitamin D3 analog, HY-11, with low potential to cause hypercalcemia." Int J Oncol 32(2): 387-396.

Yuan, C., J. Kosewick, et al. (2011). "Sensitive measurement of serum 1alpha,25-dihydroxyvitamin D by liquid chromatography/tandem mass spectrometry after removing interference with immunoaffinity extraction." Rapid Commun Mass Spectrom 25(9): 1241-1249.

18

Chemotherapy Toxicity in Patients with Acute Leukemia

Jose Manuel Vagace[1] and Guillermo Gervasini[2]
[1]*Department of Pediatric Hematology, University Hospital Infanta Cristina*
[2]*Department of Pharmacology, Medical School, University of Extremadura, Badajoz Spain*

1. Introduction

During the treatment for acute leukemia (AL) a patient may experience a wide variety of complications that mainly have three possible origins, namely the disease itself (leukemic infiltration), peripheral blood cell depression (because of hemorrhagic or infectious processes) and toxicity induced by chemotherapy.

The toxicity of chemotherapy is a common cause of morbidity and mortality in cancer patients, as well as a frequent source of sequelae at mid-long term. These adverse effects are often the consequence of direct toxicity in healthy tissue, as a result of the low specificity displayed by these drugs. Furthermore, and regardless of their specificity, these compounds may also exacerbate complications derived from the tumor growth, as it is the case of pancytopenia or the *Tumor Lysis Syndrome*. Chemotherapy toxicity becomes more frequent as the treatment is intensified, thus challenging the clinician with both diagnostic and therapeutic problems. In this chapter we will discuss the major clinical signs of toxicity produced by chemotherapy drugs in patients with AL. Hematological and gastrointestinal (mucositis, nausea and vomiting) adverse effects will not be included, as their description suits better in an *Initial Management* chapter. In the last section of this chapter we will discuss recent data on whether pharmacogenetics may help individualize the therapy for AL, thus avoiding serious toxicity.

2. Cardiotoxicity

Cardiovascular abnormalities in patients with AL usually result from derangements in metabolic, electrolyte, and pulmonary function. Because leukemic infiltration of the heart is rare, the majority of cardiovascular problems in AL patients are chemotherapy-related toxicities produce by anthracyclines (Pihan, 2009).

Anthracycline chemotherapy is associated with *acute effects* (occurring during and shortly after administration), e.g. electrocardiographic alterations including prolongation of QT interval, development of ventricular late potentials and various arrhythmias (Bagnes et al., 2010); *subacute effects* (noted within days or weeks of administration) consisting of toxic myocarditis or pericartitis and *chronic effects*, which occur weeks or months after administration and manifest as cardiomyopathy. Cardiomyopathy is a multifactorial process related to oxidative stress and myocyte induction of apoptosis. Our inability to predict and prevent anthracycline cardiotoxicity is, in part, due to the fact that the molecular and cellular mechanisms remain controversial and incompletely understood (Sawyer et al., 2010).

At a cumulative dose of 550 mg/m^2 doxorubicin more than a quarter of patients develop congestive heart failure (CHF). This complication can take place at lower doses in susceptible individuals such as elderly, children, subjects with prior cardiac disease, and those who have had previous mediastinal irradiation (Ng et al., 2006). In the pediatric population , cardiomyopaty can occur at cumulative doses of 300 mg/m^2 (given as daunorubicin equivalent) (Creutzig et al., 2007). In addition, the long-term effects of cardiac damage are more apparent in children. In a study of long term survivors of childhood cancers, cardiac mortality was shown to be the second most likely cause of death following malignancy (Creutzig et al., 2007).

There are different techniques utilized to monitor for cardiotoxicity:

1. Endomyocardial Biopsy (EB), which was traditionally viewed as the gold standard test, is actually an impractical means of monitoring due to the invasive nature of test.
2. Evaluation of left ventricular ejection fraction (LVEF) with two-dimensional echocardiography (2D-ECHO) or radionuclide ventriculography remains the most pragmatic monitoring technique. Calculation of the LVEF by 2D-ECHO is slightly more difficult; however, the fact that radiation is not used makes it more suitable for the pediatric population.
3. Other techniques have also been tested: Antimyosin antibody scintigraphy is a marker of cardiac damage, but its high sensitivity may produce positive results at very low cumulative doses of anthraciclines, thus limiting its clinical utility (Valdes Olmos et al., 2002). Cardiac troponins and natriuretic peptides, the most commonly used biomarkers of myocardial destruction and ventricular dysfunction respectively, have also been studied for this purpose (Germanakis et al., 2008).

Pretherapy baseline evaluation of LVEF is recommended for all patients with AL before starting induction therapy. However, unless the patient is known or suspected to have a cardiac disease, the treatment does not need to be delayed pending the results of LVEF (Pihan, 2009). Dose exposure should be reduced in patients with a baseline LVEF of less than 50% or in those with a 10% LVEF decline from baseline to final values below 50% (Schwartz et al., 1987).

Different anthracyclines have different patterns of toxicity (Table 1). However, changing to a different anthracyclin does not substantially modify the risk for cardiotoxicity. In an attempt to reduce this adverse effect, liposomal doxorubicin has been developed. Most studies with liposomal doxorubicin have been performed in women with metastatic breast cancer. In this population, liposomal doxorubicin has shown equivalent efficacy to doxorubicin with a reduced rate of cardiotoxicity (Batist et al., 2001).

Several meta-analysis have studied the influence of different anthracyclines or different dosage schedules on the risk of cardiotoxicity in adult patients with cancer. These studies support the administration of a 6-hour (or longer) infusion (van Dalen et al., 2009), and the use of liposomal-doxorubicin over doxorubicin (van Dalen et al., 2010). It is of note that both studies agree in that there is insufficient evidence to implement such measures in children

or in patients with leukemia. In this regard, a meta-analysis with data retrieved from trials in children with ALL that randomized anthracyclines or measures to reduce cardiotoxicity, found no significant differences regarding type of anthracycline, method of administration or use of cardioprotectants (Childhood ALL Collaborative Group, 2009).
Because one of the proposed mechanisms of anthracyclins cardiotoxicity involves the generation of free iron radicals, dexazoxane, by its iron chelating effect, confers a significant reduction in the risk of cardiotoxicity. A meta-analysis by Van Dalen et al concluded that if the risk of cardiac damage is expected to be high, it might be justified the use of dexrazoxane in patients with cancer treated with anthracyclines (van Dalen et al., 2008). In children with AL, the use of dexrazoxane seems safe and provides long-term cardioprotection without compromising oncological efficacy. Currently, in the absence of more data, the use of dexrazoxane might be justified in children if the risk of cardiac damage is expected to be high (Lipshultz et al., 2010).

2.1 Treatment of cardiomyopathy

The natural history of Anthracyclines cardiomyopathy, as well as its response to modern CHF therapy, remains poorly defined. Hence, evidence-based recommendations for the management of this form of cardiomyopathy are still lacking. Progress in treatment of cardiac failure, in particular the availability of drugs as angiotensin converting enzyme (ACE) inhibitors, spironolactone and beta-blokers and the current practice of monitoring cardiotoxicity, may explain the improved prognosis of this complication that , in early retrospective studies , had a mortality rate of more than 40%. The prophylactic use of enalapril resulted in the reduction of cardiac function deterioration. A recent study has shown that when this therapy is initiated soon after detection of LVEF impairment, there are more patients who present LVEF recovery and cardiac event reduction (Cardinale et al., 2010). These results show the importance of monitoring cardiotoxicity in all patients treated with anthracyclines in order to (i) identify early heart damage and (ii) begin treatment before the onset of CHF.
Among the newest compounds, symptomatic or asymptomatic QT aberrations have been reported with tyrosine-kinase inhibitors (Bagnes et al., 2010) and arsenic trioxide (Ohnishi et al., 2000).

Adverse effect	CTX	MTX	ADR	DNR	EPI	IDA	NOV	AMS
Cardiomyopathy			+++	+++	++	++	++	+
Myo/pericarditis	++		+	++	+			
ECG changes	++	+	++	++				+

CTX, cyclophosphamide; MTX, methotrexate; ADR, doxorubicin; DNR, daunorubicin; EPI, epirubicin; IDA, idarubicin; NOV, mitoxantrone; AMS, amsacrine.
+, rare or little clinical significance; ++, occasional or clinically relevant; +++, common or severe.

Table 1. Main cardiac toxicity for chemotherapy drugs used in acute leukemia

3. Hepatotoxicity

Hepatotoxicity is defined as an injury to the liver that is associated with impaired liver function caused by exposure to a drug. The clinical patterns of liver injury are defined as *hepatocellular*, with a predominant initial elevation of the alanine aminotransferase level

(ALT), *cholestatic*, in which the serum alkaline phosphatase concentrations are increased, or *mixed*, if both enzymes are elevated. An ALT level of more than three times the upper limit of normal values and a total bilirubin concentration of more than twice the upper limit are used to define clinically significant abnormalities on liver test. Elevation in serum enzyme levels is taken as indicator of liver injury, whereas increases in bilirrubin levels, albumin concentration and the prothrombin time are measures of overall liver function (Navarro & Senior, 2006).

Chemotherapy-induced hepatotoxicity is a common cause of abnormal liver function test in patients with AL. It mainly occurs in an idiosyncratic manner and is generally reversible and nonfatal. This toxicity is manifested in a variety of patterns. In addition to those mentioned above, we find steatosis, ductal injury fibrosis, cirrhosis, veno-occlusion, peliosis hepatis, and nodular regenerative hyperplasia. The two latter lesions appear as pseudometastatic hepatic nodules that may indicate disease progression, especially if they are multiple (Brisse et al., 2000).

Hepatotoxicity usually begins with vague clinical symptoms such as fatigue, anorexia, nausea, dark urine, right upper quadrant discomfort and jaundice. Suspected drug exposure must precede the symptoms and liver injury may improve when administration is stopped. However, the latent period is highly variable and enzyme levels may take weeks to increase. Before attributing these symptoms to a chemotherapy drug, other causes of liver injury must be ruled out (Navarro & Senior, 2006). Abnormal liver function may be due to multiple causes in patients with AL. Leukemic infiltration usually causes mild to moderate hepatomegaly with limited impact on serum transaminase levels. Transfusions increase the likelihood of viral hepatitis. Other circumstances such as sepsis, hypotension or malnutrition may contribute to liver damage (Pihan, 2009).

AL patients are treated with combination chemotherapy, making it difficult to identify the precise agent involved in the hepatic injury. Moreover, diagnosis becomes more challenging by the large number of non-chemotherapeutic drugs commonly used in those patients, some of them holding the potential of being hepatoxic, e.g. allopurinol, ondansetron and different antifungal agents (Perry, 1992).

Pre-existing liver disease can alter the metabolism and excretion of chemotherapy causing increased and persistent drug levels and hence systemic toxicity. On the other hand, chemotherapy may worsen liver disease, such as occurs with hepatitis. Severe liver dysfunction and fatal fulminant hepatitis through virus reactivation have been described in patients with viral hepatitis. Prophylactic therapy with nucleoside analogues, typically lamivudine, has been recommended for HBs Ag positive patients. This strategy has been reported to allow optimal administration of chemotherapy (Parrish et al., 2010).

3.1 Dose modification of chemotherapy with altered hepatic function

All patients with AL must undergo evaluation of baseline values before starting chemotherapy. This includes liver function test, viral hepatitis serology and, if clinically indicated, hepatic imaging. Liver function test should be reassessed before each course of therapy and known hepatotoxins should be avoided (Perry, 1992). Patients more susceptible to hepatotoxicity such as those with malnutrition or alcoholism, elderly, obese, or diabetic, should be followed up more closely. Liver response may also be abnormal in cases of previous liver disease or coexisting illnesses (Floyd et al., 2006). In cases of elevated liver test (ELT), drugs undergoing hepatic metabolism should be avoided if possible and/or dose modifications should be considered if guidelines are available. In rare instances in which ELT is caused by leukemic infiltration it is not necessary to adjust dosing (Figure 1).

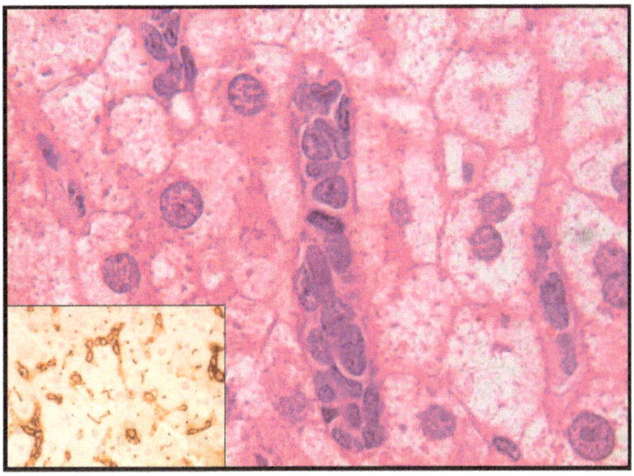

Fig. 1. Liver biopsy of a child with relapsed ALL. Lymphoblasts (C43+) infiltrate the hepatic sinusoids. Despite of abnormal liver test, chemotherapy was administered without complications.

3.2 Hepatotoxicity of major chemotherapy agents used in acute leukemia

3.2.1 6-Mercaptopurine and 6-Thioguanine

6-Mercaptopurine (6-MP) in orally daily regimen associated with weekly MTX is the backbone of maintenance chemotherapy acute lymphoblastic leukemia (ALL). Hepatotoxicity produced by this drug include both cholestatic and hepatocellular disease. Characteristic diagnostic profiles include prominently elevated serum bilirubin, typically between 3 and 7 mg/dL, accompanied by mild to moderate elevations in aminotransferases and alkaline phosphatase (Floyd et al., 2006). Liver function tests are transiently abnormal in the majority of children during maintenance of ALL, in the absence of other evidence of severe liver toxicity or viral hepatitis, it is generally not necessary to withhold or reduce the dose of continuation chemotherapy (Pui & Evans, 2006). When liver biopsies are performed in this population, inflammatory and fatty changes are common and not related with ALT levels. Early portal fibrosis is found only in patients with prolonged therapy. The risk of portal fibrosis is low after 2-3 years of continuing chemotherapy and most patients go back to normal ALT values with drug cessation. The mechanism underlying 6-MP-induced hepatotoxicity is related to its methylated metabolites and correlates with ALT levels. Indeed, ALT levels have been proposed as a surrogate marker for treatment compliance (Nygaard et al., 2004). A study by Schmiegelow et al. has shown that ALL pediatric patients with mean ALT levels above the upper normal limit (40 IU/l) who were kept on therapy had a significantly lower risk of hematological relapse compared to other children (Schmiegelow, 1991). These data support the concept of *treating to toxicity* for maintenance therapy.

6-Thioguanine as maintenance treatment in childhood ALL has also been shown to cause hepatic veno-occlusive disease (VOD) usually mild and reversible on withdrawing 6-TG or replacing it with 6-MP (Stoneham et al., 2003).

3.2.2 Methotrexate

MTX inhibits dihydrofolate reductase resulting in depletion of critical reduced folates. The net result is effective inhibition of DNA and RNA synthesis and potent cytotoxicity to rapidly dividing cells. MTX causes hepatotoxicity, fibrosis and cirrhosis, but usually after prolonged use and/or when it is used in the treatment of autoimmune diseases.

In a high percentage of patients with ALL, MTX causes isolated elevations of ALT during maintenance chemotherapy, usually transient and asymptomatic. This ALT elevations are not predictive of subsequent hepatic disease and do not require treatment modification (Farrow et al., 1997).

As in the maintenance treatment, when MTX is used in high IV doses (HD-IV MTX), the characteristic hepatotoxic pattern is transient, ALT levels are related to the dose of MTX and increase with the number of cycles received. A difference with the maintenance treatment is that in cases of altered hepatic function it is necessary to modify or suspend the administration of HD-IV MTX (Table 2). In any case, despite the usual benign character of MTX-induced hepatotoxicity, there are reports of hepatoma in association with hepatic fibrosis occurring in children following ALL treatment (Fried et al., 1987).

3.2.3 Cytarabine

Cytarabine (ara-C) have revealed a cumulative dose-dependent hepatotoxicity. Several case reports have demonstrated direct histologic evidence of a hepatotoxic role for ara-C, expressed as increased ALT levels or as intrahepatic cholestasis. Although the actual incidence of this toxicity remains to be elucidated, mild elevations of liver function in a cholestatic pattern represent the reversible, rarely fatal clinical picture (George et al., 1984). Ara-C is reported to be partially detoxified in the liver. Therefore, it is recommended that its dose be reduced in patients with liver impairment (Table 2).

3.2.4 L-Asparaginase

In addition to hypersensitivity reactions, the most common toxic effects of L-asparaginase are related to the depletion of proteins synthesized in the liver, such as clotting factor, insulin , albumin, haptoglobin and transferrin. Liver function abnormalities (including hyperbilirubinemia and elevated transaminase levels) and hyperlipidemia (hypertriglyceridemia and hypercholesterolemia) have been frequently reported in patients receiving the drug (Earl, 2009). As a result of these metabolic abnormalities, up to 7% of children with AL develop pancreatitis (Treepongkaruna et al., 2009). Another common metabolic complication of this drug is hyperglycemia, which occurs in up to 10% of children with AL during their induction therapy (Pui et al., 1981) and is associated with the synergistic effect of L-asparaginase and glucocorticoids (Spinola-Castro et al., 2009). It should be noted that the use of pegylated asparaginase does not prevent these complications (Silverman et al.).

3.2.5 Other drugs

In spite of requiring metabolic activation in the liver, cyclophosphamide, antitumor antibiotics and vinca alkaloids are uncommon hepatic toxins. Indeed, reports of severe hepatotoxicity attributed to these drugs are scarce (Floyd et al., 2006). However, dose modifications are necessary to prevent systemic toxicity in case of liver impairment (Table 2).

Agent	Bilirubin (mg/dl)	Aminotransferases	% Dose administered
Alkylating agents			
Cyclophosphamide	3.1-5	>3 x ULN	75
	>5		0
Antimetabolites			
Cytarabine		Any	50%; increase by monitoring toxicity
6-mercaptopurine			No dose reduction is necessary
Methotrexate	3.1-5.0	>3 x ULN	75
	>5.0		0
6-Thioguanine	>5.0		0
Antibiotics			
Doxorubicin		2-3 x ULN	75
	1.2-3.0	>3 x ULN	50
	3.1-5.0		25
	>5.0		0
Daunorubicin	1.2-3.0		75
	3.1-5.0		50
	>5.0		0
Epirubicin	1.2-3	2-4 x ULN	75
	>3	>4 xULN	50
Idarubicin	1.5-3.0	AST 2-3 x ULN	75
	3.1-5.0	AST>3 x ULN	50
	>5		0
Mitoxantrone	>3.0		75
Plant alkaloids			
Vincristine and	1.5-3.0	2-3 x ULN	50
Vinblastine*	>3.1	>3 x ULN	0
Etoposide	1.5-3.0	AST>3 x ULN	50
	>3	AST>3 x ULN	0
Teniposide			Evaluate if necessary
Miscellaneous			
L-asparaginase			No dose reduction is necessary

*Vincristine and vinblastine: 50% reduction if alkaline phosphatase is elevated. ULN, Upper limit of normal.

Table 2. Dosage of main chemotherapeutic agents used in AL according to liver function

4. Peripheral neuropathy

The most prevalent neurologic complication of cancer treatment is chemotherapy-induced peripheral neuropathy (CIPN). Vincristine is the main etiological agent involved in peripheral neuropathy in leukemia patients (Kannarkat et al., 2007). Virtually all ALL patients receiving vincristine have some degree of neuropathy. Neurotoxicity commonly pesents as peripheral neuropathy, which is predominantly sensory in nature. The clinical manifestations are subjective and predominantly manifest as distal and symmetrically distributed pure sensory symptoms such as paresthesias, hyperesthesias, hypoesthesias, and dysesthesias. The most common and earliest symptoms are numbness and tingling in the fingertips and feet as well as constipation due to autonomic neuropathy. Symptoms of motor weakness are observed in patients with more persistent and severe sensory findings. Isolated motor weakness with the complete absence of sensory involvement has not been reported. If such findings were observed, consideration should be given to other conditions such as steroid myopathy or diabetic neuropathy (Hausheer et al., 2006).

Sensory findings, as diminished or absent proprioception and vibration are typically diminished in the stocking-glove distribution in symptomatic patients. Loss of ankle stretch reflexes is an early and almost universal sign, and with continued therapy all reflexes may diminish or disappear. The toxicity of vincristine is believed to occur through disruption of microtubule polymerization. Neurophysiologic studies are compatible with a primarily axonal neuropathy. Symptoms develop gradually and may manifest after the first dose. As the disease progresses, muscle weakness becomes apparent, patients lose the ability to walk on their heels and lose strength in wrist extensors. Motor weakness from vincristine can become severe enough to render the patient immobile. In addition, some patients may develop impotence, postural hypotension, or an atonic bladder (Quasthoff & Hartung, 2002). When symptoms are severe, a hereditary motor and sensory neuropathy should be suspected (Mercuri et al., 1999).

Because there is no effective treatment, prevention is the only useful measure for neurotoxicity. All patients should take prophylactic stool softeners and/or laxatives. Dose level and cumulative dose are the most significant risk factors. The maximum dose of 2 mg, and cumulative doses over 15-20 mg should not be exceeded due to the considerable increase in the incidence and severity of symptoms. When symptoms of neuropathy disturb the patient a common practice is to administer vinblastine instead and even to discontinue therapy if marked weakness appears. Recovery generally occurs 1 to 3 months after treatment cessation, withholding the drug or reducing its dose, but CIPN symptoms may also persist or worsen following vincristine discontinuation (Verstappen et al., 2005).

5. Central neurotoxicity

Chemotherapy-induced central neurotoxicity can result in multiple clinical manifestations: impaired consciousness, focal deficits, seizures, headaches, etc. However, before attributing these symptoms to chemotherapy in AL patients, other causes must be ruled out first (Table 3). Furthermore, it is necessary to consider other factors such as drug-drug interactions. For instance, MTX intracellular levels may be elevated in the presence of vincristine. In addition, circumstances such as cranial irradiation or CNS affectation by leukemia may cause direct damage to the blood-brain barrier, thereby increasing MTX permeability and subsequent toxicity (Naing et al., 2005).

Metabolic disturbances (e.g. hyponatremia)
Intracerebral hemorrhage
Cerebral infarction or venous sinus thrombosis
CNS infection
Meningeal Leukemia
Epilepsy
Migraine
Drugs

Table 3. Main causes of CNS disease in patients with AL

5.1 Cerebrovascular accidents

In patients with AL, ischemic or hemorrhagic cerebrovascular accidents may be either a consequence of the disease or a complication of chemotherapy. Intracranial hemorrhage (ICH), which is the second leading cause of mortality in patients with acute myeloid leukemia (AML) (accounting for up to 70% in some series), occurs mostly during induction therapy. Brainstem, epidural and subarachnoid hemorrhage are particularly dangerous (Chen et al., 2009). In a risk score model for fatal intracranial hemorrhage, female gender, thrombocytopenia, prolonged prothrombin time, hyperleukocytosis (particularly in presence of symptoms of pulmonary leukostasis), and acute promyelocytic leukemia (APL), were significantly associated with the occurrence of this complication (Kim et al., 2006).

Thrombotic events, particularly sino-venous thrombosis, are more frequent in ALL. Therapy with L-asparaginase is considered the major risk factor for this complication in these patients. Thrombosis develops after the administration of the first doses of the drug in induction therapy. The most common symptoms are headaches and seizures which resolve without sequelae in most cases (Kieslich et al., 2003). In a previous study with 238 patients treated with L-asparaginase, 4.2% of patients showed cerebral thrombosis and 2.1% cerebral haemorrhages (Nicholson et al., 1996). In this regard, it has been shown that increased triglycerides and decreases of antithrombin III, fibrinogen, protein S, protein C, plasminogen and alpha-2-antiplasmin are associated with the dose of L-asparaginase (Hongo et al., 2002; Nowak-Göttl et al., 1994). Other factors such as central venous catheters, obesity, use of steroids and thrombophilia may contribute to thrombotic imbalance in these patients.

5.2 Aseptic meningitis

Aseptic meningitis or chemical arachnoiditis is the most common neurotoxicity induced by MTX. It affects approximately 10% of patients receiving intrathecal (IT) therapy. The onset is generally abrupt and occurs within hours of IT administration. The patient has headache, meningismus, nausea, vomiting, fever, and altered consciousness. Cerebrospinal fluid (CSF) studies demonstrate pleocytosis and elevated protein. The symptoms are self-limited and usually resolve within 72 hours. Further treatment with IT MTX is not contraindicated and patients may receive subsequent doses of chemotherapy without incident. Co-administration of MTX and IT hydrocortisone or premedication with oral corticosteroids may be useful to prevent the syndrome (Sul & Deangelis, 2006). The use of IT ara-C can also result in aseptic meningitis similar to that seen with IT MTX. The incidence has been observed to be higher with the liposomal formulation (DepoCyt®), which maintains cytotoxic concentrations of the drug in the CSF for up to 14 days. Side effects become so frequent that all patients require prophylactic corticosteroids pre and post DepoCyt® administration (Glantz et al., 1999).

5.3 Transverse myelopathy

Transverse myelopathy is an uncommon complication of IT MTX manifested by the development of back or leg pain followed by paraplegia, sensory loss, and sphincter dysfunction in the absence of a compressive lesion. The onset is usually between 30 minutes and 48 hours after treatment, although the reaction may also appear up to two weeks later. MRI may illustrate cord edema and irregular post-gadolinium enhancement. In contrast to myelopathies caused by other reasons, corticosteroids are not helpful. This is thought to be an idiosyncratic drug reaction, and therefore the identification of potentially susceptible patients is not possible. Unlike aseptic meningitis, transverse myelopathy is an absolute contraindication to further treatment with IT MTX. In addition to IT MTX, a similar transverse myelopathy was reported in two pediatric AML patients receiving IT and IV ara-C (Sul & Deangelis, 2006).

5.4 Acute encephalopathy

High doses of Cytarabine (HD-ara-C) (≥3 g/m^2 every 12 hours) may result in CNS dysfunction, especially impaired cerebellar function. The characteristic syndrome begins with somnolence and occasionally encephalopathy that develops two to five days after treatment. Immediately thereafter, cerebellar signs are noted on physical examination. Symptoms range in severity from mild ataxia to inability to sit or walk unassisted. Rarely, seizures may also develop. There may be MRI changes in the white matter and cerebellum, but the CSF is usually normal. Discontinuation of therapy generally results in partial recovery within several weeks, but complete resolution is achieved by only 30% of patients. Neurologic deficits can be permanent if treatment is continued after the onset of symptoms (Friedman & Shetty, 2001).

Since the occurrence of severe cerebellar dysfunction is greatly affected by age, patients older than 50 years should be given a reduced schedule of HD-ara-C. Furthermore, it has been shown that avoidance of very high doses of the drug in patients with renal impairment and the administration of HD-ara-C on a once-daily rather than twice-daily schedule reduce the incidence of this syndrome (Smith et al., 1997).

5.5 Subacute encephalopathy

Subacute encephalopathy is an uncommon complication of MTX therapy that generally develops within 5–14 days after the administration of IT or HD-MTX, not being observed in maintenance therapy when low doses of oral or parenteral MTX are used. The syndrome is manifest by abrupt onset of focal neurological deficits, such as aphasia or hemiparesis and presents after a median of three courses of IV or IT MTX. Typical symptoms are headache and nausea followed by stroke-like hemiparesis or bilateral weakness. Hemiparesis may be alternating and evolving over a period of minutes to hours. In addition, aphasia or expressive dysphasia, emotional lability and disorientation are also common signs. Other manifestations such as seizure, transient ataxia, choreoathetoid movements, temporary blindness or visual hallucinations are less frequent. Most neurological symptoms resolve after 1-7 days and the majority of patients can resume HD-MTX therapy without permanent neurological sequelae. Recurrence may be experienced by 10-56% patients (Inaba et al., 2008).

In the absence of histopathological data, diagnosis is based upon spinal fluid analysis and neuroimaging techniques. CFS analysis is usually normal and electroencephalogram (EEG) shows nonspecific diffuse or focal slowing. At the onset of MTX-induced encephalopathy, conventional CT scans, T1 or T2 weighted MR imaging and angiography typically show no abnormalities, whereas diffusion-weighted imaging (DWI) is able to show restricted diffusion of water in the brain that clears after resolution of the clinical symptoms. This abnormalities are consistent with cytotoxic or intramyelinic sheath edema within white matter tracts (Haykin et al., 2006). Follow-up MR imaging shows variable abnormal T2 and FLAIR signal intensity in the deep white matter, with no detectable neurological sequelae in most patients (Haykin et al., 2006) (Figure 2). The pathogenesis of MTX neurotoxicity is poorly understood and no specific risk factors for the development of this complication have been identified to date. Indeed, pharmacokinetic data are normal in most patients with MTX-induced neurotoxicity (Rubnitz et al., 1998). In this regard, there are recent data indicating that pharmacogenetics could play a significant role in the development of this complication (Mahadeo et al., 2010; Vagace et al., 2011).

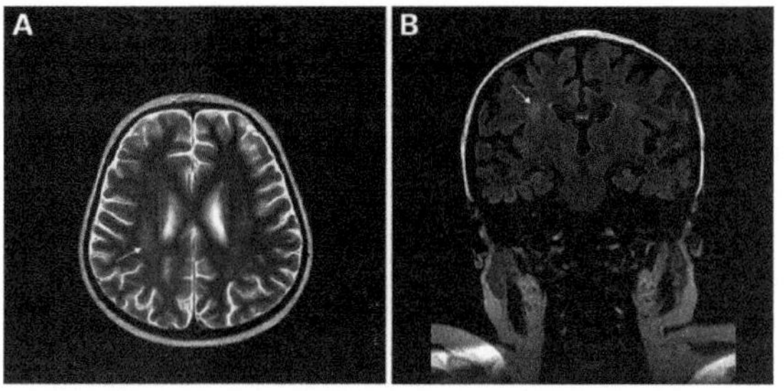

Fig. 2. MR imaging findings six weeks after an episode of subacute encephalopathy by MTX. White arrows in Axial T2 (A) and coronal FLAIR (B) sequences show deep and periventricular white matter hyperintensity, especially in the right hemisphere (Vagace et al., 2011).

5.6 Posterior reversible encephalopathy

In 1996, Hinchey et al. described a reversible syndrome of headache, altered mental functioning, seizures, and loss of vision associated with abnormalities on neuroimaging in the posterior regions of the cerebral hemispheres. The syndrome occured in patients who had renal insufficiency or hypertension or in those who were immunosuppressed. Although not previously recognized as a complication of chemotherapy, *Posterior Reversible Encephalopathy* (PRE) is now considered as one the most common abnormalities leading to seizures in children with leukemia (Norman et al., 2007). The patient usually presents with headache, altered alertness, confusion, seizures (that may begin focally but usually become generalized), vomiting and alterations of visual perception. These visual disturbances are nearly always detectable with symptoms such as blurred vision, hemianopia, visual hallucinations or cortical blindness. Hypertension and hypomagnesemia are additional diagnostic criteria but are not always present (Dicuonzo et al., 2009).

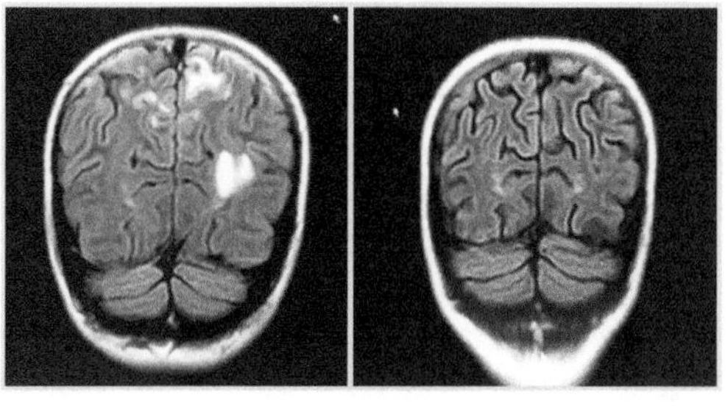

Fig. 3. *Posterior Reversible Encephalopaty*: MR imaging, Coronal T2 FLAIR, of a child with AL treated with vincristine that developed headache, hypertension and seizures. Left panel shows white matter hyperintensity in both hemispheres. After 18 days (right panel) these signs were inappreciable.

The cardinal features of PRE are both clinical and radiologic. Abnormalities are usually observed in bilateral, parietal and occipital lobes. CT scans typically show posterior cerebral white-matter hypodensities. If PRE is suspected, MRI series should be performed, including T2, DWI, and FLAIR images for the most accurate diagnosis. MR abnormalities are characterized by increased signal on T2-weighted and FLAIR sequences. DWI may appear normal or show increased diffusion consistent with vasogenic edema (Shin et al., 2001) (Fig 3).
Sudden elevations in systemic blood pressure exceeding the autoregulatory capability of the brain vasculature, leading to capillary leakage and subsequent vasogenic edema has been proposed as the underlying mechanism of PRE. The preferential involvement of the parietal and occipital lobes may be due to the observed relative reduction in the sympathetic innervation of the posterior circulation. Based on brain SPECT studies, a migraine-like mechanism has been proposed by other authors. Additionally, hypomagnesemia or vascular instability resulting from the toxicity of the chemotherapy agents on the endothelium of the blood-brain barrier may also be contributing factors (Sanchez-Carpintero et al., 2001). Most cases of PRE occur during induction chemotherapy for ALL, consequently, a variety of drugs routinely used during this phase have been linked to PRE, namely vincristine, IT MTX, HD-MTX, L-asparaginase, cyclophosphamide and ara-C (Gupta et al., 2008).
Early and aggressive therapy for hypertension and quickly control the seizures, are the only defined treatment recommendations for this syndrome. In most patients chemotherapy can be restarted without recurrence or permanent neurological sequelae. In conclusion, chemotherapy for AL should be added to the growing list of causes of PRE. However, more information is needed before a clear association can be established between PRE and specific chemotherapy agents (Titos-Arcos et al., 2011).

5.7 Chronic Leukoencephalopaty

Chronic leukoencephalopathy is a commonly described but poorly understood phenomenon, which is associated with the use of HD-MTX with inadequate leucovorin rescue and that may be exacerbated by prior cranial irradiation. This complication presents several months to years after therapy and may lead to severe neuropsychological impairment (Ziereisen et al., 2006).

6. Renal toxicity and electrolytes imbalance

The kidneys, being the elimination pathway of many antitumor drugs and their metabolites, are quite vulnerable to injury in chemotherapy. Several factors are known to contribute to the nephrotoxic potential of antineoplastic drugs in patients with AL, namely the concomitant use of other nephrotoxic drugs (e.g., amphothericin), urinary infections, intravascular volume depletion, sepsis and other comorbidities such as hypertension, diabetes mellitus or heart failure. Suggested dosing of the main chemotherapeutic drugs used in AL according to renal function is shown in Table 4.
Chemotherapy-induced nephrotoxicity may affect glomeruli, tubules, renal vasculature or excretory system depending on the drugs involved. Creatinine clearance is the usual measure to assess the glomerular filtration rate. Serum creatininine is less sensitive for this purpose and does not significantly change until the clearance is below 70 ml/min. Measurement of the tubular function is often accomplished by evaluating the fractional excretion of glucose, uric acid, calcium, phosphorous and magnesium (de Jonge & Verweij, 2006).

6.1 Hemorrhagic cystitis

Cyclophosphamide and ifosfamide are drugs with similar chemical structures that are biotransformed to acrolein. Hemorrhagic cystitis occurs subsequent to urinary excretion of this metabolite, which is capable of binding the sulfhydryl constituent within proteins of bladder epithelium causing an inflammatory process. Saline-based hyperhydration and mesna (2-mercaptoethane sulfonate), which binds acrolein preventing direct contact with the uroepithelium, are concurrently administered to reduce the incidence and severity of hemorrhagic cystitis. Hemorrhagic cystitis is usually seen in transplant recipients who are treated with doses of cyclophosphamide higher than those used in AL. When the process lasts longer than 7 days, adenovirus and polyomavirus infection (specifically BK viruria) are often responsible (Korkmaz et al., 2007).

Treatment of hemorrhagic cystitis is challenging. If blood clots form, bladder irrigation with isotonic saline may be required to break up an obstructive uropathy. Other measures that have been used include intravesical therapy with instillation of chemicals to cause mucosal fibrosis, hyperbaric oxygen therapy, and embolization or ligation of internal iliac arteries. Cystectomy is reserved for massive bladder hemorrhage, a clinical problem with a high mortality rate (Hu et al., 2008).

Agent	**CrCl (ml/min)**	**[Cr]s (mg/dl)**	**% Dose administered**
Alkylating agents			
Cyclophosphamide	10-50		75
	<10		50
Antimetabolites			
Cytarabine			Evaluate if necessary
6-mercaptopurine			No formal recommendation.
Methotrexate	30-60		50
	<30		0
Antibiotics*			
Daunorubicin		>3.0	50
Plant alkaloids			
Etoposide	10-50		75
	<10		50
Miscellaneous			
L-asparaginase	<60		0

CrCl, creatinine clearance; [Cr]s, serum creatinine
**No reduction is necessary for mitoxantrone, doxorubicin, epirubicin, idarubicin, vincristine or vinblastine*

Table 4. Dosage of main chemotherapeutic agents used in AL according to renal function

6.2 Methotrexate-induced nephrotoxicity

Nephrotoxicity is a potentially life-threatening complication of HD-MTX therapy (>1g/m^2). Both the parent drug and the 7-hydroxy-MTX metabolite may precipitate in the acidic environment of renal tubules and collecting ducts producing acute tubular necrosis. Renal dysfunction results in delayed MTX excretion and sustained elevated plasma MTX

concentrations, which in turn may lead to a marked enhancement of other toxicities of MTX, especially myelosuppression, mucositis, hepatitis, and dermatitis. Uniform institution of aggressive hydration, alkalinization (urinary pH monitoring required), and pharmacokinetically guided leucovorin rescue , significantly reduce the morbidity rate in patients receiving this therapy. Implementation of this regimen reduces the incidence of nephrotoxicity to approximately 2% of patients (Widemann & Adamson, 2006).
Delayed MTX excretion and high plasma MTX concentrations identify patients at high risk of toxicity. These subjects may benefit from supplemental leucovorin rescue or from the administration of glucarpidase (carboxypeptidase G2, CPDG2), a recombinant enzyme with cleaves MTX in inactive metabolites and is able to lower plasma MTX concentrations rapidly and efficiently. The use of CPDG2 is well-tolerated and renders a more profound, rapid, and consistent decrease in plasma MTX concentrations compared to dialysis-based methods, and should therefore be considered over dialysis in patients with HD-MTX-induced renal dysfunction (Patterson & Lee, 2010).

6.3 Syndrome of inappropriate antidiuretic hormone secretion

Hyponatremia is the most common electrolyte disorder in clinical medicine and occurs in approximately one of every three hospitalized patients. The *syndrome of inappropriate Secrection of Antidiuretic Hormone* (SIADH) is the most frequent cause of hyponatremia. Malignant diseases, pulmonary and CNS disorders and drugs are causes of SIADH. With regard to chemotherapy drugs used in AL, vincristine and cyclophosphamide have been implicated in this complication (Ellison & Berl, 2007).
The diagnosis of SIADH requires the presence of hyponatremia (Na^{+}<135 mmol/L) with a low serum osmolarity (<275 mmol/L) in the absence of other causes of hyponatremia such as oral or IV water excess, low effective circulating volume (heart or liver failure), use of thiazide diuretics, endocrine processes (hipopituitarism, adrenal insufficiency or hypothyroidism), renal failure or salt wasting. On the other hand *Cerebral Salt Wasting* is a syndrome due to the production of natriuretic factor and/or a disruption of neural input into the kidney that decreases proximal sodium reabsorption, resulting in a loss of sodium by the urine. The identification of this disorder is of considerable clinical importance because its treatment comprises vigorous sodium and volume replacement, whereas fluid restriction is the treatment of choice in SIADH (Hoorn & Zietse, 2008). Table 5 shows useful data to differentiate between these two syndromes.

	CSW	**SIADH**
Extracellular fluid volumen*	Decreased	Increased
Diuresis	Normal or increased	Normal or decreased
Hematocrit	Increased	Normal
Plasma BUN/Creatinine	Increased	Decreased
Treatment	Normal saline	Fluid restriction

*The main difference but clinical assessment of volume status is imprecise. CSW, cerebral salt wasting; SIADH, syndrome of inappropriate antidiuretic hormone secretion.

Table 5. Clinical features of CSW and SIADH [Modified from (Palmer, 2003)].

7. Pulmonary toxicity

Most pulmonary complications in AL patients are due to concurrent medical problems, such as bacteremia, sepsis, fungal infection or CHF. These patients also show an increased risk of thromboembolic disorders. Therefore, the occurrence of acute respiratory insufficiency in AL may be suspicious of pulmonary thromboembolism, especially if treatment with L-asparaginase was previously implemented. L-asparaginase reduces antithrombin III levels thereby increasing the risk for thrombosis, which may be safely prevented with the use of heparin (Meister et al., 2008).
Other chemotherapy drugs such as all-trans-retinoic acid (ATRA), imatinib and ara-C can cause a capillary leak syndrome which manifests as pulmonary edema, pleural effusions, pericardial effusions or ascites. Drug withdrawal and steroid therapy is generally recommended in this case (Meadors et al., 2006).

7.1 The Acute Promyelocytic Leukemia Differentiation Syndrome

All-trans retinoic acid (ATRA) and arsenic trioxide are agents used for the treatment of the acute promyelocytic leukemia (APL) with a unique toxicity profile. The *APL Differentiation Syndrome* or *Retinoic Acid Syndrome* is mediated by endothelial inflammation and vascular leak that occurs when leukemic blasts suddenly differentiate into mature granulocytes and adhere to pulmonary endothelium. The differentiation syndrome occurs in approximately 25% of patients with APL treated with these agents (Luesink et al., 2009; Montesinos et al., 2009).
Diagnosis should be suspected clinically in the presence of dyspnea, unexplained fever, weight gain, peripheral edema, unexplained hypotension, acute renal failure or CHF, but particularly by a chest radiograph demonstrating interstitial pulmonary infiltrates or pleuro-pericardial effusion. In this situation, dexamethasone should be started promptly and ATRA temporarily discontinued if the patient develops respiratory distress or renal failure. Prophylactic treatment with corticosteroids is recommended in patients with a WBC count greater than $5 \times 10^9/l$ to reduce mortality and morbility (Sanz et al., 2009).

8. Cutaneous toxicity

Cutaneous side effects related to chemotherapy (Table 6) may range from relatively common adverse events, such as alopecia or hyperpigmentation (which are the result of direct toxicity on skin in contact with the drugs through blood or sweat) to more unusual phenomena such as photosensitivity or hypersensitivity reactions (DeSpain, 1992).
Most chemotherapeutic agents may cause alopecia. Hair loss usually begins 7 to 10 days after the initiation of treatment and is prominent within 1 to 2 months of treatment. Once chemotherapy is finished hair grows back in the majority of the patients, although it may present a different texture or color.
Pigmentary changes involving the skin, nails, and mucous membranes are usually related to alkylating agents and antitumor antibiotics, but they may as well occur with other drugs used in AL, namely etoposide, MTX or vincristine. The latter may cause a distinctive pattern of hyperpigmentation called *Serpentine Hyperpigmentation*, which follows an underlying vein proximal to an infusion site (Payne, A.S. et al., 2006).
Eccrine Squamous Syringometaplasia is characterized by self-limited, asymptomatic erythematous papules on trunk and extremities that may be confused with erythema nodosum.
MTX can produce a phototoxic recall reaction (*Photoreactivation*) in the absence of light. It is characterized by an erythematous eruption in the distribution of UV-induced sunburns that

may have occurred months or years prior to the administration of the drug. HD-MTX is also associated with severe erythema in sun-exposed areas when the drug is given within two to five days of exposure to UV light. In contrast to *Photoreactivation*, retreatment with MTX does not usually reproduce the reaction (Payne, A.S., DMF, 2011). Patients receiving photosensitizing drugs should be counseled regarding the risk of adverse reactions to sunlight and encouraged to use UV protection with sunscreens and protective clothing.

Agent	AL	CP	ESS	PS	AE	NEH	SS	HR
Alkylating agents	+							
Cyclophosphamide	+	+	+			+		+
Ifosfamide	+							
Antimetabolites								
Cytarabine	+		+		++	++		+
6-mercaptopurine					+			
Methotrexate	+	+	+	+	+			+
Antibiotics								
Doxorubicin	+		+		+	+		+
Plant alkaloids								
Vincristine and Vinblastine*	+	+		+				
Etoposide	+		+		+			++
Tyrosine kinase inhibitors								
Imatinib		+		+			+	
Miscellaneous								
L-asparaginase								++
Tretinoin (ATRA)							+	

AL, Alopecia; CP, Cutaneous Hyper-Pigmentation; ESS, Eccrine squamous syringometaplasia; PS, Photosensibility; AE, Acral erythema; NEH, Neutrophilic eccrine hidradenitis ; SS, Sweet´s Syndrome; HR, Hypersensitivity reactions.

Table 6. Cutaneous toxicity of the main chemotherapy agents used in AL.

Acral Erythema or *Hand-Foot Syndrome*, is characterized by painful erythematous plaques on the palms and soles and heals with prominent desquamation that usually resolves within two to four weeks after discontinuation of the causative agent (Figure 4).

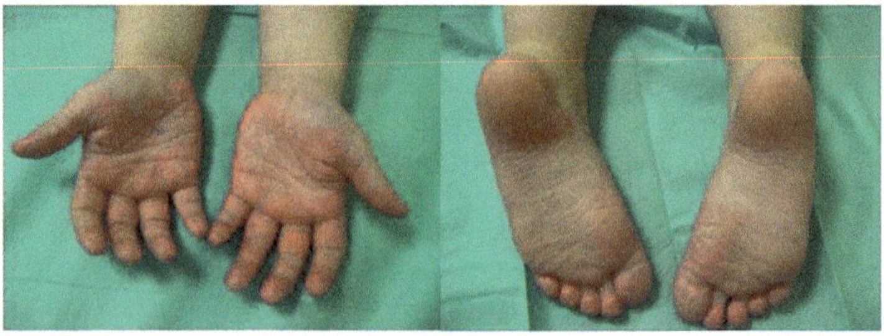

Fig. 4. Hand-Foot Syndrome in a child treated with ara-C for AL

Neutrophilic Eccrine Hidradenitis (NEH) is a reactive disorder that may occur in association with malignancy (with or without chemotherapy), infections, and certain medications. NEH is characterized by asymptomatic and self-limited violaceus plaques on the trunk and extremities. In all cases of suspected NEH, a biopsy should be performed to differentiate of septic emboli, metastatic infiltrates or *Sweet´s Syndrome* (Brehler et al., 1997).

Sweet´s Syndrome (SS), also called *Acute Febrile Neutrophilic Dermatosis*, is characterized by fever, neutrophilia, erythematous and painful skin lesions, diffuse neutrophilic infiltrate in the dermis, and rapid response to corticosteroids (Saavedra et al., 2006). Ten to twenty per cent of SS cases are related to neoplasms, especially AML, the remaining being idiopathic o drug related. In AL patients, therapy with cytokines such as granulocyte colony-stimulating factor (G-CSF) and all-trans retinoic acid (ATRA) are involved in most cases (Thompson & Montarella, 2007) (Figure 5).

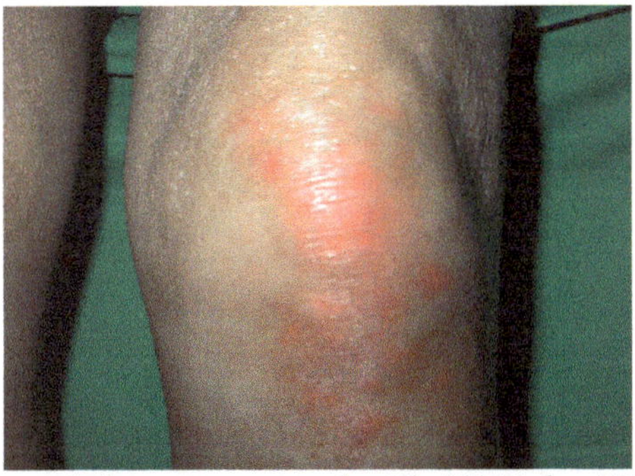

Fig. 5. *Sweet Syndrome* in an adult patient treated with ATRA for APL

Hypersensitivity reactions (HR) typically occur within an hour of drug administration and are characterized by pruritus, urticaria, swelling at the injection site, rash and in more severe cases, bronchospasm and hypotension. L-Asparaginase shows the highest risk for such reactions. The overall risk approaches 30% after four doses, but it can be also observed after the first dose. Some risk factors for this reaction are IV administration, prior exposure to L-Asparaginase and weekly intervals of administration (as opposed to daily).

There is no reliable method for determining who will sustain a HR with this drug. Skin testing is not worthwhile for this purpose. Changing to intramuscular *Erwinia* L-asparaginase instead of *E.Coli* L-asparaginase or use modified asparaginase with attached polyethylene glycol are suitable options for sensitized patients (Earl, 2009). Etopoxide is also capable of producing HR in 6-7% of patients from the first dose, especially when the drug is infused. Recommended anaphylaxis precautions for patients receiving these drugs include: blood pressure monitoring, premedication with IV diphenhydramine and having an IV access to administer epinephrine and corticosteroids in case of reaction (Shepherd, 2003).

Ara-C causes an acute reaction called the *Cytarabine Syndrome* characterized by high fever, rigors, diaphoresis, myalgia, arthralgia, conjunctivitis and maculopapular rash. This ara-C syndrome may not be a HR but a constellation of direct toxicities of the drug which is likely mediated by cytokines. Corticosteroids are the treatment of choice for this syndrome (Chng, 2003).

9. Pharmacogenetics determinants of chemotherapy toxicity in Acute Leukemia

The fact that the efficacy of chemotherapy in AL patients has significantly increased in the last twenty years, has rendered a growing body of pharmacogenetic studies focused on toxicity rather than efficiency of chemotherapy drugs. Indeed, some genetic polymorphisms have been identified to play an important role.

Most notably, polymorphisms in the thiopurine methyltransferase *(TPMT)* gene, which codes for a key enzyme in the metabolism of 6-MP, have been shown to produce a defective enzyme. Individuals homozygous for these SNPs present extremely high levels of active thioguanine nucleotides and therefore may have unacceptable, life-threatening toxicity from normal doses of 6-MP. In consequence, AL patients scheduled to receive 6-MP are regularly tested for polymorphisms in the TPMT gene in order to adjust therapy (Relling et al., 1999).

MTX, the cornerstone for therapy of ALL, has also been the focus of many pharmacogenetic studies aimed to identify genetic determinants of its toxicity. The methylenetetrahydrofolate reductase (*MTHFR*) gene has been by far the most extensively studied. Two polymorphisms, C677T and A1298C, have been associated with increased MTX toxicity, with the first likely playing a more significant role (Gervasini, 2009). Accordingly, some ALL treatment protocols in the induction phase include MTX dose reductions for subjects homozygous for the 677T variant or for those carrying both heterozygous genotypes (Badell et al., 2008). Given the complexity of the MTX mechanism of action, there are possibly polymorphisms in genes other than *MTHFR* that could be involved in the development of MTX adverse effects. Particularly, the occurrence of polymorphisms in membrane transporters that are responsible for the intake and efflux of MTX may constitute an exciting field of research (Gervasini, 2009).

There are other drugs included in the chemotherapy of AL whose toxicity may also be increased by the presence of genetic polymorphisms. In this regard, some studies have addressed the impact of polymorphisms in ATP binding cassette (ABC) transporters on the toxicity of imatinib, vincristine or mitoxantrone, albeit with contradictory results (Cotte et al., 2009; Gurney et al., 2007; Hartman et al., 2010; Plasschaert et al., 2004). In addition, polymorphisms in drug-metabolizing enzymes such cytochrome P450 (CYP) 2B6 or CYP2D6 may also be involved in the occurrence of adverse effects in response to treatments including imatinib, cyclophosphamide and etoposide (Gardner et al., 2006; Kishi et al., 2004; Rocha et al., 2009). However, these results are far from being consistently demonstrated and further studies are needed to elucidate whether these polymorphisms represent a clinical concern.

10. Conclusions

In this chapter we have aimed to describe a number of guidelines to correctly recognize and treat the main adverse effects induced by chemotherapy in AL patients. In order to identify subjects at higher risk of toxicity, a complete clinical-analytical evaluation must be performed in all patients before the administration of each chemotherapy cycle. Furthermore, clinicians should be familiar with the different metabolic pathways of each administered drug, and doses should be adjusted accordingly if necessary, especially in cases with decreased renal or liver function. However, even with these precautions, chemotherapy-induced toxicity is still an important clinical concern in AL. Indeed, at the present time the cornerstone of therapy for AL is still formed by a reduced number of drugs with a highly toxic profile.

The present challenge would therefore be to reduce the frequency and seriousness of adverse effects while maintaining efficacy and avoiding overtreatment of patients. The design of new drugs such as the so-called molecular target drugs, the further development of existing therapeutic groups, or the knowledge of genetic determinants of toxicity may help achieve these goals.

11. References

Badell, I., A. Munoz, J. Estella, et al. (2008). Long-term results of two consecutive trials in childhood acute lymphoblastic leukaemia performed by the Spanish Cooperative Group for Childhood Acute Lymphoblastic Leukemia Group (SHOP) from 1989 to 1998. *Clin Transl Oncol,* Vol.10, No 2, pp. 117-24

Bagnes, C., P. N. Panchuk & G. Recondo (2010). Antineoplastic chemotherapy induced QTc prolongation. *Curr Drug Saf,* Vol.5, No 1, pp. 93-6

Batist, G., G. Ramakrishnan, C. S. Rao, et al. (2001). Reduced cardiotoxicity and preserved antitumor efficacy of liposome-encapsulated doxorubicin and cyclophosphamide compared with conventional doxorubicin and cyclophosphamide in a randomized, multicenter trial of metastatic breast cancer. *J Clin Oncol,* Vol.19, No 5, pp. 1444-54

Brehler, R., S. Reimann, G. Bonsmann, et al. (1997). Neutrophilic hidradenitis induced by chemotherapy involves eccrine and apocrine glands. *Am J Dermatopathol,* Vol.19, No 1, pp. 73-8

Brisse, H., V. Servois, B. Bouche, et al. (2000). Hepatic regenerating nodules: a mimic of recurrent cancer in children. *Pediatr Radiol,* Vol.30, No 6, pp. 386-93

Cardinale, D., A. Colombo, G. Lamantia, et al. (2010). Anthracycline-induced cardiomyopathy: clinical relevance and response to pharmacologic therapy. *J Am Coll Cardiol,* Vol.55, No 3, pp. 213-20

Cotte, S., N. von Ahsen, N. Kruse, et al. (2009). ABC-transporter gene-polymorphisms are potential pharmacogenetic markers for mitoxantrone response in multiple sclerosis. *Brain,* Vol.132, No Pt 9, pp. 2517-30

Creutzig, U., S. Diekamp, M. Zimmermann, et al. (2007). Longitudinal evaluation of early and late anthracycline cardiotoxicity in children with AML. *Pediatr Blood Cancer,* Vol.48, No 7, pp. 651-62

Chen, C. Y., C. H. Tai, W. Tsay, et al. (2009). Prediction of fatal intracranial hemorrhage in patients with acute myeloid leukemia. *Ann Oncol,* Vol.20, No 6, pp. 1100-4

Childhood ALL Collaborative Group (2009). Beneficial and harmful effects of anthracyclines in the treatment of childhood acute lymphoblastic leukaemia: a systematic review and meta-analysis. *Br J Haematol,* Vol.145, No 3, pp. 376-88

Chng, W. J. (2003). Cytarabine syndrome revisited. *Br J Haematol,* Vol.122, No 6, pp. 875

de Jonge, M. J. & J. Verweij (2006). Renal toxicities of chemotherapy. *Semin Oncol,* Vol.33, No 1, pp. 68-73

DeSpain, J. D. (1992). Dermatologic toxicity of chemotherapy. *Semin Oncol,* Vol.19, No 5, pp. 501-7

Dicuonzo, F., A. Salvati, M. Palma, et al. (2009). Posterior reversible encephalopathy syndrome associated with methotrexate neurotoxicity: conventional magnetic resonance and diffusion-weighted imaging findings. *J Child Neurol,* Vol.24, No 8, pp. 1013-8

Earl, M. (2009). Incidence and management of asparaginase-associated adverse events in patients with acute lymphoblastic leukemia. *Clin Adv Hematol Oncol,* Vol.7, No 9, pp. 600-6

Ellison, D. H. & T. Berl (2007). Clinical practice. The syndrome of inappropriate antidiuresis. *N Engl J Med,* Vol.356, No 20, pp. 2064-72

Farrow, A. C., G. R. Buchanan, R. J. Zwiener, et al. (1997). Serum aminotransferase elevation during and following treatment of childhood acute lymphoblastic leukemia. *J Clin Oncol,* Vol.15, No 4, pp. 1560-6

Floyd, J., I. Mirza, B. Sachs, et al. (2006). Hepatotoxicity of chemotherapy. *Semin Oncol,* Vol.33, No 1, pp. 50-67

Fried, M., J. Kalra, C. F. Ilardi, et al. (1987). Hepatocellular carcinoma in a long-term survivor of acute lymphocytic leukemia. *Cancer,* Vol.60, No 10, pp. 2548-52

Friedman, J. H. & N. Shetty (2001). Permanent cerebellar toxicity of cytosine arabinoside (Ara C) in a young woman. *Mov Disord,* Vol.16, No 3, pp. 575-7

Gardner, E. R., H. Burger, R. H. van Schaik, et al. (2006). Association of enzyme and transporter genotypes with the pharmacokinetics of imatinib. *Clin Pharmacol Ther,* Vol.80, No 2, pp. 192-201

George, C. B., R. P. Mansour, J. Redmond, 3rd, et al. (1984). Hepatic dysfunction and jaundice following high-dose cytosine arabinoside. *Cancer,* Vol.54, No 11, pp. 2360-2

Germanakis, I., N. Anagnostatou & M. Kalmanti (2008). Troponins and natriuretic peptides in the monitoring of anthracycline cardiotoxicity. *Pediatr Blood Cancer,* Vol.51, No 3, pp. 327-33

Gervasini, G. (2009). Polymorphisms in methotrexate pathways: what is clinically relevant, what is not, and what is promising. *Curr Drug Metab,* Vol.10, No 6, pp. 547-66

Glantz, M. J., S. LaFollette, K. A. Jaeckle, et al. (1999). Randomized trial of a slow-release versus a standard formulation of cytarabine for the intrathecal treatment of lymphomatous meningitis. *J Clin Oncol,* Vol.17, No 10, pp. 3110-6

Gupta, A., C. Swaroop, R. Rastogi, et al. (2008). Simultaneous occurrence of posterior reversible leukoencephalopathy syndrome in two cases of childhood acute lymphoblastic leukemia induction chemotherapy. *Pediatr Hematol Oncol,* Vol.25, No 4, pp. 351-8

Gurney, H., M. Wong, R. L. Balleine, et al. (2007). Imatinib disposition and ABCB1 (MDR1, P-glycoprotein) genotype. *Clin Pharmacol Ther,* Vol.82, No 1, pp. 33-40

Hartman, A., R. H. van Schaik, I. P. van der Heiden, et al. (2010). Polymorphisms in genes involved in vincristine pharmacokinetics or pharmacodynamics are not related to impaired motor performance in children with leukemia. *Leuk Res,* Vol.34, No 2, pp. 154-9

Hausheer, F. H., R. L. Schilsky, S. Bain, et al. (2006). Diagnosis, management, and evaluation of chemotherapy-induced peripheral neuropathy. *Semin Oncol,* Vol.33, No 1, pp. 15-49

Haykin, M. E., M. Gorman, J. van Hoff, et al. (2006). Diffusion-weighted MRI correlates of subacute methotrexate-related neurotoxicity. *J Neurooncol,* Vol.76, No 2, pp. 153-7

Hongo, T., S. Okada, T. Ohzeki, et al. (2002). Low plasma levels of hemostatic proteins during the induction phase in children with acute lymphoblastic leukemia: A retrospective study by the JACLS. Japan Association of Childhood Leukemia Study. *Pediatr Int,* Vol.44, No 3, pp. 293-9

Hoorn, E. J. & R. Zietse (2008). Hyponatremia revisited: translating physiology to practice. *Nephron Physiol,* Vol.108, No 3, pp. p46-59

Hu, R. Q., H. Mehter, T. Nadasdy, et al. (2008). Severe hemorrhagic cystitis associated with prolonged oral cyclophosphamide therapy: case report and literature review. *Rheumatol Int,* Vol.28, No 11, pp. 1161-4

Inaba, H., R. B. Khan, F. H. Laningham, et al. (2008). Clinical and radiological characteristics of methotrexate-induced acute encephalopathy in pediatric patients with cancer. *Ann Oncol,* Vol.19, No 1, pp. 178-84

Kannarkat, G., E. E. Lasher & D. Schiff (2007). Neurologic complications of chemotherapy agents. *Curr Opin Neurol,* Vol.20, No 6, pp. 719-25

Kieslich, M., L. Porto, H. Lanfermann, et al. (2003). Cerebrovascular complications of L-asparaginase in the therapy of acute lymphoblastic leukemia. *J Pediatr Hematol Oncol,* Vol.25, No 6, pp. 484-7

Kim, H., J. H. Lee, S. J. Choi, et al. (2006). Risk score model for fatal intracranial hemorrhage in acute leukemia. *Leukemia,* Vol.20, No 5, pp. 770-6

Kishi, S., W. Yang, B. Boureau, et al. (2004). Effects of prednisone and genetic polymorphisms on etoposide disposition in children with acute lymphoblastic leukemia. *Blood,* Vol.103, No 1, pp. 67-72

Korkmaz, A., T. Topal & S. Oter (2007). Pathophysiological aspects of cyclophosphamide and ifosfamide induced hemorrhagic cystitis; implication of reactive oxygen and nitrogen species as well as PARP activation. *Cell Biol Toxicol,* Vol.23, No 5, pp. 303-12

Lipshultz, S. E., R. E. Scully, S. R. Lipsitz, et al. (2010). Assessment of dexrazoxane as a cardioprotectant in doxorubicin-treated children with high-risk acute lymphoblastic leukaemia: long-term follow-up of a prospective, randomised, multicentre trial. *Lancet Oncol,* Vol.11, No 10, pp. 950-61

Luesink, M., J. L. Pennings, W. M. Wissink, et al. (2009). Chemokine induction by all-trans retinoic acid and arsenic trioxide in acute promyelocytic leukemia: triggering the differentiation syndrome. *Blood,* Vol.114, No 27, pp. 5512-21

Mahadeo, K. M., G. Dhall, A. Panigrahy, et al. (2010). Subacute methotrexate neurotoxicity and cerebral venous sinus thrombosis in a 12-year-old with acute lymphoblastic leukemia and methylenetetrahydrofolate reductase (MTHFR) C677T polymorphism: homocysteine-mediated methotrexate neurotoxicity via direct endothelial injury. *Pediatr Hematol Oncol,* Vol.27, No 1, pp. 46-52

Meadors, M., J. Floyd & M. C. Perry (2006). Pulmonary toxicity of chemotherapy. *Semin Oncol,* Vol.33, No 1, pp. 98-105

Meister, B., G. Kropshofer, A. Klein-Franke, et al. (2008). Comparison of low-molecular-weight heparin and antithrombin versus antithrombin alone for the prevention of symptomatic venous thromboembolism in children with acute lymphoblastic leukemia. *Pediatr Blood Cancer,* Vol.50, No 2, pp. 298-303

Mercuri, E., J. Poulton, J. Buck, et al. (1999). Vincristine treatment revealing asymptomatic hereditary motor sensory neuropathy type 1A. *Arch Dis Child,* Vol.81, No 5, pp. 442-3

Montesinos, P., J. M. Bergua, E. Vellenga, et al. (2009). Differentiation syndrome in patients with acute promyelocytic leukemia treated with all-trans retinoic acid and anthracycline chemotherapy: characteristics, outcome, and prognostic factors. *Blood,* Vol.113, No 4, pp. 775-83

Naing, A., D. Luong & M. Extermann (2005). Methotrexate-induced status epilepticus. *Am J Hematol,* Vol.80, No 1, pp. 35-7

Navarro, V. J. & J. R. Senior (2006). Drug-related hepatotoxicity. *N Engl J Med,* Vol.354, No 7, pp. 731-9

Ng, R., N. Better & M. D. Green (2006). Anticancer agents and cardiotoxicity. *Semin Oncol,* Vol.33, No 1, pp. 2-14

Nicholson, J. C., J. M. Darmady & J. A. Kohler (1996). Superior sagittal sinus thrombosis complicating maintenance treatment for acute lymphoblastic leukemia. *Pediatr Hematol Oncol,* Vol.13, No 3, pp. 287-91

Norman, J. K., J. T. Parke, D. A. Wilson, et al. (2007). Reversible posterior leukoencephalopathy syndrome in children undergoing induction therapy for acute lymphoblastic leukemia. *Pediatr Blood Cancer,* Vol.49, No 2, pp. 198-203

Nowak-Göttl, U., J. E. A. Wolff & N. Kuhn (1994). Enhanced thrombin generation, P-von Willebrand factor, P-fibrin D-dimer and P-plasminogen activator inhibitor 1: predictive for venous thrombosis in asparaginase-treated children. *Fibrinolysis,* Vol.8, No, pp. 63-5

Nygaard, U., N. Toft & K. Schmiegelow (2004). Methylated metabolites of 6-mercaptopurine are associated with hepatotoxicity. *Clin Pharmacol Ther,* Vol.75, No 4, pp. 274-81

Ohnishi, K., H. Yoshida, K. Shigeno, et al. (2000). Prolongation of the QT interval and ventricular tachycardia in patients treated with arsenic trioxide for acute promyelocytic leukemia. *Ann Intern Med,* Vol.133, No 11, pp. 881-5

Palmer, B. F. (2003). Hyponatremia in patients with central nervous system disease: SIADH versus CSW. *Trends Endocrinol Metab,* Vol.14, No 4, pp. 182-7

Parrish, C., P. Moreton & J. Ashcroft (2010). Simultaneous acute myeloid leukaemia and de novo acute hepatitis B: A novel management strategy. *Leuk Res,* No,

Patterson, D. M. & S. M. Lee (2010). Glucarpidase following high-dose methotrexate: update on development. *Expert Opin Biol Ther,* Vol.10, No 1, pp. 105-11

Payne, A. S., DMF (2011). Cutaneous complications of conventional chemotherapy agents. *In: UpToDate, Drews, RE (Ed), UpToDate, Ofori,AO,* No,

Payne, A. S., W. D. James & R. B. Weiss (2006). Dermatologic toxicity of chemotherapeutic agents. *Semin Oncol,* Vol.33, No 1, pp. 86-97

Perry, M. C. (1992). Chemotherapeutic agents and hepatotoxicity. *Semin Oncol,* Vol.19, No 5, pp. 551-65

Pihan, K. B. M. a. G. (2009). Clinical Manifestations of Acute Myeloid Leukemia in Hoffman "Hematology Basic Principles and Practice" 5° Edition. Ch 60 , pp. 933-63

Plasschaert, S. L., E. Groninger, M. Boezen, et al. (2004). Influence of functional polymorphisms of the MDR1 gene on vincristine pharmacokinetics in childhood acute lymphoblastic leukemia. *Clin Pharmacol Ther,* Vol.76, No 3, pp. 220-9

Pui, C. H., G. A. Burghen, W. P. Bowman, et al. (1981). Risk factors for hyperglycemia in children with leukemia receiving L-asparaginase and prednisone. *J Pediatr,* Vol.99, No 1, pp. 46-50

Pui, C. H. & W. E. Evans (2006). Treatment of acute lymphoblastic leukemia. *N Engl J Med,* Vol.354, No 2, pp. 166-78

Quasthoff, S. & H. P. Hartung (2002). Chemotherapy-induced peripheral neuropathy. *J Neurol,* Vol.249, No 1, pp. 9-17

Relling, M. V., M. L. Hancock, G. K. Rivera, et al. (1999). Mercaptopurine therapy intolerance and heterozygosity at the thiopurine S-methyltransferase gene locus. *J Natl Cancer Inst,* Vol.91, No 23, pp. 2001-8

Rocha, V., R. Porcher, J. F. Fernandes, et al. (2009). Association of drug metabolism gene polymorphisms with toxicities, graft-versus-host disease and survival after HLA-identical sibling hematopoietic stem cell transplantation for patients with leukemia. *Leukemia,* Vol.23, No 3, pp. 545-56

Rubnitz, J. E., M. V. Relling, P. L. Harrison, et al. (1998). Transient encephalopathy following high-dose methotrexate treatment in childhood acute lymphoblastic leukemia. *Leukemia,* Vol.12, No 8, pp. 1176-81

Saavedra, A. P., S. C. Kovacs & S. L. Moschella (2006). Neutrophilic dermatoses. *Clin Dermatol,* Vol.24, No 6, pp. 470-81

Sanchez-Carpintero, R., J. Narbona, R. Lopez de Mesa, et al. (2001). Transient posterior encephalopathy induced by chemotherapy in children. *Pediatr Neurol,* Vol.24, No 2, pp. 145-8

Sanz, M. A., D. Grimwade, M. S. Tallman, et al. (2009). Management of acute promyelocytic leukemia: recommendations from an expert panel on behalf of the European LeukemiaNet. *Blood,* Vol.113, No 9, pp. 1875-91

Sawyer, D. B., X. Peng, B. Chen, et al. (2010). Mechanisms of anthracycline cardiac injury: can we identify strategies for cardioprotection? *Prog Cardiovasc Dis,* Vol.53, No 2, pp. 105-13

Schmiegelow, K. (1991). Prognostic significance of methotrexate and 6-mercaptopurine dosage during maintenance chemotherapy for childhood acute lymphoblastic leukemia. *Pediatr Hematol Oncol,* Vol.8, No 4, pp. 301-12

Schwartz, R. G., W. B. McKenzie, J. Alexander, et al. (1987). Congestive heart failure and left ventricular dysfunction complicating doxorubicin therapy. Seven-year experience using serial radionuclide angiocardiography. *Am J Med,* Vol.82, No 6, pp. 1109-18

Shepherd, G. M. (2003). Hypersensitivity reactions to chemotherapeutic drugs. *Clin Rev Allergy Immunol,* Vol.24, No 3, pp. 253-62

Shin, R. K., J. W. Stern, A. J. Janss, et al. (2001). Reversible posterior leukoencephalopathy during the treatment of acute lymphoblastic leukemia. *Neurology,* Vol.56, No 3, pp. 388-91

Silverman, L. B., J. G. Supko, K. E. Stevenson, et al. (2010). Intravenous PEG-asparaginase during remission induction in children and adolescents with newly diagnosed acute lymphoblastic leukemia. *Blood,* Vol.115, No 7, pp. 1351-3

Smith, G. A., L. E. Damon, H. S. Rugo, et al. (1997). High-dose cytarabine dose modification reduces the incidence of neurotoxicity in patients with renal insufficiency. *J Clin Oncol,* Vol.15, No 2, pp. 833-9

Spinola-Castro, A. M., A. A. Siviero-Miachon, S. Andreoni, et al. (2009). Transient hyperglycemia during childhood acute lymphocytic leukemia chemotherapy: an old event revisited. *Clin Adv Hematol Oncol,* Vol.7, No 7, pp. 465-72

Stoneham, S., L. Lennard, P. Coen, et al. (2003). Veno-occlusive disease in patients receiving thiopurines during maintenance therapy for childhood acute lymphoblastic leukaemia. *Br J Haematol,* Vol.123, No 1, pp. 100-2

Sul, J. K. & L. M. Deangelis (2006). Neurologic complications of cancer chemotherapy. *Semin Oncol,* Vol.33, No 3, pp. 324-32

Thompson, D. F. & K. E. Montarella (2007). Drug-induced Sweet's syndrome. *Ann Pharmacother,* Vol.41, No 5, pp. 802-11

Titos-Arcos, J. C., J. Leon-Villar, M. L. Amigo-Lozano, et al. (2011). [Posterior reversible leukoencephalopathy syndrome induced by L-asparaginase in a teenage female diagnosed with acute lymphoblastic leukemia]. *Rev Neurol,* Vol.52, No 1, pp. 58-60

Treepongkaruna, S., N. Thongpak, S. Pakakasama, et al. (2009). Acute pancreatitis in children with acute lymphoblastic leukemia after chemotherapy. *J Pediatr Hematol Oncol,* Vol.31, No 11, pp. 812-5

Vagace, J. M., C. Caceres-Marzal, M. Jimenez, et al. (2011). Methotrexate-induced subacute neurotoxicity in a child with acute lymphoblastic leukemia carrying genetic polymorphisms related to folate homeostasis. *Am J Hematol,* Vol.86, No 1, pp. 98-101

Valdes Olmos, R. A., I. Carrio, C. A. Hoefnagel, et al. (2002). High sensitivity of radiolabelled antimyosin scintigraphy in assessing anthracycline related early myocyte damage preceding cardiac dysfunction. *Nucl Med Commun,* Vol.23, No 9, pp. 871-7

van Dalen, E. C., H. N. Caron, H. O. Dickinson, et al. (2008). Cardioprotective interventions for cancer patients receiving anthracyclines. *Cochrane Database Syst Rev,* No 2, pp. CD003917

van Dalen, E. C., E. M. Michiels, H. N. Caron, et al. (2010). Different anthracycline derivates for reducing cardiotoxicity in cancer patients. *Cochrane Database Syst Rev,* No 5, pp. CD005006

van Dalen, E. C., H. J. van der Pal, H. N. Caron, et al. (2009). Different dosage schedules for reducing cardiotoxicity in cancer patients receiving anthracycline chemotherapy. *Cochrane Database Syst Rev,* No 4, pp. CD005008

Verstappen, C. C., S. Koeppen, J. J. Heimans, et al. (2005). Dose-related vincristine-induced peripheral neuropathy with unexpected off-therapy worsening. *Neurology,* Vol.64, No 6, pp. 1076-7

Widemann, B. C. & P. C. Adamson (2006). Understanding and managing methotrexate nephrotoxicity. *Oncologist,* Vol.11, No 6, pp. 694-703

Ziereisen, F., B. Dan, N. Azzi, et al. (2006). Reversible acute methotrexate leukoencephalopathy: atypical brain MR imaging features. *Pediatr Radiol,* Vol.36, No 3, pp. 205-12

Permissions

The contributors of this book come from diverse backgrounds, making this book a truly international effort. This book will bring forth new frontiers with its revolutionizing research information and detailed analysis of the nascent developments around the world.

We would like to thank Prof. Mariastefania Antica, PhD, for lending her expertise to make the book truly unique. She has played a crucial role in the development of this book. Without her invaluable contribution this book wouldn't have been possible. She has made vital efforts to compile up to date information on the varied aspects of this subject to make this book a valuable addition to the collection of many professionals and students.

This book was conceptualized with the vision of imparting up-to-date information and advanced data in this field. To ensure the same, a matchless editorial board was set up. Every individual on the board went through rigorous rounds of assessment to prove their worth. After which they invested a large part of their time researching and compiling the most relevant data for our readers. Conferences and sessions were held from time to time between the editorial board and the contributing authors to present the data in the most comprehensible form. The editorial team has worked tirelessly to provide valuable and valid information to help people across the globe.

Every chapter published in this book has been scrutinized by our experts. Their significance has been extensively debated. The topics covered herein carry significant findings which will fuel the growth of the discipline. They may even be implemented as practical applications or may be referred to as a beginning point for another development. Chapters in this book were first published by InTech; hereby published with permission under the Creative Commons Attribution License or equivalent.

The editorial board has been involved in producing this book since its inception. They have spent rigorous hours researching and exploring the diverse topics which have resulted in the successful publishing of this book. They have passed on their knowledge of decades through this book. To expedite this challenging task, the publisher supported the team at every step. A small team of assistant editors was also appointed to further simplify the editing procedure and attain best results for the readers.

Our editorial team has been hand-picked from every corner of the world. Their multi-ethnicity adds dynamic inputs to the discussions which result in innovative outcomes. These outcomes are then further discussed with the researchers and contributors who give their valuable feedback and opinion regarding the same. The feedback is then collaborated with the researches and they are edited in a comprehensive manner to aid the understanding of the subject.

Apart from the editorial board, the designing team has also invested a significant amount of their time in understanding the subject and creating the most relevant covers. They scrutinized every image to scout for the most suitable representation of the subject and create an appropriate cover for the book.

The publishing team has been involved in this book since its early stages. They were actively engaged in every process, be it collecting the data, connecting with the contributors or procuring relevant information. The team has been an ardent support to the editorial, designing and production team. Their endless efforts to recruit the best for this project, has resulted in the accomplishment of this book. They are a veteran in the field of academics and their pool of knowledge is as vast as their experience in printing. Their expertise and guidance has proved useful at every step. Their uncompromising quality standards have made this book an exceptional effort. Their encouragement from time to time has been an inspiration for everyone.

The publisher and the editorial board hope that this book will prove to be a valuable piece of knowledge for researchers, students, practitioners and scholars across the globe.

List of Contributors

Gamal Abdul-Hamid
University of Aden/Hematology Unit, Yemen

Abbas H. Abdulsalam
Al-Yarmouk Teaching Hospital, Baghdad, Iraq

Mariastefania Antica
Rudjer Boskovic Institute, Croatia

Ota Fuchs
Institute of Hematology and Blood Transfusion, Prague, Czech Republic Center of Experimental Hematology, First Medical Faculty, Charles University, Prague, Czech Republic

Xudong Ma, Shaohong Jiang, Yiqun Huang, Yong Zou, Ruiji Zheng and Liyun Xiao
Zhangzhou Affiliated Hospital of Fujian Medical University, China

Roel Polak
Department of Hematology, Erasmus MC, Rotterdam, The Netherlands

Miranda Buitenhuis
Department of Hematology, Erasmus MC, Rotterdam, The Netherlands
Erasmus MC Stem Cell Institute for Regenerative Medicine, Erasmus MC, Rotterdam, The Netherlands

Venkatasubramanian Dharmarajan and Michael S. Cosgrove
Department of Biology, Syracuse University, Syracuse, New York, USA

Seiji Fukuda
Department of Pediatrics, Shimane University School of Medicine, Japan

Chie Onishi
Department of Hematology, Shimane University School of Medicine, Japan

Louis M. Pelus
Department of Microbiology and Immunology, Indiana University School of Medicine, United States of America

Tatyana Nasedkina, Yuliya Yatsenko, Olga Gra, Natalia Guseva and Alexander Zasedatelev
Engelhardt Institute of Molecular Biology, Russian Academy of Sciences, Russia

Elena Samochatova
Engelhardt Institute of Molecular Biology, Russian Academy of Sciences, Russia
Federal Clinical Research Center of Pediatric Hematology, Oncology and Immunology, Russia

Yoshiko Hashii
Department of Developmental Medicine, Osaka University Graduate School of Medicine, Japan

C. Michel Zwaan and Marry M. van den Heuvel-Eibrink
Erasmus MC-Sophia Children's Hospital, Rotterdam, The Netherlands

Lílian Barros Queiroz, Cezar Martins de Sá and Beatriz Dolabela de Lima
Departamento de Biologia Celular, Universidade de Brasília, Brasília, DF, Brazil

Íris Ferrari and Juliana Forte Mazzeu
Departamento de Genética e Morfologia, Instituto de Ciências Biológicas, Universidade de Brasília, Brasília, DF, Brazil

Isis Quezado Magalhães
Núcleo de Oncologia e Hematologia Pediátrica, Secretaria de Saúde do DF, Brasília, DF, Brazil

C. Vandenbriele
Internal medicine, University Hospitals Gasthuisberg, Belgium

A. Vassou
Hematology Department, Belgium

G. Pentheroudakis
Oncology Department, University Hospital of Ioannina, Hellas, Belgium

K. Van Calsteren
Obstetrics, University Hospitals Gasthuisberg, Belgium

F. Amant
Leuven Cancer Institute, Gynecologic Oncology, University Hospitals Gasthuisberg, Belgium

Takaaki Konuma
Department of Cellular and Molecular Medicine, Graduate School of Medicine, Chiba University, Chiba, Tokyo

Satoshi Takahashi
Division of Molecular Therapy, Advanced Clinical Research Center, Institute of Medical Science, University of Tokyo, Tokyo, Japan

Ron Ram, Liat Vidal, Ronit Gurion, Pia Raanani and Ofer Shpilberg
Institute of Hematology, Davidoff Cancer Center, Beilinson Hospital, Rabin Medical Center and Sackler School of Medicine, Tel- Aviv University, Israel

Josep-Maria Ribera
Clinical Hematology Department, Institut Català d'Oncologia, Hospital Universitari Germans Trias i Pujol, Institut de Recerca contra la Leucemia Josep Carreras, Universitat Autònoma de Barcelona, Spain

Hun Ju Lee and Meir Wetzler
Leukemia Section, Department of Medicine, USA

Candace S. Johnson
Department of Pharmacology and Therapeutics, USA

Donald Trump
Department of Medicine, Roswell Park Cancer Institute, Buffalo, NY, USA

Jose Manuel Vagace
Department of Pediatric Hematology, University Hospital Infanta, Cristina, Spain

Guillermo Gervasini
Department of Pharmacology, Medical School, University of Extremadura, Badajoz, Spain